Current and Future Advances in Male Infertility

Ashok Agarwal • Ramadan Saleh
Florence Boitrelle • Rupin Shah
Editors

Current and Future Advances in Male Infertility

A Compendium for Clinicians and Researchers

Springer

Editors
Ashok Agarwal
Global Andrology Forum
Moreland Hills, OH, USA

Cleveland Clinic Foundation
Cleveland, OH, USA

Florence Boitrelle
Department of Reproductive Biology
Fertility Preservation, Andrology, CECOS
Poissy Hospital
Poissy, France

Department of Biology, Reproduction, Epigenetics, Environment and Development
Paris Saclay University
UVSQ, INRAE, BREED
Jouy-en-Josas, France

Global Andrology Forum
Moreland Hills, OH, France

Ramadan Saleh
Department of Dermatology, Venereology and Andrology
Faculty of Medicine
Sohag University
Sohag, Egypt

Ajyal IVF Center
Ajyal Hospital
Sohag, Egypt

Rupin Shah
Department of Urology
Lilavati Hospital and Research Centre
Mumbai, Maharashtra, India

ISBN 978-3-031-62647-0 ISBN 978-3-031-62648-7 (eBook)
https://doi.org/10.1007/978-3-031-62648-7

This Springer imprint is published by the registered company Springer Nature Switzerland AG
The registered company address is: Gewerbestrasse 11, 6330 Cham, Switzerland

In memory of my father, Professor RC Aggarwal, whose legacy of integrity, dedication, and hard work remains a guiding light. To my wife, Meenu, and sons, Rishi and Neil-Yogi, whose unwavering love sustains me. Gratitude to Professor Kevin Loughlin (Harvard Medical School), the late Professor Anthony Thomas (Cleveland Clinic), and Dr. Rupin Shah (India) for their invaluable friendship, guidance, and profound impact on my journey. To over thousand researchers, students, and the countless patients who entrusted me over four decades – your collaboration and trust have been my greatest inspiration.

***Ashok Agarwal**, MSc, PhD, HCLD (Andrology)*

To my family for your constant love and support. You have always been there for me.

To Professor Ashok Agarwal (Global Andrology Forum, USA) for your guidance and support. Thank you for believing in my dream. You were the first person to encourage me to be part of this achievement.

To the late Professor Kamal Abdel Hafez (Assiut University, Egypt) for his mentorship and guidance.

***Ramadan Saleh**, MD*

The idea for this book was born a few years ago. While the WHO manual is part of our day-to-day work as andrologists, we felt it was important to understand it better in order to use it more effectively. To improve international research in Andrology, Prof. Agarwal created the Global Andrology Forum. For me, becoming a member of this group has enabled me to get to know andrologists who are passionate about their profession, whether they live in France, Europe, or the rest of the world. I would like to thank him warmly for inviting me to edit this book with him. Dear Ashok, dear co-editors (Rupin and Ramadan), thank you for this wonderful adventure.

***Florence Boitrelle,** MD, PhD*

Foreword

The book by Agarwal et al. entitled, *Current and Future Advances in Male Infertility: A Compendium for Clinicians and Researchers* provides new insights into a series of important issues relevant for the evaluation and management of male infertility. The chapter on semen evaluation, presented as an analysis of clinical implications of semen analyses has great promise for enhancing our understanding of the value of WHO standards. Endocrine disruptor discussions are extensive and insightful, providing key insights into the conditions that may predispose to what we refer to as testicular dysgenesis. Lifestyle effects on male fertility are reviewed with an emphasis on the mechanistic basis for adverse effects of lifestyle. The complex issues of the effects of germ cell tumors on testicular function are effectively reviewed as well. Sperm DNA fragmentation is presented and the clinical implications of abnormal sperm DNA fragmentation are reviewed. The pathophysiology of seminal oxidative stress is overviewed in detail. The essence of dysfunctional spermatozoal function is well explained by observations on oxidative stress and their adverse effects on sperm as well as the propagation of damage from spermatozoal injury. Management of spermatozoal oxidative stress is a key component of patient care that is extensively reviewed. The genetic basis of male infertility is incompletely understood despite there being clinical relevance to the limited factors that have been identified as being causal of severe male infertility, including azoospermia and severe oligospermia. Novel insights into spermatozoal function are possible with new epigenetic evaluations of sperm. It is remarkable that even normal appearing sperm may have epigenetic anomalies that could predict reproductive dysfunction.

No consideration of male infertility would be complete without discussion of varicocele and its known adverse effects on sperm production, quality, and fertility potential. The controversies of varicocele and its clinical significance are also effectively presented. The controversial area of male genital infection and its relationship to fertility and infertility are provided in a balanced discussion. Sexual dysfunction is overviewed with its management. The controversies and effects of male hypogonadism and ineffective testosterone production/action are also presented. Non-obstructive azoospermia, a particular area of interest of mine, is well discussed including hormonal and surgical treatment. Certainly, this condition is one of the more challenging diagnoses in male infertility to manage. The discussion of alternative approaches to management of male infertility is also provided. Sperm optimization, a broad area of interest for andrologists is discussed in a penultimate chapter. Artificial intelligence concepts including applications for diagnosis of andrological abnormalities, improvement of surgical approaches, and the ability to optimize assisted reproductive results are reviewed.

Most of the chapters have a balanced group of authors from different institutions, including US and international contributors that help provide a more complete evaluation of existing data on factors affecting male fertility and their management. This impressive international collaboration of authors provides a unique perspective for this new book specializing in all key areas of andrology. Well worth the read.

New York Mens Health Medical
New York, NY, USA

Peter N. Schlegel,

Preface

Male factor is implicated in up to 50% of all cases of infertility. Additionally, there is growing concern about the progressive decline of men's fertility potential observed over the past 50 years. In recent years, there have been major advances in the understanding of pathophysiological mechanisms, diagnostic tools, and therapy of male infertility. However, several challenges and controversies remain, both in newer therapies and the management of common conditions like varicocele, genital tract inflammation/infection, or non-obstructive azoospermia.

This book discusses different aspects related to declining male fertility potential, including the role of endocrine-disrupting chemicals, lifestyle factors, and testicular cancer. This book provides a comprehensive review of cellular, molecular, and genetic aspects of testicular function and men's fertility and highlights the state of the art of the currently available advanced tests or newly evolving diagnostic tools for male infertility. This book discusses the management of challenging conditions, clinical dilemmas, and controversial issues of male infertility and presents recent methods for sperm optimization before its use in assisted reproductive techniques. Finally, this book highlights the potential role of artificial intelligence in the diagnosis and prognosis of male infertility and provides insights into the future of male infertility research. This book will be of great value to all clinicians involved in the management of male infertility.

Current and Future Advances in Male Infertility book has 19 chapters grouped into eight sections. Each chapter is coauthored by senior clinicians, thus bringing a truly clinically relevant perspective. Our book includes 42 contributors who were selected from 17 countries. The authors form an impressive international collaboration to provide the latest information in well-written, and meticulously researched chapters. Without their unwavering support, this book would not have been possible.

Special thanks are extended to the organizational prowess of Lillie Mae Gaurano, Springer Editor, Clinical Medicine (Books), and the day-to-day support of Production Editor Janakiraman G.

In honor of our families, mentors, and patients, this book is a dedication to those who inspire and motivate us to advance knowledge in the field of male infertility.

Moreland Hills, USA	Ashok Agarwal
Sohag, Egypt	Ramadan Saleh
Poissy, France	Florence Boitrelle
Mumbai, India	Rupin Shah

Contents

About the Editors

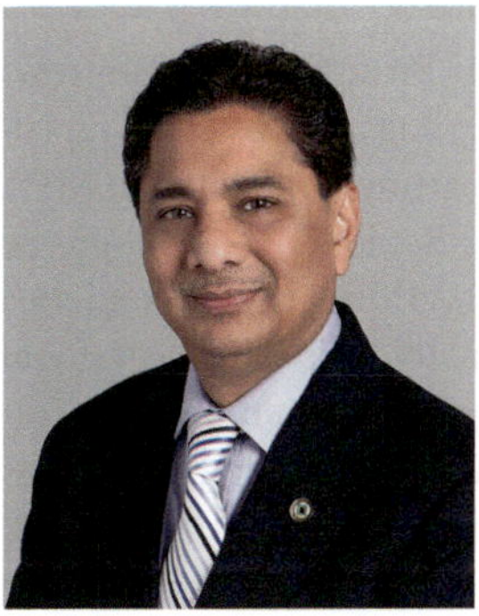

Ashok Agarwal is a highly regarded andrologist and researcher who has made significant contributions to the field of male infertility. As the founder and current President of the Global Andrology Forum (GAF) headquartered in Moreland Hills, Ohio, he leads an international coalition of 700 members from 84 countries, tirelessly propelling the advancements in male reproductive health. For nearly three decades (1993–2022), Ashok served as the Director of the Andrology Laboratory and Research in Urology at Cleveland Clinic, concurrently holding the position of Professor of Surgery at Case Western Reserve University, Cleveland. His prolific contributions encompass over 950 scientific articles and the editing of 55 medical textbooks, earning him numerous accolades in andrology and male infertility research. Beyond his groundbreaking research and clinical expertise, Ashok's dedication extends to education and mentorship. He has shared his knowledge with over 1000 clinicians and scientists from 65+ countries, shaping the future of andrology. Recognized as a foremost authority in male infertility research, Ashok has been a featured speaker at countless national and international conferences, showcasing his leadership in the global dialogue on male reproductive health.

Global Andrology Forum, Moreland Hills, OH, USA
Cleveland Clinic Foundation, Cleveland, OH, USA

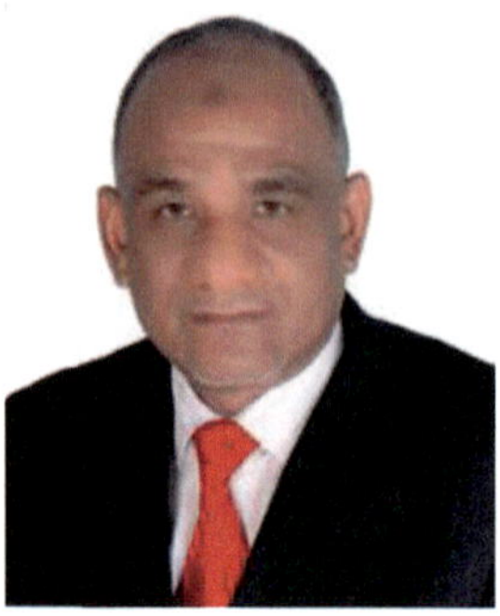

Ramadan Saleh is a Professor of Dermatology, Venereology, and Andrology, in Sohag University, Egypt. He is the founder of Ajyal IVF Center, Ajyal Hospital, Sohag, Egypt. He is a co-founder of Global Andrology Forum established in December 2021. He is a member of several professional societies and a reviewer in many international journals in the field of reproductive medicine. He has published more than 150 research articles in peer-reviewed scientific journals, and co-edited three books.

Department of Dermatology, Venereology and Andrology, Faculty of Medicine, Sohag University, Sohag, Egypt

Ajyal IVF Center, Ajyal Hospital, Sohag, Egypt

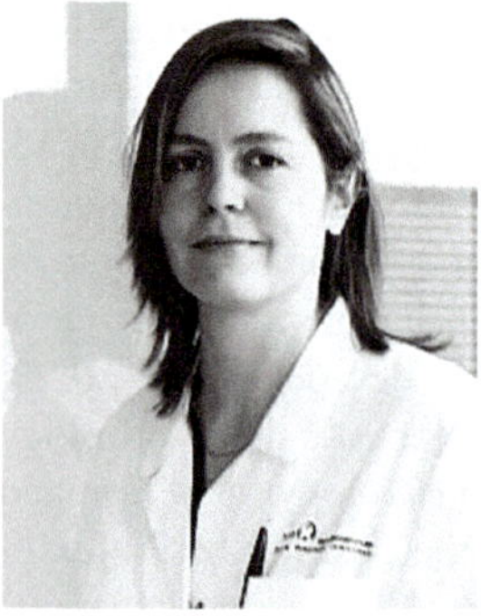

Florence Boitrelle, MD, PhD Prof. Florence Boitrelle is a doctor specializing in Andrology and assisted reproduction. She is head of the department, head of an MPA center, former president of the Société d'Andrologie de langue Française, member of various learned societies in France and internationally (ESHRE, Global Andrology Forum...). Passionate about clinical andrology and research, she is the author of over 100 articles referenced in PubMed and has participated in over 80 communications in France and abroad.

Department of Reproductive Biology, Fertility Preservation, Andrology, CECOS, Poissy Hospital, Poissy, France

Department of Biology, Reproduction, Epigenetics, Environment and Development, Paris Saclay University, UVSQ, INRAE, BREED, Jouy-en-Josas, France

Global Andrology Forum, Moreland Hills, OH, USA

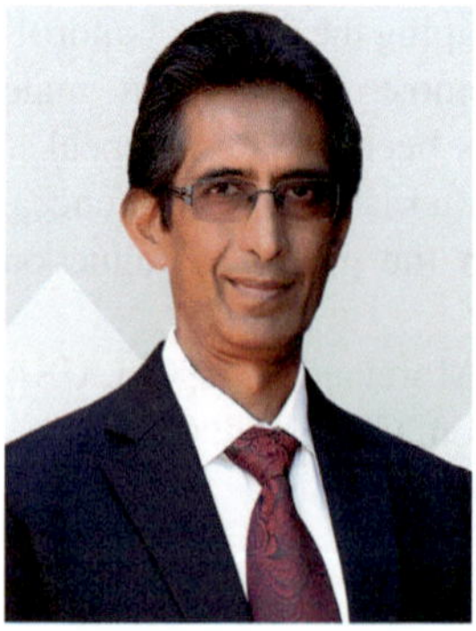

Rupin Shah is a senior uro-andrologist practicing male infertility and sexual dysfunction in Mumbai at the Lilavati Hospital and Research Centre. He is Founder-President of the South Asian Society of Sexual Medicine, Chairman of the Post-Doctoral Fellowship in Andrology of the National Board of Examinations of India, Co-Chair of the International Consultation on Sexual Medicine-2024, Associate Editor of the journal *Fertility and Reproduction,* and Senior Advisor to the Global Andrology Forum.

Part I
Declining Male Reproductive Health

Chapter 1
Clinical Implications of the WHO 6th Edition on Human Semen Analysis

Florence Boitrelle and Gökhan Çeker

Introduction

Infertility affects around 15% of couples of childbearing age, i.e., some 48 million couples and 186 million individuals worldwide [1]. In almost 50% of cases, a male factor is involved [2]. When a couple presents with infertility, it is therefore important to evaluate both the man and the woman. In men, the cornerstone of male infertility assessment is conventional semen analysis, which provides a baseline measure of the male reproductive system. This is usually the first test requested for the male partner, as it is noninvasive, informative, and relatively inexpensive.

The evaluation of semen parameters is currently based on "standards" defined in the laboratory manual for the examination and processing of human semen created by the World Health Organization (WHO). Since the 1980s, the WHO has standardized the process of conventional semen analysis and continues to update its manual on how the test should be performed [3, 4]. In 2021, the WHO published sixth edition of the "Manual for the examination and processing of human semen" [4]. The new manual essentially comprises three parts: semen examination, sperm preparation and cryopreservation, and quality control/assurance. Semen examination

F. Boitrelle (✉)
Department of Reproductive Biology, Fertility Preservation, Andrology, CECOS, Poissy Hospital, Poissy, France

Department of Biology, Reproduction, Epigenetics, Environment and Development, Paris Saclay University, UVSQ, INRAE, BREED, Jouy-en-Josas, France

Global Andrology Forum, Moreland Hills, OH, USA

G. Çeker
Department of Urology, Başakşehir Çam and Sakura City Hospital, Istanbul, Turkey

Department of Histology and Embryology, Hamidiye Institute of Health Sciences, University of Health Sciences, Istanbul, Turkey

A. Agarwal et al. (eds.), *Current and Future Advances in Male Infertility*,
https://doi.org/10.1007/978-3-031-62648-7_1

(analysis) procedures include basic (routine) examinations, extended examinations (which may be used by laboratories or clinicians in certain situations), and advanced tests (which are not currently recommended for routine use and are primarily intended for research). The sections on extended and advanced tests have been written in line with current clinical practice, with the abandonment of many older tests (such as the cervical mucus test) and the adoption of new tests. Recent scientific advances in the understanding of sperm DNA fragmentation (SDF), seminal oxidative stress (OS), and reactive oxygen species (ROS) analysis have shed further light on the prognosis of reproductive outcome in terms of natural conception and assisted reproduction techniques (ARTs). It is for this reason that the WHO manual has included SDF tests in the "extended examinations" section [3]. Given the growing awareness that chromosomal abnormalities and genetic mutations are often at the root of a wide range of male infertility cases, genetic and genomic tests also receive increased attention in this new sixth edition. Other tests such as assessment of the mitochondrial membrane potential of spermatozoa are not detailed in the latest manual probably due to scarcity of publications on the topic. It should be noted that conventional semen analysis does not measure the functional capacity of spermatozoa, which must travel an arduous path through the female reproductive tract before they can fertilize the oocytes. The diagnostic and clinical value of conventional semen analysis is modest at best, as individual semen parameters can show significant variability [5]. The major "novelty" of this sixth edition is that the concept of "norm" has been erased. Indeed, the manual no longer mentions the names of pathologies, and the terms asthenozoospermia, teratozoospermia, necrozoospermia, etc. have been removed. The manual makes it clear that the fifth percentiles given as reference values cannot be considered in isolation from the clinical aspects of the patient and should only be used as a guide in the clinical assessment of the infertile man. Extended and advanced semen tests have been developed to help predict a male partner's fertility potential more reliably. These tests are not used routinely but are indicated in certain clinical scenarios or research fields, respectively. They can help identify sperm dysfunction, abnormalities of internal sperm components, as well as markers of inflammation of the male reproductive system, all of which can reduce a man's fertility capabilities.

In this chapter, we detail the role of semen analysis in the infertility workup and review basic semen analysis as well as expanded and advanced sperm function tests. We will also review the recent recommendations of the three main male infertility guidelines, the American Urologic Association/American Society of Reproductive Medicine (AUA/ASRM), the European Association of Urology (EAU), and the European Academy of Andrology (EAA), on the clinical utility of these tests.

Sperm Analysis as Part of the Initial Workup for Infertile Couples

According to the latest recommendations for the management of infertile men and couples [6], a basic semen analysis is the first test to be prescribed for men consulting us for infertility. This examination is prescribed after interviewing the man about his history, symptoms, and sexual and reproductive history, but is prescribed before the man's clinical examination [6]. The decision tree below summarizes the recommendations for prescribing semen analysis and clinical examination in men consulting for infertility (Fig. 1.1).

Basic Sperm Parameters

The basic semen examination is a set of tests that are combined to provide an estimate of the male partner's ability to contribute to conception. Parameters include semen volume, coagulation, liquefaction, consistency, sperm count, sperm motility, sperm morphology, sperm viability, presence of round cells, and leukocyte concentration. The main aim of semen analysis is to identify patients at risk of infertility and to distinguish them from fertile patients. This methodology of studying and comparing the spontaneous fertility of couples according to sperm parameters was introduced in 2010 (fifth edition). Norms and reference intervals for sperm parameters were defined using the fifth percentile statistical method. This methodology

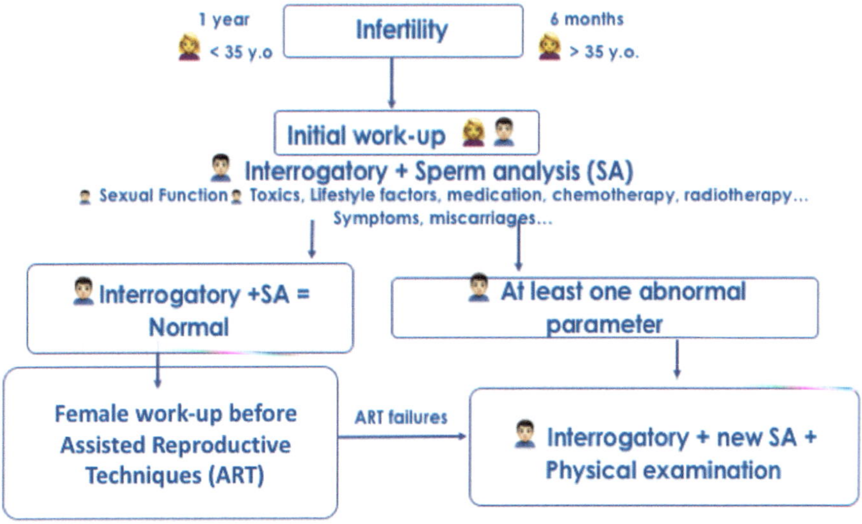

Fig. 1.1 Decision tree for the initial assessment of couples and men consulting for infertility, according to international recommendations [6]

has also been used in the latest sixth edition of the manual, albeit with some limitations which we will describe below.

The sixth edition, published in July 2021, highlights the importance of semen analysis as a tool for (1) assessing male reproductive health and function and guiding management, (2) guiding the choice of assisted reproductive procedure, (3) monitoring response to treatment, and (4) measuring the efficacy of male contraception [4].

The sixth edition also aimed to remedy the fifth edition's drawback linked to the demographic underrepresentation of certain geographical regions. The sixth edition therefore combined data from the previous fifth edition with new data on fertile men, whose partners had a delay to pregnancy ≤12 months, collected between 2010 and 2020 [7]. Thus, the sixth edition contains the results of sperm samples from 3589 fertile men (1800 subjects from the fifth edition and 1789 new subjects). The newly added data come from two Southern European countries, which were underrepresented in the fifth edition, as well as two Asian countries and one African country, which were not represented in the previous version. However, certain geographical areas, such as South America and sub-Saharan Africa, remain underrepresented in the sixth edition [3].

In the sixth edition, certain adjustments have been made to the basic semen parameters. The assessment of semen odor has been added, and the manual specifies that "odors of urine or putrefaction may be of clinical interest." It should be noted that the assessment of semen odor is subjective, which makes standardization of this parameter complicated. Furthermore, the addition of this parameter is contradicting with recommendations for the safety of laboratory personnel. It is possible that some countries will recommend the analysis of this parameter (along with all other semen parameters), which goes against the rules of personal protection against viruses and whose respiratory transmission cannot be excluded [3].

Regarding sperm motility, the sixth edition has readopted the distinction of progressive motility into two categories (grades a and b). Thus, the categorization of sperm motility has reverted to fast and progressive, slow and progressive, and non-progressive and immobile (grade a, b, c, or d, respectively) as mentioned in the fourth edition. This requires preincubation of clean microscope slides at 37 °C. To justify this choice, the WHO manual cites older articles indicating that rapid motility (grade a) is of clinical value [4].

With regard to indications for sperm vitality assessment, the sixth edition has resolved an inconsistency concerning sperm vitality assessment that existed in the previous fifth edition [3]. In the previous fifth edition, if progressive motility was below 40%, a vitality test was recommended, but the 40% threshold itself corresponded to that of total motility. In the sixth edition, sperm vitality testing is recommended when total sperm motility is below 40%.

Evaluation of sperm morphology using a systematic approach is described in the sixth edition with multiple, higher quality micrographs of sperm from untreated semen samples that are considered normal, borderline, or abnormal. These micrographs are accompanied by explanations of the classification of each evaluation, making this a useful guide. The evaluation of morphological abnormalities of the head, midpiece, and tail is described. The importance of recording the presence of large cytoplasmic droplets is emphasized.

Finally, an important change in version 6 of the manual is the abandonment of reference values. The thresholds for the fundamental sperm parameters used in the fifth edition and those described as "useful values" in the sixth edition are relatively comparable. The inclusion of additional areas and continents and the addition of a greater number of samples in the final analysis give greater statistical power to the reference ranges shown, even though the fifth percentiles are not significantly different from those in the 2010 WHO fifth edition (Table 1.1).

Although it is correct to state that reference values are not sufficient to assess the infertile man, in clinical practice, it is very likely that clinicians will be faced with some confusion in the absence of reference values. To rely on other reference values, clinicians will have to search the literature for other sources. This can be time-consuming and difficult. In addition, the latest international recommendations state that semen analysis is the cornerstone of infertility diagnosis. If sperm parameters are normal, the female partner should be evaluated for female factor infertility. If both male and female assessments are normal, the condition is considered as "unexplained infertility." In the case of normal sperm parameters and in the absence of evidence suggesting male infertility, it is not necessary to recheck the sperm results of a couple consulting for an initial fertility assessment. In the case of abnormal sperm parameters, the results of a single ejaculate examination may be sufficient to decide on the next steps in a male infertility investigation [6, 8–13]. However, due to the variability of sperm parameters from one ejaculate to another, repeated semen analysis (examination of 2 or 3 different ejaculates) can provide accurate mean values of sperm parameters [8–18]. Therefore, if one or more sperm parameters are abnormal (below fifth percentile values) [5], or if any element of the evaluation suggests male infertility, the couple should be referred for specialist care. A complete history, clinical examination, and sperm analysis are then recommended [6]. It seems difficult for clinicians to abandon the notion of "reference thresholds." The

Table 1.1 Lower fifth percentile (with 95% confidence interval) of WHO 2010 (fifth edition) and WHO 2021 (sixth edition) male semen parameters in couples initiating pregnancy within 1 year of unprotected intercourse resulting in natural conception [3, 4]

	WHO 2010	WHO 2021
Semen volume (ml)	1.5 (1.4–1.7)	1.4 (1.3–1.5)
Total number of spermatozoa (10^6 per ejaculate)	39 (33–46)	39 (35–40)
Sperm concentration (10^6/ml)	15 (12–16)	16 (15–18)
Total motility (%)	40 (38–42)	42 (40–43)
Progressive motility (%)	32 (31–34)	30 (29–31)
Nonprogressive motility (%)	1	1 (1–1)
Immobile spermatozoa (%)	22	20 (19–20)
Vitality (%)	58 (55–63)	54 (50–56)
Normal forms (%)	4 (3–4)	4 (3.9–4)

fifth percentile values will no doubt continue to be used at least to determine which additional tests should be carried out on a couple consulting us for infertility.

Extended Examination

The WHO sixth edition has brought together a series of extended semen tests that are not part of routine semen analysis but can be used to better assess sperm function and male fertility potential in certain clinical scenarios. These tests include indices of multiple sperm defects, SDF, genetic and genomic tests, tests related to immunology and immunological methods, interleukin assessment, immature germ cell assessment, sperm antibody coating test, biochemical tests for accessory gland function, and ejaculation sequence assessment [5].

Multiple Sperm Defect Indices

Multiple sperm defect indices consist of a detailed assessment of the incidence of morphological abnormalities in relation to an assessment of the percentage of morphologically normal sperm reported in the baseline sperm evaluation. These are three indices known as the teratozoospermia index (TZI), the multiple abnormalities index (MAI), and the sperm deformity index (SDI), which assess the head, middle, and main part of the spermatozoa [5]. The AUA/ASRM, EAU, and EAA guidelines on male infertility suggest the assessment of sperm Kruger morphology as part of a semen analysis and do not mention the use of multiple sperm abnormality indices [6, 19, 20]. This is due to the low sensitivity and specificity of indices of multiple sperm defects, and of morphology in general, in male infertility, except in specific situations that have a genetic basis for abnormal morphology, such as macrocephaly, globozoospermia, or fibrous sheath dysplasia [21]. However, evidence of multiple sperm abnormalities may be considered in situations where detailed evaluation of morphology is required.

Sperm DNA Fragmentation

Sperm DNA fragmentation can occur when base pairs are damaged or a break occurs in one or both strands of chromosomal DNA within spermatozoa [22, 23]. Sperm DNA fragmentation can be caused by both intrinsic and extrinsic factors, and increased SDF is associated with male infertility [24]. Abnormal SDF can affect embryonic development, implantation, and clinical pregnancies in both natural and assisted reproduction [5]. Four tests to assess SDF are described in the WHO sixth edition: terminal deoxynucleotidyl transferase biotin-dUTP labeling (TUNEL), sperm chromatin dispersion (SCD) test, comet assay, and acridine orange flow cytometry. It is not clear which of these tests best assesses SDF, and there is no consensus on thresholds for normal limits. The AUA/ASRM guidelines on male infertility suggest that SDF should be checked in male partners of couples with recurrent pregnancy loss (RPL) [6]. The UAE guidelines follow the same line and also call for testing in men with unexplained infertility, as well as in cases where ART has failed [20]. The EAA guideline states that SDF should be assessed before considering antiretroviral treatment [19]. This would allow correction of causes of SDF elevation, such as smoking cessation and other lifestyle modifications, varicocele repair, and treatment of male accessory gland infections.

Sperm Fluorescence In Situ Hybridization (FISH)

Sperm fluorescence in situ hybridization (FISH) is a cytogenetic test for detecting sperm aneuploidy. Gonadotoxic therapies, such as chemotherapy and radiotherapy, or advanced paternal age can lead to aneuploidy in spermatozoa [20]. If an aneuploid sperm fertilizes a euploid egg, it can lead to chromosomal abnormalities in the offspring, such as trisomy of an autosome, sex chromosome abnormalities such as 47 XXX or 47 XXY, or Robertsonian translocations [5]. Indications for sperm FISH testing are not detailed in the WHO manual and remain unclear, but it has been applied to couples with recurrent pregnancy losses and repeated implantation failures [25]. Additionally, the AUA/ASRM, EAU, and EAA guidelines on male infertility do not indicate when this test should be used.

Leukocytospermia

Leukocytes are normally present in most semen samples, but an abnormally high concentration is known as leukocytospermia. Leukocytospermia has been correlated with increased ROS production and elevated SDF. Leukocytospermia has several causes, including infection or inflammation of the male genitourinary tract, varicocele, urethral strictures, infrequent ejaculation, smoking and alcoholism, and autoimmune diseases. The WHO sixth edition describes two tests for identifying neutrophils in semen: cell peroxidase staining with ortho-toluidine and pan-leukocyte immunocyte staining. There are also protocols for assessing interleukins, a marker of inflammation in the male genital tract, and round cells in semen. AUA/ASRM, EAU, and EAA guidelines suggest that if leukocytospermia is identified on semen analysis, semen culture and treatment should be considered, as it may have an impact on fertility status.

Anti-sperm Antibodies (ASAs)

Anti-sperm antibodies (ASAs) are antibodies derived from an immune response directed against sperm antigens. IgA and IgG ASAs can be detected in semen, cervical mucus, and blood, while IgM is usually detected in blood. They can be identified following vasectomy, trauma, or infection involving the male reproductive system. The presence of ASAs can impair sperm motility and transit in the cervical mucus and the acrosomal response [5]. The WHO sixth edition described direct (mixed antiglobulin reaction and immunobead test) and indirect (indirect immunobead test) protocols for identifying ASAs. AUA/ASRM and EAU guidelines recognize ASA as an immunological cause of male infertility, but testing should only be performed if clinically relevant and if it alters patient management [4, 6, 19, 20].

Seminal Biochemistry

The measurement of zinc, fructose, and alpha-glucosidase in semen can provide important information on the secretory health of the prostate, seminal vesicles, and epididymides. The WHO sixth edition describes protocols for measuring levels of these substances to aid clinical diagnosis of infection or obstruction. Neither the AUA/ASRM nor the EAU guidelines mention the clinical usefulness of these tests. The EAA guideline deals only with the usefulness of seminal fructose testing [19]. History and physical examination, endocrine assessment, and acidic semen pH with low ejaculate volume are increasingly used to help identify obstructive causes of male infertility, limiting the use of these tests, which assess the secretory health of the male accessory glands.

Ejaculate Fraction

Ejaculation sequence assessment is an extended semen test based on the fact that the first third of the ejaculate contains sperm as well as prostatic secretions, and the last two-thirds contain seminal vesicular fluid [5]. This assessment is not recommended by any of the major guidelines on male infertility. The test may not be practical due to difficulty of the sample collection process, so it is mainly used for research purposes.

Advanced Tests

The WHO sixth edition identified that male infertility may be due to functional defects in sperm rather than insufficient production or impaired motility. Advanced sperm tests have been developed to better assess the ability of sperm to perform the tasks required to fertilize an egg in the female reproductive system. These tests include seminal OS and ROS analysis, acrosome reaction assessment, sperm chromatin assessment, sperm ion flow and transmembrane transport, computer-assisted sperm analysis (CASA), and other emerging technologies [5].

Seminal Oxidative Stress

There is growing evidence that seminal OS and ROS play an important role in male infertility [25–27]. Seminal ROS are produced by leukocytes and immature spermatozoa and also as a normal by-product of ATP production [28–30]. A balance between ROS and antioxidants is necessary for optimal sperm function. In the event of an imbalance between ROS and antioxidants, a state of OS occurs [31]. Oxidative stress can damage the sperm plasma membrane and lead to an increase in SDF while affecting concentration, motility, morphology, and capacitation [27, 32]. The term male oxidative stress infertility (MOSI) has been proposed to describe men with infertility and elevated OS who were previously classified as suffering from idiopathic male infertility [33]. The WHO sixth edition identifies three tests for measuring OS: luminol, oxidation reduction potential, and total antioxidant capacity. However, due to a lack of standardization and evidence from prospective trials, the EAU, AUA/ASRM, and EAA guidelines on male infertility do not recommend ROS testing in the routine assessment of male infertility [6, 19, 20]. Future studies could help shed light on this issue.

Acrosome Reaction

The physiological acrosome reaction occurs in the zona pellucida after sperm attachment. The integrity of the acrosome structure and the ability to undergo acrosomal exocytosis are required for normal fertility. The acrosome reaction is a process that occurs in vivo near the oocyte and must occur in order for the spermatozoa to penetrate the oocyte robes and fuse with the oocyte. Calcium influx is believed to be an initiating event in the normal acrosome reaction. Several different stimuli are known to induce the acrosome reaction. Among them, zona pellucida proteins and progesterone are considered possible physiological inducers of the acrosome reaction due to their high concentrations near the oocyte [34]. In the sixth edition of the WHO manual, unlike the previous edition, explanations are made with progesterone induction. After induction of the acrosome reaction in vitro, acrosome status can be assessed by microscopy or flow cytometry with fluorescently labeled lectins such as *Pisum sativum* (pea agglutinin) or *Arachis hypogaea* (peanut lectin) or monoclonal antibodies to the acrosome antigen CD46. The WHO sixth edition proposes two tests to assess sperm acrosome functionality: the acrosome status test and the induced acrosome reaction test [5]. Further validation of these tests is required before they can be recommended in guidelines and taken into account in the routine assessment of male infertility.

Sperm Chromatin Condensation

The structure of sperm chromatin is important for normal fertilization and embryonic development. The normality of sperm chromatin can be evaluated by the evaluation of DNA strand breaks or by dyes that bind to histones (aniline blue) or nucleic acid (chromomycin A3) and is evaluated histologically or by flow cytometry. Aniline blue (AB) binds to the lysine residues of histones. The percentage of AB-stained sperm can be evaluated in either whole semen or selected (swim-up or density gradient prepared) sperm. Chromomycin A3 (CMA3) competes with protamines for binding to the minor groove of the DNA helix. The percentage of CMA3-stained sperm can be evaluated in whole semen or spermatozoa selected by swim-up. Scoring for both methods is operator-dependent, so results may be subjective. Abnormal chromatin structure is associated with increased SDF [35]. As sperm chromatin structure abnormalities are closely associated with elevated SDF, they may be considered in scenarios of RPL, unexplained infertility, or failure of previous ART. Future studies are warranted to clarify whether there is an advantage to performing these tests rather than directly measuring SDF, before they are adopted by clinical guidelines.

Transmembrane Ion Flow

Transmembrane ion flow and sperm transport are emerging areas of research in male infertility. Several key sperm functions are activated by intracellular changes in pH, calcium concentration, or membrane tension [5]. Abnormalities in sperm transmembrane ion flow can potentially impact motility, capacitation, and acrosome response. Defects in the CatSper gene have been associated with male infertility due to alteration of the sperm flagellum, which ultimately affects motility and function [36]. Hence, unlike previous editions, functional analysis of transmembrane ion flow and transport in sperm is included in the sixth edition of the WHO manual. A series of physiological events, such as sperm hyperactivation, egg-directed chemotaxis, capacitation, and acrosome reaction, which are crucial for fertility, are triggered by the activation of sperm ion channels in response to various chemical uses.

The new edition discusses ion exchange and transport in two main channels: CatSper Ca channel and K channels.

These signaling events are mediated by the interaction of unique, mostly sperm-specific ion channels, exchangers, and transporters, e.g., CatSper Ca^{2+} channels, Slo3 K+ channels, Hv1 H+ channels, Na+/H+ modifiers (sNHE, NHA1, NHA2), Ca^{2+} ATPases (PMCA4), and Mg^{2+} transporters (CNNM2, CNNM4). Many as yet unexplained cases of sperm dysfunction may result from defective function of one or more of these proteins. Genetic abnormalities affecting CatSper genes, defective CatSper function or expression, and defective K+– channel function have been associated with male infertility [36]. Until now, routine diagnostic procedures to evaluate the function of ion channels, exchangers, and transporters in sperm from patients are unfortunately lacking. However, research protocols have been developed to investigate the activity of ion channels (with low to moderate efficiency) in sperm from patients within the framework of clinical studies.

The CatSper channel is confined to the principal piece of sperm flagellum as shown by localization pattern in mice and humans. The function of CatSper in human sperm can be studied by electrophysiology and kinetic Ca^{2+} fluorimetry, respectively.

Slo3 represents the principal K+ channel in human sperm. It is activated by Ca^{2+} and thus modulates the membrane potential of human sperm in a $[Ca^{2+}]$i-dependent manner. The function of Slo3 in human sperm can be studied in low and moderate yield whole-cell patch-clamp recordings and Vm fluorimetry, respectively. Functional tests are lacking for many of these proteins, and current techniques for assessing CatSper or Slo3 function are too demanding to be applied in the clinical laboratory.

CASA Systems

Computer-assisted semen analysis (CASA) technology uses electronic imaging to visualize sperm and analyze several individual semen parameters, including concentration, motility, sperm kinematics, and morphology. The main advantages of CASA analysis over conventional semen analysis are that it guarantees reliability, consistency, accuracy, and repeatability when processing multiple images of a semen sample. In addition, computerized systems are used to assess sperm hyperactivation [5]. However, the agglutination and pleomorphic morphology of human spermatozoa, generally high viscosity of human semen, and background cellular debris have limited the use of CASA in clinical andrology laboratories [37]. In addition, CASA systems generally fail on low-concentration semen, which limits their usefulness in semen analysis laboratories, since in this case, the manual technique must be performed. Furthermore, these systems are expensive and cannot be integrated into all andrology laboratories worldwide, thus limiting their use. Emerging technologies have been developed in the field of computer and technological advances to improve quality, visualization, and access to male infertility diagnostics. Some systems can be used at home. All these diagnostics should undergo a rigorous validation process before being included in male infertility guidelines.

Conclusion

The new edition of the WHO manual is technically sound and provides all the details needed to perform a semen analysis. In the current edition of the WHO manual, it is stated that semen analysis should be used to assist in:

- Diagnosis of male reproductive disorders
- Identify avenues of investigation
- Choose appropriate initial and follow-up therapy
- Choose appropriate ARTs, if necessary

However, criteria for the clinical use of these parameters are lacking, notably due to the absence of reference values. As a result, clinicians no longer know how to interpret test results or what action to take. Such limitation may be overcome in future editions of the WHO manual.

Take-Home Messages

1. When a couple is experiencing infertility, it is important to assess both partners, as a male factor is involved in 50% of cases.
2. The basic evaluation of the man should include (at least) a medical history and basic semen analysis.
3. The need for further testing, including extended semen testing, endocrine and genetic evaluation, and imaging, should be based on the results of the initial baseline evaluation.
4. The WHO sixth edition recommends the clinician to determine fertility potential of the patient based on the clinical evaluation including results of semen analysis.
5. Several advanced semen tests have been described in the WHO sixth edition. However, these tests are not incorporated into male infertility guidelines and require future studies to assess their clinical utility.

References

1. Boivin J, Bunting L, Collins JA, Nygren KG. International estimates of infertility prevalence and treatment-seeking: potential need and demand for infertility medical care. Hum Reprod Oxf Engl. 2007;22(6):1506–12.
2. Agarwal A, Baskaran S, Parekh N, Cho CL, Henkel R, Vij S, et al. Male infertility. Lancet Lond Engl. 2021;397(10271):319–33.

3. Boitrelle F, Shah R, Saleh R, Henkel R, Kandil H, Chung E, et al. The sixth edition of the WHO manual for human semen analysis: a critical review and SWOT analysis. Life Basel Switz. 2021;11(12):1368.
4. World Health Organization. WHO laboratory manual for the examination and processing of human semen. 6th ed. Geneva: World Health Organization; 2021. Available from: https://apps.who.int/iris/handle/10665/343208
5. Guzick DS, Overstreet JW, Factor-Litvak P, Brazil CK, Nakajima ST, Coutifaris C, et al. Sperm morphology, motility, and concentration in fertile and infertile men. N Engl J Med. 2001;345(19):1388–93.
6. Schlegel PN, Sigman M, Collura B, De Jonge CJ, Eisenberg ML, Lamb DJ, et al. Diagnosis and treatment of infertility in men: AUA/ASRM guideline part I. Fertil Steril. 2021;115(1):54–61.
7. Poland ML, Moghissi KS, Giblin PT, Ager JW, Olson JM. Variation of semen measures within normal men. Fertil Steril. 1985;44(3):396–400.
8. Barratt CLR, Björndahl L, De Jonge CJ, Lamb DJ, Osorio Martini F, McLachlan R, et al. The diagnosis of male infertility: an analysis of the evidence to support the development of global WHO guidance-challenges and future research opportunities. Hum Reprod Update. 2017;23(6):660–80.
9. Christman MS, Kraft KH, Tasian GE, Zderic SA, Kolon TF. Reproducibility and reliability of semen analysis in youths at risk for infertility. J Urol. 2013;190(2):683–8.
10. Francavilla F, Barbonetti A, Necozione S, Santucci R, Cordeschi G, Macerola B, et al. Within-subject variation of seminal parameters in men with infertile marriages. Int J Androl. 2007;30(3):174–81.
11. Leushuis E, van der Steeg JW, Steures P, Repping S, Bossuyt PMM, Blankenstein MA, et al. Reproducibility and reliability of repeated semen analyses in male partners of subfertile couples. Fertil Steril. 2010;94(7):2631–5.
12. Mishail A, Marshall S, Schulsinger D, Sheynkin Y. Impact of a second semen analysis on a treatment decision making in the infertile man with varicocele. Fertil Steril. 2009;91(5):1809–11.
13. Stokes-Riner A, Thurston SW, Brazil C, Guzick D, Liu F, Overstreet JW, et al. One semen sample or 2? Insights from a study of fertile men. J Androl. 2007;28(5):638–43.
14. Zhu QX, Gao ES, Pathak N, Wu JQ, Zhou WJ. Single or double semen samples: the dilemma in epidemiological studies on semen quality. Hum Reprod Oxf Engl. 2016;31(3):511–7.
15. Berman NG, Wang C, Paulsen CA. Methodological issues in the analysis of human sperm concentration data. J Androl. 1996;17(1):68–73.
16. Carlsen E, Petersen JH, Andersson AM, Skakkebaek NE. Effects of ejaculatory frequency and season on variations in semen quality. Fertil Steril. 2004;82(2):358–66.
17. Castilla JA, Alvarez C, Aguilar J, González-Varea C, Gonzalvo MC, Martínez L. Influence of analytical and biological variation on the clinical interpretation of seminal parameters. Hum Reprod Oxf Engl. 2006;21(4):847–51.
18. Keel BA. Within- and between-subject variation in semen parameters in infertile men and normal semen donors. Fertil Steril. 2006;85(1):128–34.
19. Colpi GM, Francavilla S, Haidl G, Link K, Behre HM, Goulis DG, et al. European Academy of Andrology guideline Management of oligo-astheno-teratozoospermia. Andrology. 2018;6(4):513–24.
20. Tharakan T, Bettocchi C, Carvalho J, Corona G, Jones TH, Kadioglu A, et al. European Association of Urology guidelines panel on male sexual and reproductive health: a clinical consultation guide on the indications for performing sperm DNA fragmentation testing in men with infertility and testicular sperm extraction in nonazoospermic men. Eur Urol Focus. 2022;8(1):339–50.
21. Gatimel N, Moreau J, Parinaud J, Léandri RD. Sperm morphology: assessment, pathophysiology, clinical relevance, and state of the art in 2017. Andrology. 2017;5(5):845–62.
22. Simon L, Emery B, Carrell DT. Sperm DNA fragmentation: consequences for reproduction. Adv Exp Med Biol. 2019;1166:87–105.

23. Tan J, Taskin O, Albert A, Bedaiwy MA. Association between sperm DNA fragmentation and idiopathic recurrent pregnancy loss: a systematic review and meta-analysis. Reprod Biomed Online. 2019;38(6):951–60.
24. Agarwal A, Majzoub A, Baskaran S, Panner Selvam MK, Cho CL, Henkel R, et al. Sperm DNA fragmentation: a new guideline for clinicians. World J Mens Health. 2020;38(4):412.
25. Rodrigo L, Meseguer M, Mateu E, Mercader A, Peinado V, Bori L, et al. Sperm chromosomal abnormalities and their contribution to human embryo aneuploidy. Biol Reprod. 2019;101(6):1091–101.
26. Agarwal A, Sharma RK, Nallella KP, Thomas AJ, Alvarez JG, Sikka SC. Reactive oxygen species as an independent marker of male factor infertility. Fertil Steril. 2006;86(4):878–85.
27. Agarwal A, Durairajanayagam D, Halabi J, Peng J, Vazquez-Levin M. Proteomics, oxidative stress and male infertility. Reprod Biomed Online. 2014;29(1):32–58.
28. Wagner H, Cheng JW, Ko EY. Role of reactive oxygen species in male infertility: an updated review of literature. Arab J Urol. 2018;16(1):35–43.
29. Aitken RJ, West K, Buckingham D. Leukocytic infiltration into the human ejaculate and its association with semen quality, oxidative stress, and sperm function. J Androl. 1994;15(4):343–52.
30. Cassina A, Silveira P, Cantu L, Montes JM, Radi R, Sapiro R. Defective human sperm cells are associated with mitochondrial dysfunction and oxidant production. Biol Reprod. 2015;93(5):119.
31. Walczak-Jedrzejowska R, Wolski JK, Slowikowska-Hilczer J. The role of oxidative stress and antioxidants in male fertility. Cent Eur J Urol. 2013;66(1):60–7.
32. Aitken RJ. Reactive oxygen species as mediators of sperm capacitation and pathological damage. Mol Reprod Dev. 2017;84(10):1039–52.
33. Agarwal A, Parekh N, Panner Selvam MK, Henkel R, Shah R, Homa ST, et al. Male oxidative stress infertility (MOSI): proposed terminology and clinical practice guidelines for management of idiopathic male infertility. World J Mens Health. 2019;37(3):296–312.
34. Beltrán C, Treviño CL, Mata-Martínez E, Chávez JC, Sánchez-Cárdenas C, Baker M, et al. Role of ion channels in the sperm acrosome reaction. Adv Anat Embryol Cell Biol. 2016;220:35–69.
35. Bungum M, Bungum L, Giwercman A. Sperm chromatin structure assay (SCSA): a tool in diagnosis and treatment of infertility. Asian J Androl. 2011;13(1):69–75.
36. Smith JF, Syritsyna O, Fellous M, Serres C, Mannowetz N, Kirichok Y, et al. Disruption of the principal, progesterone-activated sperm Ca^{2+} channel in a CatSper2-deficient infertile patient. Proc Natl Acad Sci U S A. 2013;110(17):6823–8.
37. Mortimer ST, van der Horst G, Mortimer D. The future of computer-aided sperm analysis. Asian J Androl. 2015;17(4):545–53.

Chapter 2
Endocrine-Disrupting Chemicals (EDCs) and Male Infertility

Lucia Rocco, Damayanthi Durairajanayagam, and Filomena Mottola

Key Points

- In this review, we will discuss endocrine-disrupting chemicals (EDCs) and their impact on the male reproductive system and semen quality.
- We will summarize main mechanisms by which EDCs disrupt sperm quality.
- Additionally, we will discuss the disorders associated with EDCs in the male and their potential transgenerational impact.
- Furthermore, we will highlight the limitations of EDC research and future research trends.

Introduction

Over the last two decades, there has been a decline in human fertility around the world. It is estimated that 9% of couples have difficulties in procreating after a year of unprotected intercourse, and in one in two cases, the hurdle in obtaining a pregnancy is related to male reproductive problems [1]. The discriminating factor appears to be a reduction in sperm count in young men, of which 10–15% have such low sperm concentration that they require fertility treatment [2, 3]. Reduced concentration of spermatozoa is most often attributable to cryptorchidism, varicocele, inflammatory and infectious states of the seminal tract, use of drugs, and altered lifestyles [4–8]. Sometimes, the cause lies in testicles' imperfect development that already occurs in the fetus due to birth defects associated with exposure to toxic environmental factors. Environmental exposures deriving from the modern lifestyle represent the most important cause of infertility etiology. External factors can influence the endocrine system of adult and act directly or through epigenetic

L. Rocco (✉) · F. Mottola
Department of Environmental, Biological and Pharmaceutical Sciences and Technologies, University of Campania "Luigi Vanvitelli", Caserta, Italy
e-mail: lucia.rocco@unicampania.it; filomena.mottola@unicampania.it

D. Durairajanayagam
Department of Physiology, Faculty of Medicine, Universiti Teknologi MARA, Sungai Buloh Campus, Shah Alam, Selangor, Malaysia

A. Agarwal et al. (eds.), *Current and Future Advances in Male Infertility*, https://doi.org/10.1007/978-3-031-62648-7_2

modifications, impacting several generations after exposure [2]. Humans can be exposed to a large number of chemicals identified as endocrine-disrupting chemicals (EDCs); the main sources of these substances such as polychlorinated biphenyls (PCBs), dichlorodiphenyltrichloroethane (DDT), bisphenol A (BPA), or phthalates (DBP, DEHP) can be products of daily use, as cosmetics, food, as well as agricultural products and industrial chemicals [9]. Effects of endocrine disruptors on testis development, male fertility, and transition age are the subject of numerous studies. Despite controversial evidence, the overall conclusion finds a positive association between EDC exposure and alterations in sperm motility, male puberty, sexual function, and gonad development [10, 11]. It has been proven that exposure to EDCs during particular stages of development such as in utero exposure, early life, or during puberty can induce organ abnormalities, behavioral disturbances, onset of cancer, and bone mass dysfunction [12].

This narrative review aims to discuss the impact of EDC exposure on male reproductive health. We reviewed extensive literature on types and sources of EDCs focusing on the mechanisms behind the damage in sperm cells, sexual hormonal dysregulation, and associated EDC disorders. Moreover, we discuss epigenetic changes and increase sperm DNA damage and sperm aneuploidy following EDC exposure, potentially capable of generating transgenerational effects in offspring. At last, we highlight limitations of the current male infertility-related EDC studies and prospects for future research on EDCs aimed to fully understand their impact on male reproductive system and semen quality and endorse measures and policies to minimize exposure to EDCs, safeguarding public health and the environment.

Endocrine-Disrupting Chemicals (EDCs)

The decline in global fertility has been exacerbated by the release into the environment of an ever-increasing number of toxic substances. A noteworthy concern is EDC exposure to which humans and animals constantly struggle. These are various or a mixture of exogenous substances, capable of interacting with the endocrine system, altering its functionality, and consequently generating adverse effects on exposed organism's health. More precisely, the US Environmental Protection Agency (EPA) has defined them as compounds that interfere with the synthesis, secretion, transport, metabolism, binding, or elimination of natural hormones responsible for homeostasis, reproduction, and development [13].

Disruption of the endocrine system can occur in several ways. The ability and the way to interfere with the endocrine system vary according to the type of EDCs. They generally act by mimicking a natural hormone, thus inducing an excessive or inappropriate response to the stimulus, blocking the effects of a hormone or causing overproduction or underproduction of hormones by directly stimulating or inhibiting the endocrine system [14].

Types and sources of EDCs are so many that it is almost impossible to escape contact with them.

A recent systematic review of 48 studies sampling the air near oil and gas extraction sites identified more than 26 substances in the air with endocrine activity or as having potential endocrine activity [15]. However, EDCs have also been found in consumer products increasing the requirement in identifying the source. An older report analyzing indoor and outdoor air samples in 40 nonsmoking homes in urban, industrial, and rural areas of California found that indoor EDC concentrations were higher than outdoor concentrations placing the concern on household chemicals [16]. The presence of compounds with endocrine-disrupting activity in indoor matrices has been confirmed by a recent toxicological evaluation of indoor pollution mixtures, where in addition to the ingestion of powders, the authors consider inhalation as a non-negligible route of exposure [17]. Water is also an important source of EDCs probably due to the intensification of anthropic activities (horticulture, boating, fishing, and agricultural activities). In southern Italy, for example, they have been detected both in sediments and in water with a frequency of over 60% [18]. High concentrations were also found around the world, such as in wastewater in Canada [19] and in California [20] and discharge in China [21].

Another major concern is the presence of EDCs in the drinking water, since the complete removal of EDCs by conventional treatments does not always occur as the treatment process was not designed for their elimination [22]. In fact, several studies find drinking water as a potential source for human exposure to EDCs. This represents an enormous risk for the health of exposed organisms as, given their hydrophobicity and lipophilicity, EDCs tend to bioconcentrate along the food chain [23]. Although scientific evidence on the presence of EDCs in food and on the interactions with food components that modulate the endocrine system is still limited [24], their presence in water is a strong indicator of their accumulation in food, so diet could also be a significant source of EDC exposure.

As mentioned above, a variety of chemicals have been found to disrupt the endocrine systems, ubiquitously distributed in the different environmental matrices; the types and sources of main ones known to interfere with male reproductive health are discussed below.

Polychlorinated Biphenyls (PCBs)

Polychlorinated biphenyls (PCBs) are mixtures of up to 209 chlorinated compounds (known as congeners). They are nonnatural oily liquids or lightly colored solids, used as coolants, lubricants, and insulators, in transformers, capacitors, and other electrical equipment. Only 12 of the 209 PCB congeners have chemical-physical and toxicological characteristics comparable to dioxins and are therefore called dioxin-like (DL-PCB). The remaining congeners are the most common in the environment indicated with the following numbers depending on the number and position of the chlorine atoms, of which PCB 28, PCB 52, PCB 101, PCB 138, PCB 153, and PCB 180 are recommended to use as indicators in monitoring studies according to the Stockholm Convention [25]. PCBs are banned in the United States since 1977 as considered potentially toxic by the US Environmental Protection Agency (EPA), so, to date, the main source of PCB exposure is the redistribution of persistent PCBs in soil and water [26]. Millions of tons of PCBs are believed to have been produced, although a complete estimate of global PCB production is still difficult today [27]. Despite more than 40 years after their withdrawal, their persistence in the environment is still a concern for health. The environmental omnipresence of PCBs is due to their resistance to chemical and biological degradation, so much so that they are still detected throughout the planet [28, 29], especially in aquatic environments [30], and therefore identified as persistent organic pollutants (POP). PCBs present in aquatic environments can be transferred to the human body through dermal contact, even if only by contact with contaminated water; through inhalation near urbanized and industrialized areas; through consumption of fruits and vegetables washed down with PCB-contaminated water; and through consumption of aquatic animals from a polluted aquatic environment. This can generate biomagnification in the food chain up to being transferred to humans where they could trigger deleterious health effects [31]. The evaluation of the effects on human health deriving from exposure to PCBs is challenging as the physicochemical properties of PCB congeners can exert different actions depending on the number of chlorine atoms. But overall, these compounds are known to exert estrogenic, antiestrogenic, hepatotoxic, immunotoxic, and neurotoxic properties [26].

Dichlorodiphenyltrichloroethane (DDT) and Its Main Metabolite (DDE)

DDT is a chlorophenylethane (1,1,1-trichloro-2,2-diphenylethane) substituted by additional chlorine substituents in the four positions of the phenyl groups. It is a nonnatural organochlorine insecticide of a colorless crystalline solid form or a whitish powder, classified by the International Agency for Research on Cancer (IARC) as a possible human carcinogen [32]. Given its lipophilicity, when absorbed through dissolution in oils or fats, DDT concentrates in the adipose tissue where it is slowly eliminated [33]. DDT was banned in the United States and in many European countries in the early 1970s. To date, it falls under the Stockholm Convention on Persistent Organic Pollutants (POPs) and the POP Protocol (CLRTAP-POP) in the Convention on Atmospheric Pollution at large distance of the United Nations Economic Commission for Europe (UNECE) [34]. However, it is still used for vector control, especially in areas affected by endemic malaria [35]. DDT and metabolites are defined as the DDT complex. Among the metabolites, DDE is mainly present as a residue in soils as it is more resistant to biodegradation and photolysis [36]. DDT complex spreads into the atmosphere following nebulization operations. About half of the DDT present in the air is adsorbed to the particulate matter; the remaining part can also accumulate in the soil and reach the aquatic system from wastewater discharges, especially if used as vector control near lakes and rivers

[36]. Even a recent study has shown its presence also in European soils managed according to the rules of organic agriculture, certified according to the EC 2008 Regulation of the European Commission. Only 26 soils out of 142 sampled soils in Poland were free of detectable DDT residues [37]. Also, high concentrations of DDT have been found in the aquatic environment around the world [38]. Consequentially, DDT took part in the phenomena of biomagnification as, accumulating in the soil and water, it reaches humans through the food chain. A growing concern is DDT accumulation in breast milk. Given the high lipid content, breast milk is a significant biomarker for the estimation of POP's residues in the human body. It was noted that infants consume 39 times DDT-tolerable lipid level of human milk of 3.1 ng/g of lipids. The consequences on human health due to exposure to the DDT mixture can be varied; mainly the effects on the reproductive system are known. Data on human health show as main effects androgen receptor antagonism, prostate cancer, pancreatic cancer, breast cancer, altered bone mineral density, non-Hodgkin's lymphoma, and neurologic effects [39, 40].

Bisphenol A (BPA)

Bisphenol A is a colorless solid, insoluble in water, derived from diphenylmethane with two hydroxyphenyl groups. It is used in the commercial plastic synthesis, found in a wide range of consumer products. Mainly used for epoxy resins and polycarbonate resins as a chemical intermediate, it can also be found in adhesives and sealant chemicals, flame retardants, paint additives, propellants, and commonly used materials such as electrical and electronic products, plastic and rubber products, toys, playground, and sporting equipment [41]. Given its wide use in the production of polycarbonate plastic, its diffusion and distribution in the environment are huge. The evidence on its carcinogenicity is limited; therefore, it is classified by the IARC as belonging to group 3 ("not classifiable as to its carcinogenicity for humans"). BPA can be released into the environment by many products during the production, use, and disposal phases. It can reach all environmental matrices: air, soil, sediments, wastewater, sewage sludge, surface water, and bioaccumulative products. In fact, high concentrations in these environments were detected [42]. Volatilization can occur but is not an important pollution process due to the low vapor pressure; however, inhalation and skin contact are important routes of exposure for workers involved in the BPA production. Ingestion through contaminated food is the main route of exposure for humans [42]. However, the highest concentration was found in preserved and ready-made canned foods compared to foods in plastic, glass, or paper containers [43]. However, the data on average concentrations of BPA in foods are highly variable, probably due to different methods of food processing and storage [44].

The effects of their accumulation in organisms can be deleterious. Environmental BPA exposure is known for impaired human development, reproduction, metabolism, and cardiac and liver functions and for inducing immune, inflammation, genotoxic, and oxidative effects [44, 45].

Phthalates (DBP, DEHP)

Phthalates are odorless diesters of phthalic acid (1,2-benzenedicarboxylic acid) liquids at room temperature with a low melting point. This feature makes them ideal compounds for the manufacture of flexible plastic products [46]. They are synthesized and used as industrial solvents, plasticizers, personal care products, and additives in polyvinyl chloride (PVC) plastics. Among the latter, diethylhexyl phthalate (DEHP) is the main phthalate on the market, used to give plastic flexibility [47], while dibutyl phthalate (DBP) is the most widely used in cosmetics and personal care products.

Between 2008 and 2009, the use of phthalates was restricted in toys in Europe (https://eur-lex.europa.eu/legal-content/EN/TXT/?uri=CELEX%3A32009L0048) and in the United States (https://www.cpsc.gov/Regulations-Laws%2D%2DStandards/Statutes/The-Consumer-Product-Security Improvement Act), given that the public health concern is their possible genotoxicity and cancer-inducing potential endorsed over the years [48]. Like the other contaminants described so far, phthalates are widely spread in the environment for their enormous use; therefore, given an ever-stronger awareness of their toxicity, concern for biota and humans increases. They reach freshwater on land by precipitation and accumulate in rivers, lakes, and sediments around the world because of their low water solubility [49]. The major exposure route is dermal absorption for their presence in cosmetics and personal care products; skin exposure is also possible during industrial production [50]. Literature evidence suggests that exposure can also occur through clothing as phthalates are readily adsorbed by cotton fabric. Carcinogenic risk assessment advises that their presence in cotton could have potential adverse health effects. Several phthalates were found in percentages of 100% for each type in 24 samples of baby cotton clothing purchased from various shopping malls in China, suggesting that the danger to children is not given only by their presence in toys [51]. Anyway, ingestion through contaminated food and water should not be underestimated. By analyzing human urine samples, data on the risk assessment of possibly contaminated water showed that the health risk from exposure to phthalates was greater by drinking tap water than by consuming bottled, filtered tap water [52]. It follows a risk to foods such as fruits and vegetables rinsed with unfiltered tap water. To date, toxicological studies have demonstrated the cytotoxicity, genotoxicity, and embryotoxicity, though phthalate toxicity target is the reproductive systems primarily [53]; therefore, the need to reduce the use of phthalates, especially in commonly used products, is getting stronger.

EDCs and Semen Quality

The accumulation in the environment of toxic substances known to target the endocrine system has become a serious threat. Inverse correlations between EDC exposure and male reproduction have been found in numerous epidemiological studies suggesting that the testis is an important target organ. Parameters such as the decrease in sperm count, motility, vitality, abnormal morphology, and damage to sperm DNA have been confirmed in some studies evaluating the influence of EDCs on male fertility [54, 55]. Several studies have shown the effect of PCBs and DTT on gonadal dysfunction and sperm motility, reporting an increase in aromatase activity and estrogen production, competitive binding to cellular estrogen receptors, and inhibition of corticosterone synthesis [56]. But some results regarding sperm concentration and morphology are conflicting. A previous study concludes that exposure of adults to PCBs or DDE has no adverse effects on sperm concentration or morphology of populations in Arctic or Europe. However, populations exposed to high PCB concentrations show 20% average reduction in sperm motility compared to the slightly exposed populations [57]. Similarly, current data indicate a significant negative association with urinary BPA concentrations and sperm motility. In particular, prolonged exposure to high doses of BPA induced a reduction in mitochondrial membrane potential with activation of the caspase and decrease in motility, genomic damage, and finally reduced number of viable spermatozoa [58]. But the observational data evaluating the link between exposure to BPA and male reproductive function remain inconsistent. Some studies show that seminal levels of BPA were negatively correlated with semen parameters and positively with reduced concentrations of circulating serum sex hormones. However, others found no association between BPA levels and sperm parameters, nor with sex hormone levels [59]. Environmental exposure to phthalates may also impair human semen quality. A cross-sectional study in China shows that phthalate metabolites found in 687 human semen samples were significantly associated with decreases in sperm volume, motility, and morphology as parameters such as abnormal heads and tails were found [60]. However, contradictory data are also available for phthalates.

Although statistically significant concentrations of phthalates and their metabolites were found in infertile males, no associations were found between their presence and reduced sperm quality except a slight inverse relationship between phthalate metabolites and normal sperm morphology [61]. The evidence for induced genomic damage is likewise variable. Although some evidence on significant positive correlation between seminal EDC level and the percentage of sperm DNA damage subsists, data affirming the opposite are consistent. A regression analysis found no statistically significant consistent associations between the sperm DNA damage and any of the PCB congeners [62]. However, Spanò et al. [63] found that human exposure to PCBs negatively impacted the sperm chromatin integrity of adult European males. Similarly, a weak association between plasma DDT/DDE concentration and the incidence of chromatin defective spermatozoa was found in young South African males professionally exposed to DDT [64]. Urinary BPA concentrations appear to be related to an increase in the sperm DNA fragmentation (SDF) index in healthy young men who typically represent the population with high reproductive prospects [65]. Interestingly, the SDF value exceeded the 30% threshold considered critical for fertility [66]. Indeed, also other investigators have found correlation between urinary concentrations of BPA and damage to spermatic DNA. But it must be pointed out that the strongest correlations were evident in patients with asthenoteratospermia, oligoasthenoteratospermia, and asthenospermia to indicate that the possibility of different contributing causes of SDF was not investigated [67]. Several tests instead show a correlation between urinary levels of phthalates, more precisely of their metabolites, and damage to the spermatic DNA in a dose-response relationship [68–70]. At present, the impairment of spermatogenesis and alteration of seminal parameters by EDCs have been demonstrated in animal models. Tests on humans are limited and conflicting given the enormous heterogeneity of populations, genetic susceptibility or predisposition, different extent of environmental exposure, and lifestyles. Therefore, epidemiological studies and targeted studies on the human model are still needed to clarify the real impact of these contaminants on male fertility and perhaps blame them for the decline in global fertility.

Mechanism(s) of Action on EDCs on the Male Reproductive System

Although the effects on testicular steroid synthesis are still under consideration, various studies on occupational exposure and environmental contamination attribute reduced male fertility to EDCs. The mechanisms of action of these chemicals have not been fully understood; however, it is commonly accepted that they interact with normal hormonal homeostasis and therefore with steroidogenesis. The best known action is the interference of EDCs with the hormonal binding to the androgen receptor (AR) or the estrogen receptor (ER) followed by either a hormonal agonistic or antagonistic response [71].

Also, depending on their structure, PCB metabolites can act as estrogen agonists or antagonists. Direct gene expression modulation dependent on nuclear steroid hormone is shown in various PCB-exposed models [72]. These disruptions may have different consequences in humans [73, 74] as interference of sperm development, testicular maturation, or epididymal function as well as it could impair the ability of sperm to move as discussed above. The mechanisms below these effects were studied in rats. Underlying impairment of sperm motility appears to be a premature acrosome reaction, and reduction of prostate-specific antigen (PSA) in sperm is associated with sperm motility [57].

A systematic review of in vitro, in vivo, and epidemiological studies reported positive associations between exposure to PCBs and increased levels of pro-inflammatory cytokines.

PCBs have been shown to modulate cytochrome P450 (CYP), contributing to the release of hydrogen peroxide and superoxide radical anion and thus inducing oxidative stress [75]. Oxidative stress is the major cause of DNA damage in spermatozoa, and it is an important factor for the etiology of male infertility as the lack of DNA repair capacity [76].

Specifically, PCBs can induce the formation of reactive oxygen species (ROS), genotoxicity, immune suppression, inflammatory response, and endocrine effects, through different pathways and depending on the PCB type. Dioxin-like PCBs bind steroid and thyroid hormones, altering the endocrine system, while less chlorinated PCBs act through metabolic activation, with the formation of carcinogenic metabolites [77]. Exposure to DDE also inhibits steroidogenic function. In particular, it has been observed that chronic lower doses have a greater ability to alter steroidogenesis and testosterone production, probably causing incomplete masculinization in puberty and impairing reproductive capacity in the adult [78].

The thesis that oxidative stress is one of the main mediators of EDC action is supported by several in vivo and in vitro studies also for pesticides. In male Wistar rats, there was an increase in lipid peroxidation (LPO), one of the main manifestations of oxidative damage promoted by ROS, and increase in the level of hydrogen peroxide (H_2O_2) after DDT injection, while the level of antioxidant enzymes such as superoxide dismutase (SOD) and catalase (CAT) was reduced [79]. This was accompanied by DNA degradation and apoptosis in testicular tissues as well as intense apoptosis in the germ cells of rats exposed to DDT. DDT-induced apoptosis in testicular cells has also been demonstrated by Song et al. [80]. The authors suggested that MAPK phosphorylation could play critical roles in DDE-induced apoptosis in the Sertoli cells.

MAPK is known to translate signals from the plasma membrane to the cell nucleus and to play important functions in controlling cell survival, proliferation, and differentiation. It was found that members of the Bax family are involved in the oxidative stress activation of the MAPK pathway. Elevated levels of Bax and Bak mRNA have been highlighted, and this upregulation could explain the pro-apoptotic effect of DDE on Sertoli cells in vitro. Detrimental effects of BPA on spermatogenesis also occur through increased oxidative stress and apoptosis in mice germ cell, decrease in glutathione peroxidase (GSH-Px) activity, and increase in ROS levels, LPO levels, and number of germ cells with fragmented DNA [81]. In addition, increased levels of malondialdehyde (MDA) in rat testicular tissues and epididymis were highlighted with increasing BPA dose, suggesting the excessive generation of free radicals [76]. As well as for BPA, phthalate alters the structure and functions of the epididymis in adult rats, decreasing SOD activity and increasing MDA level [82]. They act as an antiandrogen in fact; DBP exposure in adult male rats showed a significant decrease in testicular steroidogenic enzymes such as 3β-HSD and 17β-HSD and serum testosterone levels indicating Leydig cell damage [83]. Similar studies have shown that phthalates disrupt several gene pathways. Concerning reproductive system, DEHP can alter Vanin 1 (VNN1) gene expressions, involved in testis development and essential for proper reproductive function, alpha inhibin, normal Sertoli cell development, and insulin-like 3 (INSL3) responsible for gubernacular development [84]. Human studies elucidating the mechanism underlying EDCs' reproductive effects are still limited; nevertheless, a population study found a negative association between phthalate exposure and sperm quality and a positive association between urinary phthalate metabolites and 8-OHdG, HNE-MA, and 8-iso-PGF2α oxidative stress index. However, as the authors themselves point out, results should be extrapolated with caution to the general population as study participants were enrolled from an infertility clinic [85]. Although most of the evidence is based on an animal model, we can conclude that EDCs can cause excessive oxidative stress affecting steroidogenesis, differentiation, and vitality of the germinal epithelium as well as altering testis and epididymis structures, which results in impaired mobility and damage to the DNA of sperm cells.

Disorders Associated with EDCs in the Male

Sexual differentiation in human males is highly dependent on a balanced androgen/estrogen ratio. Exposure to exogenous estrogen, such as EDCs, could disrupt this delicate balance and consequently impair Sertoli cell and Leydig cell differentiation, germ cell proliferation, and testosterone production [86]. Among the potential disorders associated with EDC exposure during development include cryptorchidism, hypospadias, testicular germ cell cancer, and impaired semen quality, which are collectively referred to as testicular dysgenesis syndrome. Increased exposure to EDCs, particularly during the developmental period, appears to contribute toward a higher incidence of testicular dysgenesis syndrome [87].

Cryptorchidism

Cryptorchidism or undescended testis refers to the condition where the testis is absent from the scrotum, on one or both sides. It occurs when the testis fails to descend spontaneously into the scrotum during fetal development and the first 4 months of life. Instead, the testis remains suspended along the normal route of testicular descent [88]. Cryptorchidism is among the most common male congenital malformations, occurring in 2–8% of full-term male births [89]. It is also a congenital cause of primary or hypergonadotropic hypogonadism, where gonadotropin levels are high but testicular testosterone levels and spermatogenesis are impaired [90]. Besides having poor semen quality, cryptorchid males are at a higher risk of developing testicular germ cell tumors (TGCTs) in adulthood [91]. An earlier systematic review and meta-analysis found that cryptorchidism is among the perinatal variables associated with the risk of testicular cancer, with the others being inguinal hernia, twinning, gestational age, and low birth weight [92].

The risk factors underlying cryptorchidism are genetics, as well as maternal and environmental factors that could impact testicular development and descent [93]. A meta-analysis that included ten studies reporting on the associations between pre- and postnatal exposure to EDCs (such as PCBs and persistent organochlorine pesticides) and cryptorchidism in six different population groups had an OR of 1.03 (95% CI 0.72–1.47) [94]. An earlier review of epidemiological studies found no indication of an association between prenatal estrogen exposure and cryptorchidism, largely due to inconsistent evidence [95]. Males who were exposed prenatally to the synthetic nonsteroidal estrogen, diethylstilbestrol (DES), had a higher risk of cryptorchidism compared to those who were not exposed (relative risk (RR) 1.9, 95% CI 1.1–3.4), particularly when exposure began before week 11 of gestation (RR 2.9, 95% CI 1.6–5.2) compared to after (RR 1.1, 95% CI 0.5–2.5) [96]. In terms of occupational exposure to EDC-containing pesticides via agriculture-related activities by parents, a minor increase (albeit not significant) in the risk for cryptorchidism was reported [97]. Earlier studies concur that in utero exposure to pesticides in sons of women working in horticulture/farming carries a slightly increased risk of cryptorchidism [98, 99].

Hypospadias

Hypospadias is a congenital abnormality of penile development in which the urethral meatus is located ventrally instead of at the tip of the penile glans. Most hypospadias occurs without concurrent incidence of cryptorchidism, and it does not share a similar risk to testicular cancer as does cryptorchidism [100]. The precise mechanism underlying the development of hypospadias is still unclear. Normal development of the male genitalia requires androgens and functioning androgen receptors. However, males with hypospadias were found to have elevated androgen receptor mRNA and protein expression, indicating a defect in androgen receptor signaling [101]. The more severe the hypospadias, the greater the androgen receptor overexpression observed [102]. Additional studies are needed to further explore these findings.

Besides genetic risk factors, occupational or environmental exposure to EDCs that affect estrogen and androgen signaling could potentially be a risk factor for hypospadias [103]. Occupational exposure of parents to EDC-containing pesticides is linked to an almost twofold increase in hypospadias risk, particularly if the mother was exposed to EDCs during her first trimester of pregnancy [104]. A meta-analysis of seven studies examining the link between EDC exposure and hypospadias had an OR of 1.13 (95% CI 0.86–1.50) [94].

Human studies show conflicting results in the association between maternal exposure to EDCs like DES and the risk of hypospadias. For example, a cohort study of Dutch women with fertility problems reported a greatly increased risk of hypospadias in their sons following in utero exposure to DES (prevalence odds ratio 21.3, 95% CI 6.5–70.1) [105], while other studies observed much lower prevalence ratios of 5.0 (95% CI 1.2–16.8, $p = 0.02$) [106] and 2.3 (95% CI 0.7–7.9) [107], respectively. Conversely, a cohort study among US women found only a slightly increased risk (although not statistically significant) of hypospadias (prevalence odds ratio of 1.7, 95% CI 0.4–6.8) [96]. Meanwhile, a cohort study in France demonstrated that the transgenerational effects of DES and increased prevalence of hypospadias affected not only the second generation but also the third generation, including boys born to daughters of mothers exposed to DES in utero [108]. DDE, an androgen antagonist, is a metabolite of DDT (an insecticide). Subjects selected from the US birth cohort study, the Collaborative Perinatal Project (CPP), had an adjusted odds ratio of 1.2 (95% CI 0.6–2.4) for hypospadias when serum DDE levels during pregnancy were 85.6 micrograms per liter or higher [109]. Another US-based study on a different cohort, however, did not find a significant association between DDE or DDT, respectively, and increased risk for either hypospadias or cryptorchidism [110]. On the other hand, findings from another study based on the CPP cohort showed no significant association between maternal levels of PCB levels when pregnant and hypospadias [111].

Testicular Cancer

Testicular cancer is the most common cancer among males aged between 14 and 44 years, particularly among Caucasians [112]. As nearly all testicular neoplasms (~98%) are germ cell tumors, the terms testicular cancer and testicular germ cell tumor (TGCT) are often used interchangeably [113]. According to the 2016 WHO classification, testicular germ cell tumors can be broadly categorized into germ cell neoplasia in situ (type II TGCTs) and non-germ cell neoplasia in situ (type I TGCT and type III TGCT or spermatocytic seminoma) [114]. Type II TGCTs occur in adolescents and young adults and can be categorized into seminomas (originating from the seminiferous tubule germinal epithelium) and non-seminomas [112]. (Among the risk factors for testicular cancer include genetic predisposition, cryptorchidism, impaired spermatogenesis in sub- or infertility, and maternal exposure to estrogen [112].

The testicular dysgenesis syndrome hypothesis proposes that a deficit in androgen action prenatally (for example, in case of exposure to antiandrogenic EDCs) is a crucial contributor to testicular cancer etiology [115]. A US nested case-control study investigating the link between early postpartum concentrations of DDT-related compounds in maternal serum and testicular cancer risk in her son three decades later found that these mothers had a significantly higher DDT-to-DDE ratio, indicating earlier exposure to DDT and its slower elimination [116]. A meta-analysis of ten studies observed that maternal exposure to EDCs was associated with increased risk of TGCT (RR 2.16, 95% CI 1.78–2.62). However, direct (postnatal) exposure of adult males to EDCs did not show an association with increased TGCT risk. An earlier meta-analysis of six studies reporting on the associations between exposure to EDCs and testicular cancer had an OR of 1.20 (95% CI 0.78–1.89) [94].

A Swedish case-control study reported current raised blood concentrations of PCBs, hexachlorobenzene (HCB), and chlordanes (but not DDT-related compounds) among mothers of sons with testicular cancer (n = 44) compared to age-matched mothers of controls (n = 45) [117]. A matched case-control study based on participants in the US Servicemen's Testicular Tumor Environmental and Endocrine Determinants (STEED) Study reported an association between increased DDE exposure and risk of TGCTs and between chlordane exposure and risk of seminomas [118]. Similarly, a nested case-control study within the Cancer Registry of Norway (Janus Serum Bank) cohort showed an association between DDE and chlordane exposures and TGCT risk [119]. The same study also suggested a potential association between PCB congeners and risk of TGCT. However, another study among males in the US armed forces found that exposure to PCB did not increase TGCT risk, especially for non-seminomas [120]. A Spanish hospital-based case-control study also reported a significant association between raised serum levels of organochlorines from pesticide exposure and testicular cancer risk in patients (n = 50) compared to controls (n = 48) (adjusted OR 3.34, 95% CI 1.09–10.17) [121]. These studies imply that certain EDC exposures could potentially increase TGCT risk.

Transgenerational Effects of EDCs

During gestation, an adequate hormonal environment is crucial for the development of the testis and the male reproductive tract. The action of hormones, in particular androgens and anti-Müllerian, is essential for the maintenance of Wolff's duct and its differentiation into the deferens ducts and seminal vesicles, and then male sexual differentiation under the action of testosterone. An external toxic insult acting on the endocrine system genetic regulation could interfere with the normal testicle development in such a delicate phase and compromise the masculinization process with effects on fertility in adulthood.

Epigenetic Alterations to the Fetus

Prenatal exposure to EDCs, in addition to having negative effects on neuronal development, metabolism, and birth weight and increasing the risk of preterm birth, can lead to congenital abnormality of the male genitalia and thus infertility in adults [122–124].

The most worrying effects on offspring are certainly epigenetic changes with transgenerational effects. Strong evidence is emerging on a large scale that environmental induced epigenetic alterations to the fetus in gestational stage, but also to the germline in adulthood, can be passed on through generations. It is known that intense environmental stimuli are able to determine a chromatin remodeling and therefore a greater or lesser transcription of certain genes through epigenetic mechanisms. These changes arise in the DNA and histone structure, proteins that enclose DNA in nucleosomes, and modify gene expression without changing the DNA sequence. The molecular mechanisms associated with these effects are particular chemical modifications such as methylation, which occurs on lysine and arginine residues and inhibits gene expression; acetylation, which occurs on lysine residues and activates transcription; and phosphorylation, which takes place on serine residues and promotes acetylation with highly transcribed chromatin. EDCs can methylate DNA by adding a methyl group to the 5' position of the pyrimidine ring of the cytosine residues located in the cytosine-phosphate-guanine (CpG) dinucleotides. The modification of histones often occurs in association with DNA methylation and results in impaired chromatin accessibility and therefore alteration of transcriptional activities [125]. During gametogenesis and early preimplantation development, an epigenetic reprogramming erases the parental genomic footprint and avoids the inheritance of epimutations from generation to generation [126]. An external disturbance in this phase can compromise the correct embryonic development. Low-dose bisphenol A (BPA) exposure in the prenatal phase can cause epigenetic effects and impaired expression of noncoding RNA, such as microRNA with long-term effects in adult life [127], and even reproductive disorders in males; in fact, a correlation between maternal serum levels of PCBs, DDT, and DDE and children born with undescended testicles and hypospadias was found [128]. This is because during pregnancy, and in particular in the first trimester, there is an overload of the aerobic metabolism with a greater energy demand which increases ROS production rate, appropriately balanced by the endogenous antioxidant system. Exposure to highly oxidizing substances during this sensitive phase could contribute to pregnancy disorders and fetal harm [129].

Exposure to phthalates during pregnancy can modify DNA methylation and chromatin and gene expression. In particular, exposure to DEHP in pregnant rats downregulates the expression of glucose transporter (Glut4), causing testicular dysfunction in the offspring. It also induces a downregulation of Insl3 and methylation of imprinted genes, such as insulin-like growth factor receptor 2 (Igf2r) and paternally expressed 3 (Peg3) gene influencing pubertal abnormalities and testis functions in adulthood [123]. It has been shown that DDE alters the paternally transcribed Igf2 gene and maternally transcribed H19 gene, as well as transgenerational sperm function. Ancestral exposure to DDE reduced sperm concentration, motility, and elongated spermatids in seminiferous tubules in the F3 generation of Sprague-Dawley rats [130].

Genetic Disruptions of Spermatogenesis

A wide variety of environmental and lifestyle stressors can affect sperm epigenome in adults. Epigenetic dysregulation by EDC stimuli can have negative effects on sperm quality. Endocrine interference during the epigenetic reprogramming phase demonstrated a greater increase in spermatogenic cell apoptosis up to the fourth generation [131].

Genetic disruptions of spermatogenesis through the activation of endogenous endonucleases and then apoptosis mediate the fragmentation of germ cell DNA. Although spermatozoa with damaged DNA show a lower fertilization capacity, the possibility of pregnancy is not excluded, leading to an increased risk of transmitting genetic defects to offspring. Although too few epidemiological studies have been conducted to draw a conclusive correlation between EDC exposure and disturbance of sperm chromatin integrity, animal studies have shown an association between spermatozoa damaged by exposure to toxic substances and genetic alterations in the offspring [132]. A recent literature review compared SDF to a mutagen. In fact, these are real mutations in the paternal genome which, if not properly repaired, can generate infantile tumors, high levels of genomic instability in somatic cells and germ cells, or even imprinting defects and early postnatal death in the offspring in animal models [133]. Considering as described above, a transgenerational effect of SDF-mediated EDCs is certainly possible; however, this aspect still needs experimental confirmation.

In view of the impact on spermatogenesis, an increase in sperm aneuploidies due to meiotic interference following exposure to EDCs and responsible for inherited chromosomal abnormalities is plausible; however, at present, there are no concrete and consistent data in this regard. An overview of the epidemiological evidence found that only a few studies have demonstrated a negative association between exposure to EDCs and sperm chromosome ratio [134]. Also, in this case, the lack of evidence could be due to confounding factors such as lifestyles and contemporary exposure to different environmental components not adequately taken into consideration.

Limitations of Research on EDCs

Although the relationship between EDCs and male fertility potential has been extensively explored, currently the literature data is still controversial. This is because most of the studies evaluating the association between exposure to EDCs and fertility are cross-sectional epidemiological studies that do not take into account seasonal geographic variation [71], differences in sample size, study design, life stage, and different toxicokinetics and toxicogenomics, which combine to determine different effects on different tissues, organs, and biological systems. Moreover, the large differences in the approaches to data analysis and/or in the strategies for obtaining exposure data and the different and nonhomogeneous endpoints investigated make it very difficult to draw a single and complete general verdict on the effects of EDCs on reproductive health. Probably the most important aspect to point out is that humans are constantly exposed to a combination of several toxic substances acting in synergy or antagonism, so the role of the single contaminant is challenging to clarify.

It is known that environmental co-exposure to toxic molecules influences pollutant toxicity [135]. A recent zebra fish model study demonstrated that titanium dioxide nanoparticles (TiO_2-NPs), which are widely spread in the environment, increase the body burden of BPA, leading to greater adverse effects on the thyroid endocrine system across generations [136], as well as combined exposure to multiple pesticides can cause adverse effects on male sexual development, even if doses of individual compounds did not induce any biological damage [137]. On the other hand, the toxicity of BPA and nonylphenol (NP) in combination was reduced compared to the single exposure to BPA/NP in the rat, indicating an antagonistic effect resulting from their combination [138]. However, most of the studies aimed at clarifying the effects of EDC mixtures are based on animal models; at present, studies in this direction on human models are still scarce.

Lastly, despite the difficulties to identify a biomarker for each individual EDC, DNA methylation studies are still necessary to establish a universal epigenetic marker. Despite the identification of factors such as alteration of the expression of insulin-like genes, growth factor receptors, and imprinted genes as markers of damage by EDCs in the animal model, human trials are either still scarce or absent.

Future Research on EDCs and Male Infertility

It is almost impossible to escape exposure to EDCs as they are widespread in all environmental districts. Their elimination would require both technological-scientific and commercial efforts, but to date, there are still no pollutant abatement systems capable of solving the problem globally, and their widespread use both in industries and as products in common use makes it difficult to adopt a prohibition policy. The goal in preventing the harmful effect on health by EDCs could be identifying early-stage biomarkers of EDC exposure to reduce the incidence of adult-onset infertile phenotype. Methylation and sequence analysis of human genes involved in sperm function in exposed males and comparative studies on human models exposed in vitro to single and a combination of multiple EDCs could be the turning point to define their molecular mechanisms of action and establish an epigenetic damage marker.

Additionally, it is important to clarify the effects of a mixture of EDCs on spermatogenesis as compared to single exposures so as to be able to interpret the conflicting epidemiological data. Hence, future research in this direction on human and animal models is still needed. Of course, defining the type of harm induced by EDCs does not represent a defense strategy, while the integration of antioxidants capable of counteracting sperm DNA damage induced by environmental contaminants may be the solution to effectively treat EDC-exposed patients. Oral administration of vitamin C is known to have positive effects on sperm chromatin maturation [139], as well as ellagic acid, alone and in combination with vitamin C, has shown genoprotective effects against damage induced by environmental contaminants, in terms of improvement of seminal parameters, restoration of oxidative balance, and reduction of induced sperm DNA damage [140, 141]. But, once again, more studies are needed to establish their doses, the type of antioxidant molecule to use, and the duration of any therapy.

Summary

Exposure to environmental contaminants has been an important cause of the decline in male fertility in the last 20 years. The most serious threat is represented by substances released into the environment from chemical industries, agriculture, or constituents of various personal care products, capable of interfering with the endocrine system. The so-called endocrine-disrupting chemicals (EDCs) can come into contact with humans through various routes such as inhalation or ingestion of contaminated food and water. Urinary and blood concentrations of EDCs are correlated with a lower quality of semen parameters. Alteration of sperm quality is due to effects on steroidogenesis, oxidative stress induction, and causative epigenetic effects. Furthermore, the effects that EDCs can have on the male reproductive system already in intrauterine life should not be overlooked, resulting in a higher incidence of congenital anomalies and testicular neoplasms. This narrative literature review analyzes the impact of EDC exposure on male reproductive potential. The effects on hormonal regulation and consequent alteration in the normal number, morphology, and motility of spermatozoa were taken into consideration, as well as effects on sperm nuclear maturity associated with epigenetic alterations transmissible through generations and EDCs' implication in the pathogenesis of reproductive system diseases. The limitations of studies on male reproduction effects of EDCs and new research perspectives to overcome them are also discussed.

References

1. Fainberg J, Kashanian JA. Recent advances in understanding and managing male infertility. F1000Research. 2019;8:F1000 Faculty Rev-670. https://doi.org/10.12688/f1000research.17076.1.
2. Skakkebaek NE, Rajpert-De Meyts E, Buck Louis GM, Toppari J, Andersson AM, Eisenberg ML, Jensen TK, Jørgensen N, Swan SH, Sapra KJ, et al. Male reproductive disorders and fertility trends: influences of environment and genetic susceptibility. Physiol Rev. 2016;96:55. https://doi.org/10.1152/PHYSREV.00017.2015.
3. Punab M, Poolamets O, Paju P, Vihljajev V, Pomm K, Ladva R, Korrovits P, Laan M. Causes of male infertility: a 9-year prospective monocentre study on 1737 patients with reduced total sperm counts. Hum Reprod. 2017;32:18–31. https://doi.org/10.1093/humrep/dew284.
4. van Brakel J, Dinkelman-Smit M, de Muinck Keizer-Schrama SMPF, Hazebroek FWJ, Dohle GR. Sperm DNA damage measured by sperm chromatin structure assay in men with a history of undescended testes. Andrology. 2017;5:838–43. https://doi.org/10.1111/andr.12384.
5. Panner Selvam MK, Ambar RF, Agarwal A, Henkel R. Etiologies of sperm DNA damage and its impact on male infertility. Andrologia. 2021;53:1–15. https://doi.org/10.1111/and.13706.

6. Haidl F, Haidl G, Oltermann I, Allam JP. Seminal parameters of chronic male genital inflammation are associated with disturbed sperm DNA integrity. Andrologia. 2015;47:464–9. https://doi.org/10.1111/and.12408.
7. Pourmasumi S, Sabeti P, Rahiminia T, Mangoli E, Tabibnejad N, Talebi AR. The etiologies of sperm DNA abnormalities in male infertility: an assessment and review. Int J Reprod Biomed. 2017;15:331–44. https://doi.org/10.29252/ijrm.15.6.331.
8. Finelli R, Mottola F, Agarwal A. Impact of alcohol consumption on male fertility potential: a narrative review. Int J Environ Res Public Health. 2022;19:328. https://doi.org/10.3390/ijerph19010328.
9. Oncology TL. Endocrine disruptors—the lessons (not) learned. Lancet Oncol. 2021;22:1483. https://doi.org/10.1016/S1470-2045(21)00597-0.
10. Lombó M, Herráez P. The effects of endocrine disruptors on the male germline: an intergenerational health risk. Biol Rev. 2021;96:1243–62. https://doi.org/10.1111/brv.12701.
11. Cargnelutti F, Di Nisio A, Pallotti F, Sabovic I, Spaziani M, Tarsitano MG, Paoli D, Foresta C. Effects of endocrine disruptors on fetal testis development, male puberty, and transition age. Endocrine. 2021;72:358–74. https://doi.org/10.1007/s12020-020-02436-9.
12. Turan S. Endocrine disrupting chemicals and bone. Best Pract Res Clin Endocrinol Metab. 2021;35:101495. https://doi.org/10.1016/j.beem.2021.101495.
13. Diamanti-Kandarakis E, Bourguignon JP, Giudice LC, Hauser R, Prins GS, Soto AM, Zoeller RT, Gore AC. Endocrine-disrupting chemicals: an endocrine society scientific statement. Endocr Rev. 2009;30:293. https://doi.org/10.1210/ER.2009-0002.
14. Harding AK, Daston GP, Boyd GR, Lucier GW, Safe SH, Stewart J, Tillitt DE, Van Der Kraak G. Endocrine disrupting chemicals research program of the U.S. Environmental Protection Agency: summary of peer-review report. Environ Health Perspect. 2006;114:1276–82. https://doi.org/10.1289/ehp.8875.
15. Bolden AL, Schultz K, Pelch KE, Kwiatkowski CF. Exploring the endocrine activity of air pollutants associated with unconventional oil and gas extraction. Environ Health. 2018;17:1–17. https://doi.org/10.1186/S12940-018-0368-Z.
16. Rudel RA, Dodson RE, Perovich LJ, Morello-Frosch R, Camann DE, Zuniga MM, Yau AY, Just AC, Brody JG. Semivolatile endocrine-disrupting compounds in paired indoor and outdoor air in two northern California communities. Environ Sci Technol. 2010;44:6583. https://doi.org/10.1021/ES100159C.
17. Nováková Z, Novák J, Bittner M, Čupr P, Přibylová P, Kukučka P, Smutná M, Escher BI, Demirtepe H, Miralles-Marco A, et al. Toxicity to bronchial cells and endocrine disruptive potentials of indoor air and dust extracts and their association with multiple chemical classes. J Hazard Mater. 2022;424:127306. https://doi.org/10.1016/J.JHAZMAT.2021.127306.
18. Russo G, Laneri S, Di Lorenzo R, Ferrara L, Grumetto L. The occurrence of selected endocrine-disrupting chemicals in water and sediments from an urban lagoon in Southern Italy. Water Environ Res. 2021;93:1944–58. https://doi.org/10.1002/wer.1566.
19. Aborkhees G, Raina-Fulton R, Thirunavokkarasu O. Determination of endocrine disrupting chemicals in water and wastewater samples by liquid chromatography-negative ion electrospray ionization-tandem mass spectrometry. Molecules. 2020;25:1–15. https://doi.org/10.3390/molecules25173906.
20. Jackson J, Sutton R. Sources of endocrine-disrupting chemicals in urban wastewater, Oakland, CA. Sci Total Environ. 2008;405:153–60. https://doi.org/10.1016/j.scitotenv.2008.06.033.
21. Lu J, Wu J, Zhang C, Zhang Y. Possible effect of submarine groundwater discharge on the pollution of coastal water: occurrence, source, and risks of endocrine disrupting chemicals in coastal groundwater and adjacent seawater influenced by reclaimed water irrigation. Chemosphere. 2020;250:126323. https://doi.org/10.1016/j.chemosphere.2020.126323.
22. Wee SY, Aris AZ, Yusoff FM, Praveena SM. Occurrence of multiclass endocrine disrupting compounds in a drinking water supply system and associated risks. Sci Rep. 2020;10:1–12. https://doi.org/10.1038/s41598-020-74061-5.
23. Wee SY, Aris AZ. Endocrine disrupting compounds in drinking water supply system and human health risk implication. Environ Int. 2017;106:207–33. https://doi.org/10.1016/j.envint.2017.05.004.

24. Baldi F, Mantovani A. A new database for food safety: EDID (endocrine disrupting chemicals—diet interaction database). Ann Ist Supe Sanita. 2008;44:57–63. https://doi.org/10.1016/j.reprotox.2008.05.005.
25. Lallas PL. The Stockholm Convention on persistent organic pollutants. Am J Int Law. 2001;95(3):692–708.
26. Christensen K, Carlson LM, Lehmann GM. The role of epidemiology studies in human health risk assessment of polychlorinated biphenyls. Environ Res. 2021;194:110662. https://doi.org/10.1016/J.ENVRES.2020.110662.
27. Breivik K, Sweetman A, Pacyna JM, Jones KC. Towards a global historical emission inventory for selected PCB congeners—a mass balance approach. 3. An update. Sci Total Environ. 2007;377:296–307. https://doi.org/10.1016/j.scitotenv.2007.02.026.
28. Barcauskaitė K. Gas chromatographic analysis of polychlorinated biphenyls in compost samples from different origin. Waste Manag Res Sage J. 2019;37:556–62. https://doi.org/10.1177/0734242X19828156.
29. Grimm FA, Hu D, Kania-Korwel I, Lehmler HJ, Ludewig G, Hornbuckle KC, Duffel MW, Bergman A, Robertson LW, Robertson LW. Metabolism and metabolites of polychlorinated biphenyls (PCBs) corresponding author and complete contact info HHS Public Access. Crit Rev Toxicol. 2015;45:245–72. https://doi.org/10.3109/10408444.2014.999365.
30. Wang W, Bai J, Zhang G, Jia J, Wang X, Liu X, Cui B. Occurrence, sources and ecotoxicological risks of polychlorinated biphenyls (PCBs) in sediment cores from urban, rural and reclamation-affected rivers of the Pearl River Delta, China. Chemosphere. 2019;218:359–67. https://doi.org/10.1016/j.chemosphere.2018.11.046.
31. Ngoubeyou PSK, Wolkersdorfer C, Ndibewu PP, Augustyn W. Toxicity of polychlorinated biphenyls in aquatic environments—a review. Aquat Toxicol. 2022;251:106284. https://doi.org/10.1016/j.aquatox.2022.106284.
32. IARC Working Group on the Evaluation of Carcinogenic Risks to Humans. DDT, Lindane, and 2,4-D. Lyon (FR): International Agency for Research on Cancer; 2018. PMID: 29912510.
33. Daglioglu N, Gulmen MK, Akcan R, Efeoglu P, Yener F, Ünal I. Determination of organochlorine pesticides residues in human adipose tissue, data from Cukurova, Turkey. Bull Environ Contam Toxicol. 2010;85:97–102. https://doi.org/10.1007/s00128-010-0057-2.
34. Gusev A, MacLeod M, Bartlett P. Intercontinental transport of persistent organic pollutants: a review of key findings and recommendations of the task force on hemispheric transport of air pollutants and directions for future research. Atmos Pollut Res. 2012;3:463–5. https://doi.org/10.5094/APR.2012.053.
35. Fiedler H, Van der Veen I, de Boer J. Assessment of four rounds of interlaboratory tests within the UNEP-coordinated POPs projects, 2022. Chemosphere 288, 132441.
36. Turci R, Clinici I, Maugeri S, Businaro J. Insecticides: DDT, DDE, DDD. G Ital Med Lav Ergon. 2010;32(2):93–144.
37. Malusá E, Tartanus M, Danelski W, Miszczak A, Szustakowska E, Kicińska J, Furmanczyk EM. Monitoring of DDT in agricultural soils under organic farming in poland and the risk of crop contamination. Environ Manag. 2020;66:916–29. https://doi.org/10.1007/s00267-020-01347-9.
38. Vasseghian Y, Hosseinzadeh S, Khataee A, Dragoi EN. The concentration of persistent organic pollutants in water resources: a global systematic review, meta-analysis and probabilistic risk assessment. Sci Total Environ. 2021;796:149000. https://doi.org/10.1016/j.scitotenv.2021.149000.
39. Beard J. DDT and human health. Sci Total Environ. 2006;355:78–89. https://doi.org/10.1016/j.scitotenv.2005.02.022.
40. Longnecker MP, Rogan WJ, Lucier G. The human health effects of DDT (dichlorodiphenyltrichloroethane) and PCBs (polychlorinated biphenyls) and an overview of organochlorines in public health. Annu Rev Public Health. 1997;18:211–44. https://doi.org/10.1146/annurev.publhealth.18.1.211.
41. Abraham A, Chakraborty P. A review on sources and health impacts of bisphenol A. Rev Environ Health. 2019;35:201–10. https://doi.org/10.1515/REVEH-2019-0034/MACHINEREADABLECITATION/RIS.

42. Careghini A, Filippo Mastorgio A, Saponaro S, Sezenna E. Bisphenol A, nonylphenols, benzophenones, and benzotriazoles in soils, groundwater, surface water, sediments, and food: a review. Environ Sci Pollut Res. 2015;22:5711–41. https://doi.org/10.1007/s11356-014-3974-5.
43. Andújar N, Gálvez-Ontiveros Y, Zafra-Gómez A, Rodrigo L, Álvarez-Cubero MJ, Aguilera M, Monteagudo C, Rivas A. Bisphenol A analogues in food and their hormonal and obesogenic effects: a review. Nutrients. 2019;11:2136. https://doi.org/10.3390/NU11092136.
44. Ma Y, Liu H, Wu J, Yuan L, Wang Y, Du X, Wang R, Marwa PW, Petlulu P, Chen X, et al. The adverse health effects of bisphenol A and related toxicity mechanisms. Environ Res. 2019;176:108575. https://doi.org/10.1016/j.envres.2019.108575.
45. Rochester JR. Bisphenol A and human health: a review of the literature. Reprod Toxicol. 2013;42:132–55. https://doi.org/10.1016/j.reprotox.2013.08.008.
46. Gani KM, Tyagi VK, Kazmi AA. Occurrence of phthalates in aquatic environment and their removal during wastewater treatment processes: a review. Environ Sci Pollut Res. 2017;24:17267–84. https://doi.org/10.1007/s11356-017-9182-3.
47. Wang Y, Zhu H, Kannan K. A review of biomonitoring of phthalate exposures. Toxics. 2019;7(2):21. https://doi.org/10.3390/toxics7020021.
48. Wang YC, Chen HS, Long CY, Tsai CF, Hsieh TH, Hsu CY, Tsai EM. Possible mechanism of phthalates-induced tumorigenesis. Kaohsiung J Med Sci. 2012;28:22–7. https://doi.org/10.1016/j.kjms.2012.05.006.
49. Gao DW, Wen ZD. Phthalate esters in the environment: a critical review of their occurrence, biodegradation, and removal during wastewater treatment processes. Sci Total Environ. 2016;541:986–1001. https://doi.org/10.1016/j.scitotenv.2015.09.148.
50. Olkowska E, Gržinić G. Skin models for dermal exposure assessment of phthalates. Chemosphere. 2022;295:133909. https://doi.org/10.1016/j.chemosphere.2022.133909.
51. Li HL, Ma WL, Liu LY, Zhang Z, Sverko E, Zhang ZF, Song WW, Sun Y, Li YF. Phthalates in infant cotton clothing: occurrence and implications for human exposure. Sci Total Environ. 2019;683:109–15. https://doi.org/10.1016/j.scitotenv.2019.05.132.
52. Li J, Zhao H, Xia W, Zhou Y, Xu S, Cai Z. Nine phthalate metabolites in human urine for the comparison of health risk between population groups with different water consumptions. Sci Total Environ. 2019;649:1532–40. https://doi.org/10.1016/j.scitotenv.2018.08.294.
53. Zhang YJ, Guo JL, Xue JC, Bai CL, Guo Y. Phthalate metabolites: characterization, toxicities, global distribution, and exposure assessment. Environ Pollut. 2021;291:118106. https://doi.org/10.1016/j.envpol.2021.118106.
54. Cai J, Wang C, Wu T, Moreno JML, Zhong Y, Huang X, Chen Y, Zuo Z. Disruption of spermatogenesis and differential regulation of testicular estrogen receptor expression in mice after polychlorinated biphenyl exposure. Toxicology. 2011;287:21–8. https://doi.org/10.1016/j.tox.2011.05.010.
55. Jenardhanan P, Panneerselvam M, Mathur PP. Effect of environmental contaminants on spermatogenesis. Semin Cell Dev Biol. 2016;59:126–40. https://doi.org/10.1016/j.semcdb.2016.03.024.
56. Czarnywojtek A, Jaz K, Ochmanska A, Zgorzalewicz-Stachowiak M, Czarnocka B, Sawicka-Gutaj N, ZioŁkowska P, Krela-Kazmierczak I, Gut P, Florek E, et al. The effect of endocrine disruptors on the reproductive system—current knowledge. Eur Rev Med Pharmacol Sci. 2021;25:4930–40. https://doi.org/10.26355/eurrev_202108_26450.
57. Toft G, Rignell-Hydbom A, Tyrkiel E, Shvets M, Giwercman A, Lindh CH, Pedersen HS, Ludwicki JK, Lesovoy V, Hagmar L, et al. Semen quality and exposure to persistent organochlorine pollutants. Epidemiology. 2006;17:450–8. https://doi.org/10.1097/01.ede.0000221769.41028.d2.
58. Castellini C, Muselli M, Parisi A, Totaro M, Tienforti D, Cordeschi G, Giorgio Baroni M, Maccarrone M, Necozione S, Francavilla S, et al. Association between urinary bisphenol A concentrations and semen quality: a meta-analytic study. Biochem Pharmacol. 2022;197:114896. https://doi.org/10.1016/j.bcp.2021.114896.

59. Cannarella R, Gül M, Rambhatla A, Agarwal A. Temporal decline of sperm concentration: role of endocrine disruptors. Endocrine. 2023;79:1–16. https://doi.org/10.1007/s12020-022-03136-2.
60. Wang YX, Zeng Q, Sun Y, Yang P, Wang P, Li J, Huang Z, You L, Huang YH, Wang C, et al. Semen phthalate metabolites, semen quality parameters and serum reproductive hormones: a cross-sectional study in China. Environ Pollut. 2016;211:173–82. https://doi.org/10.1016/j.envpol.2015.12.052.
61. Rana R, Joon S, Kumar Jain A, Kumar Mohanty N. A study on the effect of phthalate esters and their metabolites on idiopathic infertile males. Andrologia. 2020;52:1–9. https://doi.org/10.1111/and.13720.
62. Hauser R, Singh NP, Chen Z, Pothier L, Altshul L. Lack of an association between environmental exposure to polychlorinated biphenyls and p,p′-DDE and DNA damage in human sperm measured using the neutral comet assay. Hum Reprod. 2003;18:2525–33. https://doi.org/10.1093/humrep/deg508.
63. Spanò M, Toft G, Hagmar L, Eleuteri P, Rescia M, Rignell-Hydbom A, Tyrkiel E, Zvyezday V, Bonde JP, Bizzaro D, et al. Exposure to PCB and p,p′-DDE in European and Inuit populations: impact on human sperm chromatin integrity. Hum Reprod. 2005;20:3488–99. https://doi.org/10.1093/humrep/dei297.
64. De Jager C, Aneck-Hahn NH, Bornman MS, Farias P, Leter G, Eleuteri P, Rescia M, Spanò M. Sperm chromatin integrity in DDT-exposed young men living in a malaria area in the Limpopo Province, South Africa. Hum Reprod. 2009;24:2429–38. https://doi.org/10.1093/humrep/dep249.
65. Kiwitt-Cárdenas J, Adoamnei E, Arense-Gonzalo JJ, Sarabia-Cos L, Vela-Soria F, Fernández MF, Gosálvez J, Mendiola J, Torres-Cantero AM. Associations between urinary concentrations of bisphenol A and sperm DNA fragmentation in young men. Environ Res. 2021;199:111289. https://doi.org/10.1016/j.envres.2021.111289.
66. Rex AS, Wu C, Aagaard J, Fedder J. DNA fragmentation in human spermatozoa and pregnancy rates after intrauterine insemination. Should the DFI threshold be lowered? J Clin Med. 2021;10:1–13. https://doi.org/10.3390/jcm10061310.
67. Omran GA, Gaber HD, Mostafa NAM, Abdel-Gaber RM, Salah EA. Potential hazards of bisphenol A exposure to semen quality and sperm DNA integrity among infertile men. Reprod Toxicol. 2018;81:188–95. https://doi.org/10.1016/j.reprotox.2018.08.010.
68. Jurewicz J, Radwan M, Sobala W, Ligocka D, Radwan P, Bochenek M, Hawuła W, Jakubowski L, Hanke W. Human urinary phthalate metabolites level and main semen parameters, sperm chromatin structure, sperm aneuploidy and reproductive hormones. Reprod Toxicol. 2013;42:232–41. https://doi.org/10.1016/j.reprotox.2013.10.001.
69. Hauser R, Meeker JD, Singh NP, Silva MJ, Ryan L, Duty S, Calafat AM. DNA damage in human sperm is related to urinary levels of phthalate monoester and oxidative metabolites. Hum Reprod. 2007;22:688–95. https://doi.org/10.1093/humrep/del428.
70. Duty SM, Singh NP, Silva MJ, Barr DB, Brock JW, Ryan L, Herrick RF, Christiani DC, Hauser R. The relationship between environmental exposures to phthalates and DNA damage in human sperm using the neutral comet assay. Environ Health Perspect. 2003;111:1164–9. https://doi.org/10.1289/ehp.5756.
71. Sifakis S, Androutsopoulos VP, Tsatsakis AM, Spandidos DA. Human exposure to endocrine disrupting chemicals: effects on the male and female reproductive systems. Environ Toxicol Pharmacol. 2017;51:56–70. https://doi.org/10.1016/j.etap.2017.02.024.
72. Hamers T, Kamstra JH, Cenijn PH, Pencikova K, Palkova L, Simeckova P, Vondracek J, Andersson PL, Stenberg M, Machala M. In vitro toxicity profiling of ultrapure non-dioxin-like polychlorinated biphenyl congeners and their relative toxic contribution to PCB mixtures in humans. Toxicol Sci. 2011;121:88–100. https://doi.org/10.1093/toxsci/kfr043.
73. Crinnion W. Polychlorinated biphenyls: persistent pollutants with immunological, neurological, and endocrinological consequences. Altern Med Rev J Clin Ther. 2011;16(1):5–13.

74. Fucic A, Gamulin M, Ferencic Z, Katic J, Krayer Von Krauss M, Bartonova A, Merlo DF. Environmental exposure to xenoestrogens and oestrogen related cancers: reproductive system, breast, lung, kidney, pancreas, and brain. Environ Health. 2012;11(Suppl. 1):S8. https://doi.org/10.1186/1476-069X-11-S1-S8.
75. Peinado FM, Artacho-Cordón F, Barrios-Rodríguez R, Arrebola JP. Influence of polychlorinated biphenyls and organochlorine pesticides on the inflammatory milieu. A systematic review of in vitro, in vivo and epidemiological studies. Environ Res. 2020;186:109561. https://doi.org/10.1016/j.envres.2020.109561.
76. Tiwari D, Vanage G. Bisphenol A induces oxidative stress in bone marrow cells, lymphocytes, and reproductive organs of Holtzman rats. Int J Toxicol. 2017;36:142–52. https://doi.org/10.1177/1091581817691224.
77. Lauby-Secretan B, Loomis D, Baan R, El Ghissassi F, Bouvard V, Benbrahim-Tallaa L, Guha N, Grosse Y, Straif K. Use of mechanistic data in the IARC evaluations of the carcinogenicity of polychlorinated biphenyls and related compounds. Environ Sci Pollut Res. 2016;23:2220–9. https://doi.org/10.1007/s11356-015-4829-4.
78. Molina EM, Kavazis AN, Mendonça MT, Akingbemi BT. Effects of different DDE exposure paradigms on testicular steroid hormone secretion and hepatic oxidative stress in male Long-Evans rats. Gen Comp Endocrinol. 2022;317:113963. https://doi.org/10.1016/j.ygcen.2021.113963.
79. Marouani N, Hallegue D, Sakly M, Benkhalifa M, Ben Rhouma K, Tebourbi O. p,p'-DDT induces testicular oxidative stress-induced apoptosis in adult rats. Reprod Biol Endocrinol. 2017;15:1–10. https://doi.org/10.1186/s12958-017-0259-0.
80. Song Y, Shi Y, Yu H, Hu Y, Wang Y, Yang K. p,p′-Dichlorodiphenoxydichloroethylene induced apoptosis of Sertoli cells through oxidative stress-mediated p38 MAPK and mitochondrial pathway. Toxicol Lett. 2011;202:55–60. https://doi.org/10.1016/j.toxlet.2011.01.020.
81. Kaur S, Saluja M, Bansal MP. Bisphenol A induced oxidative stress and apoptosis in mice testes: modulation by selenium. Andrologia. 2018;50:1–8. https://doi.org/10.1111/and.12834.
82. Sedha S, Kumar S, Shukla S. Role of oxidative stress in male reproductive dysfunctions with reference to phthalate compounds. Urol J. 2015;12:2304–16.
83. Nelli G, Pamanji SR. Di-n-butyl phthalate prompts interruption of spermatogenesis, steroidogenesis, and fertility associated with increased testicular oxidative stress in adult male rats. Environ Sci Pollut Res. 2017;24:18563–74. https://doi.org/10.1007/s11356-017-9478-3.
84. Latini G, Del Vecchio A, Massaro M, Verrotti A, De Felice C. Phthalate exposure and male infertility. Toxicology. 2006;226:90–8. https://doi.org/10.1016/j.tox.2006.07.011.
85. Liu C, Duan P, Chen YJ, Deng YL, Luo Q, Miao Y, Cui SH, Liu EN, Wang Q, Wang L, et al. Mediation of the relationship between phthalate exposure and semen quality by oxidative stress among 1034 reproductive-aged Chinese men. Environ Res. 2019;179:108778. https://doi.org/10.1016/j.envres.2019.108778.
86. Skakkebæk NE, Rajpert-De Meyts E, Main KM. Testicular dysgenesis syndrome: an increasingly common developmental disorder with environmental aspects. Hum Reprod. 2001;16:972–8. https://doi.org/10.1093/humrep/16.5.972.
87. Gore AC, Chappell VA, Fenton SE, Flaws JA, Nadal A, Prins GS, Toppari J, Zoeller RT. Executive summary to EDC-2: the Endocrine Society's second scientific statement on endocrine-disrupting chemicals. Endocr Rev. 2015;36:593–602. https://doi.org/10.1210/er.2015-1093.
88. Foresta C, Zuccarello D, Garolla A, Ferlin A. Role of hormones, genes, and environment in human cryptorchidism. Endocr Rev. 2008;29:560–80. https://doi.org/10.1210/er.2007-0042.
89. Brucker-Davis F, Wagner-Mahler K, Delattre I, Ducot B, Ferrari P, Bongain A, Kurzenne JY, Mas JC, Fénichel P, Pacini P, et al. Cryptorchidism at birth in Nice area (France) is associated with higher prenatal exposure to PCBs and DDE, as assessed by colostrum concentrations. Hum Reprod. 2008;23:1708–18. https://doi.org/10.1093/humrep/den186.
90. Gurung P, Yetiskul E, Jialal I. Physiology, male reproductive system. StatPearls; 2023.

91. Rodprasert W, Virtanen HE, Mäkelä JA, Toppari J. Hypogonadism and cryptorchidism. Front Endocrinol (Lausanne). 2020;10:1–27. https://doi.org/10.3389/fendo.2019.00906.
92. Cook MB, Akre O, Forman D, Patricia Madigan M, Richiardi L, McGlynn KAA. Systematic review and meta-analysis of perinatal variables in relation to the risk of testicular cancer-experiences of the son. Int J Epidemiol. 2010;39:1605–18. https://doi.org/10.1093/ije/dyq120.
93. Leslie SW, Sajjad H, Villanueva CA. Cryptorchidism. StatPearls; 2023.
94. Bonde JP, Flachs EM, Rimborg S, Glazer CH, Giwercman A, Ramlau-Hansen CH, Hougaard KS, Høyer BB, Hærvig KK, Petersen SB, et al. The epidemiologic evidence linking prenatal and postnatal exposure to endocrine disrupting chemicals with male reproductive disorders: a systematic review and meta-analysis. Hum Reprod Update. 2016;23:104–25. https://doi.org/10.1093/HUMUPD/DMW036.
95. Storgaard L, Bonde JP, Olsen J. Male reproductive disorders in humans and prenatal indicators of estrogen exposure: a review of published epidemiological studies. Reprod Toxicol. 2006;21:4–15. https://doi.org/10.1016/j.reprotox.2005.05.006.
96. Palmer JR, Herbst AL, Noller KL, Boggs DA, Troisi R, Titus-Ernstoff L, Hatch EE, Wise LA, Strohsnitter WC, Hoover RN. Urogenital abnormalities in men exposed to diethylstilbestrol in utero: a cohort study. Environ Heal A Glob Access Sci Source. 2009;8:4–9. https://doi.org/10.1186/1476-069X-8-37.
97. Carbone P, Giordano F, Nori F, Mantovani A, Taruscio D, Lauria L, Figà-Talamanca I. The possible role of endocrine disrupting chemicals in the aetiology of cryptorchidism and hypospadias: a population-based case-control study in rural Sicily. Int J Androl. 2007;30:3–13. https://doi.org/10.1111/j.1365-2605.2006.00703.x.
98. Biggs ML, Baer A, Critchlow CW. Maternal, delivery, and perinatal characteristics associated with cryptorchidism: a population-based case-control study among births in Washington State. Epidemiology. 2002;13:197–204. https://doi.org/10.1097/00001648-200203000-00015.
99. Weidner IS, Møller H, Jensen TK, SkakkebÆk NE. Risk factors for cryptorchidism and hypospadias. J Urol. 1999;161:1606–9. https://doi.org/10.1016/S0022-5347(05)68992-6.
100. Raghavan R, Romano ME, Karagas MR, Penna FJ. Pharmacologic and environmental endocrine disruptors in the pathogenesis of hypospadias: a review. Curr Environ Heal Rep. 2018;5:499–511. https://doi.org/10.1007/s40572-018-0214-z.
101. Pichler R, Djedovic G, Klocker H, Heidegger I, Strasak A, Loidl W, Bektic J, Skradski V, Horninger W, Oswald J. Quantitative measurement of the androgen receptor in prepuces of boys with and without hypospadias. BJU Int. 2013;112:265–70. https://doi.org/10.1111/j.1464-410X.2012.11731.x.
102. Balaji D, Reddy G, Babu R, Paramaswamy B, Ramasundaram M, Agarwal P, Joseph L, D'cruze L, Sundaram S. Androgen receptor expression in hypospadias. J Indian Assoc Pediatr Surg. 2020;25:6. https://doi.org/10.4103/JIAPS.JIAPS_166_18.
103. Mattiske DM, Pask AJ. Endocrine disrupting chemicals in the pathogenesis of hypospadias, developmental and toxicological perspectives. Curr Res Toxicol. 2021;2:179–91. https://doi.org/10.1016/j.crtox.2021.03.004.
104. Das D, Dutta HK, Borbora D, Brahma RC, Das JM. Assessing the relationship between hypospadias risk and parental occupational exposure to potential endocrine-disrupting chemicals. Occup Environ Med. 2023;80:93–6. https://doi.org/10.1136/OEMED-2022-108594.
105. Klip H, Verloop J, Van Gool JD, Koster META, Burger CW, Van Leeuwen FE. Hypospadias in sons of women exposed to diethylstilbestrol in utero: a cohort study. Lancet. 2002;359:1102–7. https://doi.org/10.1016/S0140-6736(02)08152-7.
106. Pons JC, Papiernik E, Billon A, Hessabi M, Duyme M. Hypospadias in sons of women exposed to diethylstilbestrol in utero. Prenat Diagn. 2005;25:418–9. https://doi.org/10.1002/PD.1136.
107. Brouwers MM, Feitz WFJ, Roelofs LAJ, Kiemeney LALM, de Gier RPE, Roeleveld N. Hypospadias: a transgenerational effect of diethylstilbestrol? Hum Reprod. 2006;21:666–9. https://doi.org/10.1093/humrep/dei398.

108. Kalfa N, Paris F, Soyer-Gobillard MO, Daures JP, Sultan C. Prevalence of hypospadias in grandsons of women exposed to diethylstilbestrol during pregnancy: a multigenerational national cohort study. Fertil Steril. 2011;95:2574–7. https://doi.org/10.1016/j.fertnstert.2011.02.047.
109. Longnecker MP, Klebanoff MA, Brock JW, Zhou H, Gray KA, Needham LL, Wilcox AJ. Maternal serum level of 1,1-dichloro-2,2-bis(p-chlorophenyl)ethylene and risk of cryptorchidism, hypospadias, and polythelia among male offspring. Am J Epidemiol. 2002;155:313–22. https://doi.org/10.1093/aje/155.4.313.
110. Bhatia R, Shiau R, Petreas M, Weintraub JM, Farhang L, Eskenazi B. Organochlorine pesticides and male genital anomalies in the child health and development studies. Environ Health Perspect. 2005;113:220–4. https://doi.org/10.1289/ehp.7382.
111. McGlynn KA, Guo X, Graubard BI, Brock JW, Klebanoff MA, Longnecker MP. Maternal pregnancy levels of polychlorinated biphenyls and risk of hypospadias and cryptorchidism in male offspring. Environ Health Perspect. 2009;117:1472–6. https://doi.org/10.1289/ehp.0800389.
112. Cheng L, Albers P, Berney DM, Feldman DR, Daugaard G, Gilligan T, Looijenga LHJ. Testicular cancer. Nat Rev Dis Prim. 2018;4(1):29. https://doi.org/10.1038/s41572-018-0029-0.
113. McGlynn KA, Trabert B. Adolescent and adult risk factors for testicular cancer. Nat Rev Urol. 2012;9:339–49. https://doi.org/10.1038/nrurol.2012.61.
114. Moch H, Cubilla AL, Humphrey PA, Reuter VE, Ulbright TM. The 2016 WHO classification of tumours of the urinary system and male genital organs—Part A: Renal, penile, and testicular tumours. Eur Urol. 2016;70:93–105. https://doi.org/10.1016/j.eururo.2016.02.029.
115. Bräuner EV, Lim Y-H, Koch T, Uldbjerg CS, Gregersen LS, Pedersen MK, Frederiksen H, Petersen JH, Coull BA, Andersson A-M, et al. Endocrine disrupting chemicals and risk of testicular cancer: a systematic review and meta-analysis. J Clin Endocrinol Metab. 2021;106:4834–60. https://doi.org/10.1210/clinem/dgab523.
116. Cohn BA, Cirillo PM, Christianson RE. Prenatal DDT exposure and testicular cancer: a nested case-control study. Arch Environ Occup Health. 2010;65:127–34. https://doi.org/10.1080/19338241003730887.
117. Hardell L, van Bavel B, Lindström G, Calberg M, Dreifaldt AC, Wijkström H, Starkhammar H, Eriksson M, Hallquist A, Kolmert T. Increased concentrations of polychlorinated biphenyls, hexachlorobenzene, and chlordanes in mothers of men with testicular cancer. Environ Health Perspect. 2003;111:930–4. https://doi.org/10.1289/ehp.5816.
118. McGlynn KA, Quraishi SM, Graubard BI, Weber JP, Rubertone MV, Erickson RL. Persistent organochlorine pesticides and risk of testicular germ cell tumors. J Natl Cancer Inst. 2008;100:663–71. https://doi.org/10.1093/jnci/djn101.
119. Purdue MP, Engel LS, Langseth H, Needham LL, Andersen A, Barr DB, Blair A, Rothman N, McGlynn KA. Prediagnostic serum concentrations of organochlorine compounds and risk of testicular germ cell tumors. Environ Health Perspect. 2009;117:1514–9. https://doi.org/10.1289/ehp.0800359.
120. McGlynn KA, Quraishi SM, Graubard BI, Weber JP, Rubertone MV, Erickson RL. Polychlorinated biphenyls and risk of testicular germ cell tumors. Cancer Res. 2009;69:1901–9. https://doi.org/10.1158/0008-5472.CAN-08-3935.
121. Giannandrea F, Gandini L, Paoli D, Turci R, Figà-Talamanca I. Pesticide exposure and serum organochlorine residuals among testicular cancer patients and healthy controls. J Environ Sci Health B. 2011;46:780–7. https://doi.org/10.1080/03601234.2012.597704.
122. Preston EV, Fruh V, Quinn MR, Hacker MR, Wylie BJ, O'Brien K, Mahalingaiah S, James-Todd T. Endocrine disrupting chemical-associated hair product use during pregnancy and gestational age at delivery: a pilot study. Environ Heal A Glob Access Sci Source. 2021;20:1–9. https://doi.org/10.1186/s12940-021-00772-5.

123. Lucaccioni L, Trevisani V, Passini E, Righi B, Plessi C, Predieri B, Iughetti L. Perinatal exposure to phthalates: from endocrine to neurodevelopment effects. Int J Mol Sci. 2021;22(8):4063. https://doi.org/10.3390/ijms22084063.
124. Qian Y, Shao H, Ying X, Huang W, Hua Y. The endocrine disruption of prenatal phthalate exposure in mother and offspring. Front Public Heal. 2020;8:548585. https://doi.org/10.3389/fpubh.2020.00366.
125. Plunk EC, Richards SM. Epigenetic modifications due to environment, ageing, nutrition, and endocrine disrupting chemicals and their effects on the endocrine system. Int J Endocrinol. 2020;2020(1):9251980. https://doi.org/10.1155/2020/9251980.
126. Amoako AA, Nafee TM, Ola B. Epigenetic influences during the periconception period and assisted reproduction. Adv Exp Med Biol. 2017;1014:15–39. https://doi.org/10.1007/978-3-319-62414-3_2/COVER.
127. De Felice B, Manfellotto F, Palumbo A, Troisi J, Zullo F, Di Carlo C, Sardo ADS, De Stefano N, Ferbo U, Guida M, et al. Genome-wide microRNA expression profiling in placentas from pregnant women exposed to BPA. BMC Med Genet. 2015;8:1–13. https://doi.org/10.1186/s12920-015-0131-z.
128. Ünüvar T, Büyükgebiz A. Fetal and neonatal endocrine disruptors. J Clin Res Pediatr Endocrinol. 2012;4(2):51–60. https://doi.org/10.4274/Jcrpe.569.
129. Ramiro-Cortijo D, de la Calle M, Rodríguez-Rodríguez P, López de Pablo ÁL, López-Giménez MR, Aguilera Y, Martín-Cabrejas MA, González MDC, Arribas SM. Maternal antioxidant status in early pregnancy and development of fetal complications in twin pregnancies: a pilot study. Antioxidants. 2020;9(4):269. https://doi.org/10.3390/antiox9040269.
130. Brehm E, Flaws JA. Transgenerational effects of endocrine-disrupting chemicals on male and female reproduction. Endocrinology. 2019;160:1421–35. https://doi.org/10.1210/en.2019-00034.
131. Rajender S, Avery K, Agarwal A. Epigenetics, spermatogenesis and male infertility. Mutat Res Rev Mutat Res. 2011;727:62–71. https://doi.org/10.1016/j.mrrev.2011.04.002.
132. Lewis SEM, Aitken RJ. DNA damage to spermatozoa has impacts on fertilization and pregnancy. Cell Tissue Res. 2005;322:33–41. https://doi.org/10.1007/s00441-005-1097-5.
133. Qiu Y, Yang H, Li C, Xu C. Progress in research on sperm DNA fragmentation. Med Sci Monit. 2020;26:1–11. https://doi.org/10.12659/MSM.918746.
134. Zamkowska D, Karwacka A, Jurewicz J, Radwan M. Environmental exposure to non-persistent endocrine disrupting chemicals and semen quality: an overview of the current epidemiological evidence. Int J Occup Med Environ Health. 2018;31:377–414. https://doi.org/10.13075/ijomeh.1896.01195.
135. Mottola F, Santonastaso M, Iovine C, Frenzilli G, Picchietti S, Genualdo V, Rocco L. TiO_2-NPs and cadmium co-exposure: in vitro assessment of genetic and genomic DNA damage on Dicentrarchus labrax embryonic cells. Environ Sci Pollut Res. 2022;29:62208–18. https://doi.org/10.1007/S11356-021-17645-6/METRICS.
136. Guo Y, Chen L, Wu J, Hua J, Yang L, Wang Q, Zhang W, Lee JS, Zhou B. Parental co-exposure to bisphenol A and nano-TiO_2 causes thyroid endocrine disruption and developmental neurotoxicity in zebrafish offspring. Sci Total Environ. 2019;650:557–65. https://doi.org/10.1016/J.SCITOTENV.2018.09.007.
137. Jacobsen PR, Christiansen S, Boberg J, Nellemann C, Hass U. Combined exposure to endocrine disrupting pesticides impairs parturition, causes pup mortality and affects sexual differentiation in rats. Int J Androl. 2010;33:434–42. https://doi.org/10.1111/J.1365-2605.2009.01046.X.
138. Shi R, Liu Z, Liu T. The antagonistic effect of bisphenol A and nonylphenol on liver and kidney injury in rats. Immunopharmacol Immunotoxicol. 2021;43:527–35. https://doi.org/10.1080/08923973.2021.1950179.
139. Hamidian S, Talebi AR, Fesahat F, Bayat M, Mirjalili AM, Ashrafzadeh HR, Rajabi M, Montazeri F, Babaei S. The effect of vitamin C on the gene expression profile of sperm

protamines in the male partners of couples with recurrent pregnancy loss: a randomized clinical trial. Clin Exp Reprod Med. 2020;47:68–76. https://doi.org/10.5653/cerm.2019.03188.

140. Mottola F, Iovine C, Carannante M, Santonastaso M, Rocco L. In vitro combination of ascorbic and ellagic acids in sperm oxidative damage inhibition. Int J Mol Sci. 2022;23:14751. https://doi.org/10.3390/ijms232314751.
141. Iovine C, Mottola F, Santonastaso M, Finelli R, Agarwal A, Rocco L. In vitro ameliorative effects of ellagic acid on vitality, motility and DNA quality in human spermatozoa. Mol Reprod Dev. 2021;88:167–74. https://doi.org/10.1002/mrd.23455.

Chapter 3
Lifestyle Modifications and Male Infertility

Nguyen Quang and Tuncay Toprak

Key Points

- In this review, we will consider the effects of lifestyle factors such as psychological stress, alcohol consumption, smoking, obesity, performance-enhancing and recreational substance abuse, and diet and physical exercise on male infertility.
- Also, we will discuss the effects of lifestyle change intervention on sperm parameters.
- In addition, we will provide guidance on lifestyle changes and what needs to be done for the management of infertile couples.

Introduction

Infertility is the inability of a couple to achieve pregnancy for more than 1 year despite unprotected, regular, and well-timed sexual intercourse [1]. Approximately, 15% of couples who want to conceive will experience infertility, and 50% of these couples will have male-related problems [2, 3]. Nearly 30% of infertility is due to male only, and this rises to 50% when considered as a combination of male and female factors [2]. Male infertility affects 1 in 20 men and is thought to affect an estimated 80 million men worldwide [4, 5].

N. Quang (✉)
Center for Andrology and Sexual Medicine, Viet Duc University Hospital, Hanoi, Vietnam

Department of Urology—Andrology and Sexual Medicine, University of Medicine and Pharmacy (UMP), Vietnam National University, Hanoi, Vietnam

T. Toprak
Department of Urology, University of Health Sciences, Hamidiye Faculty of Medicine, FSM Health Practice & Research Center, Istanbul, Turkey

A. Agarwal et al. (eds.), *Current and Future Advances in Male Infertility*,
https://doi.org/10.1007/978-3-031-62648-7_3

Occupational, environmental, and modifiable lifestyle factors may contribute to the decline in sperm count and quality [6]. The desire to identify and treat modifiable causes of male infertility remains an important issue. Semen quality is affected by environmental factors and lifestyle changes [6]. Alcohol [7], cigarette smoke [7], testis heat stress [8], electromagnetic radiation exposure [9], obesity [10], psychological stress [7], and diet applications and coffee consumption [11] are some examples that affect male infertility. Lifestyle modifications associated with male fertility are defined as cessation or limitation of unhealthy lifestyle-related factors, proper nutrition, weight loss, and appropriate exercise regimen combined with psychological comfort that may help a man father a child [12].

In this review, we aim to describe the effects of lifestyle factors on male infertility and the potential mechanisms underlying these effects.

Lifestyle Factors Affecting Male Infertility

Obesity

Obesity, which is an increasing health problem worldwide, is defined by the World Health Organization (WHO) as "excessive fat accumulation that can impair health" [13]. The WHO estimates that one in ten adult people in the world is obese [13]. The decrease in sperm quality with global increase of obesity has led many scientists to investigate the effect of obesity on sperm parameters. Hammoud et al. and Sallmen et al. (2008, 2006) found that body mass index (BMI) is associated with lower sperm motility and count and concentration [14, 15]. Martini et al. (2010) reported a negative relationship of BMI with sperm motility, but there was no relationship with sperm concentration [16]. Hofny et al. (2010) reported that BMI has a negative correlation with sperm concentration, normal morphology, and motility [17]. Stewart and Tunc et al. (2009, 2011) reported that obese men had lower sperm concentration [18, 19]. There have been other studies reporting impairment of certain semen parameters with obesity [20–23]. When the results of 250 couples who underwent intracytoplasmic sperm injection (ICSI) were analyzed, sperm motility and concentration were negatively affected by BMI [24]. There are also studies that do not find a relationship between sperm parameters and increased BMI [25–27]. A meta-analysis of 30 studies with over 115,000 men reported that obesity was associated with lower semen parameters, with an increased likelihood of DNA fragmentation, abnormal morphology, and infertility [28]. Another meta-analysis examining 13,077 males has reported that obese males were more likely to be azoospermic or oligozoospermic [29]. It has been reported that for every 9 kg overweight, there is a 10% higher risk of infertility in men [15]. A study suggested that lowering BMI helps improve sperm parameters in some men, but not all of them [30].

Diet

Diet and nutrition have a significant effect on semen quality. Although there was limited data, several studies have described the association between low vitamin/mineral concentration and subfertility [31, 32]. A comprehensive systematic review concluded that a balanced and healthy diet can improve fertility rates and semen quality [33]. For example, the Mediterranean diet rich in antioxidants, vitamins, and omega-3 fatty acids and low in trans-fatty acids was found to be directly proportional to semen quality [33]. A healthy diet has been reported to improve semen parameters [34]. Fish, poultry, vegetables, fruits, grains, and low-fat dairy were positively associated with semen quality. However, diets consisting of coffee, alcohol, full-fat dairy products, processed meats, and sugar-sweetened beverages have been associated with poor sperm quality [33]. Among 701 Danish men who underwent routine premilitary screening, those who received a higher intake of saturated fat were found to have lower sperm counts [35]. Legume and cereal consumption positively affects semen parameters [36]. Rato et al. (2013) evaluated the fertility parameters of rats fed with high-fat diet and showed a decrease in normal morphology and increase in oxidative stress (OS) markers [37]. In conclusion, diet is important for the quality of sperm parameters.

Smoking

The harmful effects of smoking on overall health are well known. However, its association with male infertility is the subject of debate. Cigarette smoke is important, as one-third of people over the age of 15 smoke worldwide, and it is common among young adult males of reproductive age [38]. It contains >7000 chemicals from different classes [39]. Although there is a consensus that smoking is a risk factor for infertility, current evidence cannot clearly demonstrate a causal relationship between smoking and male reproduction [40]. This is because it is largely unknown which chemicals cause infertility. Smoking is associated with leukocytospermia, a source of reactive oxygen species (ROS). Also, cigarette smoke contains ROS, and increased levels of seminal ROS expose the sperm to OS and impair sperm function. A meta-analysis concluded that smoking causes decreased sperm quality in both infertile and fertile men [7]. One study reported that smokers had 13–17% lower sperm concentration than nonsmokers [41]. Tobacco smoking has also been found to be responsible for aneuploidies and increases in DNA damage [42]. Therefore, smoking can cumulatively affect male fertility by affecting oxidative stress, DNA damage, and cell apoptosis. Many studies have shown that smokers have lower sperm counts [43–45], lower motility [44–46], significantly lower sperm concentrations [47–49], and lower normal morphology [47, 48, 50]. Factors that cause these effects include levels of nicotine, cotinine, and cadmium [51].

Seminal Zn level was significantly decreased in fertile smokers compared with fertile nonsmokers being correlated with daily number of smoked cigarettes and smoking duration [52]. The total quantity of Zn in the ejaculate of smokers was significantly lower than nonsmokers, jeopardizing the content of chromatin zinc and the stability of the sperm chromatin contributing to reproductive failures [53]. There was a negative effect of smoking on seminal Zn levels, which was correlated with quantity and duration of cigarette smoking [49]. Cigarette smoking affects both Ca^{2+}-ATPase activity and sperm motility attributed to reduced seminal Zn level [54]. A correlated decreased seminal Zn in smokers and the extent of smoking was found, suggesting a part of associated increased seminal OS that is also responsible for the impaired sperm motility, vitality, and sperm DNA integrity [52]. Also, it was found that deterioration of semen parameters, semen pH, and semen viscosity is correlated with decreased seminal Zn level [55].

Alcohol Consumption

Substance abuse, especially alcohol addiction, is a rapidly increasing health problem in the world. The World Health Organization estimates that there are close to two billion people in the world who use alcoholic beverages. Many people are unaware of the harmful effects of drinking alcohol [56]. However, many people experience the social, physical, and psychological effects of alcohol, which is associated with more than 60 types of illness and injury. There are a limited number of studies reporting conflicting results on the effect of alcohol on semen quality in adults with some suggesting a harmful effect [57], while others suggesting that moderate use is not harmful or even protective [58]. A meta-analysis of 29,914 men found a significant association between alcohol intake and low semen volume [7]. However, another meta-analysis involving 16,395 men reported a detrimental effect of alcohol intake on semen volume and sperm morphology [59]. Since testicular membranes are rich in polyenoic fatty acids, it is conceivable that alcohol abuse may lead to testicular lipid peroxidation, resulting in negative endocrine and reproductive outcomes. Consistent with such a mechanism, polyenoic fatty acids have been shown to be reduced in the testicles of alcohol-fed animals. In a follow-up study, 347 young adult boys were selected from a cohort of pregnant women who consumed alcohol during pregnancy. The results of the latter study indicated that sperm concentration decreased with increasing prenatal alcohol exposure [60]. It is suggested that alcohol intake leads to sperm morphological changes such as curling of the tail, swelling of the middle part, and breakage of the head. In addition, people who consume alcohol often have degenerated spermatids in their seminiferous tubules, resulting in azoospermia [61]. It has been shown that direct exposure of spermatozoa to alcohol at doses corresponding to serum levels after moderate and heavy alcohol intake impairs sperm motility and morphology in a dose-dependent manner [62]. Spermatogenesis has been shown to decrease gradually with increasing alcohol intake [63]. Sertoli cell-only syndrome and spermatogenic arrest have been shown to be more common in heavy alcohol drinkers [64]. In conclusion, men should be informed of the negative impact of chronic alcohol intake on fertility and advised to avoid chronic alcohol consumption.

Caffeine

Many studies have reported no association between moderate caffeine intake and male fertility [65]. A meta-analysis evaluating 29,914 men showed that coffee consumption did not have a significant effect on sperm quality [7]. Another study also found no association between reduced semen quality and moderate caffeine intake [66]. There are studies reporting a relationship between sperm DNA damage and caffeine intake. A meta-analysis reported that caffeine intake may be associated with sperm aneuploidy and sperm double-stranded DNA breaks [67]. Conversely, there are studies reporting that there is lower risk of DNA fragmentation with caffeine intake [68]. A study linked caffeine intake with a lower probability of live birth per assisted reproductive technique (ART) cycle [69]. Another study reported that male coffee consumption is negatively associated with intracytoplasmic sperm injection (ICSI) fertilization rate, but not implantation, pregnancy, and miscarriage rates [24]. However, it is not possible to establish a definitive potential association between caffeine intake and male infertility based on the available data.

Performance-Enhancing Drug Usage

Recreational drugs such as anabolic-androgenic steroids, marijuana, opiates, cocaine, and methamphetamines have a negative impact on male fertility. These drugs can impair testicular architecture, hypothalamic-pituitary gonadal (HPG) axis, and spermatozoa function [70]. There is accumulated evidence that drug use adversely affects male reproductive function [71, 72].

Testosterone and testosterone derivatives contain a family of hormones that are called anabolic-androgenic steroids (AASs). These are mainly used by men to improve their general performance or personal well-being and appearance [73]. Increased exogenous testosterone levels due to AAS use suppress spermatogenesis with negative feedback to HPG axis and cause testicular atrophy and infertility. Some studies have argued that the use of AAS may have a permanent effect on male fertility, so they did not recommend the use of AAS [74].

Recreational Substance Abuse

Marijuana is the most abused illicit drug worldwide [75]. Total sperm count and sperm concentration were found to be lower in young men who regularly use marijuana [76]. It has been shown that if the endogenous cannabinoid system is disrupted, spermatogenesis is affected and total sperm count and motility are reduced [77].

Opioids such as morphine, hydrocodone, and oxycodone are a class of analgesic drugs used to treat pain, cough, or diarrhea [78]. Heroin is synthesized from morphine and has a high addictive potential. Opioids are the third most commonly abused drugs worldwide [79]. Opioids affect testicular function through changes in hormonal levels. Sperm function is affected both indirectly by altered reproductive hormone levels and directly by affecting opioid receptors found on spermatozoa [80–82]. However, the evidence regarding the effects of opioids on sperm concentration, viability, and motility is conflicting.

Cocaine is a powerful stimulant with high addictive potential. Long-term cocaine users have decreased sperm motility, concentration, and normal morphology [83]. Methamphetamine and MDMA have been shown to reduce sperm motility, sperm concentration, and sperm DNA integrity in rats [84, 85].

Sport/Physical Activity

Among lifestyle factors, sport/physical activity has been demonstrated to improve general and reproductive health, while excessive intensity of physical activity results in enhanced male-related infertility problems [86]. Sport/physical activity is recommended by medical practitioners to improve general health [87, 88]. It has also been recommended by the WHO that adults (between 18 and 64 years old) should perform aerobic physical activity for at least 150 min weekly with moderate intensity or combine a 75 min per week of moderate activity with vigorous intensity training to maintain their general health [87].

A comprehensive, controlled trial study was done to examine the effect of exercise intensity and duration, using two moderate-intensity (60% of VO_2 max) and high-intensity (80% of VO_2 max—maximum oxygen uptake) training protocols [89]. The results revealed a remarkable decline in the level of LH, FSH, testosterone, and free testosterone after 12 weeks of training in both moderate- and high-intensity training groups. After 60 weeks of training, followed by 36 weeks of low-intensity training as a recovery period, all evaluated parameters were restored.

The effect of exercise on sex hormone-binding globulin (SHBG) was also evaluated. Although there is no consensus about this protein's alteration in training conditions, a study reported a significant increment in the level of SHBG in both moderate- and high-intensity training. Indeed, a higher level of SHBG resulted in lower serum-free testosterone levels [89] and bioavailability [90, 91].

It has been reported that the most important molecular alteration underlying endocrine dysfunction following exercise is related to ROS generation in the whole body and specifically in the testicular tissue [92, 93]. In addition to excess oxygen consumption due to exercise, diminished microvascular oxygen partial pressure has been revealed as another underlying mechanism leading to ROS generation [94]. Clinical findings have demonstrated that higher intensity of exercise results in a lower level of total and free testosterone levels in serum.

However, ROS generation directly increases apoptosis in Leydig cells, which in turn leads to lower testosterone secretion. A decreased testosterone could be related to 3β-hydroxysteroid dehydrogenase (3β-HSD) and 17β-hydroxysteroid dehydrogenase (17β-HSD), which are also diminished due to exercise [95, 96]. There is a possible link between training intensity and decreased 3β-HSD and 17β-HSD levels, leading to diminished testosterone production [95, 96].

Additionally, a randomized controlled trial revealed a remarkable increase in inflammatory cytokines in chronic moderate- and high-intensity trained men [96]. The authors of the latter study revealed a significant increment in the level of interleukin (IL)-1β, IL-6, IL-8, and tumor necrosis factor-alpha (TNF-α) in semen samples [97]. In another randomized controlled trial study, the same researchers illustrated IL-1β, IL-6, IL-8, and TNF-α upregulation in semen samples of men submitted to resistance training and of combined treadmill plus resistance trained men [98]. The IL-6 directly inhibits LH-specific receptors in Leydig cells resulting in testosterone production decrement [99, 100]. Moreover, TNF-α inhibits cholesterol availability content for Leydig cell mitochondria and diminishes steroidogenesis in Leydig cells [101]. IL-1 has been recognized as a cytochrome p450c17 inhibitor in Leydig cells [102]. Based on current findings, pro-inflammatory cytokine alteration due to exercise is another potential mechanism leading to dysfunction of hypothalamic-pituitary-gonadal axis [98, 103].

Electromagnetic/Radiofrequency Exposure

Laptops, cell phones, and microwave ovens are frequently used in our life. These devices use microwaves, which are a type of electromagnetic wave (EMW). It is unclear how EMW radiation affects male fertility. In a study by Agarwal et al. (2008), semen analyses of 361 men were correlated with cell phone use duration. The authors reported a decrease in sperm motility, normal morphology, and viability with an increase in cell phone use duration [104]. In a similar study, a reduction in sperm motility and normal morphology depending on cell phone use was found [105]. Fejes and colleagues reported a decrease in sperm motility with increased cell phone use [106]. In a study, semen samples were exposed to mobile phone, and a decrease in sperm viability and motility was found [107]. In another study, it was found that there was a decrease in sperm motility as a result of exposure to mobile phones [108].

To date, few studies have focused on thermal and nonthermal effects of Wi-Fi and laptop use. Thermal toxicity has been associated with male infertility [109, 110]. Sheynkin et al. [111, 112] investigated the effect of laptop usage on the legs of young men on scrotal hyperthermia and found an approximately 3 °C increase in scrotal temperature with 60 min of seated laptop use. However, in these studies, semen parameters or pregnancy status were not investigated. The available literature is devoid of any studies investigating secondary thermal toxicity from laptop Wi-Fi use. Therefore, it is unclear with laptop usage whether the increase in scrotal temperature is clinically significant. Due to the lack of literature, the nonthermal effects of EMWs are still unclear. Oni et al. [113] investigated the effects of EMWs from Wi-Fi on the ejaculate. Ten samples were separated and placed 60 cm away from each laptop for 1 h and compared with unexposed samples. The authors found reductions in morphology and motility of the exposed samples. Nevertheless, in the latter study, it is difficult to distinguish the nonthermal effects of EMW from the thermal effects. There are no human studies on male reproductive health and microwave oven leakage. However, animal studies generally mention harmful effects [114–116]. Although EMW exposure appears to affect semen quality, the underlying mechanism remains unclear.

Heat Stress

Male testis is 1–2 °C lower than body temperature. So, scrotal hyperthermia may disrupt the intratesticular oxidative balance, leading to oxidative stress, perm DNA damage, and cell apoptosis [117, 118]. It has been shown that tight underwear, that could keep the testicles in the groin position, increased the scrotal temperature by 2 °C and if this temperature increase was maintained for more than 20 days, a significant increase in DNA damage was demonstrated [110]. Fever was shown to cause sperm DNA fragmentation, which peaks 1 month after illness and lasts for at least 79 days [119]. There are studies showing that the higher the scrotal temperature, the more the sperm quality deteriorates [120]. An increase of 1 °C suppresses spermatogenesis by 14% [121]. It was found that sperm with abnormal morphology doubled on average 6–8 months after exposure to high temperature [121]. Consequently, hyperthermia is likely to impair semen parameters.

Psychological Stress and Anxiety

A man's inability to get his partner pregnant naturally leads to a stressful situation. Psychological stress is a natural consequence of male infertility [122]. However, it is unclear whether stress causes infertility. While most studies do not consider psychological stress alone as a factor of male infertility, it may act as an additional risk factor. In an experimental study, acute stress has been shown to decrease sperm motility [123]. A meta-analysis of 29,914 participants and 57 cross-sectional studies reported that psychological stress can reduce sperm progressive motility, concentration, and normal sperm morphology [7]. A study evaluated the associations between stressful life events, perceived stress, and work-related stress on sperm parameters [124]. Of these, stressful life events and perceived stress were negatively associated with sperm parameters, especially sperm morphology and motility. However, the relationship between work-related stress and semen parameters was not observed. Another study among healthy volunteers reported that examination stress negatively affected seminal antioxidant content and sperm quality [125]. In a study of 225 infertile men, it was reported that stress was negatively correlated with semen parameters [126]. It has also been reported that there is an inverse relationship between psychological stress and sperm parameters in couples undergoing in vitro fertilization [127, 128]. In conclusion, while infertility leads to stress, stress may contribute to infertility and thus the condition falls into a vicious cycle.

Mechanisms by Which Lifestyle Factors Affect Male Fertility

The pathophysiology of male infertility could be explained by cascades of molecular, biochemical, and physiological events, which are mostly represented by abnormal semen quality parameters.

Seminal Oxidative Stress

Imbalance in ROS and antioxidant defenses in the cell thereby leading to a state of oxygen paradox is defined by a cellular condition known as OS, which interferes with the essential cellular processes, inactivates essential metabolic enzymes, and disrupts various cellular signaling pathways [129]. It has been suggested that insufficient antioxidants and increased OS may contribute to the risk of declining semen quality [130]. Both catalase activity and total antioxidant capacity (TAC) were significantly correlated with sperm motility and morphology [131].

Oxidative stress impairs the structural and functional integrity of spermatozoa leading to peroxidative damage to the sperm plasma membrane, DNA fragmentation in sperm nuclear/mitochondrial genome, and dysregulation in levels of mRNAs/transcripts [132]. Reactive oxygen species which include superoxide anion ($O_2^{\cdot}$), hydrogen peroxide (H_2O_2), peroxyl ($ROO^{\cdot}$), and hydroxyl ($OH^{\cdot}$) radicals are the highly reactive oxidizing agents, and their major source of production in spermatozoa includes activated leukocytes in the seminal plasma and the mitochondria in the spermatozoa itself. Low/moderate levels of ROS are required by spermatozoa for the activation of several redox-sensitive physiological processes, such as sperm capacitation and hyperactivation, whereas supraphysiological ROS levels impede sperm membrane fluidity and permeability and cause sperm DNA damage [133].

Significance of ROS in sperm hyperactivation was further supported by a study which demonstrated that in vitro incubation of spermatozoa with low concentration of OH triggered sperm hyperactivation [134].

The exact mechanism of how OS negatively affects the sperm function is largely unknown but is mainly attributed to peroxidative damage to axoneme and depletion of intracellular ATP levels, followed by generation of 4-hydroxynonenal and malondialdehyde owing to oxidation of lipid membrane components and fragmentation of both nuclear and mitochondrial DNA [135]. Sperm plasma membrane is most accessible to OS-induced injury because of the high content of polyunsaturated fatty acids (PUFAs), which provides exuberant sites for free radical-induced damage [136]. It also has a limited cytosolic space with minimal antioxidants post-spermiogenesis. Sperm harbors a truncated DNA damage detection and repair system, which makes sperm further vulnerable to accumulate oxidatively induced damage to both mitochondrial and nuclear DNA [137]. Seminal plasma is well endowed with enzymatic antioxidants (such as superoxide dismutase and catalase) and nonenzymatic antioxidants (such as pyruvate and ascorbic acid), which scavenge ROS and protect spermatozoa from OS, specifically after leaving the testicles.

Antioxidants act to reduce the amount of ROS, including hydroxyl radicals, superoxide anions, and hydrogen peroxide [138]. The free radical scavenging system, superoxide dismutase (SOD), and catalase are present in all oxygen-metabolizing cells, and their function is to provide a defense against the potentially damaging activities of superoxide and H_2O_2 [139]. Depletion in the enzymatic activity observed in the study of Kumar et al. [140] may be explained due to decreased synthesis of enzyme or oxidative inactivation of enzyme protein. Decrease in the SOD activity indicated an incomplete removal of the free superoxide radical generated by various lifestyle habits and/or toxicant exposure. Further, reduction in catalase activity also reflected the inability to eliminate H_2O_2 produced by lifestyle and/or toxicant exposure. All these could contribute to the imbalance of ROS.

Reactive oxygen species play an important role in modulating the essential functions of sperm, e.g., capacitation, hyperactivation, and acrosomal reaction; however, imbalances between ROS production and semen antioxidant capacity will result in oxidation of membrane polyunsaturated fatty acids [141, 142], loss of mitochondrial membrane potential [143], and single- and double-strand DNA fragmentation [144].

Sperm plasma membrane integrity is necessary for motility and fertilization. Spermatozoa are highly sensitive to injuries caused by generations of ROS concentration such as superoxide anion, hydrogen peroxide, and hydroxyl radical, which can result in the damage to cell membrane [145] and lead to deterioration in sperm motility and functional capacity. Oxidative stress in semen leads to peroxidative injury to the sperm membrane, resulting in consequent impairment of related functional properties, such as sperm motility [141].

Studies on the peroxidation of phospholipids in mammalian sperm have demonstrated that peroxidation reaction causes membrane damage, which leads to loss of motility and membrane integrity [146]. Lipid peroxide levels were higher in the seminal plasma of subjects who had lifestyle habits and/or were exposed to environmental factors, which might be due to increased oxidative stress, exerted by these factors [140].

There is a strong association between decreased sperm motility and OS [147, 148]. Sperm motility is generated through constant ATP production by mitochondria localized in the sperm midpiece. To produce ATP through oxidative phosphorylation, the mitochondrial membrane must have selective permeability, which maintains an electrolytic gradient between the inner and outer mitochondrial environments. Excessive ROS will alter phospholipid membranes, and thus disrupt membrane selectivity, and will also inhibit oxidative phosphorylation, ultimately leading to decreased ATP production [149, 150].

Direct Testicular Toxicity

Toxicant damage directly affects the testicular tissues, which can result in various adverse effects, namely reduced sperm count, production of defective spermatozoa, and impaired androgen production [140, 151]. An agent which affects the testis without endocrine mediation will be classified as a direct reproductive toxicant. The site of biotransformation of direct-acting compounds may determine the extent of their testicular toxicity. Highly reactive intermediates produced in the liver are not likely to reach the testes in significant concentration because of their short biological half-lives. Conversely, less reactive metabolic products of hepatic metabolism may attain significant concentrations in the testes and, presumably, be further metabolized to more toxic forms. The testes contain measurable amounts of cytochrome P450, mixed-function oxidases, epoxide hydrolases, aryl hydrocarbon hydrolases, and various transferases necessary for the biotransformation of many exogenous compounds, although these enzymes and cofactors are often present at only a fraction of their concentration in the liver. Nonetheless, these enzymatic activities are present in close proximity to the germ cells and may, therefore, be of particular importance in the biotransformation of testicular toxicants. In fact, the interaction between gonadal activation and hepatic detoxification of xenobiotics likely plays a significant role in the modulation of testicular toxicity [152].

Germ Cell Changes

The exercise-induced inflammatory condition can directly or indirectly disrupt spermatogenesis, for instance, due to increased IL-1β, IL-6, IL-8, and TNF-α, reported in high-intensity runner's semen samples [97]. Consistent with this issue, a previously conducted study reported TNF-α's key role in extrinsic apoptosis induction through their specific receptor [153], explaining this fact that TNF-α increment in exercise condition can induce germ cell apoptosis in seminiferous tubules. These pro-inflammatory cytokines not only induce spermatogenesis arrest through increasing apoptosis, but may also act more specifically. For instance, Huang et al. [154] reported that TL-6 regulates the gene expression of spermatogonial stem cell's self-renewal genes, such as Sox-2. Considering IL-6 increment in excessive exercise condition [97, 98], it may explain the exercise-induced germ cell arrest in exercise condition [93, 155].

Histopathological Changes

Histopathological changes can range from germ cells, Sertoli cells, and Leydig cells to changes in structures such as seminiferous tubules and testicular connective tissue, leading to a decrease in volume and weight of a testicle. For example, bromuconazole also caused a decrease in relative testis and epididymis weights and degenerative changes in seminiferous tubules.

A recently conducted study using low (50–60% VO_2 max), moderate (60–70% VO_2 max), and high (80–85% VO_2 max) intensity continuous training (running 45 min/day for 8 weeks) illustrated various pathological effects of HICT in rats, while low- and moderate-intensity running conditions showed no statistically significant changes versus the control group (non-trained animals). In HICT-induced rat's histopathological examinations, germ cell dissociation, and depletion, increased negative tubular differentiation (TDI) and increased negative spermiogenesis (SPI) indices were observed. Moreover, testicular Sertoli cell numbers were also diminished in the HICT-induced rat's testicular tissues [156]. Simultaneously, 8-week HICT resulted in a significant reduction in Johnsen score, meiotic index (MI), and seminiferous tubule diameter in C57BL6 mice model testis [157].

Soudmand and colleagues in 2021 illustrated a significant decrease in lactate dehydrogenase (LDH) level and germ cell cytoplasmic carbohydrate storage following HICT. Moreover, the authors showed that HICT results in reduced glucose transporter-1 (Glut-1) and MCT-4 expression in Sertoli and germ cells, which resulted in increased Sertoli and germ cell loss in the testicular tissue [156]. Samaneh and colleagues [158] reported that glucose, LDH, lactate, intracytoplasmic carbohydrate, and lipid reduction in HICT (running 45 min/day for 8 weeks) results in autophagia induction as a possible mechanism for depletion of Sertoli and germ cells in the exercise-performed rat's testicular tissue [159].

Hormonal Mechanisms

Spermatogenesis is hampered if the body does not produce enough androgens. In addition to testicular shrinkage and fibrosis, these men often have significantly diminished germ cell numbers, which contributes to an unusually reduced rate of spermatogenesis in the testicles. It has already been mentioned that testosterone's capacity to limit GnRH release at the hypothalamus is mediated by the hormone's conversion into estrogen. A primary excess of estrogens can work in a similar manner to have an inhibitory effect on the HPG axis, resulting in lower fertility (Table 3.1, Fig. 3.1).

The neuroendocrine regulation by the hypothalamic-pituitary-gonadal (HPG) axis plays a crucial role in maintaining the intricate balance of male reproductive hormone secretion and function. Gonadotropin-releasing hormone (GnRH) from hypothalamus initiates this cascade by stimulating the anterior pituitary to release luteinizing hormone (LH) and follicle-stimulating hormone (FSH). While LH acts on Leydig cells to support steroidogenesis, FSH aids spermatogenesis by acting on Sertoli cells. Leydig cells are the primary source of testosterone or androgens in males that drive maturation of Sertoli cells. Sertoli cells then secrete activin and inhibin, contributing to the feedback loop that regulates the HPG axis. Disruptions in this delicate hormonal cross talk, which is often caused by endocrinopathies, can lead to dysfunction. Conditions like obesity, thyroid hormone imbalance, and diabetes mellitus cause oxidative stress that leads to impairment of the normal endocrine control of male reproductive functions. Hyperprolactinemia is characterized by elevated prolactin levels that impede GnRH release from hypothalamus, leading to reduced gonadotropin secretion and perhaps inhibiting gonadotropin actions on gonads (testis). In addition, upregulation of aromatase CYP19 results in heightened estrogen levels, which can inhibit the HPG axis. Besides, the hypothalamus-pituitary-adrenal (HPA) axis regulates both production and secretion of cortisol released by the adrenal glands. High cortisol levels can inhibit LH and FSH release from anterior pituitary. Cortisol also plays an important role in the stress response. Some research has found that men with higher levels of anxiety and stress have lower sperm concentration and counts. Therefore, loss of HPA axis regulation can lead to cortisol excess disorders that can result in reduced male fertility.

Table 3.1 Reports on endocrinopathies and their impact on male reproduction

Endocrinopathy	Changes in male reproduction
Hypogonadotropic hypogonadism (genetic: Kallmann syndrome)	Delayed puberty and infertility caused by a malfunction of GnRH-secreting neurons to migrate; cessation of gonadotropin secretion
Hypergonadotropic hypogonadism	Increased FSH/LH, normal or ↓testis volume, decreased pubic hair and penis size, infertility
Androgen excess	Inhibition to GnRH secretion, normal or ↓FSH, ↓LH
Estrogen excess	↓T:E2, ↓semen parameters
Hyperprolactinemia	Normal or ↓FSH/LH, ↓testosterone
Insulin disorders	↓Spermatogenesis, ↓reduced vacuolization in the Sertoli cells, ↓fertility, ↓semen parameters, ↓Leydig cell count, ↓testosterone

↓ = decrease, T:E2 = testosterone-to-estradiol ratio

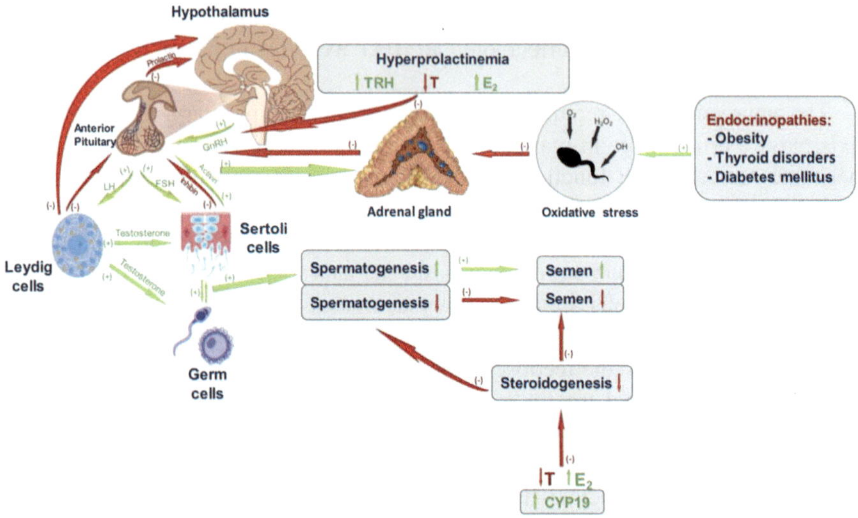

Fig. 3.1 Endocrinopathies and male reproduction

Nutritional Imbalances

Recent literature supports the hypothesis that certain nutritional factors (saturated fats, omega-3 fats, soy, beef consumption, zinc, and antioxidants) can affect semen quality (sperm concentration, morphology, motility, sperm aneuploidy).

The study by Attaman et al. [160] of dietary fat and semen quality reported that high intake of saturated fats was negatively related to sperm concentration, whereas higher intake of omega-3 fats was positively related to sperm morphology (Fig. 3.2).

Low intake of antioxidant nutrients was associated with poor semen quality in a case-control study in Spain [161].

Commonly studied supplemental and dietary antioxidants include vitamin D, vitamin E, vitamin C, β-carotene, and coenzyme Q10. The lack of these agents in the body can lead to male infertility. For example, in a prospective pilot study of infertile men, the incidence of low vitamin D was 76.9% (mean serum vitamin D level of 23.6 ng/mL). After treatment with vitamin D supplements, the rate of low sperm motility (<40%) improved [162].

Coenzyme Q10 is a component of the mitochondrial respiratory chain that is required for energy metabolism. CoQ10 is an antioxidant, an energy-promoting agent, a membrane stabilizer, and a regulator of mitochondrial permeability transition pores. Given these actions, it is theorized that this added cellular energy may improve sperm count and motility. The amount of CoQ10 in the seminal fluid shows a direct correlation with semen parameters. A strong correlation between sperm count, motility, and ubiquinol (reduced form of CoQ10) has been reported [163, 164]. Reduced levels of CoQ10 were noted in infertile men with idiopathic and varicocele-associated asthenozoospermia [165]. There was deterioration of semen

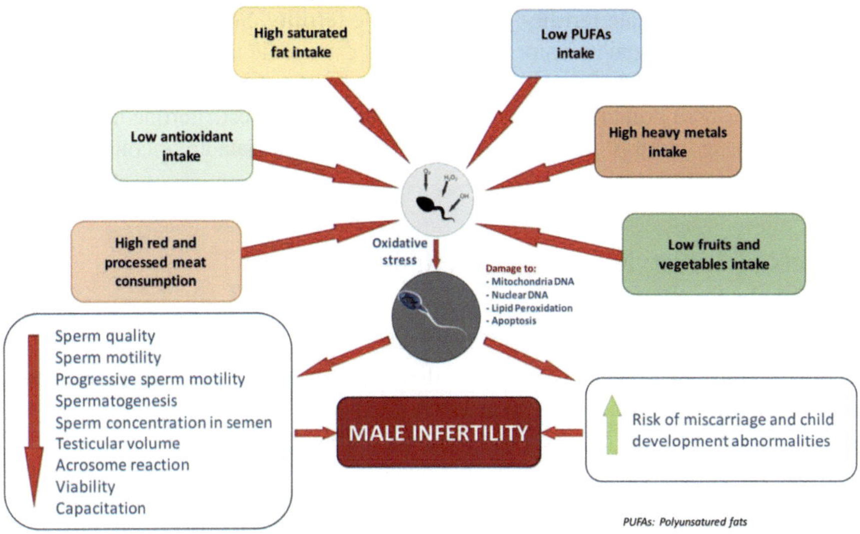

Fig. 3.2 Nutritional imbalances related to oxidative stress and male infertility

parameters, semen pH, and semen viscosity correlated with decreased seminal Zn level [55].

Genetic Mechanisms

The integrity of sperm chromatin structure is influenced by certain endogenous and exogenous factors, such as peroxidative damage of DNA, which may arise from infectious or toxic agents [166]. Sperm DNA integrity has been extensively researched recently as a marker of male factor infertility. Initially, ROS usually alters the sperm lipid bilayer by oxidation of methylene groups in polyunsaturated fatty acids. The process ultimately leads to the production of lipid degradation by-products, of which malonaldehyde is one of the most common. Malonaldehyde is an alkylating agent with the ability to covalently bind to nucleophilic groups of DNA, peptides, and proteins, modifying their molecular function [149]. In the second stage of excessive ROS production, guanosine is oxidized to 8′-OH guanosine, a pre-mutagenic effect that leads to altered pairing of DNA bases. In the third stage, excess ROS will directly interact with DNA and cause single- and double-strand nonspecific breaks in the DNA molecule [147].

Reduced testicular specific heat shock protein-70-2 (HSP-70-2) has been reported following high-intensity training [92]. Considering this protein-specific role in response to heat and oxidative stress conditions [167], as well as in DNA packing process [168], reduced HSP-70 in excessive exercise conditions can be another cause of spermatogenesis arrest.

Soy may help female fertility yet hinder male fertility. Soy contains isoflavones that bind to the estrogen receptor and have mild estrogenic activity [169, 170]. It is theorized that this mild estrogenic activity may affect spermatogenesis, induce capacitation and a premature acrosome reaction, or lower testosterone levels [171]. However, these findings are from animal models, and the data are inconsistent.

Effects of Lifestyle Changes on Semen Quality and Male Fertility

Men who consume a "health-conscious" diet (high intakes of fruits, vegetables, fish, and whole grains) have lower sperm DNA damage [172]. Human nutrition affects semen quality and the level of reproductive hormones. Men who consume fish, chicken, fruits, cruciferous vegetables, tomatoes, leafy green vegetables, legumes, and whole grains had a lower sperm DNA damage and higher sperm concentration and testosterone level [173]. Semen parameters may be improved by diets consisting of limited processed meats and cheese and by increased low-fat dairy and fish [174].

Supplementing with certain vitamins and CoQ10 has been shown to play a role in improving fertility in men. For example, after 6 months of supplementation with CoQ10 (200 mg/day twice daily), there was an increase in seminal plasma, sperm cells, and sperm cell motility [175]. In a randomized trial between placebo and 300 mg coenzyme Q10 supplementation, the men who were supplemented with the CoQ10 had improved sperm count (57.8 vs. 47.8 million, $p < 0.01$), motility (27.6 vs. 23.1%, $p < 0.01$), and morphology (9.6 vs. 7.8%, $p < 0.07$) [89]. Reducing or giving up bad habits can also improve men's chances of having a baby. Smoking cessation improves fecundity and sperm parameters [176].

While excessive exercise adversely affects testosterone biogenesis, spermatogenesis, and semen quality, low- and moderate-intensity exercise (during lifetime or as a sperm booster) increases sperm production and semen quality. One of the positive impacts of sport is associated with an improved oxygen consumption in inflammation, cardiac, and other conditions [177]. Moreover, it has been illustrated that exercise positively increased LDH activity [168] and lactate dehydrogenase C (LDHC) and ODF1 [178, 179] protein expression in the testis of exercise experimental models, resulting in oxygen efficiency usage in Sertoli and sperm cells. Regarding these two contradictory impacts, it seems that individual health status as well as exercise volume, intensity, and duration are effectively involved cofactors in the outcomes.

Conclusion

Several studies suggest the role of lifestyle factors in the deterioration of semen quality. Several mechanisms are proposed to explain the impairment of semen parameters and men's fertility potential due to lifestyle factors including OS, hormonal alterations, and direct reproductive toxicant pathway among others. This data is useful in advocating for adopting a healthy lifestyle in order to reduce the male reproductive health problems.

Physicians can help the patient identify modifiable risk factors, especially given the cost and time commitment associated with infertility treatments. If patients are made aware of simple lifestyle changes that could impact their fertility, they are generally receptive to making those adjustments. All patients should be encouraged to strive for a healthy, sustainable lifestyle. In areas where there is clear evidence that a lifestyle behavior may impact fertility, such as smoking, the patient should be encouraged to modify behavior. When the recommendations are less clear, the limitations of evidence should be discussed with the patients.

References

1. Isidori A, Latini M, Romanelli F. Treatment of male infertility. Contraception. 2005;72(4):314–8.
2. Thonneau P, et al. Incidence and main causes of infertility in a resident population (1850000) of three French regions (1988–1989). Hum Reprod. 1991;6(6):811–6.
3. Attia AM, Al-Inany HG, Proctor ML. Gonadotrophins for idiopathic male factor subfertility: a Cochrane systematic review. Middle East Fertil Soc J. 2007;12(2):77–85.
4. Mosher WD. Fecundity and infertility in the United States. Am J Public Health. 1988;78(2):181–2.
5. Hull M, et al. Population study of causes, treatment, and outcome of infertility. Br Med J (Clin Res Ed). 1985;291(6510):1693–7.
6. Montano L, et al. Effects of a lifestyle change intervention on semen quality in healthy young men living in highly polluted areas in Italy: the FASt randomized controlled trial. Eur Urol Focus. 2022;8(1):351–9.
7. Li Y, Lin H, Li Y, Cao J. Association between socio-psycho-behavioral factors and male semen quality: systematic review and meta-analyses. Fertil Steril. 2011;95(1):116–23.
8. Durairajanayagam D, Sharma RK, du Plessis SS, Agarwal A. Testicular heat stress and sperm quality. In: Male infertility: a complete guide to lifestyle and environmental factors; 2014. p. 105–25.
9. McGill JJ, Agarwal A. The impact of cell phone, laptop computer, and microwave oven usage on male fertility. In: Male infertility: a complete guide to lifestyle and environmental factors; 2014. p. 161–77.
10. Khullar K, Agarwal A, du Plessis SS. BMI and obesity. In: Male infertility: a complete guide to lifestyle and environmental factors; 2014. p. 31–45.
11. Trost LW, Gudeloglu A, Ko EY, Parekattil SJ. The importance of diet, vitamins, malnutrition, and nutrient deficiencies in male fertility. In: Male infertility: a complete guide to lifestyle and environmental factors; 2014. p. 61–82.
12. Yao DF, Mills JN. Male infertility: lifestyle factors and holistic, complementary, and alternative therapies. Asian J Androl. 2016;18(3):410.

13. World Health Organization. Office of health communications and public relations. Obesity and overweight. Geneva: World Health Organization; 2006.
14. Hammoud AO, et al. Male obesity and alteration in sperm parameters. Fertil Steril. 2008;90(6):2222–5.
15. Sallmén M, et al. Reduced fertility among overweight and obese men. Epidemiology. 2006;17(5):520–3.
16. Martini AC, et al. Overweight and seminal quality: a study of 794 patients. Fertil Steril. 2010;94(5):1739–43.
17. Hofny ER, et al. Semen parameters and hormonal profile in obese fertile and infertile males. Fertil Steril. 2010;94(2):581–4.
18. Stewart T, et al. Associations between andrological measures, hormones and semen quality in fertile Australian men: inverse relationship between obesity and sperm output. Hum Reprod. 2009;24(7):1561–8.
19. Tunc O, Bakos H, Tremellen K. Impact of body mass index on seminal oxidative stress. Andrologia. 2011;43(2):121–8.
20. Shayeb AG, Harrild K, Mathers E, Bhattacharya S. An exploration of the association between male body mass index and semen quality. Reprod Biomed Online. 2011;23(6):717–23.
21. Fariello RM, et al. Association between obesity and alteration of sperm DNA integrity and mitochondrial activity. Br J Urol. 2012;110(6):863.
22. Hammiche F, et al. Body mass index and central adiposity are associated with sperm quality in men of subfertile couples. Hum Reprod. 2012;27(8):2365–72.
23. La Vignera S, Condorelli RA, Vicari E, Calogero AE. Negative effect of increased body weight on sperm conventional and nonconventional flow cytometric sperm parameters. J Androl. 2012;33(1):53–8.
24. Braga DP, Halpern G, Rita de Cássia SF, Setti AS, Iaconelli A Jr, Borges E Jr. Food intake and social habits in male patients and its relationship to intracytoplasmic sperm injection outcomes. Fertil Steril. 2012;97(1):53–9.
25. Aggerholm AS, et al. Is overweight a risk factor for reduced semen quality and altered serum sex hormone profile? Fertil Steril. 2008;90(3):619–26.
26. Pauli EM, et al. Diminished paternity and gonadal function with increasing obesity in men. Fertil Steril. 2008;90(2):346–51.
27. Chavarro JE, et al. Body mass index in relation to semen quality, sperm DNA integrity, and serum reproductive hormone levels among men attending an infertility clinic. Fertil Steril. 2010;93(7):2222–31.
28. Campbell JM, Lane M, Owens JA, Bakos HW. Paternal obesity negatively affects male fertility and assisted reproduction outcomes: a systematic review and meta-analysis. Reprod Biomed Online. 2015;31(5):593–604.
29. Sermondade N, et al. BMI in relation to sperm count: an updated systematic review and collaborative meta-analysis. Hum Reprod Update. 2013;19(3):221–31.
30. Kahn BE, Brannigan RE. Obesity and male infertility. Curr Opin Urol. 2017;27(5):441–5.
31. Benedetti S, et al. Differences in blood and semen oxidative status in fertile and infertile men, and their relationship with sperm quality. Reprod Biomed Online. 2012;25(3):300–6.
32. Kaushal N, Bansal M. Diminished reproductive potential of male mice in response to selenium-induced oxidative stress: involvement of HSP70, HSP70-2, and MSJ-1. J Biochem Mol Toxicol. 2009;23(2):125–36.
33. Salas-Huetos A, Bulló M, Salas-Salvadó J. Dietary patterns, foods and nutrients in male fertility parameters and fecundability: a systematic review of observational studies. Hum Reprod Update. 2017;23(4):371–89.
34. Giahi L, Mohammadmoradi S, Javidan A, Sadeghi MR. Nutritional modifications in male infertility: a systematic review covering 2 decades. Nutr Rev. 2016;74(2):118–30.
35. Jensen TK, et al. High dietary intake of saturated fat is associated with reduced semen quality among 701 young Danish men from the general population. Am J Clin Nutr. 2013;97(2):411–8.

36. Trost LW, Gudeloglu A, Ko EY, Parekattil SJ. The importance of diet, vitamins, malnutrition, and nutrient deficiencies in male fertility. In: Male infertility. Springer; 2014. p. 61–82.
37. Rato L, et al. High-energy diets may induce a pre-diabetic state altering testicular glycolytic metabolic profile and male reproductive parameters. Andrology. 2013;1(3):495–504.
38. Saleh RA, et al. Effect of cigarette smoking on levels of seminal oxidative stress in infertile men: a prospective study. Fertil Steril. 2002;78(3):491–9.
39. Centers for Disease Control and Prevention (US); National Center for Chronic Disease Prevention and Health Promotion (US); Office on Smoking and Health (US). How tobacco smoke causes disease: the biology and behavioral basis for smoking-attributable disease: a report of the Surgeon General. Atlanta (GA): Centers for Disease Control and Prevention (US), 2010. PMID: 21452462.
40. Practice Committee of the American Society for Reproductive Medicine. Smoking and infertility. Fertil Steril. 2008;90(5):S254–9.
41. Adashi EY, et al. Cigarette smoking and sperm density: a meta-analysis. Fertil Steril. 1994;61(1):35–43.
42. Beal MA, Yauk CL, Marchetti F. From sperm to offspring: assessing the heritable genetic consequences of paternal smoking and potential public health impacts. Mutat Res/Rev Mutat Res. 2017;773:26–50.
43. Close CE, Roberts PL, Berger RE. Cigarettes, alcohol and marijuana are related to pyospermia in infertile men. J Urol. 1990;144(4):900–3.
44. Künzle R, et al. Semen quality of male smokers and nonsmokers in infertile couples. Fertil Steril. 2003;79(2):287–91.
45. Ramlau-Hansen C, et al. Is smoking a risk factor for decreased semen quality? A cross-sectional analysis. Hum Reprod. 2007;22(1):188–96.
46. Hassa H, et al. Effect of smoking on semen parameters of men attending an infertility clinic. Clin Exp Obstetr Gynecol. 2006;33(1):19–22.
47. Bouvet R, Paparella V, Feldman N. Effect of tobacco consumption on the spermatogenesis in males with idiopathic infertility. Arch Esp Urol. 2007;60(3):273–7.
48. Merino G, Lira SC, Martinez-Chequer J. Effects of cigarette smoking on semen characteristics of a population in Mexico. Arch Androl. 1998;41(1):11–5.
49. Zhang J-P, et al. Effect of smoking on semen quality of infertile men in Shandong, China. Asian J Androl. 2000;2(2):143–6.
50. Moskova P, Popov I. Sperm quality in smokers and nonsmokers among infertile families. Akush Ginekol. 1993;32(1):28–30.
51. Dai J-B, Wang Z-X, Qiao Z-D. The hazardous effects of tobacco smoking on male fertility. Asian J Androl. 2015;17(6):954.
52. Liu R, et al. Seminal plasma zinc level may be associated with the effect of cigarette smoking on sperm parameters. J Int Med Res. 2010;38(3):923–8.
53. Oldereid N, Rui H, Clausen O, Purvis K. Cigarette smoking and human sperm quality assessed by laser–Doppler spectroscopy and DNA flow cytometry. Reproduction. 1989;86(2):731–6.
54. Kumosani T, Elshal MF, Al-Jonaid A, Abduljabar H. The influence of smoking on semen quality, seminal microelements and Ca2+-ATPase activity among infertile and fertile men. Clin Biochem. 2008;41(14–15):1199–203.
55. Dissanayake D, Wijesinghe P, Ratnasooriya W, Wimalasena S. Relationship between seminal plasma zinc and semen quality in a subfertile population. J Hum Reprod Sci. 2010;3(3):124.
56. Borges E Jr, Pasqualotto FF. The effect of alcohol consumption on male infertility. In: Male infertility: a complete guide to lifestyle and environmental factors. Springer; 2014. p. 83–92.
57. La Vignera S, et al. Does alcohol have any effect on male reproductive function? A review of literature. Asian J Androl. 2013;15(2):221.
58. Marinelli D, Gaspari L, Pedotti P, Taioli E. Mini-review of studies on the effect of smoking and drinking habits on semen parameters. Int J Hyg Environ Health. 2004;207(3):185–92.
59. Ricci E, et al. Semen quality and alcohol intake: a systematic review and meta-analysis. Reprod Biomed Online. 2017;34(1):38–47.

60. Ramlau-Hansen C, et al. Maternal alcohol consumption during pregnancy and semen quality in the male offspring: two decades of follow-up. Hum Reprod. 2010;25(9):2340–5.
61. Hadi HA, Hill JA, Castillo RA. Alcohol and reproductive function: a review. Obstet Gynecol Surv. 1987;42(2):69–74.
62. Donnelly G, McClure N, Kennedy M, Lewis S. Direct effect of alcohol on the motility and morphology of human spermatozoa. Andrologia. 1999;31(1):43–7.
63. Pajarinen J, et al. Moderate alcohol consumption and disorders of human spermatogenesis. Alcohol Clin Exp Res. 1996;20(2):332–7.
64. Pajarinen J, Karhunen P. Spermatogenic arrest and 'Sertoli cell-only' syndrome—common alcohol-induced disorders of the human testis. Int J Androl. 1994;17(6):292–9.
65. Durairajanayagam D. Lifestyle causes of male infertility. Arab J Urol. 2018;16(1):10–20.
66. Jensen TK, et al. Caffeine intake and semen quality in a population of 2554 young Danish men. Am J Epidemiol. 2010;171(8):883–91.
67. Ricci E, et al. Coffee and caffeine intake and male infertility: a systematic review. Nutr J. 2017;16(1):1–14.
68. Belloc S, et al. Caffeine intake and sperm parameters. Analysis of a cohort of 4474 consecutive semen samples. Fertil Steril. 2013;100(3):S212.
69. Karmon AE, et al. Male caffeine and alcohol intake in relation to semen parameters and in vitro fertilization outcomes among fertility patients. Andrology. 2017;5(2):354–61.
70. Fronczak CM, Kim ED, Barqawi AB. The insults of illicit drug use on male fertility. J Androl. 2012;33(4):515–28.
71. Boyadjiev N, Georgieva K, Massaldjieva R, Gueorguiev S. Reversible hypogonadism and azoospermia as a result of anabolic-androgenic steroid use in a body builder with personality disorder: a case report. J Sports Med Phys Fitness. 2000;40(3):271.
72. Dohle G, Smit M, Weber R. Androgens and male fertility. World J Urol. 2003;21(5):341–5.
73. Kanayama G, Hudson JI, Pope HG Jr. Illicit anabolic–androgenic steroid use. Horm Behav. 2010;58(1):111–21.
74. de Souza GL, Hallak J. Anabolic steroids and male infertility: a comprehensive review. BJU Int. 2011;108(11):1860–5.
75. Di Marzo V. A brief history of cannabinoid and endocannabinoid pharmacology as inspired by the work of British scientists. Trends Pharmacol Sci. 2006;27(3):134–40.
76. Gundersen TD, et al. Association between use of marijuana and male reproductive hormones and semen quality: a study among 1,215 healthy young men. Am J Epidemiol. 2015;182(6):473–81.
77. Lewis MSE, et al. Long-term use of HU210 adversely affects spermatogenesis in rats by modulating the endocannabinoid system. Int J Androl. 2012;35(5):731–40.
78. Melzack R. The tragedy of needless pain. Sci Am. 1990;262(2):27–33.
79. Laxmaiah Manchikanti M, Bert Fellows M, Hary Ailinani M. Therapeutic use, abuse, and nonmedical use of opioids: a ten-year perspective. Pain Physician. 2010;13:401–35.
80. Agirregoitia E, et al. Expression and localization of δ-, κ-, and μ-opioid receptors in human spermatozoa and implications for sperm motility. J Clin Endocrinol Metabol. 2006;91(12):4969–75.
81. Kalra PS, Sahu A, Kalra SP. Opiate-induced hypersensitivity to testosterone feedback: pituitary involvement. Endocrinology. 1988;122(3):997–1003.
82. Safarinejad MR, et al. The effects of opiate consumption on serum reproductive hormone levels, sperm parameters, seminal plasma antioxidant capacity and sperm DNA integrity. Reprod Toxicol. 2013;36:18–23.
83. Bracken MB, et al. Association of cocaine use with sperm concentration, motility, and morphology. Fertil Steril. 1990;53(2):315–22.
84. Dickerson SM, et al. The recreational drug ecstasy disrupts the hypothalamic-pituitary-gonadal reproductive axis in adult male rats. Neuroendocrinology. 2008;88(2):95–102.
85. Nudmamud-Thanoi S, Thanoi S. Methamphetamine induces abnormal sperm morphology, low sperm concentration and apoptosis in the testis of male rats. Andrologia. 2011;43(4):278–82.

86. Di Luigi L, Romanelli F, Sgrò P, Lenzi A. Andrological aspects of physical exercise and sport medicine. Endocrine. 2012;42:278–84.
87. World Health Organization T. Global recommendations on physical activity for health. World Health Organization; 2010.
88. Jóźków P, Rossato M. The impact of intense exercise on semen quality. Am J Mens Health. 2017;11(3):654–62.
89. Safarinejad MR. Efficacy of coenzyme Q10 on semen parameters, sperm function and reproductive hormones in infertile men. J Urol. 2009;182(1):237–48.
90. Priskorn L, et al. Is sedentary lifestyle associated with testicular function? A cross-sectional study of 1210 men. Am J Epidemiol. 2016;184(4):284–94.
91. Grandys M, et al. Endurance training of moderate intensity increases testosterone concentration in young, healthy men. Int J Sports Med. 2009;30(7):489–95.
92. Matos B, Howl J, Ferreira R, Fardilha M. Exploring the effect of exercise training on testicular function. Eur J Appl Physiol. 2019;119:1–8.
93. Samadian Z, et al. Moderate-intensity exercise training ameliorates the diabetes-suppressed spermatogenesis and improves sperm parameters: Insole and simultaneous with insulin. Andrologia. 2019;51(11):e13457.
94. Dominguez JM 2nd, et al. Aging and exercise training reduce testes microvascular PO_2 and alter vasoconstrictor responsiveness in testicular arterioles. Am J Phys Regul Integr Comp Phys. 2011;301(3):R801–10.
95. Manna I, Jana K, Samanta P. Effect of intensive exercise-induced testicular gametogenic and steroidogenic disorders in mature male Wistar strain rats: a correlative approach to oxidative stress. Acta Physiol Scand. 2003;178(1):33–40.
96. Manna, I., K. Jana, P. Samanta, Effect of different intensities of swimming exercise on testicular oxidative stress and reproductive dysfunction in mature male albino Wistar rats; 2004.
97. Maleki BH, Tartibian B, Chehrazi M. The effects of three different exercise modalities on markers of male reproduction in healthy subjects: a randomized controlled trial. Reproduction. 2017;153(2):157–74.
98. Maleki BH, Tartibian B, Chehrazi M. Effects of aerobic, resistance, and combined exercise on markers of male reproduction in healthy human subjects: a randomized controlled trial. J Strength Cond Res. 2019;33(4):1130–45.
99. Hassani-Bafrani H, Najaran H, Razi M, Rashtbari H. Berberine ameliorates experimental varicocele-induced damages at testis and sperm levels; evidences for oxidative stress and inflammation. Andrologia. 2019;51(2):e13179.
100. Tsigos C, et al. Dose-dependent effects of recombinant human interleukin-6 on the pituitary-testicular axis. J Interferon Cytokine Res. 1999;19(11):1271–6.
101. Lister A, Van Der Kraak G. Modulation of goldfish testicular testosterone production in vitro by tumor necrosis factor α, interleukin-1β, and macrophage conditioned media. J Exp Zool. 2002;292(5):477–86.
102. Svechnikov KV, Sultana T, Söder O. Age-dependent stimulation of Leydig cell steroidogenesis by interleukin-1 isoforms. Mol Cell Endocrinol. 2001;182(2):193–201.
103. Bornstein S, Rutkowski H, Vrezas I. Cytokines and steroidogenesis. Mol Cell Endocrinol. 2004;215(1–2):135–41.
104. Agarwal A, et al. Effect of cell phone usage on semen analysis in men attending infertility clinic: an observational study. Fertil Steril. 2008;89(1).124–8.
105. Wdowiak A, Wdowiak L, Wiktor H. Evaluation of the effect of using mobile phones on male fertility. Ann Agric Environ Med. 2007;14(1):169–72.
106. Fejes I, et al. Is there a relationship between cell phone use and semen quality? Arch Androl. 2005;51(5):385–93.
107. Agarwal A, et al. Effects of radiofrequency electromagnetic waves (RF-EMW) from cellular phones on human ejaculated semen: an in vitro pilot study. Fertil Steril. 2009;92(4):1318–25.
108. Erogul O, et al. Effects of electromagnetic radiation from a cellular phone on human sperm motility: an in vitro study. Arch Med Res. 2006;37(7):840–3.

109. Dada R, Gupta NP, Kucheria K. Spermatogenic arrest in men with testicular hyperthermia. Teratog Carcinog Mutagen. 2003;23(S1):235–43.
110. Ahmad G, et al. Mild induced testicular and epididymal hyperthermia alters sperm chromatin integrity in men. Fertil Steril. 2012;97(3):546–53.
111. Sheynkin Y, Welliver R, Winer A, Hajimirzaee F, Ahn H, Lee K. Protection from scrotal hyperthermia in laptop computer users. Fertil Steril. 2010;95:647–51. https://doi.org/10.1016/j.fertnstert.2010.10.013.
112. Sheynkin Y, et al. Increase in scrotal temperature in laptop computer users. Hum Reprod. 2005;20(2):452–5.
113. Oni OM, Amuda DB, Gilbert CE. Effects of radiofrequency radiation from WiFi devices on human ejaculated semen. Int J Res Rev Appl Sci. 2011;9(2):292–4.
114. Kesari KK, Behari J. Microwave exposure affecting reproductive system in male rats. Appl Biochem Biotechnol. 2010;162(2):416–28.
115. Saygin M, et al. Testicular apoptosis and histopathological changes induced by a 2.45 GHz electromagnetic field. Toxicol Ind Health. 2011;27(5):455–63.
116. Kumar S, Kesari KK, Behari J. The therapeutic effect of a pulsed electromagnetic field on the reproductive patterns of male Wistar rats exposed to a 2.45-GHz microwave field. Clinics. 2011;66(7):1237–45.
117. Banks S, King SA, Irvine DS, Saunders PT. Impact of a mild scrotal heat stress on DNA integrity in murine spermatozoa. Reproduction. 2005;129(4):505–14.
118. Shiraishi K, Takihara H, Matsuyama H. Elevated scrotal temperature, but not varicocele grade, reflects testicular oxidative stress-mediated apoptosis. World J Urol. 2010;28(3):359–64.
119. Sergerie M, et al. High risk of temporary alteration of semen parameters after recent acute febrile illness. Fertil Steril. 2007;88(4):970. e1-970. e7
120. Mieusset R, et al. Association of scrotal hyperthermia with impaired spermatogenesis in infertile men. Fertil Steril. 1987;48(6):1006–11.
121. Wang C, et al. Effect of increased scrotal temperature on sperm production in normal men. Fertil Steril. 1997;68(2):334–9.
122. Lenzi A, et al. Stress, sexual dysfunctions, and male infertility. J Endocrinol Investig. 2003;26(Suppl. 3):72–6.
123. Li X, et al. Effects of acute restraint stress on sperm motility and secretion of pituitary, adrenocortical, and gonadal hormones in adult male rats. J Vet Med Sci. 2010;72(11):1501–6.
124. Jurewicz J, et al. Occupational, life stress and family functioning: does it affect semen quality? Ann Hum Biol. 2014;41(3):220–8.
125. Eskiocak S, et al. Glutathione and free sulphydryl content of seminal plasma in healthy medical students during and after exam stress. Hum Reprod. 2005;20(9):2595–600.
126. Eskiocak S, Gozen AS, Kilic AS, Molla S. Association between mental stress & some antioxidant enzymes of seminal plasma. Indian J Med Res. 2005;122(6):491.
127. Pook M, Krause W, Röhrle B. Coping with infertility: distress and changes in sperm quality. Hum Reprod. 1999;14(6):1487–92.
128. Clarke RN, Klock SC, Geoghegan A, Travassos DE. Relationship between psychological stress and semen quality among in-vitro fertilization patients. Hum Reprod. 1999;14(3):753–8.
129. Valko M, et al. Free radicals and antioxidants in normal physiological functions and human disease. Int J Biochem Cell Biol. 2007;39(1):44–84.
130. Shiva M, et al. Association between sperm quality, oxidative stress, and seminal antioxidant activity. Clin Biochem. 2011;44(4):319–24.
131. Khosrowbeygi A, Zarghami N, Deldar Y. Correlation between sperm quality parameters and seminal plasma antioxidants status. Iran J Reprod Med. 2012;2:58–64.
132. Agarwal A, Virk G, Ong C, du Plessis SS. Effect of oxidative stress on male reproduction. World J Mens Health. 2014;32(1):1–17.
133. Mishra S, et al. Mild oxidative stress is beneficial for sperm telomere length maintenance. World J Methodol. 2016;6(2):163–70.

134. Desai N, et al. Physiologic and pathologic levels of reactive oxygen species in neat semen of infertile men. Fertil Steril. 2009;92(5):1626–31.
135. Aitken RJ, et al. Sperm motility is lost in vitro as a consequence of mitochondrial free radical production and the generation of electrophilic aldehydes but can be significantly rescued by the presence of nucleophilic thiols. Biol Reprod. 2012;87(5):110.
136. Henkel RR. Leukocytes and oxidative stress: dilemma for sperm function and male fertility. Asian J Androl. 2011;13(1):43–52.
137. Evgeni E, Charalabopoulos K, Asimakopoulos B. Human sperm DNA fragmentation and its correlation with conventional semen parameters. J Reprod Infertil. 2014;15(1):2–14.
138. Combelles CM, Gupta S, Agarwal A. Could oxidative stress influence the in-vitro maturation of oocytes? Reprod Biomed Online. 2009;18(6):864–80.
139. Gupta PC, Ray CS. Epidemiology of betel quid usage. Ann Acad Med Singap. 2004;33(Suppl. 4):31–6.
140. Kumar S, Murarka S, Mishra VV, Gautam AK. Environmental & lifestyle factors in deterioration of male reproductive health. Indian J Med Res. 2014;140(Suppl. 1):S29–35.
141. Sharma RK, Agarwal A. Role of reactive oxygen species in male infertility. Urology. 1996;48(6):835–50.
142. Alvarez JG, Storey BT. Differential incorporation of fatty acids into and peroxidative loss of fatty acids from phospholipids of human spermatozoa. Mol Reprod Dev. 1995;42(3):334–46.
143. Wang X, et al. Alterations in mitochondria membrane potential and oxidative stress in infertile men: a prospective observational study. Fertil Steril. 2003;80(Suppl. 2):844–50.
144. Kodama H, et al. Increased oxidative deoxyribonucleic acid damage in the spermatozoa of infertile male patients. Fertil Steril. 1997;68(3):519–24.
145. Aitken RJ, Clarkson JS. Cellular basis of defective sperm function and its association with the genesis of reactive oxygen species by human spermatozoa. J Reprod Fertil. 1987;81(2):459–69.
146. Engel S, Schreiner T, Petzoldt R. Lipid peroxidation in human spermatozoa and maintenance of progressive sperm motility. Andrologia. 1999;31(1):17–22.
147. Blumer CG, et al. Sperm nuclear DNA fragmentation and mitochondrial activity in men with varicocele. Fertil Steril. 2008;90(5):1716–22.
148. Agarwal A, Saleh RA, Bedaiwy MA. Role of reactive oxygen species in the pathophysiology of human reproduction. Fertil Steril. 2003;79(4):829–43.
149. Turner RM. Tales from the tail: what do we really know about sperm motility? J Androl. 2003;24(6):790–803.
150. Bourgeron T. Mitochondrial function and male infertility. Results Probl Cell Differ. 2000;28:187–210.
151. Oliva A, Spira A, Multigner L. Contribution of environmental factors to the risk of male infertility. Hum Reprod. 2001;16(8):1768–76.
152. Working PK. Mechanistic approaches in the study of testicular toxicity: agents that directly affect the testis. Toxicol Pathol. 1989;17(2):452–6.
153. Kantapan J, et al. Pentagalloyl glucose- and ethyl Gallate-rich extract from Maprang seeds induce apoptosis in MCF-7 breast cancer cells through mitochondria-mediated pathway. Evid Based Complement Alternat Med. 2020;2020:5686029.
154. Huang G, Yuan M, Zhang J, Li J, Gong D, Li Y, Zhang J, Lin P, Huang L. IL-6 mediates differentiation disorder during spermatogenesis in obesity-associated inflammation by affecting the expression of Zfp637 through the SOCS3/STAT3 pathway. Sci Rep. 2016;6:28012. https://doi.org/10.1038/srep28012. PMID: 27329259; PMCID: PMC4916425.
155. Tolouei Azar J, Habibi Maleki A, Moshari S, Razi M. The effect of different types of exercise training on diet-induced obesity in rats, cross-talk between cell cycle proteins and apoptosis in testis. Gene. 2020;754:144850.
156. Soudmand P, et al. Different continuous exercise training intensities induced effect on sertoli-germ cells metabolic interaction; implication on GLUT-1, GLUT-3 and MCT-4 transporting proteins expression level. Gene. 2021;783:145553.

157. Bahadorani M, et al. Effects of branched-chain amino acid supplementation and/or aerobic exercise on mouse sperm quality and testosterone production. Andrologia. 2019;51(2):e13183.
158. Samaneh F-D, Reza H, Mina S, Mahnaz K. A review on antidiabetic activity of centaurea spp.: a new approach for developing herbal remedies. J Evid Based Complementary Altern Med. 2021:1–23. https://doi.org/10.1155/2021/5587938.
159. Akbar Gharehbagh S, Tolouei Azar J, Razi M. ROS and metabolomics-mediated autophagy in rat's testicular tissue alter after exercise training; Evidence for exercise intensity and outcomes. Life Sci. 2021;277:119585.
160. Attaman JA, Toth TL, Furtado J, Campos H, Hauser R, Chavarro JE. Dietary fat and semen quality among men attending a fertility clinic. Hum Reprod. 2012;27(5):1466–74. https://doi.org/10.1093/humrep/des065. Epub 2012 Mar 13. PMID: 22416013; PMCID: PMC3329193.
161. Mendiola J, et al. A low intake of antioxidant nutrients is associated with poor semen quality in patients attending fertility clinics. Fertil Steril. 2010;93(4):1128–33.
162. Waud K, Bocca S. Role of vitamin D deficiency in male fertility. Fertil Steril. 2015;103:e39.
163. Mancini A, et al. Seminal antioxidants in humans: preoperative and postoperative evaluation of coenzyme Q10 in varicocele patients. Horm Metab Res. 2005;37(7):428–32.
164. Alleva R, et al. The protective role of ubiquinol-10 against formation of lipid hydroperoxides in human seminal fluid. Mol Asp Med. 1997;18:S221–8.
165. Balercia G, et al. Coenzyme Q10 levels in idiopathic and varicocele-associated asthenozoospermia. Andrologia. 2002;34(2):107–11.
166. Irvine DS, et al. DNA integrity in human spermatozoa: relationships with semen quality. J Androl. 2000;21(1):33–44.
167. Afiyani AA, et al. Evaluation of heat-shock protein A2 (HSPA2) in male rats before and after varicocele induction. Mol Reprod Dev. 2014;81(8):766–76.
168. Aeeni M, Razi M, Alizadeh A, Alizadeh A. The molecular mechanism behind insulin protective effects on testicular tissue of hyperglycemic rats. Life Sci. 2021;277:119394.
169. Harris HA, Bapat AR, Gonder DS, Frail DE. The ligand binding profiles of estrogen receptors alpha and beta are species dependent. Steroids. 2002;67(5):379–84.
170. Thomas P, Dong J. Binding and activation of the seven-transmembrane estrogen receptor GPR30 by environmental estrogens: a potential novel mechanism of endocrine disruption. J Steroid Biochem Mol Biol. 2006;102(1–5):175–9.
171. Adeoya-Osiguwa SA, et al. 17β-Estradiol and environmental estrogens significantly affect mammalian sperm function. Hum Reprod. 2003;18(1):100–7.
172. Vujkovic M, et al. Associations between dietary patterns and semen quality in men undergoing IVF/ICSI treatment. Hum Reprod. 2009;24(6):1304–12.
173. Jurewicz J, et al. Dietary patterns and their relationship with semen quality. Am J Mens Health. 2018;12(3):575–83.
174. Afeiche MC, et al. Processed meat intake is unfavorably and fish intake favorably associated with semen quality indicators among men attending a fertility clinic. J Nutr. 2014;144(7):1091–8.
175. Balercia G, et al. Coenzyme Q(10) supplementation in infertile men with idiopathic asthenozoospermia: an open, uncontrolled pilot study. Fertil Steril. 2004;81(1):93–8.
176. Prentki Santos E, et al. Impact of spontaneous smoking cessation on sperm quality: case report. Andrologia. 2011;43(6):431–5.
177. Koch LG, Britton SL. Development of animal models to test the fundamental basis of gene-environment interactions. Obesity (Silver Spring). 2008;16(Suppl 3):S28–32.
178. Odet F, et al. Expression of the gene for mouse lactate dehydrogenase C (Ldhc) is required for male fertility. Biol Reprod. 2008;79(1):26–34.
179. Torma F, et al. Exercise increases markers of spermatogenesis in rats selectively bred for low running capacity. PLoS One. 2014;9(12):e114075.

Chapter 4
Impact of Testicular Cancer on Male Fertility

Fotios Dimitriadis

Key Points

- Patients presented with testicular cancer have altered semen parameters before orchidectomy and before other antineoplastic treatments due to cancer-related causes including intrinsic testicular damage, systemic effects, endocrine disruption, possible autoimmune effects, and possible congenital abnormalities in the maturation of the testis.
- Orchidectomy and further antineoplastic treatment including radiation therapy and chemotherapy increase oxidative stress and DNA fragmentation and affect sperm parameters and sexual function.
- Sperm cryopreservation is the mainstay of the fertility potential preservation in testicular cancer patients and should be strongly advised to all patients in reproductive age and their families before treatment.
- The potential recovery from the effects of chemotherapy is about 1–4 years after treatment, whereas the effect of radiation therapy is dose dependent.
- Testicular cancer survivors have lower 10-year paternity rate in comparison to the general population, but the majority of them will have their own biological children without medical assistance.

Introduction

Testicular cancer (TC) is relatively uncommon as it represents 1% of adult neoplasms and 5% of urological tumors [1]. However, TC is the most common solid tumor among males 20–34 years of age [2]. Over the past several decades, its incidence has increased and continues to rise, particularly in industrialized countries [3, 4] for unclear reasons. Importantly, the current diagnostic and therapeutic strategies offer to TC patients a 5-year relative survival rate more than 95% [5].

Testicular cancer alone may affect fertility, which is a severe consequence considering that TC patients usually have unfinished family plans, particularly in industrialized countries. Djaladat et al. in a systematic review investigated the association

F. Dimitriadis (✉)
Department of Urology, Aristotle University, Thessaloniki, Greece

A. Agarwal et al. (eds.), *Current and Future Advances in Male Infertility*,
https://doi.org/10.1007/978-3-031-62648-7_4

between TC and semen abnormalities before orchidectomy and found that up to 50% of patients with TC have already semen abnormalities during the diagnosis of the disease [6]. Moreover, the surgical treatment of TC per se as well as the collateral effects of chemotherapy and radiation therapy also carry significant risks of future fertilizing potential. In addition, retroperitoneal lymph node dissection (RPLND), whenever needs to be included in the therapeutic strategy, may also have fertility-related consequences due to retrograde ejaculation or anejaculation, although recent advances in surgical techniques have significantly reduced this risk [7]. Among TC survivors, the percentage that successfully has children after the treatment of cancer ranges between 48% and 92%, often with the aid of assisted reproductive techniques (ARTs) [8]. Therefore, sperm banking should be offered to these patients and to their families early in the course of treatment [9] although recent evidence shows that this recommendation is often not followed due to private practice settings and lack of multidisciplinary team planning among other reasons [10]. Male infertility as a consequence of TC has likely multifactorial etiology [11, 12]. In this chapter, we provide a comprehensive review of the relationship of TC cancer and male infertility.

Mechanisms of Infertility in TC

Direct Parenchymal Damage and Replacement by the Tumor

It is well documented that some men present with TC already have poor semen quality and diminished fertility before any treatment related to their disease [13–15]. This leads to the conclusion that the presence of tumor interferes with spermatogenesis. The impaired spermatogenesis at regions adjacent to the tumor could be explained by direct parenchymal damage due to tumor compression of seminiferous tubules or by direct invasion of tubules. Another direct mechanism could be the presence of paracrine and autocrine factors produced by the tumor [16]. The type of TC concerning the local testicular damage might also be of importance as in cases of non-seminoma tumors, the semen quality of the patients is more severely affected [17]. Although spermatogenesis is more pronounced adjacent to the tumor, this impairment extends over much of the testicular parenchyma in regions distant from the tumor and often appears as areas of tubules with depressed spermatogenesis in otherwise relatively normal tissue, particularly in men with embryonal carcinoma [17, 18]. In these cases, the impairment may result from the production of tumor-related factors such as alpha-fetoprotein (AFP) [18] and/or from an immune response to tumor mediated by cytokines, such as tumor necrosis factor and interleukin-1 [18]. In addition, tumor production of human chorionic gonadotrophin (hCG) is related to diminished fertility in men with TC [19, 20]. The biological action of hCG is very similar to the action of luteinizing hormone (LH); thus, the elevated intratesticular levels of hCG may influence the secretory function of Leydig cells and ultimately disturb the local spermatogenesis.

Correlative Etiologies

Cryptorchidism

Cryptorchidism occurs worldwide in a range between 1% and 4% of full-term newborn boys [21], whereas in prematurely born males, it is much more common, occurring in up to 45% of them [22]. Cryptorchidism is a well-established risk factor for both testicular neoplasms and infertility, although the mechanisms behind these pathologies are not fully elucidated yet [23]. About 10% of the males with infertility problems have also a history of cryptorchidism [24]. The increased temperature in the cryptorchid testis may lead to an aberrant transformation of neonatal germ cells, which may ultimately cause increased rates of both cancer and infertility [25]. Male germ cells, as progenitors of gametes, follow a long and complex journey towards the haploid male gamete able to fertilize the oocyte. The complexity of this journey and the unique characteristics that neonatal germ cells possess make them very vulnerable to environmental factors such as heat stress under the state of cryptorchidism, and failure in any stage may lead to infertility, malignancy, or both. A crucial factor for the future fertility of the male is the hormonal surge of mini puberty. In the cryptorchid testis, this process is largely deranged, and consequently, there is a disturbed transforming gonocyte leading to a lack of Ad spermatogonia [26]. Therefore, males with undescended testes are reported to have deficient spermatogonia stem cells, lower sperm concentrations, and decreased paternal rates [27–29].

Testicular Dysgenesis Syndrome

Skakkebaek in 1993 proposed the term "testicular dysgenesis syndrome" (TDS) as a condition than includes low-quality sperm, undescended testes, hypospadias, abnormal testicular differentiation, and finally TC. In their study, they hypothesized that increased estrogen exposure in utero, mainly diethylstilbestrol (DES), a powerful synthetic estrogen, could be the cause of all these aberrations presented in the male embryos [30]. Furthermore, biopsy material from the contralateral "healthy" testis has revealed that 24% of the patients presenting with unilateral TC have also irreversibly impaired spermatogenesis in the contralateral testis [19]. Thus, according to the TDS theory, TC and male infertility are some of the symptoms [31, 32] of an external independent factor and not the direct cause of TC to male infertility or vice versa. Further histological studies have confirmed the presence of dysgenetic features, including poorly differentiated spermatic tubules with immature Sertoli cells or hyaline bodies and often TC [31–33]. Since then, a growing list of endocrine disruptors including chemical and xenoestrogen products has been shown to exert an antiandrogenic action and increased estrogen levels in the male embryo with subsequent inhibition of the hypothalamus-pituitary-gonadal (HPG) axis. Disturbance of the HPG results in decreased secretion of follicle-stimulating hormone (FSH) with detrimental effects on the amount of Sertoli cells between the fetal phase and prepubertal phase [34]. However, at this point, it is important to underline that not all cases of male infertility and TC are part of TDS; only cases associated with poor fetal testicular development can be regarded as part of this syndrome [32, 35].

Causative Mechanisms

Endocrine Disruption and Hypogonadism

Review and meta-analytic studies report an increased risk of testosterone deficiency (TD) following treatment for TC [36, 37]. On the other hand, there is evidence suggesting that testosterone (T) production is already declined before TC diagnosis and TDS might be one of the factors that explain this finding [31]. However, alterations because of TDS might be limited according to Bandak et al. [38] who found no significant differences in LH and T levels between healthy men and hCG-negative patients with unilateral stage I TC before orchidectomy. The same author, however, reported a significant increase in LH level 1 year after orchidectomy [38]. In addition, two small studies presented evidence that the TD preexists and is associated with testicular microlithiasis and testicular atrophy [39, 40], and thus the risk of TD in TC patients is not influenced by the treatment. The function of Leydig cells before any treatment for TC has scarcely been studied. Only limited studies have investigated pre-orchidectomy Leydig cell function in TC patients [38, 41]. Thus, it remains unclear whether preexisting Leydig cell dysfunction is more prevalent in patients with advanced stages of the disease.

Previous studies in Leydig cell tumors reported G-protein-coupled estrogen receptor signaling and estrogen-level disturbances [42, 43]. In fact, it has been demonstrated that the biochemical properties of human Leydig cell tumors involve the disruption of the estrogen signalization with canonical and noncanonical estrogen receptors and the altered expression of the peroxisome proliferator-activated receptor, a multi-level-acting lipid balance- and steroidogenesis-controlling protein [42, 43]. Moreover, light and transmission electron microscopy studies, western blotting, and immunohistochemical studies in samples of human Leydig cell tumors showed significantly enhanced expression of leptin, adiponectin, and their receptors, aromatase, phospholipase C, and kinases Raf, ERK which are part of adipokine transductional pathways [44]. Thus, it appears that estrogen level and signaling, together with lipid status and Leydig cell tumors, are related to each other, and increased aromatase activity leads to disturbed androgen/estrogen balance and infertility.

Primary testicular hypogonadism presents as a first sign, with elevated levels of LH in order to stimulate the secretory function of Leydig cells. Elevated LH levels indicate critical Leydig cell potential for proper function. If this stimulus is not enough, testosterone levels start to decline, and clinical symptoms of hypogonadism begin to appear including loss of libido, fatigue, osteoporosis, anemia, and metabolic syndrome [36]. In long term, deterioration of hypogonadism may appear in TC survivors. This could be explained by several contributing factors such as the status of having only one gonad, TDS, and aging [36]. In fact, among TC survivors, those who were older than 45 years corresponded to a 1.4-fold increase in odds ratio (OR) for hypogonadism [45]. All TC patients who are suspected to present early symptoms of hypogonadism need laboratory evaluation, including T, LH, and FSH measurements, in order to diagnose this condition as early as possible and stay in close follow-up. For the moment, there is a lack of consensus on the screening and follow-up plan that TC survivors with hypogonadism should follow. Limited data suggest, however, that the quality of life in these patients does not differ significantly between normo- and hypogonadal survivors [37].

Systemic Inflammation due to TC

Evidence suggests that infection and inflammation are relevant entities of male reproductive disorders that contribute significantly to male infertility [46]. Damage to the testis is associated with increased levels of leukocytic infiltration among edema formation, fibrosis, germ cell loss, and a relative hypoandrogenic status. Increased levels of reactive oxygen species (ROS) and pro-inflammatory cytokines and the subsequent increased oxidative stress are thought to elicit negative effects on spermatogenesis. These cytokines have physiological functions when present at lower levels and under physiologic conditions. Increased levels, however, as in the case of cancer are harmful to the endocrine and exocrine functions of the testis [47]. T cells represent the major component of inflammatory infiltrates associated with TC, and increased infiltration of immune cells into the testicular parenchyma with subsequent impairment in testicular functions is associated with cancer [48]. Moreover, there is also evidence that B cells are involved within infiltrates of testes present with seminoma [48]. Hasan et al. investigated the specific immune cell and cytokine characteristics of human testicular germ cell neoplasia and reported within germ cell neoplasia in situ (GCNIS) and seminoma, the presence of T cells and dendritic cells. They also found B cells organized in cell clusters, whereas they could not detect any mast cells [48]. Importantly, they also noticed that in testicular samples of germ cell neoplasia, there was the presence of a pro-tumorigenic environment composed of increased levels of transcripts encoding pro-inflammatory cytokines (IL-1β, IL-6, and TNF-α), anti-inflammatory cytokines (TGF-β1), Th1-driven cytokines (IL-2 and IFN-γ), as well as chemokines (CXCL-13, CXCL-10, and CCL-5) [48]. On the contrary, testicular samples with normal spermatogenesis or hypospermatogenesis were characterized by the presence of Th2-related cytokines including IL-5, IL-13, and IL-23a [48]. They highlighted the crucial role of

IL-6 in TC as a potential novel diagnostic and/or immune therapeutic tool in the perspective of TC [48]. Finally, elevated temperature caused by fever associated with metastatic malignancy or chemotherapy also represents a direct threat to spermatogenesis [49].

Antisperm Antibodies

The testis is considered an immune-privileged organ because it does not elicit any inflammatory immune response after the introduction of sperm autoantigens at the onset of puberty [50]. This physiological but "bizarre" immune behavior is crucial for the maintenance of normal spermatogenesis of the male throughout his entire life and is based fundamentally on the formation of the blood-testis barrier (BTB) between adjacent Sertoli cells. BTB among the other complex physiologic actions also possesses the ability to seclude most of the developing germ cells from the interstitial compartment and thus from the introduction to the leukocytes [46, 50]. Regulatory T cells (also called Tregs) play a pivotal role in regulating or suppressing other cells in the immune system, and they are crucial for preventing organ-specific autoimmunity [51]. Sertoli cells and BTB prevent the transcellular leakage of antigens via transcytosis into the interstitial space where antigen-presenting cells (dendritic cells, macrophages) reside, and thus, Sertoli cells help to maintain Treg tolerance to meiotic antigens. Reduction of the Treg contributes to autoimmune orchitis underlining the importance of the Sertoli cell-macrophage-Treg axis in maintaining immune privilege [52]. It is believed that testicular tumors disrupt the BTB followed by the formation of antisperm antibodies and long lymphocytic infiltrates into the parenchyma adjacent to tumor germ cells. This could have a negative impact on spermatogenesis as antisperm antibodies are linked with decreased count and motility and increased morphological anomalies of the sperm [13].

Elevated DNA Fragmentation

Prior to the Treatment with Chemotherapy and/or Radiation Therapy

In 1984, Evenson et al. using flow cytometric analyses were the first to show that sperm chromatin condensation in patients with TC was abnormal after orchidectomy and before any antineoplastic treatment [53]. They also demonstrated that these abnormalities in sperm chromatin condensation can last up to 1 year post-orchidectomy [53]. This finding has been later confirmed by similar studies by Fossa et al. who demonstrated a significant increase in the percentage of non-condensed haploid sperm cells in patients presented with TC after orchidectomy and before any other antineoplastic treatment in comparison with healthy donors [54]. In the following decades, the methods to study chromatin integrity have greatly evolved, and thus the interest in sperm DNA damage has increased, especially in TC patients.

The sperm chromatin structure assay (SCSA) is a reliable flow cytometric test where sperm DNA breaks can be evaluated indirectly through DNA denaturability revealing possible strand breaks or protamine-histone replacement defects [55]. Most studies using SCSA found increased, but moderate, levels of sperm DNA damage in TC patients compared to healthy controls [56–59]. However, in comparison with infertile patients without TC, TC patients may have comparable levels of chromatin damage. This finding supports the hypothesis that TC affects semen quality only temporarily [56].

The alkaline Comet assay and terminal deoxynucleotidyl transferase (TdT) dUTP nick-end labeling (TUNEL) assay are also reliable and widely used methods to identify double- and single-strand DNA breaks [55, 60]. TUNEL studies investigating the sperm of TC patients found increased levels of sperm DNA fragmentation, suggesting disturbed apoptotic control equilibrium due to TC [57, 59, 61]. Corroborating to these findings, studies employing Comet assay also found more sperm damage, in patients with TC than in controls [60, 62, 63].

Posttreatment with Radiation Therapy and/or Chemotherapy

Radiation therapy and chemotherapy are important causes of iatrogenic sperm DNA damage [64] with a major damaging effect on reproductive function through both cytological and molecular effects. The deleterious effects can last up to 18–24 months after the end of the therapy or even permanently and include oligozoospermia or azoospermia [65] and increased rates of aneuploidies [66, 67].

The testicles are one of the most radiosensitive tissues, and they are especially vulnerable to damage from direct radiation [68]. Sperm DNA is particularly sensitive to radiation therapy, and radiotoxicity may induce permanent damage according to the dose (see later in this chapter) or transient damage from 6 months after the end of the treatment but normalizes within 2–5 years [56]. The ionization effect on the organ can be direct through the excitation of the atoms making up the DNA molecule or indirect through its interaction with non-DNA molecules, which induce the ionization of the genetic material through the emission of secondary electrons [69].

Chemotherapeutic agents, on the other hand, have a different mechanism of action, and their gonadotoxic effect is less clear-cut than that of radiation therapy. Chemotherapeutic drugs can penetrate the BTB and damage germ cells, particularly the actively proliferating type B spermatogonia, which are for this reason extremely susceptible to cytotoxic agents [56]. Type A spermatogonia are mitotically less active and, for this reason, less affected and could survive the treatment up to a threshold of cumulative cytostatic doses [70]. The negative effect of chemotherapy on sperm chromatin can last up to 2 years after the end of the therapy. Importantly different chemotherapeutic drugs modify various components of the chromatin structure, affecting this way not only fragmentation but also chromatin compaction [71]. Therefore, it may take different times to be repaired after chemotherapy, and the extent of sperm DNA impairment may also differ. At this point, it should be emphasized that the studies investigating pre- and post-therapy chromatin integrity are mostly small caseloads and highly heterogeneous regarding the methodology used. Importantly, the degree of sperm chromatin damage does not appear to be correlated with the patient's age or the histology of the TC but with the advanced stages of TC as well as with the type and intensity of treatment. This is also another factor that can explain the divergent results on the impact of chemotherapy on sperm DNA integrity among the studies so far.

Relationship of Testicular Cancer Treatment and Infertility

Orchidectomy/RPLND and Fertility

The mainstay of treatment for a suspected TC is radical inguinal orchidectomy. This therapeutical approach is mandatory but often does not come without a cost in terms of fertility. Several studies have shown that radical unilateral orchidectomy has a detrimental impact on semen parameters and endocrinologic profile [16, 72, 73]. Petersen et al. demonstrated that patients that underwent radical unilateral orchidectomy for TC presented low sperm concentration, total sperm count, and serum inhibin B levels, increased LH and FSH, but unchanged serum testosterone levels [16]. In addition, they noticed that although the contralateral testis was apparently normal, 85% of patients had impaired semen parameters and 9% of them ultimately developed azoospermia after unilateral orchidectomy [16]. In another small caseload study, Andrade et al. investigated the sperm parameters (ejaculated volume, sperm concentration, motility, and morphology) in patients before and after orchidectomy, and they reported a significant decrease in all parameters [74]. In this context and considering that many of these patients are still in reproductive age, it is mandatory to preserve their fertility potential and thus their chance to future parenthood even through ARTs [74, 75]. Sperm cryopreservation before or after orchidectomy and prior to any other antineoplastic treatment is a valid and recommended option [76, 77]. In patients with severe oligozoospermia or cryptozoospermia, intraoperative testicular sperm extraction (once-TESE) from the same and the contralateral testis should be advised and attempted in specialized centers [77, 78].

Given the potential consequences of radical orchidectomy, the concept of testis-sparing surgery (TSS) has gained increasing interest. According to the European guidelines, TSS is a valid treatment option as it may prevent the sequela of orchidectomy such as hypogonadism, lifelong testosterone supplementation, and infertility in young men. This procedure is feasible in synchronous bilateral tumors, in tumors in solitary testis [79], or in cases of small or indeterminate testicular masses with normal contralateral testis and negative tumor markers preserving this way the testicular function and avoiding overtreatment of potentially benign lesions [79, 80]. Importantly, in these cases, the surgeon needs to be experienced with careful adherence to oncologically sound principles and close follow-up of the patient.

Finally, in cases of contralateral testicular volume <12 mL, and/or a history of cryptorchidism, it is strongly recommended to collect at least two additional testicular biopsies from the contralateral testis to exclude germ cell neoplasia in situ (GCNIS) [81]. In any case, during the enucleation of the lesion, frozen section examination (FSE) should also be offered as it has shown to be reliable and highly accordant with the final histopathologic result [80, 82].

Following radical inguinal orchidectomy, retroperitoneal lymph node dissection (RPLND) represents a valid option in cases of stage I non-seminomatous germ cell tumors alternatively to active surveillance and chemotherapy. Likewise, RPLND can be performed in residual masses (>1 cm) after chemotherapy in patients with stage II (or higher) non-seminomatous germ cell tumors and finally for only selected cases of seminomatous tumors [83]. However, sexual dysfunction after this treatment is very common. Capogrosso et al. investigated the erectile dysfunction in patients treated with orchidectomy for TC and receiving adjuvant antineoplastic treatment plus RPLND or RPLND alone [84]. The mean follow-up lasted for 86 months, and they reported that 25.5% of patients experienced erectile dysfunction (ED) of any grade, and the median time to erectile function recovery was 70 months after RPLND [84]. In another study, full bilateral non-nerve-sparing post-chemotherapy RPLND resulted in dry orgasms after surgery and significantly impaired orgasmic function and intercourse and overall sexual satisfaction after the operation. However, no significant difference was noticed in erectile function before and after the operation [85]. In order to minimize the consequences of primary RPLND, the nerve-sparing RPLND and minimally invasive (laparoscopic or robot-assisted) approaches have been introduced. Both are feasible but with higher recurrence and complication rates in comparison with the non-nerve-sparing RPLND [86, 87] and thus are recommended only in highly specialized and high-volume RPLND centers [88–90].

Chemotherapy and Fertility

The gonadotoxic effects of chemotherapy have been well-recognized [91]. However, the effect of the various chemotherapeutic approaches on fertility in men presenting with TC is not completely enlightened. The fate of fertility after chemotherapy for TC largely depends on the gonadal function prior to the treatment, the age of the patient, and the type/cycles of the therapy [92]. Late-stage germ cells are less rapidly dividing and thus less sensitive to cytotoxic treatment than the rapidly dividing early-stage germ cells. So, it may take weeks until an effect on spermatogenesis is observable in semen analysis. The most frequent chemotherapeutic approach applied in patients with TC includes bleomycin, etoposide, and cisplatin (BEP) [93].

Platinum-based chemotherapy agents form DNA cross-linking and pose an intermediate level of risk for persistent azoospermia. It has been shown that TC patients with normal pretreatment sperm concentration, when treated with platinum-based chemotherapy, presented a rapid decrease in sperm concentration, and the recovery period was 48% at the end of the second year of follow-up and 80% after the fifth year [94]. Moreover, patients exposed to carboplatin had a better recovery rate in comparison with the patients treated with cisplatin [94].

Alkylating agents such as cyclophosphamide and ifosfamide disrupt the DNA synthesis and RNA transcription in cancer cells and have the highest risk for persistent azoospermia. The most vulnerable germ cells are the rapidly dividing spermatocytes [95], and permanent azoospermia appears in up to 25% of men 5 years after the treatment with these agents [96].

Vinca alkaloids inhibit the microtubule formation in the dividing cell and subsequently lead to disruption of mitosis and thus usually result in temporary oligo- or azoospermia [97]. However, when administrated together with alkylating agents or platinum analogs, the effect on spermatogenesis is more permanent [97]. The number of cycles of chemotherapies is important regarding fertility. Patients who received three or four courses of BEP had a spermatogenesis recovery within 24 months [59].

Radiation Therapy and Fertility

Radiation therapy is commonly used in the treatment of TC or retroperitoneal metastases. The function of the testis is typically affected by radiation therapy in a dose-dependent fashion. The mechanism of action behind the damaging effect of radiation therapy in biological systems is based mainly upon the generation of ROS, the subsequent lipid peroxidation in the cellular membrane, and ultimately the induction of DNA damage in immature germ cells such as in primary spermatocytes, but it is still present in mature spermatozoa too [98]. Moreover, radiation therapy leads to increased apoptosis in the germinal epithelium [99]. In fact, experimental studies have shown that irradiation-mediated oxidative stress induces germ cell apoptosis [100–102], which depends on the activation of caspase-3 with increased expression of caspase-8 in adult rats [102] and decreased expression of caspase-9 in prepubertal mice [102].

In humans, radiation doses as low as 0.1 Gy have temporary effects on standard semen parameters (concentration and morphology) [103]. Greater radiation doses (>4 Gy) can cause irreversible damage to the germinal epithelium, and therefore in men with germ cell neoplasia in situ, radiation therapy with 16–20 Gy is commonly associated with permanent azoospermia. In comparison with the rapidly dividing germ cells, Leydig cells are more resistant to the damaging effect of radiation therapy. Doses over 20–30 Gy may impair Leydig cell secretory function and cause, for this reason, primary hypogonadism [104]. Even in these cases, the patients that ultimately need testosterone replacement therapy range from 15% to 25%. Therefore, all patients after radiation therapy have to be in close follow-up for adequate evaluation of their androgen levels [105]. Importantly, when designing the follow-up protocol, clinicians should be aware of the damaging effects of radiation therapy on fertility in order to avoid unnecessary ionizing radiation such as chest X-ray or computed tomography in reproductive-aged men.

Sexual Dysfunction in Survivors of TC

TC survivors are more likely to experience ED, decreased libido, and poor body image in comparison with men of the general population [106]. Although psychogenic causes represent a primary etiologic factor [107], the whole pathogenesis of sexual dysfunction in these patients is likely multifactorial. The incidence of ED in TC survivors ranges from 12% to 40%, and it is not related to the treatment protocol of TC [106], whereas according to Pühse et al., 42% of them have decreased sexual activity, and 35% of them report decreased libido [108]. In addition, data from a systematic review indicate that RPLND is definitely related to ejaculatory complaints [109], while others report that 85% of TC survivors present retrograde ejaculation, anejaculation, and premature ejaculation, and 95% of them report decreased overall sexual satisfaction [108]. However, long-lasting sexual problems after therapy for TC are present in approximately 20% of patients undergoing treatment for TC [110]. Importantly, during the follow-up protocol, clinicians should investigate the sexual function of TC survivors in order to promptly diagnose any complain and address the symptoms with appropriate therapies.

Contraception During Treatment: Paternity After Treatment

Men under chemotherapy for TC are uncertain and concerned about the chemotherapy-associated genome instability and the consequent repercussions for any offspring. Solid data and comprehensive guidelines on the risks of the various radio- and chemotherapy protocols to transmit a defective genome to their offspring are actually missing [111]. The grade of sperm aneuploidies, oxidative stress, and DNA fragmentation during radio- or chemotherapy is uncertain, but the effects generally persist for 3 months posttreatment [92]. The international literature offers extremely limited data on human spermatozoa, but there are extensive experimental genetic studies defining sensitivities for specific drugs and times. For example, it has been shown in rodents that alkylating agents carry higher risk of genetic damage as soon as 1 day after the start of the treatment [111]. On the other hand, nucleoside analogs and antimetabolites show a lower risk. Exposure of spermatids or spermatocytes to 5-fluorouracil may result in chromosomal aberrations in embryos, but there is no significant postimplantation loss [111]. Likewise, the effects of bleomycin on differentiating spermatogonia are related mainly with gene mutations rather than chromosomal mutations and are observable in spermatozoa 9 weeks after initiation of the treatment [111]. Radiation, when administrated in daily fraction to the tumor of 2 Gy or less, usually takes about a week to produce a high risk for the spermatozoa collected for pregnancy [111]. The potential recovery from the effects of chemotherapy is about 1–4 years posttreatment [59, 94, 112], whereas contraception must be used during treatment and for at least 6 months after its completion [113]. In their study, Bujan et al. reported elevated effects of radiation therapy on chromatin alterations at 6 months posttreatment [59]. They also reported an increased aneuploidy during the 17 months following treatment with BEP [59]. These findings are in line with the results of other studies, following the first 2 years posttreatment [114, 115].

TC survivors have a 30% lower 10-year paternity rate in comparison with the general population [116]. However, the majority of them will have their own biological children without medical assistance [116], while the rest of them have a significantly improved opportunity for paternity with the use of ART. In a cross-sectional study, paternity was achieved spontaneously in 77% of the cases or with the use of ART in 23% [117]. Finally, significant independent predictors for post-treatment paternity appear to be dry ejaculation, treatment received, pretreatment fatherhood, and marital status, with ejaculation disorders being the most important negative factor [116].

Summary

This chapter discusses the impact of testicular cancer and its treatment on male fertility, covering mechanisms such as direct testicular damage, endocrine disruption, and systemic inflammation. It emphasizes the importance of sperm cryopreservation for preserving fertility potential in patients of reproductive age. Additionally, the chapter addresses the influence of cancer treatments on fertility and sexual function, the need for contraception during treatment, and the potential for paternity after treatment.

References

1. Park JS, Kim J, Elghiaty A, Ham WS. Recent global trends in testicular cancer incidence and mortality. Medicine (Baltimore). 2018;97(37):e12390. https://doi.org/10.1097/MD.0000000000012390.
2. Gilligan T, Lin DW, Aggarwal R, Chism D, Cost N, Derweesh IH, et al. Testicular Cancer, Version 2.2020, NCCN Clinical Practice Guidelines in Oncology. J Natl Compr Cancer Netw. 2019;17(12):1529–54. https://doi.org/10.6004/jnccn.2019.0058.
3. Nigam M, Aschebrook-Kilfoy B, Shikanov S, Eggener S. Increasing incidence of testicular cancer in the United States and Europe between 1992 and 2009. World J Urol. 2015;33(5):623–31. https://doi.org/10.1007/s00345-014-1361-y.
4. Gurney JK, Florio AA, Znaor A, Ferlay J, Laversanne M, Sarfati D, et al. International trends in the incidence of testicular cancer: lessons from 35 years and 41 countries. Eur Urol. 2019;76(5):615–23. https://doi.org/10.1016/j.eururo.2019.07.002.

5. Travis LB, Beard C, Allan JM, Dahl AA, Feldman DR, Oldenburg J, et al. Testicular cancer survivorship: research strategies and recommendations. J Natl Cancer Inst. 2010;102(15):1114–30. https://doi.org/10.1093/jnci/djq216.
6. Djaladat H, Burner E, Parikh PM, Beroukhim Kay D, Hays K. The association between testis cancer and semen abnormalities before orchiectomy: a systematic review. J Adolesc Young Adult Oncol. 2014;3(4):153–9. https://doi.org/10.1089/jayao.2014.0012.
7. Ostrowski KA, Walsh TJ. Infertility with Testicular Cancer. Urol Clin North Am. 2015;42(3):409–20. https://doi.org/10.1016/j.ucl.2015.05.003.
8. Baird DC, Meyers GJ, Hu JS. Testicular cancer: diagnosis and treatment. Am Fam Physician. 2018;97(4):261–8.
9. Minhas S, Bettocchi C, Boeri L, Capogrosso P, Carvalho J, Cilesiz NC, et al. European Association of Urology Guidelines on Male Sexual and Reproductive Health: 2021 update on male infertility. Eur Urol. 2021;80(5):603–20. https://doi.org/10.1016/j.eururo.2021.08.014.
10. Patel P, Kohn TP, Cohen J, Shiff B, Kohn J, Ramasamy R. Evaluation of reported fertility preservation counseling before chemotherapy using the quality oncology practice initiative survey. JAMA Netw Open. 2020;3(7):e2010806. https://doi.org/10.1001/jamanetworkopen.2020.10806.
11. Girasole CR, Cookson MS, Smith JA Jr, Ivey BS, Roth BJ, Chang SS. Sperm banking: use and outcomes in patients treated for testicular cancer. BJU Int. 2007;99(1):33–6. https://doi.org/10.1111/j.1464-410X.2006.06537.x.
12. Sonnenburg DW, Brames MJ, Case-Eads S, Einhorn LH. Utilization of sperm banking and barriers to its use in testicular cancer patients. Support Care Cancer. 2015;23(9):2763–8. https://doi.org/10.1007/s00520-015-2641-9.
13. Ping P, Gu BH, Li P, Huang YR, Li Z. Fertility outcome of patients with testicular tumor: before and after treatment. Asian J Androl. 2014;16(1):107–11. https://doi.org/10.4103/1008-682X.122194.
14. Berthelsen JG. Sperm counts and serum follicle-stimulating hormone levels before and after radiotherapy and chemotherapy in men with testicular germ cell cancer. Fertil Steril. 1984;41(2):281–6. https://doi.org/10.1016/s0015-0282(16)47605-3.
15. Fossa SD, Abyholm T, Aakvaag A. Spermatogenesis and hormonal status after orchiectomy for cancer and before supplementary treatment. Eur Urol. 1984;10(3):173–7. https://doi.org/10.1159/000463782.
16. Petersen PM, Skakkebaek NE, Rorth M, Giwercman A. Semen quality and reproductive hormones before and after orchiectomy in men with testicular cancer. J Urol. 1999;161(3):822–6.
17. Fraietta R, Spaine DM, Bertolla RP, Ortiz V, Cedenho AP. Individual and seminal characteristics of patients with testicular germ cell tumors. Fertil Steril. 2010;94(6):2107–12. https://doi.org/10.1016/j.fertnstert.2009.12.021.
18. Ho GT, Gardner H, DeWolf WC, Loughlin KR, Morgentaler A. Influence of testicular carcinoma on ipsilateral spermatogenesis. J Urol. 1992;148(3):821–5. https://doi.org/10.1016/s0022-5347(17)36732-0.
19. Berthelsen JG, Skakkebaek NE. Gonadal function in men with testis cancer. Fertil Steril. 1983;39(1):68–75.
20. Tenhunen JD, Weber JA, Yocum CS, Gates DM. Solubility of gases and the temperature dependency of whole leaf affinities for carbon dioxide and oxygen: an alternative perspective. Plant Physiol. 1979;63(5):916–23. https://doi.org/10.1104/pp.63.5.916.
21. Goel P, Rawat JD, Wakhlu A, Kureel SN. Undescended testicle: an update on fertility in cryptorchid men. Indian J Med Res. 2015;141(2):163–71. https://doi.org/10.4103/0971-5916.155544.
22. Sijstermans K, Hack WW, Meijer RW, van der Voort-Doedens LM. The frequency of undescended testis from birth to adulthood: a review. Int J Androl. 2008;31(1):1–11. https://doi.org/10.1111/j.1365-2605.2007.00770.x.
23. Ferguson L, Agoulnik AI. Testicular cancer and cryptorchidism. Front Endocrinol (Lausanne). 2013;4:32. https://doi.org/10.3389/fendo.2013.00032.

24. Mieusset R, Bujan L, Massat G, Mansat A, Pontonnier F. Clinical and biological characteristics of infertile men with a history of cryptorchidism. Hum Reprod. 1995;10(3):613–9. https://doi.org/10.1093/oxfordjournals.humrep.a135998.
25. Hutson JM, Balic A, Nation T, Southwell B. Cryptorchidism. Semin Pediatr Surg. 2010;19(3):215–24. https://doi.org/10.1053/j.sempedsurg.2010.04.001.
26. Loebenstein M, Thorup J, Cortes D, Clasen-Linde E, Hutson JM, Li R. Cryptorchidism, gonocyte development, and the risks of germ cell malignancy and infertility: a systematic review. J Pediatr Surg. 2020;55(7):1201–10. https://doi.org/10.1016/j.jpedsurg.2019.06.023.
27. Lee PA, Coughlin MT. Fertility after bilateral cryptorchidism. Evaluation by paternity, hormone, and semen data. Horm Res. 2001;55(1):28–32. https://doi.org/10.1159/000049960.
28. van Brakel J, Kranse R, de Muinck Keizer-Schrama SM, Hendriks AE, de Jong FH, Bangma CH, et al. Fertility potential in men with a history of congenital undescended testes: a long-term follow-up study. Andrology. 2013;1(1):100–8. https://doi.org/10.1111/j.2047-2927.2012.00024.x.
29. Chung E, Brock GB. Cryptorchidism and its impact on male fertility: a state of art review of current literature. Can Urol Assoc J. 2011;5(3):210–4. https://doi.org/10.5489/cuaj.10106.
30. Sharpe RM, Skakkebaek NE. Are oestrogens involved in falling sperm counts and disorders of the male reproductive tract? Lancet. 1993;341(8857):1392–5. https://doi.org/10.1016/0140-6736(93)90953-e.
31. Skakkebaek NE, Rajpert-De Meyts E, Main KM. Testicular dysgenesis syndrome: an increasingly common developmental disorder with environmental aspects. Hum Reprod. 2001;16(5):972–8. https://doi.org/10.1093/humrep/16.5.972.
32. Skakkebaek NE, Rajpert-De Meyts E, Buck Louis GM, Toppari J, Andersson AM, Eisenberg ML, et al. Male Reproductive disorders and fertility trends: influences of environment and genetic susceptibility. Physiol Rev. 2016;96(1):55–97. https://doi.org/10.1152/physrev.00017.2015.
33. Jorgensen A, Lindhardt Johansen M, Juul A, Skakkebaek NE, Main KM, Rajpert-De ME. Pathogenesis of germ cell neoplasia in testicular dysgenesis and disorders of sex development. Semin Cell Dev Biol. 2015;45:124–37. https://doi.org/10.1016/j.semcdb.2015.09.013.
34. Burns WR, Sabanegh E, Dada R, Rein B, Agarwal A. Is male infertility a forerunner to cancer? Int Braz J Urol. 2010;36(5):527–36. https://doi.org/10.1590/s1677-55382010000500002.
35. Jorgensen N, Rajpert-De Meyts E, Main KM, Skakkebaek NE. Testicular dysgenesis syndrome comprises some but not all cases of hypospadias and impaired spermatogenesis. Int J Androl. 2010;33(2):298–303. https://doi.org/10.1111/j.1365-2605.2009.01050.x.
36. Oldenburg J. Hypogonadism and fertility issues following primary treatment for testicular cancer. Urol Oncol. 2015;33(9):407–12. https://doi.org/10.1016/j.urolonc.2015.01.014.
37. Bandak M, Jorgensen N, Juul A, Vogelius IR, Lauritsen J, Kier MG, et al. Testosterone deficiency in testicular cancer survivors—a systematic review and meta-analysis. Andrology. 2016;4(3):382–8. https://doi.org/10.1111/andr.12177.
38. Bandak M, Aksglaede L, Juul A, Rorth M, Daugaard G. The pituitary-Leydig cell axis before and after orchiectomy in patients with stage I testicular cancer. Eur J Cancer. 2011;47(17):2585–91. https://doi.org/10.1016/j.ejca.2011.05.026.
39. Puhse G, Secker A, Kemper S, Hertle L, Kliesch S. Testosterone deficiency in testicular germ-cell cancer patients is not influenced by oncological treatment. Int J Androl. 2011;34(5 Pt 2):e351–7. https://doi.org/10.1111/j.1365-2605.2010.01123.x.
40. Eberhard J, Stahl O, Cwikiel M, Cavallin-Stahl E, Giwercman Y, Salmonson EC, et al. Risk factors for post-treatment hypogonadism in testicular cancer patients. Eur J Endocrinol. 2008;158(4):561–70. https://doi.org/10.1530/EJE-07-0684.
41. Petersen PM, Skakkebaek NE, Vistisen K, Rorth M, Giwercman A. Semen quality and reproductive hormones before orchiectomy in men with testicular cancer. J Clin Oncol. 1999;17(3):941–7. https://doi.org/10.1200/JCO.1999.17.3.941.

42. Carpino A, Rago V, Pezzi V, Carani C, Ando S. Detection of aromatase and estrogen receptors (ERalpha, ERbeta1, ERbeta2) in human Leydig cell tumor. Eur J Endocrinol. 2007;157(2):239–44. https://doi.org/10.1530/EJE-07-0029.
43. Gorowska-Wojtowicz E, Duliban M, Kudrycka M, Dutka P, Pawlicki P, Milon A, et al. Leydig cell tumorigenesis—implication of G-protein coupled membrane estrogen receptor, peroxisome proliferator-activated receptor and xenoestrogen exposure. In vivo and in vitro appraisal. Tissue Cell. 2019;61:51–60. https://doi.org/10.1016/j.tice.2019.08.001.
44. Duliban M, Gorowska-Wojtowicz E, Tworzydlo W, Rak A, Brzoskwinia M, Krakowska I, et al. Interstitial Leydig cell tumorigenesis-leptin and adiponectin signaling in relation to aromatase expression in the human testis. Int J Mol Sci. 2020;21(10) https://doi.org/10.3390/ijms21103649.
45. Nord C, Bjoro T, Ellingsen D, Mykletun A, Dahl O, Klepp O, et al. Gonadal hormones in long-term survivors 10 years after treatment for unilateral testicular cancer. Eur Urol. 2003;44(3):322–8. https://doi.org/10.1016/s0302-2838(03)00263-x.
46. Fijak M, Pilatz A, Hedger MP, Nicolas N, Bhushan S, Michel V, et al. Infectious, inflammatory and 'autoimmune' male factor infertility: how do rodent models inform clinical practice? Hum Reprod Update. 2018;24(4):416–41. https://doi.org/10.1093/humupd/dmy009.
47. Hasan H, Bhushan S, Fijak M, Meinhardt A. Mechanism of inflammatory associated impairment of sperm function, spermatogenesis and steroidogenesis. Front Endocrinol (Lausanne). 2022;13:897029. https://doi.org/10.3389/fendo.2022.897029.
48. Klein B, Haggeney T, Fietz D, Indumathy S, Loveland KL, Hedger M, et al. Specific immune cell and cytokine characteristics of human testicular germ cell neoplasia. Hum Reprod. 2016;31(10):2192–202. https://doi.org/10.1093/humrep/dew211.
49. Jung A, Schuppe HC. Influence of genital heat stress on semen quality in humans. Andrologia. 2007;39(6):203–15. https://doi.org/10.1111/j.1439-0272.2007.00794.x.
50. Fijak M, Meinhardt A. The testis in immune privilege. Immunol Rev. 2006;213:66–81. https://doi.org/10.1111/j.1600-065X.2006.00438.x.
51. Sakaguchi S, Yamaguchi T, Nomura T, Ono M. Regulatory T cells and immune tolerance. Cell. 2008;133(5):775–87. https://doi.org/10.1016/j.cell.2008.05.009.
52. Tung KS, Harakal J, Qiao H, Rival C, Li JC, Paul AG, et al. Egress of sperm autoantigen from seminiferous tubules maintains systemic tolerance. J Clin Invest. 2017;127(3):1046–60. https://doi.org/10.1172/JCI89927.
53. Evenson DP, Klein FA, Whitmore WF, Melamed MR. Flow cytometric evaluation of sperm from patients with testicular carcinoma. J Urol. 1984;132(6):1220–5. https://doi.org/10.1016/s0022-5347(17)50109-3.
54. Fossa SD, Melvik JE, Juul NO, Pettersen EO, Theodorsen L. DNA flow cytometry in sperm cells from unilaterally orchiectomized patients with testicular cancer before further treatment. Cytometry. 1989;10(3):345–50. https://doi.org/10.1002/cyto.990100315.
55. Agarwal A, Said TM. Role of sperm chromatin abnormalities and DNA damage in male infertility. Hum Reprod Update. 2003;9(4):331–45. https://doi.org/10.1093/humupd/dmg027.
56. Paoli D, Pallotti F, Lenzi A, Lombardo F. Fatherhood and sperm DNA damage in testicular cancer patients. Front Endocrinol (Lausanne). 2018;9:506. https://doi.org/10.3389/fendo.2018.00506.
57. Stahl O, Eberhard J, Jepson K, Spano M, Cwikiel M, Cavallin-Stahl E, et al. Sperm DNA integrity in testicular cancer patients. Hum Reprod. 2006;21(12):3199–205. https://doi.org/10.1093/humrep/del292.
58. Stahl O, Eberhard J, Jepson K, Spano M, Cwikiel M, Cavallin-Stahl E, et al. The impact of testicular carcinoma and its treatment on sperm DNA integrity. Cancer. 2004;100(6):1137–44. https://doi.org/10.1002/cncr.20068.
59. Bujan L, Walschaerts M, Moinard N, Hennebicq S, Saias J, Brugnon F, et al. Impact of chemotherapy and radiotherapy for testicular germ cell tumors on spermatogenesis and sperm DNA: a multicenter prospective study from the CECOS network. Fertil Steril. 2013;100(3):673–80. https://doi.org/10.1016/j.fertnstert.2013.05.018.

60. Kumar K, Lewis S, Vinci S, Riera-Escamilla A, Fino MG, Tamburrino L, et al. Evaluation of sperm DNA quality in men presenting with testicular cancer and lymphoma using alkaline and neutral Comet assays. Andrology. 2018;6(1):230–5. https://doi.org/10.1111/andr.12429.
61. Gandini L, Lombardo F, Paoli D, Caponecchia L, Familiari G, Verlengia C, et al. Study of apoptotic DNA fragmentation in human spermatozoa. Hum Reprod. 2000;15(4):830–9. https://doi.org/10.1093/humrep/15.4.830.
62. O'Donovan M. An evaluation of chromatin condensation and DNA integrity in the spermatozoa of men with cancer before and after therapy. Andrologia. 2005;37(2–3):83–90. https://doi.org/10.1111/j.1439-0272.2005.00658.x.
63. O'Flaherty C, Vaisheva F, Hales BF, Chan P, Robaire B. Characterization of sperm chromatin quality in testicular cancer and Hodgkin's lymphoma patients prior to chemotherapy. Hum Reprod. 2008;23(5):1044–52. https://doi.org/10.1093/humrep/den081.
64. O'Flaherty C. Iatrogenic genetic damage of spermatozoa. Adv Exp Med Biol. 2014;791:117–35. https://doi.org/10.1007/978-1-4614-7783-9_8.
65. Trost LW, Brannigan RE. Oncofertility and the male cancer patient. Curr Treat Options in Oncol. 2012;13(2):146–60. https://doi.org/10.1007/s11864-012-0191-7.
66. Martin RH, Ernst S, Rademaker A, Barclay L, Ko E, Summers N. Analysis of sperm chromosome complements before, during, and after chemotherapy. Cancer Genet Cytogenet. 1999;108(2):133–6. https://doi.org/10.1016/s0165-4608(98)00125-3.
67. De Mas P, Daudin M, Vincent MC, Bourrouillou G, Calvas P, Mieusset R, et al. Increased aneuploidy in spermatozoa from testicular tumour patients after chemotherapy with cisplatin, etoposide and bleomycin. Hum Reprod. 2001;16(6):1204–8. https://doi.org/10.1093/humrep/16.6.1204.
68. Bieri S, Rouzaud M, Miralbell R. Seminoma of the testis: is scrotal shielding necessary when radiotherapy is limited to the para-aortic nodes? Radiother Oncol. 1999;50(3):349–53. https://doi.org/10.1016/s0167-8140(99)00023-7.
69. Gandini L, Sgro P, Lombardo F, Paoli D, Culasso F, Toselli L, et al. Effect of chemo- or radiotherapy on sperm parameters of testicular cancer patients. Hum Reprod. 2006;21(11):2882–9. https://doi.org/10.1093/humrep/del167.
70. Trottmann M, Becker AJ, Stadler T, Straub J, Soljanik I, Schlenker B, et al. Semen quality in men with malignant diseases before and after therapy and the role of cryopreservation. Eur Urol. 2007;52(2):355–67. https://doi.org/10.1016/j.eururo.2007.03.085.
71. O'Flaherty CM, Chan PT, Hales BF, Robaire B. Sperm chromatin structure components are differentially repaired in cancer survivors. J Androl. 2012;33(4):629–36. https://doi.org/10.2164/jandrol.111.015388.
72. Lin WW, Kim ED, Quesada ET, Lipshultz LI, Coburn M. Unilateral testicular injury from external trauma: evaluation of semen quality and endocrine parameters. J Urol. 1998;159(3):841–3. https://doi.org/10.1016/s0022-5347(01)63748-0.
73. Arap MA, Vicentini FC, Cocuzza M, Hallak J, Athayde K, Lucon AM, et al. Late hormonal levels, semen parameters, and presence of antisperm antibodies in patients treated for testicular torsion. J Androl. 2007;28(4):528–32. https://doi.org/10.2164/jandrol.106.002097.
74. Andrade MBR, Bertolla RP, Intasqui P, Antoniassi MP, Tibaldi DS, Belardin LB, et al. Effect of orchiectomy on sperm functional aspects and semen oxidative stress in men with testicular tumours. Andrologia. 2019;51(3):e13205. https://doi.org/10.1111/and.13205.
75. Lass A, Akagbosu F, Brinsden P. Sperm banking and assisted reproduction treatment for couples following cancer treatment of the male partner. Hum Reprod Update. 2001;7(4):370–7. https://doi.org/10.1093/humupd/7.4.370.
76. Hotaling JM, Patel DP, Vendryes C, Lopushnyan NA, Presson AP, Zhang C, et al. Predictors of sperm recovery after cryopreservation in testicular cancer. Asian J Androl. 2016;18(1):35–8. https://doi.org/10.4103/1008-682X.155535.
77. Nangia AK, Krieg SA, Kim SS. Clinical guidelines for sperm cryopreservation in cancer patients. Fertil Steril. 2013;100(5):1203–9. https://doi.org/10.1016/j.fertnstert.2013.08.054.

78. Schrader M, Muller M, Sofikitis N, Straub B, Krause H, Miller K. "Onco-tese": testicular sperm extraction in azoospermic cancer patients before chemotherapy-new guidelines? Urology. 2003;61(2):421–5. https://doi.org/10.1016/s0090-4295(02)02264-1.
79. Nason GJ, Aditya I, Leao R, Anson-Cartwright L, Jewett MAS, O'Malley M, et al. Partial orchiectomy: the Princess Margaret cancer centre experience. Urol Oncol. 2020;38(6):605:e19–24. https://doi.org/10.1016/j.urolonc.2020.03.012.
80. Fankhauser CD, Roth L, Kranzbuhler B, Eberli D, Bode P, Moch H, et al. The role of frozen section examination during inguinal exploration in men with inconclusive testicular tumors: a systematic review and meta-analysis. Eur Urol Focus. 2021;7(6):1400–2. https://doi.org/10.1016/j.euf.2020.06.019.
81. Dieckmann KP, Kulejewski M, Pichlmeier U, Loy V. Diagnosis of contralateral testicular intraepithelial neoplasia (TIN) in patients with testicular germ cell cancer: systematic two-site biopsies are more sensitive than a single random biopsy. Eur Urol. 2007;51(1):175–83.; discussion 83-5. https://doi.org/10.1016/j.eururo.2006.05.051.
82. Matei DV, Vartolomei MD, Renne G, Tringali VML, Russo A, Bianchi R, et al. Reliability of frozen section examination in a large cohort of testicular masses: what did we learn? Clin Genitourin Cancer. 2017;15(4):e689–e96. https://doi.org/10.1016/j.clgc.2017.01.012.
83. Heidenreich A, Paffenholz P, Nestler T, Pfister D. European Association of Urology Guidelines on Testis Cancer: important take home messages. Eur Urol Focus. 2019;5(5): 742–4. https://doi.org/10.1016/j.euf.2019.08.002.
84. Capogrosso P, Boeri L, Ferrari M, Ventimiglia E, La Croce G, Capitanio U, et al. Long-term recovery of normal sexual function in testicular cancer survivors. Asian J Androl. 2016;18(1):85–9. https://doi.org/10.4103/1008-682X.149180.
85. Dimitropoulos K, Karatzas A, Papandreou C, Daliani D, Zachos I, Pisters LL, et al. Sexual dysfunction in testicular cancer patients subjected to post-chemotherapy retroperitoneal lymph node dissection: a focus beyond ejaculation disorders. Andrologia. 2016;48(4):425–30. https://doi.org/10.1111/and.12462.
86. Heidenreich A, Albers P, Hartmann M, Kliesch S, Kohrmann KU, Krege S, et al. Complications of primary nerve sparing retroperitoneal lymph node dissection for clinical stage I nonseminomatous germ cell tumors of the testis: experience of the German Testicular Cancer Study Group. J Urol. 2003;169(5):1710–4. https://doi.org/10.1097/01.ju.0000060960.18092.54.
87. Albers P, Siener R, Krege S, Schmelz HU, Dieckmann KP, Heidenreich A, et al. Randomized phase III trial comparing retroperitoneal lymph node dissection with one course of bleomycin and etoposide plus cisplatin chemotherapy in the adjuvant treatment of clinical stage I Nonseminomatous testicular germ cell tumors: AUO trial AH 01/94 by the German Testicular Cancer Study Group. J Clin Oncol. 2008;26(18):2966–72. https://doi.org/10.1200/JCO.2007.12.0899.
88. Pearce SM, Golan S, Gorin MA, Luckenbaugh AN, Williams SB, Ward JF, et al. Safety and early oncologic effectiveness of primary robotic retroperitoneal lymph node dissection for nonseminomatous germ cell testicular cancer. Eur Urol. 2017;71(3):476–82. https://doi.org/10.1016/j.eururo.2016.05.017.
89. Rodrigues GJ, Guglielmetti GB, Orvieto M, Seetharam Bhat KR, Patel VR, Coelho RF. Robot-assisted retroperitoneal lymphadenectomy: the state of art. Asian J Urol. 2021;8(1):27–37. https://doi.org/10.1016/j.ajur.2020.09.002.
90. Calaway AC, Einhorn LH, Masterson TA, Foster RS, Cary C. Adverse surgical outcomes associated with robotic retroperitoneal lymph node dissection among patients with testicular cancer. Eur Urol. 2019;76(5):607–9. https://doi.org/10.1016/j.eururo.2019.05.031.
91. Ghafouri-Fard S, Shoorei H, Abak A, Seify M, Mohaqiq M, Keshmir F, et al. Effects of chemotherapeutic agents on male germ cells and possible ameliorating impact of antioxidants. Biomed Pharmacother. 2021;142:112040. https://doi.org/10.1016/j.biopha.2021.112040.
92. Lee SJ, Schover LR, Partridge AH, Patrizio P, Wallace WH, Hagerty K, et al. American Society of Clinical Oncology recommendations on fertility preservation in cancer patients. J Clin Oncol. 2006;24(18):2917–31. https://doi.org/10.1200/JCO.2006.06.5888.

93. Hinton S, Catalano PJ, Einhorn LH, Nichols CR, David Crawford E, Vogelzang N, et al. Cisplatin, etoposide and either bleomycin or ifosfamide in the treatment of disseminated germ cell tumors: final analysis of an intergroup trial. Cancer. 2003;97(8):1869–75. https://doi.org/10.1002/cncr.11271.
94. Lampe H, Horwich A, Norman A, Nicholls J, Dearnaley DP. Fertility after chemotherapy for testicular germ cell cancers. J Clin Oncol. 1997;15(1):239–45. https://doi.org/10.1200/JCO.1997.15.1.239.
95. Abram McBride J, Lipshultz LI. Male fertility preservation. Curr Urol Rep. 2018;19(7):49. https://doi.org/10.1007/s11934-018-0803-2.
96. Bokemeyer C, Schmoll HJ, van Rhee J, Kuczyk M, Schuppert F, Poliwoda H. Long-term gonadal toxicity after therapy for Hodgkin's and non-Hodgkin's lymphoma. Ann Hematol. 1994;68(3):105–10. https://doi.org/10.1007/BF01727413.
97. Kelleher S, Wishart SM, Liu PY, Turner L, Di Pierro I, Conway AJ, et al. Long-term outcomes of elective human sperm cryostorage. Hum Reprod. 2001;16(12):2632–9. https://doi.org/10.1093/humrep/16.12.2632.
98. Cordelli E, Fresegna AM, Leter G, Eleuteri P, Spano M, Villani P. Evaluation of DNA damage in different stages of mouse spermatogenesis after testicular X irradiation. Radiat Res. 2003;160(4):443–51. https://doi.org/10.1667/rr3053.
99. Pinon-Lataillade G, Velez de la Calle JF, Viguier-Martinez MC, Garnier DH, Folliot R, Maas J, et al. Influence of germ cells upon Sertoli cells during continuous low-dose rate gamma-irradiation of adult rats. Mol Cell Endocrinol. 1988;58(1):51–63. https://doi.org/10.1016/0303-7207(88)90053-6.
100. Lee K, Park JS, Kim YJ, Soo Lee YS, Sook Hwang TS, Kim DJ, et al. Differential expression of Prx I and II in mouse testis and their up-regulation by radiation. Biochem Biophys Res Commun. 2002;296(2):337–42. https://doi.org/10.1016/s0006-291x(02)00801-x.
101. Ma Y, Nie H, Sheng C, Chen H, Wang B, Liu T, et al. Roles of oxidative stress in synchrotron radiation X-ray-induced testicular damage of rodents. Int J Physiol Pathophysiol Pharmacol. 2012;4(2):108–14.
102. Silva AM, Correia S, Casalta-Lopes JE, Mamede AC, Cavaco JE, Botelho MF, et al. The protective effect of regucalcin against radiation-induced damage in testicular cells. Life Sci. 2016;164:31–41. https://doi.org/10.1016/j.lfs.2016.09.003.
103. Howell S, Shalet S. Gonadal damage from chemotherapy and radiotherapy. Endocrinol Metab Clin N Am. 1998;27(4):927–43. https://doi.org/10.1016/s0889-8529(05)70048-7.
104. Shalet SM, Tsatsoulis A, Whitehead E, Read G. Vulnerability of the human Leydig cell to radiation damage is dependent upon age. J Endocrinol. 1989;120(1):161–5. https://doi.org/10.1677/joe.0.1200161.
105. Heidenreich WF, Atkinson M, Paretzke HG. Radiation-induced cell inactivation can increase the cancer risk. Radiat Res. 2001;155(6):870–2. https://doi.org/10.1667/0033-7587(2001)155[0870:ricici]2.0.co;2.
106. Wiechno P, Demkow T, Kubiak K, Sadowska M, Kaminska J. The quality of life and hormonal disturbances in testicular cancer survivors in Cisplatin era. Eur Urol. 2007;52(5):1448–54. https://doi.org/10.1016/j.eururo.2007.05.012.
107. Tal R, Stember DS, Logmanieh N, Narus J, Mulhall JP. Erectile dysfunction in men treated for testicular cancer. BJU Int. 2014;113(6):907–10. https://doi.org/10.1111/bju.12331.
108. Puhse G, Wachsmuth JU, Kemper S, Husstedt IW, Evers S, Kliesch S. Chronic pain has a negative impact on sexuality in testis cancer survivors. J Androl. 2012;33(5):886–93. https://doi.org/10.2164/jandrol.110.012500.
109. Nazareth I, Lewin J, King M. Sexual dysfunction after treatment for testicular cancer: a systematic review. J Psychosom Res. 2001;51(6):735–43. https://doi.org/10.1016/s0022-3999(01)00282-3.
110. Hartmann JT, Albrecht C, Schmoll HJ, Kuczyk MA, Kollmannsberger C, Bokemeyer C. Long-term effects on sexual function and fertility after treatment of testicular cancer. Br J Cancer. 1999;80(5–6):801–7. https://doi.org/10.1038/sj.bjc.6690424.

111. Meistrich ML. Risks of genetic damage in offspring conceived using spermatozoa produced during chemotherapy or radiotherapy. Andrology. 2020;8(3):545–58. https://doi.org/10.1111/andr.12740.
112. Chatziparasidou A, Christoforidis N, Samolada G, Nijs M. Sperm aneuploidy in infertile male patients: a systematic review of the literature. Andrologia. 2015;47(8):847–60. https://doi.org/10.1111/and.12362.
113. Arnon J, Meirow D, Lewis-Roness H, Ornoy A. Genetic and teratogenic effects of cancer treatments on gametes and embryos. Hum Reprod Update. 2001;7(4):394–403. https://doi.org/10.1093/humupd/7.4.394.
114. Li Z, Yang J, Huang H. Oxidative stress induces H2AX phosphorylation in human spermatozoa. FEBS Lett. 2006;580(26):6161–8. https://doi.org/10.1016/j.febslet.2006.10.016.
115. Paoli D, Gallo M, Rizzo F, Spano M, Leter G, Lombardo F, et al. Testicular cancer and sperm DNA damage: short- and long-term effects of antineoplastic treatment. Andrology. 2015;3(1):122–8. https://doi.org/10.1111/j.2047-2927.2014.00250.x.
116. Brydoy M, Fossa SD, Klepp O, Bremnes RM, Wist EA, Wentzel-Larsen T, et al. Paternity following treatment for testicular cancer. J Natl Cancer Inst. 2005;97(21):1580–8. https://doi.org/10.1093/jnci/dji339.
117. Huddart RA, Norman A, Moynihan C, Horwich A, Parker C, Nicholls E, et al. Fertility, gonadal and sexual function in survivors of testicular cancer. Br J Cancer. 2005;93(2):200–7. https://doi.org/10.1038/sj.bjc.6602677.

Part II
Sperm Chromatin Integrity and Fertility

Chapter 5
Impact of Sperm DNA Fragmentation on Natural and Assisted Conception

Nguyen Ho Vinh Phuoc and Ramadan Saleh

Key Points
The main highlights of this chapter include the following:

- The natural repair mechanisms of sperm DNA and the pathophysiological mechanisms underlying sperm DNA fragmentation (SDF) include insufficient sperm chromatin packaging, apoptosis, and high seminal oxidative stress.
- Causes and risk factors of SDF include advanced paternal age, varicocele, male genital tract infections, exposure to toxins, and lifestyle factors such as smoking.
- The potential impact of high SDF is seen on natural fertility and assisted reproduction.
- Management of infertile couples in whom the husband suffers high SDF is discussed.
- The procedures commonly used for SDF assessment, their general principles, advantages and limitations, and the potential for implementing SDF testing into clinical practice are also elaborated.
- Insights are provided for refining the diagnostic and predictive potentials of the SDF test and optimizing its utility in clinical practice.

Introduction

Basic semen analysis is the cornerstone for evaluating subfertile/infertile men [1]. However, basic semen analysis does not provide information on the functional competence of sperm, and therefore it is not adequate for an accurate assessment of male fertility potential [2]. Additionally, the finding of normal semen parameters does not exclude infertile male as it can be reported in up to 15% of infertile men [3]. Testing

N. H. V. Phuoc
Department of Andrology, Binh Dan Hospital, Ho Chi Minh City, Vietnam

R. Saleh (✉)
Department of Dermatology, Venereology and Andrology, Faculty of Medicine, Sohag University, Sohag, Egypt

Ajyal IVF Center, Ajyal Hospital, Sohag, Egypt

A. Agarwal et al. (eds.), *Current and Future Advances in Male Infertility*,
https://doi.org/10.1007/978-3-031-62648-7_5

sperm DNA integrity may help predict male fertility potential [4]. Sperm DNA fragmentation (SDF) can be caused by several factors, including varicocele [5], male genital tract infections [6], advanced paternal age [7], and other factors such as smoking, exposure to radiation or harmful chemicals, obesity, diabetes, and cancer [8]. High SDF has been correlated with recurrent pregnancy loss (RPL) and is found in cases classified as unexplained or idiopathic infertility [9]. Additionally, high SDF has been linked with poor outcomes of assisted reproductive technologies (ARTs), including low embryo quality [10] and increased risk of miscarriage [10, 11] in couples undergoing intracytoplasmic sperm injection (ICSI).

In this chapter, we highlight the natural repair mechanisms of sperm DNA and discuss the pathophysiological aspects, types, and causes of SDF. We also review the impact of SDF on natural fertility and ART outcomes. Additionally, we provide information on the currently available techniques of SDF testing and summarize the advantages and limitations of those tests. Further, we discuss the utility of SDF tests in clinical practice and strategies to manage cases of high SDF and provide insights for future research on the topic.

Sperm DNA Natural Repair Mechanisms

Sperm DNA is organized as loops, which are subsequently attached in the nuclear matrix to specific attachment sites [12]. Sperm maturation during spermiogenesis involves an essential step of sperm chromatin packaging, where histones are replaced mainly by protamines [13, 14]. Protamines are arginine-rich structural elements present in two forms, protamines 1 and 2. The majority of sperm DNA is bound to protamines (85–90%), while only a tiny proportion is bound to histones (10–15%) [15]. Protamines condense the genetic material, resulting in transcriptional inactivation [16, 17]. The process of protamine-related DNA-dense packaging protects the sperm genome, which involves a complex series of structural and molecular changes [18]. The method of protamination initiated during spermiogenesis is continued during sperm transport in the epididymis with the formation of disulfide bonds, which add further compaction to the DNA [14]. During chromatin decondensation, the disulfide bonds are lost, resulting in an approximately tenfold increase in nuclear volume [19].

Notably, the natural repair of sperm DNA can occur in early development, while it is impossible in mature sperm. Such restoration is limited to small breaks and does not include larger ones. Therefore, the mature sperm relies on oocyte and early embryonic DNA repair systems [20–22]. Evidence suggests that the oocyte's expression of DNA repair genes is correlated negatively with maternal age [23]. Effective oocyte repair can help the recovery of sperm genetic material during and after fertilization. However, the damage to the paternal sperm DNA may be beyond the repairing capacity of the oocyte, thus resulting in miscarriage [22, 23]. Recurrent ART failure has also been correlated with high SDF levels despite the absence of noticeable zygotic or cleavage abnormalities [22].

Origin of SDF

Three mechanisms have been proposed to explain the pathogenesis of SDF, including defective sperm chromatin packaging, abortive apoptosis, and oxidative stress (OS) (Fig. 5.1).

Defective Sperm Chromatin Packaging

During the compaction process, topoisomerase enzymes relieve downstream torsional stress in DNA, resulting in the creation of nicks in the DNA strands [24]. The subsequent failure to repair these nicks leads to persistent breaks in the sperm DNA strands. Defective sperm chromatin condensation increases the susceptibility of sperm DNA to damage by various insults and stressors [25]. Immature sperm with high SDF contains a more significant proportion of histones due to incomplete exchange with protamine [24].

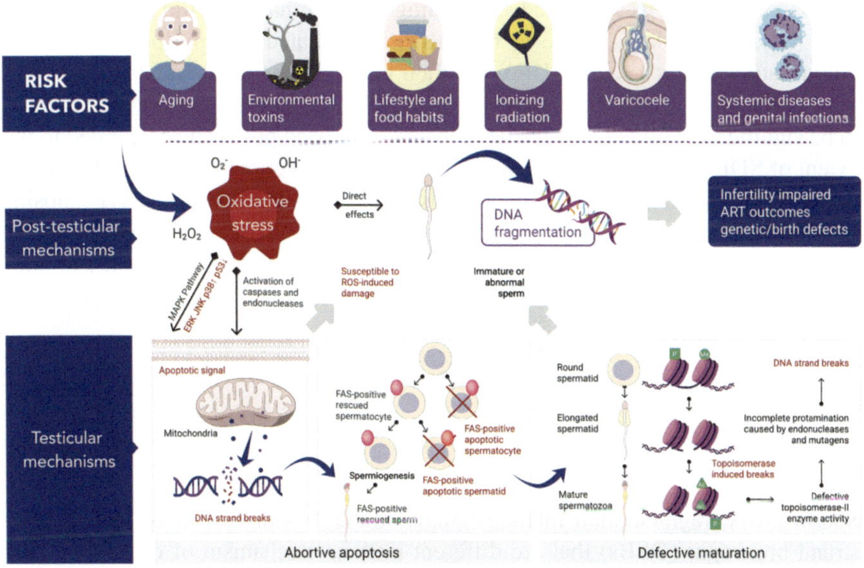

Fig. 5.1 The origin of sperm DNA fragmentation (SDF). SDF may result from underlying mechanisms such as defective maturation, abortive apoptosis, and oxidative stress. Moreover, clinical (advanced paternal age, infection, cancer, obesity, diabetes) and environmental (heat exposure, environmental toxins, radiation, smoking, drug abuse, diet) risk factors can lead to SDF. *MAPK* mitogen-activated protein kinase, *ERK* extracellular signal-regulated kinase, *JNK* c-JUN N-terminal kinase, *ROS* reactive oxygen species, *ART* assisted reproductive technique

Abortive Apoptosis

Apoptosis is a physiological phenomenon, and within the testes, it helps remove abnormal germ cells and maintain an appropriate germ cell population [26]. Apoptosis is mediated through two pathways: (1) intrinsic pathways involving mitochondria and (2) extrinsic pathway that involves cell surface receptor interactions, such as the Fas, both leading to activation of caspases followed by endonucleases, which cause DNA fragmentation as part of the cell death [27]. Failure to complete the cascade of apoptosis in spermatozoa leads to the release of sperm with fragmented DNA, a process described as abortive apoptosis [28]. As a marker of apoptosis, the activity of caspase was found to be significantly higher among the sperm population with increased DNA fragmentation [24]. Additionally, abortive apoptosis was higher among men with abnormal semen parameters [29]. Magnetic-activated cell sorting technique has been used with success to reduce SDF by removing apoptotic spermatozoa [30].

Oxidative Stress-Mediated Damage

Oxidative stress due to an imbalance between reactive oxygen species (ROS) and antioxidants has been established as a leading cause of male infertility and increased SDF [31]. Sperm damage due to high ROS is mediated by lipid peroxidation of polyunsaturated fatty acids (PUFAs) in their cell surface membrane, forming cytotoxic aldehydes such as malondialdehyde (MDA) [32]. Levels of MDA were found to be significantly higher in infertile men and have been positively correlated to the extent of SDF [33]. Additionally, ROS can cause direct damage to sperm DNA and activate the intrinsic process of apoptosis [32, 34]. 8-Hydroxydeoxyguanosine (8-OHdG) is a known indicator of oxidative sperm DNA damage and has long been associated with infertility and abnormal semen parameters [35]. Further, a significant positive correlation was found between the amount of 8-OHdG in sperm and levels of SDF [36].

Types of SDF

Sperm DNA fragmentation includes single-strand breakages (SSBs) and double-strand breakages (DSBs) that are different in their mechanism of occurrence and their impact on the development of the future embryo based on site, extent, and severity of the breaks [37, 38]. While DSBs are mainly due to inadequate sperm chromatin packaging, SSBs are caused mainly by OS [38, 39]. However, it is not easy to differentiate between DSBs and SSBs using the currently available SDF tests [38]. Both DSBs and SSBs are correlated with poor reproductive outcomes

[32]. The DSBs can lead to nonviable cells and pregnancy failure, recurrent miscarriages, embryo implantation failures following ICSI, and abnormalities in post-ICSI embryonic kinetics [38]. On the other hand, SSBs are associated with a greater probability of embryonic survival [38]. Although SSBs are generally considered less severe, they can lead to the same consequences as DSBs if present in high numbers. Types of DNA damage include mismatch of bases, loss of base, base modifications, DNA adducts and cross-link, pyrimidine dimers, and SSBs and DSBs (Fig. 5.2).

What Causes SDF?

Sperm DNA fragmentation can be caused by extrinsic factors (e.g., heat exposure, smoking, environmental pollutants, and chemotherapeutics) and/or intrinsic factors (e.g., defective germ cell maturation, abortive apoptosis, and OS) [40]. State-of-the-art evidence demonstrates that OS majorly contributes to male infertility [41]. Reactive oxygen species are vital for physiological processes such as apoptosis and capacitation, but an overproduction leads to various harmful consequences, including SDF [42].

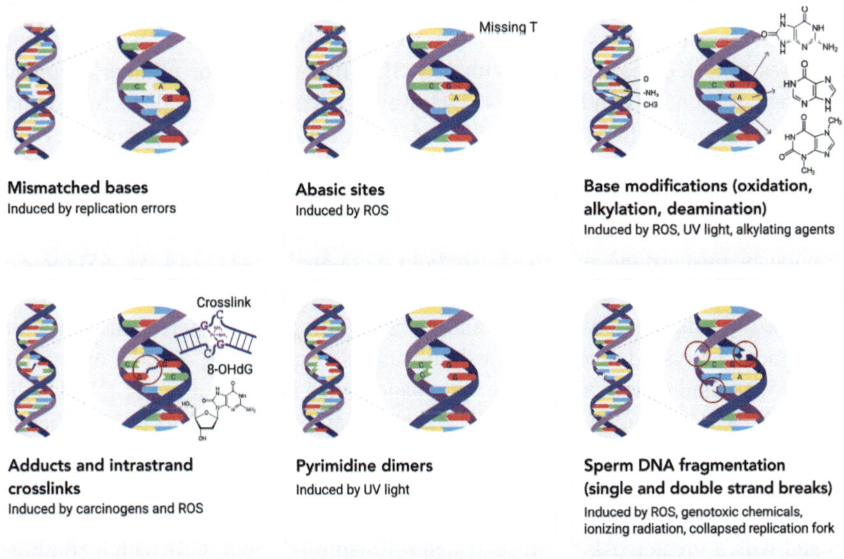

Fig. 5.2 Types of DNA damage: mismatched bases, abasic sites, base modifications (oxidation, alkylation, deamination), adducts and intra-strand cross-links, pyrimidine dimers, and single- and double-strand fragmentation. *ROS* reactive oxygen species, *UV* ultraviolet

Impact of SDF on Fertility Outcome

Spontaneous Pregnancy Outcomes

Sperm DNA integrity is crucial in fertilization and early embryo development, directly influencing the likelihood of natural conception. Reports have linked SDF to low cleavage rates [43, 44] and the arrest of embryonic development after the second cleavage state [45]. Spanò et al. [46] used the SCSA on 215 Danish first-pregnancy planners to find an inverse relationship between the level of SDF and the probability of natural pregnancy. Besides, a meta-analysis including 3 studies (616 couples) found an association between failure to achieve natural pregnancy and high SDF (has been found with an odds ratio (OR) of 7.01 (95% confidence interval [CI] = 3.68–13.36)) [43].

Outcomes of Assisted Reproductive Techniques

Studies investigating the predictive role of SDF on ART outcomes showed contradictory results [11, 43, 47–62]. This controversy can be attributed to several factors, such as the study selection methods used, differences in the SDF testing methods, and female age and fertility status. With regard to intrauterine insemination (IUI), Chen et al. [49] demonstrated that high SDF levels were associated with significantly lower pregnancy (relative risk [RR] = 0.34, 95% CI = 0.22–0.52; $p < 0.001$) and delivery rates (RR = 0.14, 95% CI = 0.04–0.56; $p < 0.001$). Two other meta-analyses reported that patients with low SDF had an OR for clinical pregnancy ranging between 7.01 and 16 [41, 43]. However, a recent meta-analysis by Sugihara et al. [50] reported that while low SDF was associated with better pregnancy rates with an RR of 3.30 (95% CI = 1.16–9.39), the test performance was inadequate due to a low positive predictive value (17%).

In IVF/ICSI, various meta-analyses have been published assessing the rates of pregnancy, miscarriage, and live birth. Four meta-analyses [11, 43, 51, 55] reported that high SDF was associated with lower pregnancy rates with conventional IVF, with the OR ranging between 0.68 and 1.7. Regarding ICSI, whereas the remaining three meta-analyses failed to find a significant association [11, 43, 51], only Simon et al. [55] found significantly lower pregnancy rates in cases of high SDF. The live birth rate was examined by one meta-analysis and was found to be significantly lower in men with high SDF following both IVF and ICSI with a combined OR of 1.17 (95% CI = 1.07–1.28; $p = 0.0005$) [56]. Three meta-analyses examined the miscarriage rate following ART concerning SDF [11, 43, 52]. High SDF was associated with a greater risk for miscarriage following IVF and ICSI with a combined OR between 2.28 and 2.48.

Cissen et al. [11] analyzed 30 studies to assess the value of SDF in predicting the chance of ongoing pregnancy with IVF or ICSI. The authors reported acceptable predictive performance for TUNEL and comet assays, while the predictive power for SCSA and SCD was found to be poor. The authors concluded that the current SDF testing methods had limited ability to predict the chance of pregnancy in the context of ART. Furthermore, Collins et al. [54] analyzed 13 studies with extensive heterogeneity and found that sperm DNA integrity was significantly associated with pregnancy following IVF and ICSI with an OR of 1.44, 95% CI = 1.03–2.03, $p = 0.04$. In the latter study, the likelihood ratios (LR(+) = 1.23, LR(−) = 0.81) were in a range suggesting that testing did not alter the outcome and was hence not clinically relevant. Subgroup analyses showed that the testing method (TUNEL or SCSA) or the ART modality (IVF or ICSI) did not materially affect the test accuracy.

Selecting a Test for SDF Evaluation

The latest sixth edition of the WHO laboratory manual of human semen analysis provides a detailed description of four assays for SDF testing, namely, terminal deoxynucleotidyl transferase deoxyuridine triphosphate (dUTP) nick end labeling (TUNEL), acridine orange flow cytometry, sperm chromatin dispersion (SCD) test, and single-cell gel electrophoresis assay [1]. However, there is no consensus as to the best technique used for the assessment of SDF. The latest sixth edition of the WHO manual of semen analysis recommends that the choice of a test is based on the availability of the tools and the expertise of the laboratory personnel. In this section, we provide a brief summary of the general principles, advantages, and limitations of SDF techniques that are in common use nowadays.

Terminal Deoxynucleotidyl Transferase-Mediated Deoxyuridine Triphosphate Nick End Labeling (TUNEL) Assay

The TUNEL assay is a direct method of SDF assessment that can rapidly evaluate up to 10,000 cells using flow cytometry [63]. A value of 20% SDF has been suggested as a threshold to distinguish between fertile and infertile populations using the TUNEL technique [64, 65]. Results of a meta-analysis comparing different DNA tests found the TUNEL assay to be most predictive of miscarriage [66].

Sperm Chromatin Structure Assay (SCSA)

The sperm chromatin structure assay (SCSA) is an indirect test of SDF using flow cytometry to measure the susceptibility of sperm DNA to in situ acid-induced denaturation by quantifying the metachromatic shift of acridine orange stain fluorescence from green (native DNA) to red (denatured DNA) [67]. The SCSA can analyze up to 10,000 cells in a few seconds using a flow cytometer and is characterized by low interlaboratory variability [68]. A study including a large sample of 1316 infertile couples that underwent IVF, and 266 that underwent ICSI, explored the predictive potential of SCSA for reproductive outcomes using DNA fragmentation index (DFI) [69]. The results of the latter study indicated that a DFI threshold <11.3% was predictive of pregnancy success after IVF with 56.1% sensitivity and 60% specificity, and threshold <30.3% was predictive of pregnancy success after ICSI with 50.6% sensitivity and 68.8% specificity.

Sperm Chromatin Dispersion (SCD) Test

The sperm chromatin dispersion (SCD) test evaluates the emission of the typical DNA halos in sperm with intact DNA after immersion in a layer of agarose and then a lysing medium to remove the nuclear proteins [70]. Levels of SDF, measured by SCD, were found to be significantly correlated with those measured by SCSA and TUNEL assay in a population of infertile and fertile men [71]. However, the results of SCD were not associated with pregnancy outcome following IUI [72].

Comet Assay

The comet assay, also known as the single-cell gel electrophoresis assay, is based on the migration of the broken strands of the DNA towards the anode during electrophoresis, generating the characteristic dispersion pattern that resembles a comet tail. In contrast, the intact DNA constitutes the comet's head [73]. The automated high-throughput comet helps visualize a patient's sperm chromatin damage profile by plotting the percentage of DNA in the tail against tail length [74]. A two-dimensional, two-tailed comet assay has been developed to differentiate between SSBs and DSBs in the same comet in sperm [75]. Although the comet technique can locate break-points and thus differentiate SSBs from DSBs, it has several limitations, including complex methodology, need for high level of expertise, and considerable interlaboratory variation [38, 76].

Implementing SDF Test into Clinical Practice

The SDF Test in the WHO Manual of Semen Analysis

The editors of the sixth edition of the WHO manual for semen analysis acknowledge that SDF testing "could represent an important addition in the workup of male infertility, becoming one of the most discussed and promising biomarkers in basic and clinical andrology" [1]. The sixth edition described four methods of SDF testing, including the TUNEL assay, SCD assay, comet assay, and acridine orange flow cytometry assay. The editors of the sixth edition stated, "Except for the Comet assay, these tests are helpful for clinical testing." However, the sixth edition of the WHO manual provides no thresholds of SDF, so the reader is uncertain as to how to use the results in a clinically meaningful way.

The SDF Test in the Guidelines of Professional Societies

The first society to advocate SDF testing was the Society for Translational Medicine (STM) in 2017, which has discussed the indications for SDF testing and provided recommendations and also examined the tests for SDF and management strategies [77]. This served as the base upon which recommendations for SDF testing were further elaborated and expanded.

The European Society of Human Reproduction and Embryology (ESHRE) discussed the role of SDF testing as a means to explain RPL [78]. The European Academy of Andrology (EAA) suggests adding SDF testing to initial basic semen analysis in men with oligo-astheno-teratozoospermia who are considered for ART [79].

The European Association of Urology (EAU) recommends SDF testing only for men with unexplained infertility or after RPL [80]. Recently, the American Urological Association (AUA) and the American Society for Reproductive Medicine (ASRM) published a guideline on male infertility, and they recommend against SDF testing in the initial evaluation of fertility but advocate its use and importance in couples experiencing RPL [81].

Limitations of SDF Test

The currently available SDF tests are often criticized for their inability to differentiate the exact type and nature of DNA breaks. Since sperm DNA cracks also occur in fertile males during chromatin condensation [82], the unknown identity of a particular sperm DNA break may impair the clinical significance of the test result. Moreover, the correlation between SDF and natural pregnancy, ART, and miscarriage has been demonstrated despite a wide variety of testing methods employed [83]. In fact, there is no single gold standard test for SDF at the moment.

Nevertheless, SDF testing provides important information on the general status of sperm quality [84] and sperm DNA content [85]. Given the complex nature of human reproduction, it is unlikely that SDF assay alone can accurately predict pregnancy outcomes that are greatly influenced by concomitant female factors [82, 86]. Although the negative impact of SDF on time to pregnancy was illustrated by the Longitudinal Investigation of Fertility and Environment (LIFE) [87] and the Danish First Pregnancy Planner [46] studies, other semen measures and male age were also identified [87], indicating that SDF should not be used in isolation.

Lastly, the current SDF tests are incapable of assessing the DNA content of a single sperm and thus selecting the best spermatozoon for injection in ICSI procedures. Nevertheless, SDF testing may play a pivotal role in altering the management plan in selected groups of patients [88].

Strategies to Reduce SDF

Limiting Exposures and Lifestyle Change

Exposure to environmental and lifestyle factors has negative implications on male fertility. Current data has consistently associated smoking with higher SDF values than nonsmokers [89–92]. However, no study has yet evaluated the impact of smoking cessation on SDF. Numerous environmental factors, such as airborne pollutants, ionizing radiation, and pesticides, have also been linked with increased SDF values [93–97]. A recent meta-analysis found no robust association between body mass index and SDF [98]. No concrete evidence of lifestyle modification impact on SDF exists [99]. However, weight loss and dietary changes have been proposed to benefit SDF indices in patients [100, 101].

The negative impact of prolonged ejaculatory abstinence on SDF has been reported without significant detrimental effects on conventional semen parameters [102, 103]. Therefore, short-term recurrent ejaculation may be a simple, noninvasive maneuver to reduce SDF. Although the beneficial effect of short ejaculatory abstinence on natural conception is unclear, applying the technique to assisted reproduction may have value [104–106]. In addition to higher pregnancy rates in ICSI, recurrent ejaculation has been associated with a significantly lower SDF [107].

Control of Male Genital Tract Infections/Inflammation

Among infertile men, the incidence of infection ranges from 2% to 18% [107]. Sexually transmitted diseases or prostatitis is associated with elevated OS and leukocytospermia, which may result in elevated SDF and impaired fertility [108, 109]. Antibiotic therapy has been reported to be effective in treating infection-induced high SDF levels [110]. Moreover, empirical antibiotic treatment for leukocytospermia may improve natural pregnancy rates [111].

Varicocele Repair

Studies indicated that varicocele repair can improve OS markers, reduce SDF indices [112], and improve fertility [113]. In a systematic review of 21 studies evaluating the effect of varicocelectomy on SDF, all studies reported a significant decrease in SDF by an average of approximately 8% [114]. Moreover, varicocele repair has improved pregnancy success in natural conception and assisted reproduction through improved SDF indices [115]. Given these observations, varicocelectomy should be discussed with patients as a potential solution to improving fertility [113].

Antioxidant Supplementation

Antioxidants play an essential role in general health by scavenging excess free radicals and, thus, preventing oxidative damage to macromolecules. However, the benefits of exogenous antioxidant therapy could be more precise [116]. Clinicians commonly use antioxidant therapy to maintain redox balance by scavenging ROS [117]. Several clinical trials have demonstrated the positive effects of antioxidants on SDF in infertile men [118–122]. However, with lack of clear guidelines on antioxidant supplementation, they are empirically used. Antioxidants can be easily purchased over the counter and are commonly considered safe. However, excess antioxidant supplementation may paradoxically affect OS and SDF, a condition referred to as reductive stress [123]. As a result, the indiscriminate use of oral antioxidants in men without elevated OS should be avoided [124].

Management of Persistently High SDF

Use of Testicular Sperm

Testicular sperm has been explored as a treatment option for high SDF based on the finding of lower SDF in testicular sperm than ejaculated sperm [125, 126] and better ICSI outcome [127–129]. However, this may be limited by risks of anesthesia and complications of surgical sperm retrieval [130]. Furthermore, a possible higher aneuploidy rate in testicular sperm is a concern [131] despite a recent report of opposing view [132]. Therefore, the use of testicular sperm in the clinical management of non-azoospermic patients with high SDF is still debated.

Use of Sperm Selection Techniques

Laboratory conditions (i.e., prolonged incubation, centrifugation, cryopreservation, and use of different media) can significantly impact SDF by increasing OS-mediated DNA damage [133–136]. Conventional (swim-up and density gradient) and advanced techniques can help select sperm with low levels of SDF [137–140]. Magnetic-activated cell sorting based on the detection of phosphatidylserine [141] showed a better selection alone [142, 143] or in combination with density gradient technique [144–147]. Intracytoplasmic morphologically selected sperm injection uses high magnification to choose the most morphologically normal sperm, as vacuoles in the nuclear region have been associated with high SDF [148, 149]. Other approaches include the physiological intracytoplasmic sperm injection, based on sperm binding to hyaluronic acid, and microfluidic devices, allowing sperm migration along microchannels [150–153].

Summary

Evidence suggests negative impact of high SDF on reproductive outcomes under natural and ART conditions. Several factors, including advanced paternal age, varicocele, male genital tract infections, lifestyle habits, and toxic exposure, may cause high SDF. The procedures commonly used for SDF assessment include the TUNEL, SCSA, SCD, and comet. Currently, the choice of an assay for SDF testing depends on the availability of the instruments, tools, and trained personnel. The latest sixth edition of the WHO manual of human semen analysis recommends the performing laboratory to determine and validate the diagnostic thresholds of the selected SDF test [1]. Strategies that may help reduce SDF in infertile men attempting natural or assisted conception include dietary and weight control, stopping smoking, reducing environmental and occupational exposure to gonadotoxins, antibiotic therapy for male genital tract infection, repair of clinical varicocele, and antioxidant supplementation [154]. Some sperm selection techniques such as magnetic-activated cell sorting, intracytoplasmic morphologically selected sperm injection, and physiological intracytoplasmic sperm injection can be used before ICSI in cases with persistently high SDF. Future research is warranted to address issues related to establishing clinical indications of SDF testing, standardizing the currently available SDF assays, determining reliable cutoff values, introducing novel SDF tests, and exploring new effective treatment options for infertile men with persistently elevated SDF.

References

1. WHO. WHO laboratory manual for the examination and processing of human semen. 6th ed. Geneva: World Health Organization; 2021.
2. Wang C, Swerdloff RS. Limitations of semen analysis as a test of male fertility and anticipated needs from newer tests. Fertil Steril. 2014;102(6):1502–7. https://doi.org/10.1016/j.fertnstert.2014.10.021. Epub 2014 Nov 25. PMID: 25458617; PMCID: PMC4254491.
3. Agarwal A, Allamaneni SS. Sperm DNA damage assessment: a test whose time has come. Fertil Steril. 2005;84(4):850–3. https://doi.org/10.1016/j.fertnstert.2005.03.080.
4. Winkle T, Rosenbusch B, Gagsteiger F, Paiss T, Zoller N. The correlation between male age, sperm quality and sperm DNA fragmentation in 320 men attending a fertility center. J Assist Reprod Genet. 2009;26(1):41–6. https://doi.org/10.1007/s10815-008-9277-3.
5. Saleh AR, Agarwal A, Sharma RK, Nelson David R, Thomas AJ Jr. Evaluation of nuclear DNA damage in spermatozoa from infertile men with varicocele. Fertil Steril. 2003;80(6):1431–6.
6. Pagliuca C, Cariati F, Bagnulo F, Scaglione E, Carotenuto C, Farina F, D'Argenio V, Carraturo F, D'Aprile P, Vitiello M, Strina I, Alviggi C, Colicchio R, Tomaiuolo R, Salvatore P. Microbiological evaluation and sperm DNA fragmentation in semen samples of patients undergoing fertility investigation. Genes (Basel). 2021;12(5):654. https://doi.org/10.3390/genes12050654.
7. Albani E, Castellano S, Gurrieri B, Arruzzolo L, Negri L, Borroni EM, Levi-Setti PE. Male age: negative impact on sperm DNA fragmentation. Aging (Albany NY). 2019;11(9):2749–61. https://doi.org/10.18632/aging.101946.
8. Panner Selvam MK, Ambar RF, Agarwal A, Henkel R. Etiologies of sperm DNA damage and its impact on male infertility. Andrologia. 2021;53(1):e13706. https://doi.org/10.1111/and.13706.
9. Farkouh A, Finelli R, Agarwal A. Beyond conventional sperm parameters: the role of sperm DNA fragmentation in male infertility. Minerva Endocrinol (Torino). 2022;47(1):23–37. https://doi.org/10.23736/S2724-6507.21.03623-X.
10. Deng C, Li T, Xie Y, Guo Y, Yang Q, Liang X, Deng C, Liu G. Sperm DNA fragmentation index influences assisted reproductive technology outcome: a systematic review and meta-analysis combined with a retrospective cohort study. Andrologia. 2019;51:e13263.
11. Zhao J, Zhang Q, Wang Y, Li Y. Whether sperm deoxyribonucleic acid fragmentation has an effect on pregnancy and miscarriage after in vitro fertilization/intracytoplasmic sperm injection: a systematic review and meta-analysis. Fertil Steril. 2014;102:998–1005.e8.
12. Kramer JA, Krawetz SA. Nuclear matrix interactions within the sperm genome. J Biol Chem. 1996;271:11619–22.
13. O'Doherty AM, McGettigan PA. Epigenetic processes in the male germline. Reprod Fertil Dev. 2015;27:725–38.
14. Shamsi MB, Kumar R, Dada R. Evaluation of nuclear DNA damage in human spermatozoa in men opting for assisted reproduction. Indian J Med Res. 2008;127:115–23.

15. Huser T, Orme CA, Hollars CW, Corzett MH, Balhorn R. Raman spectroscopy of DNA packaging in individual human sperm cells distinguishes normal from abnormal cells. J Biophotonics. 2009;2:322–32.
16. Filatov MV, Semenova EV, Vorob'eva OA, Leont'eva OA, Drobchenko EA. Relationship between abnormal sperm chromatin packing and IVF results. Mol Hum Reprod. 1999;5:825–30.
17. Steger K, Balhorn R. Sperm nuclear protamines: a checkpoint to control sperm chromatin quality. J Vet Med Ser C Anat Histol Embryol. 2018;47:273–9.
18. Bjorndahl L. Human sperm chromatin stabilization: a proposed model including zinc bridges. Mol Hum Reprod. 2010;16:23–9.
19. Smit M, Wissenburg OG, Hutchison JM, Rau DC, JE DR. Role of disulfide bonds on DNA packaging forces in bull sperm chromatin. Biophys J. 2017;113:1925–33.
20. Dada R. Sperm DNA damage diagnostics: when and why. Transl Androl Urol. 2017;6:S691–4.
21. González-Marín C, Gosálvez J, Roy R. Types, causes, detection and repair of DNA fragmentation in animal and human sperm cells. Int J Mol Sci. 2012;13:14026–52.
22. Gunes S, Sertyel S. Sperm DNA damage and oocyte repair capability. In: A Clinician's guide to sperm DNA chromatin damage; 2018. p. 321–46.
23. Horta F, Catt S, Ramachandran P, Vollenhoven B, Temple-Smith P. Female aging affects the DNA repair capacity of oocytes in IVF using a controlled model of sperm DNA damage in mice. Hum Reprod. 2020;35:529–44.
24. Muratori M, Marchiani S, Tamburrino L, Baldi E. Sperm DNA fragmentation: mechanisms of origin. Adv Exp Med Biol. 2019;1166:75–85.
25. Björndahl L, Kvist U. Structure of chromatin in spermatozoa. Adv Exp Med Biol. 2014;791:1–11.
26. Shukla KK, Mahdi AA, Singh R. Apoptosis, spermatogenesis and male infertility. Front Biosci Elite. 2012;4:746–54.
27. Elmore S. Apoptosis: a review of programmed cell death. Toxicol Pathol. 2007;35:495–516.
28. Muratori M, Tamburrino L, Marchiani S, Cambi M, Olivito B, Azzari C, et al. Investigation on the origin of sperm DNA fragmentation: role of apoptosis, immaturity and oxidative stress. Mol Med. 2015;21:109–22.
29. Sakkas D, Mariethoz E, St. John JC. Abnormal sperm parameters in humans are indicative of an abortive apoptotic mechanism linked to the Fas-mediated pathway. Exp Cell Res. 1999;251:350–5.
30. Troya J, Zorrilla I. Annexin V-MACS in infertile couples as method for separation of sperm without DNA fragmentation. J Bras Reprod Assist. 2015;19:66–9.
31. Dutta S, Majzoub A, Agarwal A. Oxidative stress and sperm function: a systematic review on evaluation and management. Arab J Urol. 2019;17:87–97.
32. Agarwal A, Virk G, Ong C, du Plessis SS. Effect of oxidative stress on male reproduction. World J Mens Health. 2014;32:1.
33. Dorostghoal M, Kazeminejad SR, Shahbazian N, Pourmehdi M, Jabbari A. Oxidative stress status and sperm DNA fragmentation in fertile and infertile men. Andrologia. 2017;49:1–9.
34. Maneesh M, Jayalekshmi H. Role of reactive oxygen species and antioxidants on pathophysiology of male reproduction. Indian J Clin Biochem. 2006;21:80–9.
35. Shen HM, Chia SE, Ong CN. Evaluation of oxidative DNA damage in human sperm and its association with male infertility. J Androl. 1999;20:718–23.
36. Aitken RJ, De Iuliis GN, Finnie JM, Hedges A, McLachlan RI. Analysis of the relationships between oxidative stress, DNA damage and sperm vitality in a patient population: development of diagnostic criteria. Hum Reprod. 2010;25:2415–26.
37. García-Rodríguez A, Gosálvez J, Agarwal A, Roy R, Johnston S. DNA damage and repair in human reproductive cells. Int J Mol Sci. 2019;20(1):31.
38. Ribas-Maynou J, Benet J. Single and double strand sperm DNA damage: different reproductive effects on male fertility. Genes (Basel). 2019;10(2):105.
39. Laberge RM, Boissonneault G. On the nature and origin of DNA strand breaks in elongating spermatids. Biol Reprod. 2005;73:289–96.

40. Baskaran S, Cho CL, Agarwal A. Role of sperm DNA damage in male infertility assessment. In: Rizk B, Agarwal A, Sabanegh Jr ES, editors. Male infertility in reproductive medicine: diagnosis and management. Boca Raton: CRC Press; 2019. p. 205.
41. Agarwal A, Prabakaran S, Allamaneni S. What an andrologist/urologist should know about free radicals and why. Urology. 2006;67:2–8.
42. Aitken RJ, Curry BJ. Redox regulation of human sperm function: from the physiological control of sperm capacitation to the etiology of infertility and DNA damage in the germ line. Antioxid Redox Signal. 2011;14:367–81.
43. Zini A. Are sperm chromatin and DNA defects relevant in the clinic? Syst Biol Reprod Med. 2011;57:78–85.
44. Borges E Jr, Zanetti BF, Setti AS, Braga DPAF, Provenza RR, Iaconelli A Jr. Sperm DNA fragmentation is correlated with poor embryo development, lower implantation rate, and higher miscarriage rate in reproductive cycles of non-male factor infertility. Fertil Steril. 2019;112:483–90.
45. Ruvolo G, Fattouh RR, Bosco L, Brucculeri AM, Cittadini E. New molecular markers for the evaluation of gamete quality. J Assist Reprod Genet. 2013;30:207–12.
46. Spanò M, Bonde JP, Hjøllund HI, Kolstad HA, Cordelli E, Leter G. Sperm chromatin damage impairs human fertility. The Danish First Pregnancy Planner Study Team. Fertil Steril. 2000;73:43–50.
47. Bungum M, Humaidan P, Spano M, Jepson K, Bungum L, Giwercman A. The predictive value of sperm chromatin structure assay (SCSA) parameters for the outcome of intrauterine insemination, IVF and ICSI. Hum Reprod. 2004;19:1401–8.
48. Sun JG, Jurisicova A, Casper RF. Detection of deoxyribonucleic acid fragmentation in human sperm: correlation with fertilization in vitro. Biol Reprod. 1997;56:602–7.
49. Chen Q, Zhao JY, Xue X, Zhu GX. The association between sperm DNA fragmentation and reproductive outcomes following intrauterine insemination, a meta analysis. Reprod Toxicol. 2019;86:50–5.
50. Sugihara A, Van Avermaete F, Roelant E, Punjabi U, De Neubourg D. The role of sperm DNA fragmentation testing in predicting intra-uterine insemination outcome: a systematic review and meta-analysis. Eur J Obstet Gynecol Reprod Biol. 2020;244:8–15.
51. Li Z, Wang L, Cai J, Huang H. Correlation of sperm DNA damage with IVF and ICSI outcomes: a systematic review and meta-analysis. J Assist Reprod Genet. 2006;23:367–76.
52. Zini A, Boman JM, Belzile E, Ciampi A. Sperm DNA damage is associated with an increased risk of pregnancy loss after IVF and ICSI: systematic review and meta-analysis. Hum Reprod. 2008;23:2663–8.
53. Cissen M, Wely MV, Scholten I, Mansell S, Bruin JP, Mol BW, et al. Measuring sperm DNA fragmentation and clinical outcomes of medically assisted reproduction: a systematic review and meta-analysis. PLoS One. 2016;11:e0165125.
54. Collins JA, Barnhart KT, Schlegel PN. Do sperm DNA integrity tests predict pregnancy with in vitro fertilization? Fertil Steril. 2008;89:823–31.
55. Simon L, Zini A, Dyachenko A, Ciampi A, Carrell DT. A systematic review and meta-analysis to determine the effect of sperm DNA damage on in vitro fertilization and intracytoplasmic sperm injection outcome. Asian J Androl. 2017;19:80–90.
56. Osman A, Alsomait H, Seshadri S, El-Toukhy T, Khalaf Y. The effect of sperm DNA fragmentation on live birth rate after IVF or ICSI: a systematic review and meta-analysis. Reprod Biomed Online. 2015;30:120–7.
57. Green KA, Patounakis G, Dougherty MP, Werner MD, Scott RT Jr, Franasiak JM. Sperm DNA fragmentation on the day of fertilization is not associated with embryologic or clinical outcomes after IVF/ICSI. J Assist Reprod Genet. 2020;37:71–6.
58. Uppangala S, Pudakalakatti S, D'souza F, Salian SR, Kalthur G, Kumar P, et al. Influence of sperm DNA damage on human preimplantation embryo metabolism. Reprod Biol. 2016;16:234–41.
59. Huang CC, Lin DP, Tsao HM, Cheng TC, Liu CH, Lee MS. Sperm DNA fragmentation negatively correlates with velocity and fertilization rates but might not affect pregnancy rates. Fertil Steril. 2005;84:130–40.

60. Boe-Hansen GB, Fedder J, Ersbøll AK, Christensen P. The sperm chromatin structure assay as a diagnostic tool in the human fertility clinic. Hum Reprod. 2006;21:1576–82.
61. Nasr-Esfahani MH, Salehi M, Razavi S, Anjomshoa M, Rozbahani S, Moulavi F, et al. effect of sperm DNA damage and sperm protamine deficiency on fertilization and embryo development post-ICSI. Reprod Biomed Online. 2005;11:198–205.
62. Simon L, Proutski I, Stevenson M, Jennings D, McManus J, Lutton D, et al. Sperm DNA damage has a negative association with live-birth rates after IVF. Reprod Biomed Online. 2013;26:68–78.
63. Sharma R, Iovine C, Agarwal A, Henkel R. TUNEL assay—standardized method for testing sperm DNA fragmentation. Andrologia. 2021;53:e13738.
64. Santi D, Spaggiari G, Simoni M. Sperm DNA fragmentation index as a promising predictive tool for male infertility diagnosis and treatment management—meta-analyses. Reprod Biomed Online. 2018;37:315–26.
65. Agarwal A, Barbăroşie C, Ambar R, Finelli R. The impact of single-and double-strand DNA breaks in human spermatozoa on assisted reproduction. Int J Mol Sci. 2020;21:1–14.
66. Robinson L, Gallos ID, Conner SJ, Rajkhowa M, Miller D, Lewis S, et al. The effect of sperm DNA fragmentation on miscarriage rates: a systematic review and meta-analysis. Hum Reprod. 2012;27:2908–17.
67. Evenson DP, Larson KL, Jost LK. Sperm chromatin structure assay: its clinical use for detecting sperm DNA fragmentation in male infertility and comparisons with other techniques. J Androl. 2002;23(1):25–43.
68. Bungum M, Bungum L, Giwercman A. Sperm chromatin structure assay (SCSA): a tool in Diagnosis and treatment of infertility. Asian J Androl. 2011;13:69–75.
69. Zhang Z, Zhu LL, Jiang HS, et al. Predictors of pregnancy outcome for infertile couples attending IVF and ICSI programmes. Andrologia. 2016;48(9):874–81.
70. Fernández JL, Muriel L, Rivero MT, Goyanes V, Vazquez R, Alvarez JG. The sperm chromatin dispersion test: a simple method for the determination of sperm DNA fragmentation. J Androl. 2003;24:59–66.
71. Chohan KR, Griffin JT, Lafromboise M, De Jonge CJ, Carrell DT. Comparison of chromatin assays for DNA fragmentation evaluation in human sperm. J Androl. 2006;27:53–9.
72. Muriel L, Meseguer M, Fernández JL, Alvarez J, Remohí J, Pellicer A, et al. Value of the sperm chromatin dispersion test in predicting pregnancy outcome in intrauterine insemination: a blind prospective study. Hum Reprod. 2006;21:738–44.
73. Klaude M, Eriksson S, Nygren J, Ahnström G. The Comet assay: mechanisms and technical considerations. Mutat Res. 1996;363:89–96.
74. Albert O, Reintsch WE, Chan P, Robaire B. HT-COMET: a novel automated approach for high throughput assessment of human sperm chromatin quality. Hum Reprod. 2016;31:938–46.
75. Cortés-Gutiérrez EI, López-Fernández C, Fernández JL, Dávila-Rodríguez MI, Johnston SD, Gosálvez J. Interpreting sperm DNA damage in a diverse range of mammalian sperm by means of the two-tailed comet assay. Front Genet. 2014;5:404.
76. Cortés-Gutiérrez EI, Fernández JL, Dávila-Rodríguez MI, López-Fernández C, Gosálvez J. Two-tailed comet assay (2T-Comet): simultaneous detection of DNA single and double-strand breaks. Methods Mol Biol. 2017;1560:285–93.
77. Agarwal A, Cho CL, Majzoub A, Esteves SC. The Society for Translational Medicine: clinical practice guidelines for sperm DNA fragmentation testing in male infertility. Transl Androl Urol. 2017;6(Suppl 4):S720–33.
78. ESHRE Guideline Group on RPL, Bender Atik R, Christiansen OB, Elson J, Kolte AM, Lewis S, et al. ESHRE guideline: recurrent pregnancy loss. Hum Reprod Open. 2018;2018:hoy004.
79. Colpi GM, Francavilla S, Haidl G, Link K, Behre HM, Goulis DG, et al. European Academy of Andrology guideline management of oligo-astheno-teratozoospermia. Andrology. 2018;6:513–24.
80. Tharakan T, Bettocchi C, Carvalho J, Corona G, Jones TH, Kadioglu A, EAU Working Panel on Male Sexual Reproductive Health, et al. European Association of Urology guidelines panel on male sexual and reproductive health: a clinical consultation guide on the indications

for performing sperm DNA fragmentation testing in men with infertility and testicular sperm extraction in nonazoospermic men. Eur Urol Focus. 2021;8(1):331–50.
81. Schlegel PN, Sigman M, Collura B, De Jonge CJ, Eisenberg ML, Lamb DJ, et al. Diagnosis and treatment of infertility in men: AUA/ASRM guideline. Linthicum (MD): American Urological Association; 2020. [cited 2021 Mar 31]
82. Balhorn R. Sperm chromatin: an overview. In: Zini A, Agarwal A, editors. Sperm chromatin: biological and clinical applications in male infertility. New York, USA: Springer; 2011. p. 3–18.
83. Agarwal A, Cho CL, Esteves SC. Should we evaluate and treat sperm DNA fragmentation? Curr Opin Obstet Gynecol. 2016;28:164–71.
84. Irvine DS, Twigg JP, Gordon EL, et al. DNA integrity in human spermatozoa: relationships with semen quality. J Androl. 2000;21:33–44.
85. Agarwal A, Cho CL, Esteves SC, Majzoub A. Current limitation and future perspective of sperm DNA fragmentation tests. Transl Androl Urol. 2017;6(Suppl. 4):S549–52.
86. Esteves SC, Sharma RK, Gosálvez J, et al. A translational medicine appraisal of specialized andrology testing in unexplained male infertility. Int Urol Nephrol. 2014;46:1037–52.
87. Buck Louis GM, Sundaram R, Schisterman EF, et al. Semen quality and time to pregnancy: the Longitudinal Investigation of Fertility and the Environment Study. Fertil Steril. 2014;101:453–62.
88. Agarwal A, Majzoub A, Esteves SC, et al. Clinical utility of sperm DNA fragmentation testing: practice recommendations based on clinical scenarios. Transl Androl Urol. 2016;5(6):935.
89. Sharma R, Harlev A, Agarwal A, Esteves SC. Cigarette smoking and semen quality: a new meta-analysis examining the effect of the 2010 World Health Organization laboratory methods for the examination of human semen. Eur Urol. 2016;70:635–45.
90. Aboulmaouahib S, Madkour A, Kaarouch I, Sefrioui O, Saadani B, Copin H, et al. Impact of alcohol and cigarette smoking consumption in male fertility potential: looks at lipid peroxidation, enzymatic antioxidant activities and sperm DNA damage. Andrologia. 2018;50(3):e12926.
91. Ranganathan P, Rao KA, Thalaivarasai BS. Deterioration of semen quality and sperm-DNA integrity as influenced by cigarette smoking in fertile and infertile human male smokers—a prospective study. J Cell Biochem. 2019;120:11784–93.
92. Mostafa RM, Nasrallah YS, Hassan MM, Farrag AF, Majzoub A, Agarwal A. The effect of cigarette smoking on human seminal parameters, sperm chromatin structure and condensation. Andrologia. 2018;50(3):e12910.
93. Rubes J, Selevan SG, Evenson DP, Zudova D, Vozdova M, Zudova Z, et al. Episodic air pollution is associated with increased DNA fragmentation in human sperm without other changes in semen quality. Hum Reprod. 2005;20:2776–83.
94. Sánchez-Peña LC, Reyes BE, López-Carrillo L, Recio R, Morán-Martínez J, Cebrián ME, et al. Organophosphorous pesticide exposure alters sperm chromatin structure in Mexican agricultural workers. Toxicol Appl Pharmacol. 2004;196:108–13.
95. Zhou DD, Hao JL, Guo KM, Lu CW, Liu XD. Sperm quality and DNA damage in men from Jilin Province, China, who are occupationally exposed to ionizing radiation. Genet Mol Res. 2016;15:gmr8078.
96. Jamal F, Haque QS, Singh S, Rastogi SK. The influence of organophosphate and carbamate on sperm chromatin and reproductive hormones among pesticide sprayers. Toxicol Ind Health. 2016;32:1527–36.
97. Lafuente R, García-Blàquez N, Jacquemin B, Checa MA. Outdoor air pollution and sperm quality. Fertil Steril. 2016;106:880–96.
98. Sepidarkish M, Maleki-Hajiagha A, Maroufizadeh S, Rezaeinejad M, Almasi-Hashiani A, Razavi M. The effect of body mass index on sperm DNA fragmentation: a systematic review and meta-analysis. Int J Obes. 2020;44:549–58.
99. Samavat J, Cantini G, Lotti F, Di Franco A, Tamburrino L, Degl'Innocenti S, et al. Massive weight loss obtained by bariatric surgery affects semen quality in morbid male obesity: a preliminary prospective double-armed study. Obes Surg. 2018;28:69–76.

100. Carette C, Levy R, Eustache F, Baron G, Coupaye M, Msika S, et al. Changes in total sperm count after gastric bypass and sleeve gastrectomy: the BARIASPERM prospective study. Surg Obes Relat Dis. 2019;15:1271–9.
101. Faure C, Dupont C, Baraibar MA, Ladouce R, Cedrin-Durnerin I, Wolf JP, et al. In subfertile couple, abdominal fat loss in men is associated with improvement of sperm quality and pregnancy: a case-series. PLoS One. 2014;9:e86300.
102. Agarwal A, Gupta S, Du Plessis S, Sharma R, Esteves SC, Cirenza C, et al. Abstinence time and its impact on basic and advanced semen parameters. Urology. 2016;94:102–10.
103. Mayorga-Torres BJ, Camargo M, Agarwal A, du Plessis SS, Cadavid ÁP, Cardona Maya WD. Influence of ejaculation frequency on seminal parameters. Reprod Biol Endocrinol. 2015;13:47.
104. Jurema MW, Vieira AD, Bankowski B, Petrella C, Zhao Y, Wallach E, et al. Effect of ejaculatory abstinence period on the pregnancy rate after intrauterine insemination. Fertil Steril. 2005;84:678–81.
105. Marshburn PB, Alanis M, Matthews ML, Usadi R, Papadakis MH, Kullstam S, et al. A short period of ejaculatory abstinence before intrauterine insemination is associated with higher pregnancy rates. Fertil Steril. 2010;93:286–8.
106. Bahadur G, Almossawi O, Illahibuccus A, Al-Habib A, Okolo S. Factors leading to pregnancies in stimulated intrauterine insemination cycles and the use of consecutive ejaculations within a small clinic environment. J Obstet Gynaecol India. 2016;66(Suppl 1):513–20.
107. Sánchez-Martín P, Sánchez-Martín F, González-Martínez M, Gosálvez J. Increased pregnancy after reduced male abstinence. Syst Biol Reprod Med. 2013;59:256–60.
108. Pasqualotto FF, Sharma RK, Potts JM, Nelson DR, Thomas AJ, Agarwal A. Seminal oxidative stress in patients with chronic prostatitis. Urology. 2000;55:881–5.
109. Aitken RJ, De Iuliis GN. Origins and consequences of DNA damage in male germ cells. Reprod Biomed Online. 2007;14:727–33.
110. Gallegos G, Ramos B, Santiso R, Goyanes V, Gosálvez J, Fernández JL. Sperm DNA fragmentation in infertile men with genitourinary infection by Chlamydia trachomatis and Mycoplasma. Fertil Steril. 2008;90:328–34.
111. Hamada A, Agarwal A, Sharma R, French DB, Ragheb A, Sabanegh ES. Jr Empirical treatment of low-level leukocytospermia with doxycycline in male infertility patients. Urology. 2011;78:1320–5.
112. Esteves SC, Santi D, Simoni M. An update on clinical and surgical interventions to reduce sperm DNA fragmentation in infertile men. Andrology. 2020;8:53–81.
113. Agarwal A, Majzoub A, Baskaran S, et al. Sperm DNA fragmentation: a new guideline for clinicians. World J Mens Health. 2020;38(4):412–71.
114. Roque M, Esteves SC. Effect of varicocele repair on sperm DNA fragmentation: a review. Int Urol Nephrol. 2018;50:583–603.
115. Smit M, Romijn JC, Wildhagen MF, Veldhoven JL, Weber RF, Dohle GR. Decreased sperm DNA fragmentation after surgical varicocelectomy is associated with increased pregnancy rate. J Urol. 2013;189(Suppl. 1):S146–50.
116. Stenqvist A, Oleszczuk K, Leijonhufvud I, Giwercman A. Impact of antioxidant treatment on DNA fragmentation index: a double-blind placebo-controlled randomized trial. Andrology. 2018;6:811–6.
117. Showell MG, Mackenzie-Proctor R, Brown J, Yazdani A, Stankiewicz MT, Hart RJ. Antioxidants for male subfertility. Cochrane Database Syst Rev. 2014;(12):CD007411.
118. Amar E, Cornet D, Cohen M, Ménézo Y. Treatment for high levels of sperm DNA fragmentation and nuclear decondensation: sequential treatment with a potent antioxidant followed by stimulation of the one-carbon cycle vs one-carbon cycle back-up alone. Austin J Reprod Med Infertil. 2015;2:1006.
119. Ménézo YJ, Hazout A, Panteix G, Robert F, Rollet J, Cohen-Bacrie P, et al. Antioxidants to reduce sperm DNA fragmentation: an unexpected adverse effect. Reprod Biomed Online. 2007;14:418–21.

120. Micic S, Lalic N, Djordjevic D, Bojanic N, Bogavac-Stanojevic N, Busetto GM, et al. Double-blind, randomized, placebo-controlled trial on the effect of L-carnitine and L-acetylcarnitine on sperm parameters in men with idiopathic oligo asthenozoospermia. Andrologia. 2019;51:e13267.
121. Tunc O, Thompson J, Tremellen K. Improvement in sperm DNA quality using an oral antioxidant therapy. Reprod Biomed Online. 2009;18:761–8.
122. Greco E, Iacobelli M, Rienzi L, Ubaldi F, Ferrero S, Tesarik J. Reduction of the incidence of sperm DNA fragmentation by oral antioxidant treatment. J Androl. 2005;26:349–53.
123. Henkel R, Sandhu IS, Agarwal A. The excessive use of antioxidant therapy: a possible cause of male infertility? Andrologia. 2019;51:e13162.
124. Schisterman EF, Sjaarda LA, Clemons T, Carrell DT, Perkins NJ, Johnstone E, et al. Effect of folic acid and zinc supplementation in men on semen quality and live birth among couples undergoing infertility treatment: a randomized clinical trial. JAMA. 2020;323:35–48.
125. Xie P, Keating D, Parrella A, Cheung S, Rosenwaks Z, Goldstein M, et al. Sperm genomic integrity by TUNEL varies throughout the male genital tract. J Urol. 2020;203:802–8.
126. Moskovtsev SI, Jarvi K, Mullen JB, Cadesky KI, Hannam T, Lo KC. Testicular spermatozoa have statistically significantly lower DNA damage than ejaculated spermatozoa in patients with unsuccessful oral antioxidant treatment. Fertil Steril. 2010;93:1142–6.
127. Esteves SC, Roque M, Bradley CK, Garrido N. Reproductive outcomes of testicular versus ejaculated sperm for intracytoplasmic sperm injection among men with high levels of DNA fragmentation in semen: systematic review and meta-analysis. Fertil Steril. 2017;108:456–467.e1.
128. Greco E, Scarselli F, Iacobelli M, Rienzi L, Ubaldi F, Ferrero S, et al. Efficient treatment of infertility due to sperm DNA damage by ICSI with testicular spermatozoa. Hum Reprod. 2005;20:226–30.
129. Bradley CK, McArthur SJ, Gee AJ, Weiss KA, Schmidt U, Toogood L. Intervention improves assisted conception intracytoplasmic sperm injection outcomes for patients with high levels of sperm DNA fragmentation: a retrospective analysis. Andrology. 2016;4:903–10.
130. Lopushnyan NA, Walsh TJ. Surgical techniques for the management of male infertility. Asian J Androl. 2012;14:94–102.
131. Mehta A, Esteves SC, Schlegel PN, Niederberger CI, Sigman M, Zini A, et al. Use of testicular sperm in nonazoospermic males. Fertil Steril. 2018;109:981–7.
132. Cheung S, Schlegel PN, Rosenwaks Z, Palermo GD. Revisiting aneuploidy profile of surgically retrieved spermatozoa by whole exome sequencing molecular karyotype. PLoS One. 2019;14:e0210079.
133. Muratori M, Maggi M, Spinelli S, Filimberti E, Forti G, Baldi E. Spontaneous DNA fragmentation in swim-up selected human spermatozoa during long term incubation. J Androl. 2003;24:253–62.
134. Di Santo M, Tarozzi N, Nadalini M, Borini A. Human sperm cryopreservation: update on techniques, effect on DNA integrity, and implications for ART. Adv Urol. 2012;2012:854837.
135. Ahmed I, Abdelateef S, Laqqan M, Amor H, Abdel-Lah MA, Hammadeh ME. Influence of extended incubation time on human sperm chromatin condensation, sperm DNA strand breaks and their effect on fertilization rate. Andrologia. 2018;50(4):e12960.
136. Raad G, Lteif L, Lahoud R, Azoury J, Azoury J, Tanios J, et al. Cryopreservation media differentially affect sperm motility, morphology and DNA integrity. Andrology. 2018;6:836–45.
137. Volpes A, Sammartano F, Rizzari S, Gullo S, Marino A, Allegra A. The pellet swim-up is the best technique for sperm preparation during in vitro fertilization procedures. J Assist Reprod Genet. 2016;33:765–70.
138. Vozdova M, Kasikova K, Oracova E, Prinosilova P, Rybar R, Horinova V, et al. The effect of the swim-up and hyaluronan-binding methods on the frequency of abnormal spermatozoa detected by FISH and SCSA in carriers of balanced chromosomal translocations. Hum Reprod. 2012;27:930–7.

139. Oguz Y, Guler I, Erdem A, Mutlu MF, Gumuslu S, Oktem M, et al. The effect of swim-up and gradient sperm preparation techniques on deoxyribonucleic acid (DNA) fragmentation in subfertile patients. J Assist Reprod Genet. 2018;35:1083–9.
140. Zini A, Finelli A, Phang D, Jarvi K. Influence of semen processing technique on human sperm DNA integrity. Urology. 2000;56:1081–4.
141. Rawe VY, Boudri HU, Alvarez Sedó C, Carro M, Papier S, Nodar F. Healthy baby born after reduction of sperm DNA fragmentation using cell sorting before ICSI. Reprod Biomed Online. 2010;20:320–3.
142. Lee TH, Liu CH, Shih YT, Tsao HM, Huang CC, Chen HH, et al. Magnetic-activated cell sorting for sperm preparation reduces spermatozoa with apoptotic markers and improves the acrosome reaction in couples with unexplained infertility. Hum Reprod. 2010;25:839–46.
143. Gil M, Sar-Shalom V, Melendez Sivira Y, Carreras R, Checa MA. Sperm selection using magnetically activated cell sorting (MACS) in assisted reproduction: a systematic review and meta-analysis. J Assist Reprod Genet. 2013;30:479–85.
144. Tavalaee M, Deemeh MR, Arbabian M, Nasr-Esfahani MH. Density gradient centrifugation before or after magnetic-activated cell sorting: which technique is more useful for clinical sperm selection? J Assist Reprod Genet. 2012;29:31–8.
145. Delbes G, Herrero MB, Troeung ET, Chan PT. The use of complementary assays to evaluate the enrichment of human sperm quality in asthenoteratozoospermic and teratozoospermia samples processed with Annexin-V magnetic activated cell sorting. Andrology. 2013;1:698–706.
146. Bucar S, Gonçalves A, Rocha E, Barros A, Sousa M, Sá R. DNA fragmentation in human sperm after magnetic-activated cell sorting. J Assist Reprod Genet. 2015;32:147–54.
147. Zhang H, Xuan X, Yang S, Li X, Xu C, Gao X. Selection of viable human spermatozoa with low levels of DNA fragmentation from an immotile population using density gradient centrifugation and magnetic-activated cell sorting. Andrologia. 2018;50(1):e12821.
148. Franco JG Jr, Baruffi RL, Mauri AL, Petersen CG, Oliveira JB, Vagnini L. Significance of large nuclear vacuoles in human spermatozoa: implications for ICSI. Reprod Biomed Online. 2008;17:42–5.
149. Garolla A, Fortini D, Menegazzo M, De Toni L, Nicoletti V, Moretti A, et al. High-power microscopy for selecting spermatozoa for ICSI by physiological status. Reprod Biomed Online. 2008;17:610–6.
150. Quinn MM, Jalalian L, Ribeiro S, Ona K, Demirci U, Cedars MI, et al. Microfluidic sorting selects sperm for clinical use with reduced DNA damage compared to density gradient centrifugation with swim-up in split semen samples. Hum Reprod. 2018;33:1388–93.
151. Parmegiani L, Cognigni GE, Bernardi S, Troilo E, Ciampaglia W, Filicori M. "Physiologic ICSI": hyaluronic acid (HA) favors selection of spermatozoa without DNA fragmentation and with normal nucleus, resulting in improvement of embryo quality. Fertil Steril. 2010;93:598–604.
152. Mongkolchaipak S, Vutyavanich T. No difference in high-magnification morphology and hyaluronic acid binding in the selection of euploid spermatozoa with intact DNA. Asian J Androl. 2013;15:421–4.
153. Nosrati R, Vollmer M, Eamer L, San Gabriel MC, Zeidan K, Zini A, et al. Rapid selection of sperm with high DNA integrity. Lab Chip. 2014;14:1142–50.
154. Agarwal A, Farkouh A, Parekh N, Zini A, Arafa M, Kandil H, et al. Sperm DNA fragmentation: a critical assessment of clinical practice guidelines. World J Mens Health. 2022;40(1):30–7.

Part III
Male Oxidative Stress Infertility (MOSI)

Chapter 6
Pathophysiology of Seminal Oxidative Stress

Marlon Martinez and Lucia Rocco

Key Points

- In this chapter, we review the mechanisms that in male infertility underlay the so-called oxidative paradox, defined as a delicate balance between oxidative stress and antioxidant ability.
- Also, we discuss the different roles of ROS on sperm pathophysiology, with particular attention to their effects on sperm functions.
- Additionally, we focus on the techniques available to evaluate the redox status in semen and on the clinical use of redox biomarkers for the diagnosis and management of male infertility.
- Finally, we describe new oxidative biomarkers to better study male infertility, predict reproductive success, and modify assisted reproductive technologies to minimize oxidative stress.

Introduction

Oxidative stress (OS) is a condition that occurs when oxidants overcome the antioxidant defense systems of cells. Several studies have confirmed the production of a whole range of oxidants by different cell types. They are commonly referred to as reactive oxygen species (ROS) and include the hydroxyl (OH), superoxide anion (O_2^-), and hydrogen peroxide (H_2O_2) radicals [1].

The excess oxidants can take part in specific and nonspecific reactions with nearby cellular components such as unsaturated lipids, proteins, and DNA, consequently compromising normal cellular processes. Oxidative stress has been associated with various diseases such as cardiovascular disease, diabetes, brain disorders (for example, Alzheimer's), as well as female and male infertility [2].

M. Martinez
Section of Urology, University of Santo Tomas Hospital, Manila, Philippines

L. Rocco (✉)
Department of Environmental, Biological and Pharmaceutical Sciences and Technologies (DiSTABiF), University of Campania "L. Vanvitelli", Caserta, Italy
e-mail: lucia.rocco@unicampania.it

A. Agarwal et al. (eds.), *Current and Future Advances in Male Infertility*,
https://doi.org/10.1007/978-3-031-62648-7_6

Currently, OS is believed to be an important and plausible cause of idiopathic male infertility. The involvement of ROS in male infertility derives from their ability to induce harmful chemical and structural changes to sperm DNA, as well as to proteins and lipids of plasma and mitochondrial membranes [3] (Fig. 6.1).

Of the four bases of DNA, guanine is the most susceptible to oxidation, and the most common oxidative lesions of DNA are 8-hydroxy-2′-deoxyguanosine (8-OHdG), which is highly mutagenic. 8-OHdG is repaired by 8-oxoguanine DNA glycosylase-1 (OGG1) during the DNA base excision repair (BER) pathway [4]. Furthermore, DNA fragmentation can damage the paternal genetic contribution to the development of the embryo [5].

In the past decade, significant improvements have been made in our understanding of sperm cell biology and ability to diagnose and treat male infertility. This is the result of combined approaches of advanced proteomics, biochemistry, and functional genomics. However, research approaches focusing on single genes or omics levels have so far yielded limited results. While many contributing factors have been identified with these methods, the complex mechanism of male infertility remains unclear. For this purpose, an integrated multi-omics approach may be more beneficial in understanding the disease process [6].

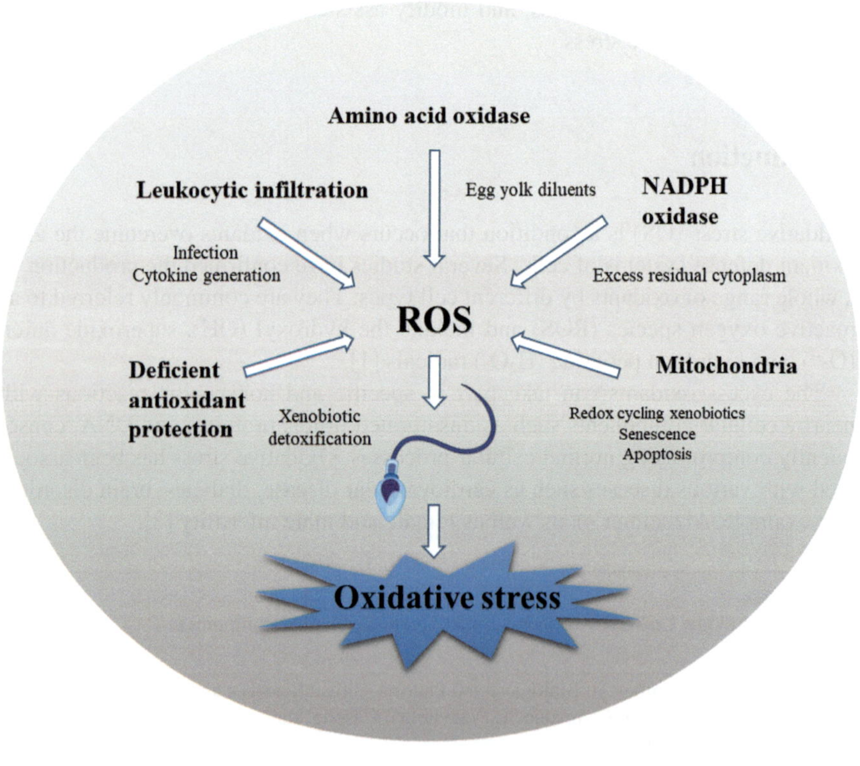

Fig. 6.1 The main factors leading to the formation of reactive oxygen species (ROS) that cause oxidative stress in sperm

In this review, we focus on the role of ROS and OS in male infertility. Additionally, we summarize the techniques available to evaluate the redox status in semen and the clinical use of redox biomarkers for the diagnosis and management of male infertility. Further, we describe new oxidative biomarkers and multi-omics approaches to better study the relationship of OS and male infertility.

Role of Reactive Oxygen Species and Oxidative Stress in Male Infertility

Reactive oxygen species (ROS) are natural by-products of oxygen metabolism. The biologically important ROS include superoxide anions, hydrogen peroxide, and hydroxyl radicals [7]. In order to achieve ground state, two complementary electrons should be moving in an opposite direction in its outer orbit. Addition of extra electron to oxygen can result in the formation of superoxide anion radical, which can be converted to other forms of ROS [8]. Sequential transfer of electrons from complete reduction to water leads to generation of hydroperoxide and hydroxyl radical (Fig. 6.2). Reactive oxygen species can act as free radicals due to unpaired electrons in their outer orbit. These will transform them into unstable and highly reactive molecules with a very short half-life of nanosecond to millisecond range [9]. They will steal electrons from surrounding molecules to maintain a stable ground state. However, during this course, this other molecule loses an electron with subsequent formation of new radical leading to radical chain reactions. This can induce cellular damage by acting as oxidants leading to oxidation of lipids, proteins,

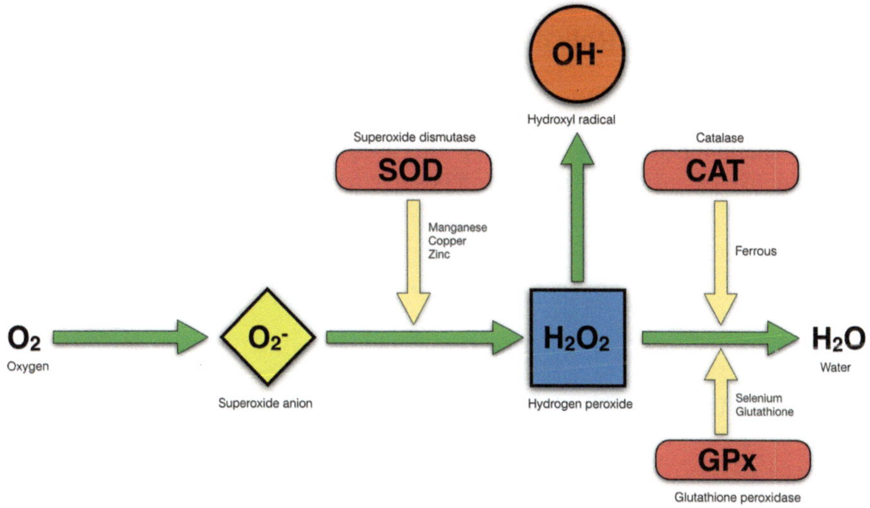

Fig. 6.2 Generation of ROS from sequential transfer of electrons from complete reduction to water

and amino acids [5]. They can only become stable once they obtain electrons from nearby molecules.

Biological homeostasis is achieved through a balance between ROS and antioxidants, which act as reducing agents that react and buffer with ROS [10]. These antioxidants can be categorized as enzymatic and nonenzymatic [7]. There are several antioxidants, such as superoxide dismutase (SOD), catalase (CAT), and glutathione peroxidase (GPx), that act as first body defense against the attack of ROS [11]. SOD, with cofactors manganese, copper, or zinc, converts the superoxide anion into hydrogen peroxide, which can be further eliminated by CAT and GPx [12]. Catalase converts hydrogen peroxide into water and molecular oxygen. On the other hand, GPx, with cofactor selenium, catalyzes the reduction of hydrogen peroxide and other organic peroxides into water and alcohol.

When there are overproduction and overactivity of ROS against antioxidants, this will result in biological imbalance called OS (Fig. 6.3) [13]. Sperm can become highly susceptible to the threat of OS once they lose their capabilities to scavenge these free radicals. In addition, deficient cellular repair systems and scarce antioxidant defenses expose them to its detrimental effects [14].

These most relevant ROS are believed to play a vital role in the so-called free radical theory of infertility [8]. Generation of ROS entails several processes resulting in negative impact on reproductive potential [15]. About 30–80% of cases of male factor infertility are believed to have an elevated ROS level in seminal plasma [16]. A novel descriptor termed as male oxidative stress infertility (MOSI) was introduced to describe infertile men with abnormal semen parameters, positive evidence of OS, and normal female partner evaluation [17]. This includes men previously classified under idiopathic male factor infertility.

The Physiological Role of ROS in Sperm Cells

Several studies have shown that physiological amounts of ROS are necessary for normal sperm functions (Fig. 6.4) [18]. This integral role warrants understanding of the oxidative balance that will result in positive fertilizing ability of the sperm.

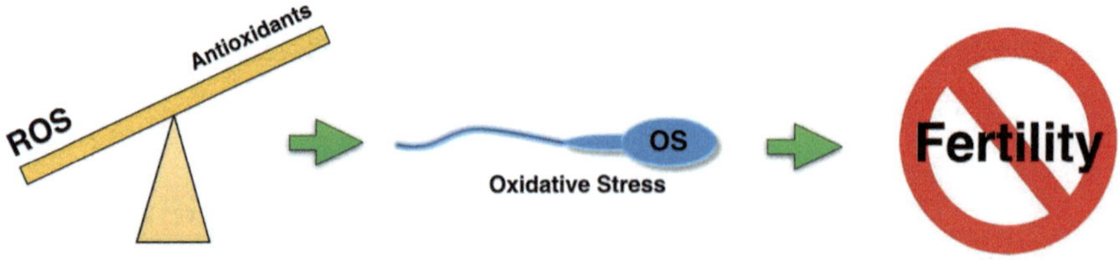

Fig. 6.3 Overproduction and overactivity of ROS against antioxidants will lead to OS. This will eventually result in poor reproductive potential in males

Maturation

Sperm acquire their full maturation while on transit along the epididymal tubules [14]. This is highly influenced by a physiological amount of ROS. Their presence is essential in the formation of disulfide bonds securing densely packed chromatin stability and protecting sperm DNA from any insult.

Capacitation

A prerequisite event before sperm achieve their fertilizing ability is capacitation [19]. Reactive oxygen species plays significant role in this process by converting adenosine triphosphate (ATP) into cyclic adenosine monophosphate (cAMP), which is activated by bicarbonate and calcium. This results in stimulation of the protein kinase A phosphorylation cascade, regulation of the tyrosine phosphorylation in the tail of the sperm, and induction of sterol oxidation.

Acrosome Reaction

Reactive oxygen species facilitate the penetration and fusion of sperm with oocyte by phosphorylation of the tyrosine proteins of the plasma membrane [18]. This enables the sperm to travel across the cumulus oophorus and attach itself to the zone pellucida wherein they can release the proteolytic enzymes necessary to achieve fertilization.

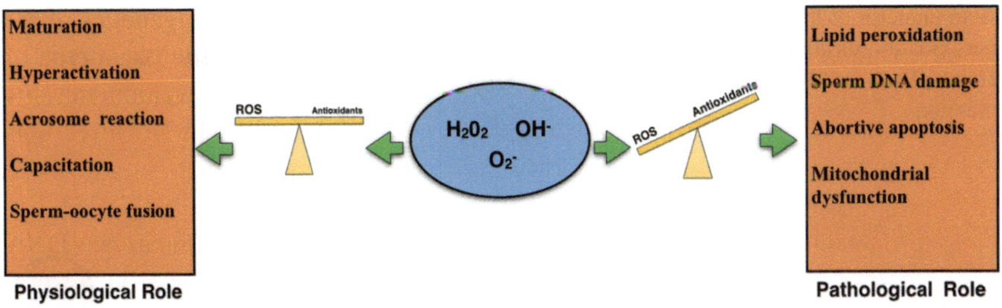

Fig. 6.4 Physiological and pathological roles of ROS

Sperm-Oocyte Fusion

A favorable outcome on the interaction between the sperm and oocyte can be expected after an uneventful capacitation and acrosome reaction as being facilitated by ROS. They increase sperm plasma membrane fluidity necessary for fusion of these two cellular components [20]. This is achieved by preventing the deactivation of phospholipase A2, thereby allowing this to cleave the polyunsaturated fatty acids (PUFAs) of the sperm plasma membrane.

Pathological Role of ROS in Sperm Cells

The pathological impact of ROS on reproductive potential is due to imbalance between OS and antioxidant capacity. These include lipid peroxidation (LPO), sperm DNA damage, mitochondrial dysfunction, and abortive apoptosis (Fig. 6.4).

Lipid Peroxidation

The effect of OS on human sperm plasma membrane through LPO was first introduced by Jones et al. [21]. Due to high abundance of PUFA in their plasma membrane, sperm are vulnerable to the attack of ROS. Reduction in the fluidity of the plasma membrane caused by insult to the double bonds in the PUFA affects the normal sperm physiologic functions like capacitation, acrosome reaction, and sperm-oocyte fusion [22]. Hydroxyl radical is an inductor of LPO through two significant reactions (Fig. 6.5). In Haber-Weiss reaction, ferric ion is reduced to ferrous ion in the presence of superoxide radical [23]. This is followed by Fenton reaction wherein the ferrous ion reacts with hydrogen peroxide forming back the ferric ion and the hydroxyl radical. Malondialdehyde (MDA) is a known mutagenic product of LPO, which is an essential indirect marker of OS [24].

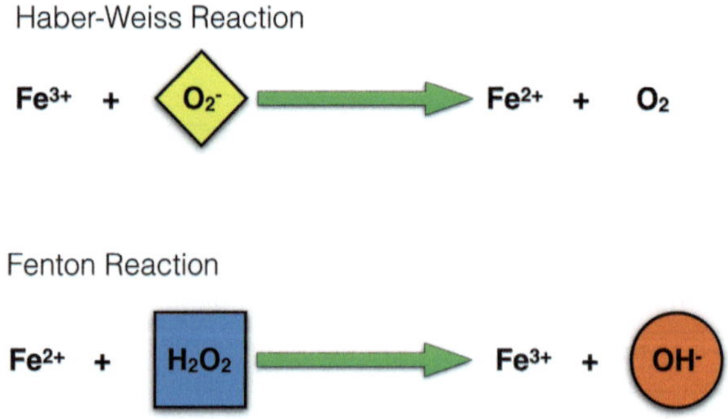

Fig. 6.5 Hydroxyl radical is an inductor of lipid peroxidation through Haber-Weiss and Fenton reaction

Sperm DNA Fragmentation

Due to less compact fashion of packaging of mitochondrial DNA and absent DNA repair systems of nuclear DNA, these make the sperm highly susceptible to the attack of ROS leading to DNA damage [9]. Most of the sperm DNA damage are ROS induced. They inflict DNA damage through single- and double-stranded DNA breaks, DNA mutations, and direct oxidation of DNA bases [25].

Apoptosis

Apoptosis is a physiological event which involves cellular mechanism responsible for controlled cell death. Tight control in this process is necessary to secure that only intact germ cells become mature sperm with normal genetic compositions and functions. Abundant levels of ROS leading to OS activate the cascading steps of apoptosis pathways [26]. These pathways lead to activation of caspase-3 responsible for cross-linking of proteins [27]. In addition, other processes, such as cytoskeletal and nuclear degradation, sperm DNA fragmentation, and expression of phagocytic receptors, also lead to phagocytosis of the cells and their components.

Mitochondrial Dysfunction

The entire development of the sperm from production to maturation requires high-energy-demanding processes [28]. Mitochondria, as the site of production of ATP through aerobic respiration and electron transport chain, might serve as a tool for the generation of excessive ROS causing abnormal sperm parameters.

ROS Sources in Seminal Plasma

There are several endogenous sources of ROS in seminal plasma [14, 29]. These include leukocytes and immature sperm.

Leukocytes are usually present in semen, mainly composed of macrophages and polymorphonuclear leukocytes which are the main source of ROS [30]. One of the significant contributors to the generation of ROS is the activated leukocytes [18]. Activated seminal leukocytes can produce 1000 times more ROS than aerobic metabolism [31]. There are several studies that link a negative relationship between seminal leukocytes and male fertility potential. Activation of leukocytes can be triggered as response to infection or inflammation [32]. Reaction to these stimuli causes the nicotinamide adenine dinucleotide phosphate (NADPH) oxidase to catalyze the formation of free radicals necessary to control the infection. This is facilitated, through the hexose monophosphate shunt, with subsequent formation of reduced NADPH and production of superoxide anion [33].

Immature spermatozoa with excess cytoplasm around the midpiece contribute to the bulk of seminal OS [34]. Reactive oxygen species are generated by immature sperm by the production of superoxide anion, and oxidation-reduction in mitochondria generate ROS.

There are several exogenous etiologies that can induce OS [35]. These include alcohol consumption, cigarette smoking, obesity, diabetes, physical exercise, psychological stress, aging, environmental factors, infections, toxins, chemotherapy, and radiation. Testicular hyperthermia is a known pathologic reason causing the detrimental effect of varicocele on reproductive outcome through production of excessive amount of ROS [36]. This also inactivates enzymes and proteins necessary for sperm production.

Redox Status in Semen

Methods to Assess Redox Status

Despite the established role of ROS in male infertility, literature still lacks consensus on selection of patients for ROS testing, ideal ROS test, and treatment options, which can result in good reproductive outcome [7].

In a routine semen analysis, there are certain basic abnormal parameters that might suggest the presence of OS [14]. These include the findings of asthenozoospermia, teratozoospermia, hyperviscosity, and leukocytospermia. However, these may represent indirect signs of OS and are therefore nonconclusive. In the latest sixth edition of the World Health Organization (WHO) laboratory manual for semen analysis, tests for OS and ROS were described under advanced examination [37]. Therefore, these tests are still not recommended in the routine evaluation of infertile men [38]. In a global online survey joined by 1327 reproductive specialists on the use of OS testing, 65.7% of respondents stated that they are not requesting these tests [39]. Presence of lifestyle factors and sperm abnormalities are the most common indications of those respondents who are ordering the tests. There are several tests to measure OS [7, 40–42] (Table 6.1). Direct tests, such as chemiluminescence, flow cytometry, electron spin resonance, cytochrome c reduction, and nitroblue tetrazolium, measure ROS production and sperm cell oxidation. On the other hand, indirect tests, such as lipid peroxidation, evaluate oxidation by measuring the markers of insult from the ROS.

A novel method called male infertility oxidative system (MiOXSYS) was introduced to measure oxidation reduction potential (ORP) levels in semen and seminal plasma [43]. The transfer of electrons from a reductant to an oxidant can be analyzed through this galvanostat-based technology. The ORP cutoff value of

Table 6.1 Direct and indirect measurement of OS in human semen

Direct assay	
Chemiluminescence	Quantifies both intracellular and extracellular ROS using sensitive probes such as luminol and lucigenin Threshold values <102.2 RLU/s/10^6 sperm/ml are used to differentiate infertile from fertile population
Flow cytometry	Quantities the amount of fluorescence per cell emitted by dyes or monoclonal antibodies used to bind selected molecules Based on the ROS-mediated dye oxidation with fluorescence compound Green and red fluorescence
Nitroblue tetrazolium (NBT)	Based on the conversion of NBT into a blue pigment called diformazan after the interaction with superoxide released from sperm or leukocytes Threshold value of 24 μg formazan/10^7 is used to differentiate fertility status
Electron spin resonance	Obtains absorption spectra of the spin energy of unpaired electrons
Cytochrome c reduction	Identification of reduction of superoxide radicals to ferricytochrome
Indirect assay	
MDA-thiobarbituric acid (TBA) adduct detection assay	MDA forms a 1:2 adduct with TBA producing colored substance that can be measured by fluorometry and spectrophotometry LPO marker Results are expressed as nmol MDA/10^7 sperm
ORP (MiOYSYS)	Based on galvanostatic measure of electron transfer during reductive reactions from antioxidants to oxidants Cutoff value of 1.34 mV/106 sperm/ml
Myeloperoxidase test	Identification of granulocytes in seminal fluid using benzidine to buffer and assess samples for peroxidase activity
Total antioxidant capacity	Evaluation of antioxidant status in seminal plasma

1.34 mV/10^6 sperm/ml can be used to differentiate between abnormal semen parameters with OS and those without abnormality [41, 44]. This threshold value provided a sensitivity of 98.1%, specificity of 40.6%, positive predictive value of 94.7%, and negative predictive value of 66.6%.

Redox Biomarkers of Male Infertility

New approach in the evaluation of infertile men includes the use of the different redox biomarkers. Some of the established biomarkers of OS are free thiols and MDA [45]. In a study of 50 infertile men, there was a significant correlation between free thiol levels and sperm concentration and progressive motility. Likewise, negative correlation was observed between MDA level and sperm concentration. Several seminal plasma proteomic biomarkers of OS were identified in patients with OS [46]. Overexpression of seminal proteins was observed in infertile men with increased OS. These proteins include the aldose reductase, 1-chymotrypsin, DJ-1, haptoglobin, mucin 5B, peroxiredoxin 4, prolactin-induced protein, protein S100A9, and tubulin folding cofactor B. In addition, 23 proteins were demonstrated differently in conditions induced by ROS such as varicocele, male accessory gland infection, smoking, and obesity. In a comparative study between infertile (n = 15) and fertile men (n = 15), the former had significantly higher MDA levels [47]. In contrast, levels of total redox antioxidant potential and glutathione were significantly lower in infertile men. In a meta-analysis involving 65 studies, infertile men had significantly higher concentrations of MDA, nitric oxide, and carbonyl proteins in their seminal plasma [48]. On the contrary, significant lower concentrations of glutathione (GSH), vitamin C, and vitamin E and lower activities of CAT, GPx, and glutathione S-transferase were observed in same set of patients.

Measurement of ORP is a new technique to assess OS in seminal fluid. Oxidation-reduction potential is the measure of transfer of electrons from a reductant to an oxidant [49]. This reflects the existing balance between oxidants and antioxidants in a biological system. Management of men with elevated ORP should be guided by the initial OS status [44]. It is believed that eradicating the underlying etiologies of OS will result in reduction of the ORP levels and favorable reproductive outcomes [2].

Also, the standardization of probes to detect DNA oxidation in the form of 8-OHdG has also been used as a biomarker of oxidative stress in a reproductive context, in particular to assess oxidative stress in sperm [50].

Treatment of OS-Related Male Infertility

Treatment options for infertile men should directly address specific etiologies induced by OS. Further studies are warranted to develop strategies that will determine the real impact of ROS on fertility potential and the consequence of its management to reproductive outcomes [12].

There are several antioxidants that are known to improve semen parameters, sperm functions, and reproductive outcomes [51]. A recent Cochrane database systematic review indicated that antioxidant supplementation for infertile men is significantly associated with increased pregnancy rate (OR 1.89), increased live birth rate (OR 1.43), and decreased miscarriage rate (OR 1.46) [52]. However, it is associated with increased chance of gastrointestinal discomfort (2.70). Despite the positive effects, most of the included studies provided low-certainty evidence. In an online survey conducted globally, eight out of ten respondents stated that they are prescribing antioxidants to infertile men [39]. Majority of participants indicated that they give these supplements for 3 months (43.7%). There is still no recommendation for specific supplements to use for infertile men [53].

Varicocele does not only affect the basic semen parameters, but it also has a negative impact on advanced sperm functions resulting in increased SDF and OS in semen [54]. Varicocele is known to cause OS, leading to poor reproductive potential [42]. Sperm are susceptible to the effect of OS by varicocele due to limited capacity of DNA repair system [55]. The American Urological Association (AUA) and the American Society for Reproductive Medicine (ASRM) recommend varicocelectomy in infertile males who are not azoospermic but exhibit abnormal seminal parameters. These recommendations are based on two meta-analyses, which report a statistically significant improvement in seminal parameters, particularly an increase in sperm concentration, total sperm count, and total sperm motility, especially progressive motility [56]. However, following surgical repair of varicocele, a non-statistically significant reduction in sperm vitality has been observed, although there are no studies on this marker of sperm quality [57]. Therefore, these meta-analyses provide additional evidence in favor of the role of varicocelectomy in infertile men.

Varicocelectomy has been associated with a reduction in 8-hydroxy-2′-deoxyguanosine (8-OHdG) content in spermatozoa DNA and increases in seminal plasma protein thiols and ascorbic acid in 30 infertile men 6 months after the surgery [58]. Likewise, varicocelectomy increases the antioxidant activity of seminal plasma. In a study of 68 infertile men with varicoceles, there was a significant increase in the seminal levels of SOD, CAT, GPx, and vitamin C after 3 months of surgical correction of varicocele [59]. Another prospective study of 60 men with varicocele and abnormal semen parameters found significant reduction in ROS levels and significant increase in TAC 3–6 months postoperatively [60]. In addition, varicocelectomy can improve static ORP [61]. In a prospective clinical trial involving 49 subjects, there was significant improvement of static ORP after 3 months of surgery compared to its preoperative level.

Male accessory gland infection is known to cause detrimental effect on the altered secretory functions of the epididymis, seminal vesicles, and prostate [62]. This leads to reduction of the scavenging properties of the seminal plasma along the reproductive tract. Treatment with antibiotics and anti-inflammatories aids in the reduction of the excessive amount of these ROS-producing leukocytes in the seminal plasma [63]. Other therapeutic options, such as low-dose corticosteroids, mast cell blockers, and other immune modulatory compounds, are believed to decrease pathogenic bacteria in the ejaculate [64].

Lifestyle modifications are also recommended to improve OS in men suffering from poor reproductive potential [17]. These include exercise, weight loss, and cessation of smoking and healthy balanced diet.

Insights into Future Redox Biomarker Research

Omics studies include several study areas: genomics (at the gene level), transcriptomics (at the level of transcription products), proteomics (at the protein level), and metabolomics (at the metabolite level) [65].

Certainly, omics approach will allow the identification of unknown genetic factors and the diagnosis of male fertility in the near future [6]. Among them, metabolomics is expected to become a very powerful tool for diagnostic testing [66]. The metabolomic studies by Minai-Tehrani and co-workers [67] have associated altered levels of OS, glycerylphosphorylcholine, citrate, and lactate with male infertility. Furthermore, disciplines such as glycomics and lipidomics were found capable to identify other diagnostic targets, such as increased levels of arachidonic acid and other fatty acids in sperm [68]. Furthermore, it has been suggested that the seminal plasma glycome profile may be associated with male reproductive potential [69].

Summary

Seminal ROS are necessary for normal sperm physiological functions. However, overproduction of these natural by-products of oxygen metabolism can lead to OS. There are endogenous and exogenous sources of ROS in seminal plasma, which is known to cause detrimental effects to sperm, which can lead to poor male fertility potential and subsequent undesirable reproductive outcomes. This may lead to decreased fertilization, implantation, and pregnancy and live birth rates while increase in miscarriage rate.

Although semen analysis is considered as the cornerstone in the initial evaluation of infertile men, it cannot directly detect the presence of OS. There is still lack of data as to which ideal ROS test to use to determine seminal ROS. Significant evidences showed that measurement of ORP can be utilized to assess OS in seminal fluid. There are novel approaches to evaluate different redox biomarkers involved in OS. However, future studies should be conducted to determine its use in infertile men with ROS-induced OS.

Treatment of infertile men with OS should directly address the identifiable etiologies. Newer strategies should be developed to counteract the real impact of ROS on reproductive potential.

References

1. Tohru F, Ushio-Fukai M. Superoxide dismutases: role in redox signaling, vascular function, and diseases. Antioxid Redox Signal. 2011;15(6):1583–606. https://doi.org/10.1089/ars.2011.3999.

2. Mannucci A, Argento FR, Fini E, et al. The Impact of oxidative stress in male infertility. Front Mol Biosci. 2022;8:799294.
3. Agarwal A, Sengupta P. Oxidative stress and its association with male infertility. In: Parekattil S, Esteves S, Agarwal A, editors. Male infertility. Cham: Springer; 2020. https://doi.org/10.1007/978-3-030-32300-4_6.
4. Markkanen E. Not breathing is not an option: how to deal with oxidative DNA damage. DNA Repair (Amst). 2017;59:82–105.
5. Tremellen K. Oxidative stress and male infertility—a clinical perspective. Hum Reprod Update. 2008;14(3):243–58.
6. Ogrinc WA, Turk A, Kunej T. Towards a multi-Omics of male infertility. World J Mens Health. 2023;41(2):272–88. https://doi.org/10.5534/wjmh.220186.
7. Wagner H, Cheng JW, Ko EY. Role of reactive oxygen species in male infertility: an updated review of literature. Arab J Urol. 2017;16(1):35–43.
8. Evans EPP, Scholten JTM, Mzyk A, et al. Male subfertility and oxidative stress. Redox Biol. 2021;46:102071.
9. Henkel R, Samanta L, Agarwal A. Oxidants, antioxidants, and impact of the oxidative status in male reproduction. London, UK: Elsevier; 2018.
10. Sies H. Oxidative stress: from basic research to clinical application. Am J Med. 1991;91(3C):S31–8.
11. Barati E, Nikzad H, Karimian M. Oxidative stress and male infertility: current knowledge of pathophysiology and role of antioxidant therapy in disease management. Cell Mol Life Sci. 2020;77(1):93–113.
12. Ritchie C, Ko EY. Oxidative stress in the pathophysiology of male infertility. Andrologia. 2021;53(1):e13581.
13. Sies H. Oxidative stress: a concept in redox biology and medicine. Redox Biol. 2015;4:180–3. https://doi.org/10.1016/j.redox.2015.01.002.
14. Dutta S, Majzoub A, Agarwal A. Oxidative stress and sperm function: A systematic review on evaluation and management. Arab J Urol. 2019;17(2):87–97.
15. Agarwal A, Virk G, Ong C, du Plessis SS. Effect of oxidative stress on male reproduction. World J Mens Health. 2014;32(1):1–17.
16. Bui AD, Sharma R, Henkel R, Agarwal A. Reactive oxygen species impact on sperm DNA and its role in male infertility. Andrologia. 2018;50(8):e13012.
17. Agarwal A, Parekh N, Panner Selvam MK, et al. Male oxidative stress infertility (MOSI): proposed terminology and clinical practice guidelines for management of idiopathic male infertility. World J Mens Health. 2019;37(3):296–312.
18. Du Plessis SS, Agarwal A, Halabi J, Tvrda E. Contemporary evidence on the physiological role of reactive oxygen species in human sperm function. J Assist Reprod Genet. 2015;32(4):509–20.
19. Aitken RJ. Reactive oxygen species as mediators of sperm capacitation and pathological damage. Mol Reprod Dev. 2017;84(10):1039–52. https://doi.org/10.1002/mrd.22871.
20. Khosrowbeygi A, Zarghami N. Fatty acid composition of human spermatozoa and seminal plasma levels of oxidative stress biomarkers in subfertile males. Prostaglandins Leukot Essent Fatty Acids. 2007;77(2):117–21.
21. Jones R, Mann T, Sherins R. Peroxidative breakdown of phospholipids in human spermatozoa, spermicidal properties of fatty acid peroxides, and protective action of seminal plasma. Fertil Steril. 1979;31(5):531–7.
22. Moazamian R, Polhemus A, Connaughton H, et al. Oxidative stress and human spermatozoa: diagnostic and functional significance of aldehydes generated as a result of lipid peroxidation. Mol Hum Reprod. 2015;21(6):502–15.
23. Koppenol WH. The Haber-Weiss cycle—70 years later. Redox Rep. 2001;6(4):229–34.
24. Łuczaj W, Skrzydlewska E. DNA damage caused by lipid peroxidation products. Cell Mol Biol Lett. 2003;8(2):391–413.

25. Sharma RK, Said T, Agarwal A. Sperm DNA damage and its clinical relevance in assessing reproductive outcome. Asian J Androl. 2004;6(2):139–48.
26. Zamzami N, Marchetti P, Castedo M, et al. Sequential reduction of mitochondrial transmembrane potential and generation of reactive oxygen species in early programmed cell death. J Exp Med. 1995;182(2):367–77.
27. Elmore S. Apoptosis: a review of programmed cell death. Toxicol Pathol. 2007;35(4):495–516.
28. Amaral A, Lourenço B, Marques M, Ramalho-Santos J. Mitochondria functionality and sperm quality. Reproduction. 2013;146(5):R163–74. Published 2013 Oct 1
29. Das A, Roychoudhury S. Reactive oxygen species in the reproductive system: sources and physiological roles. Adv Exp Med Biol. 2022;1358:9–40.
30. Wolff H. The biologic significance of white blood cells in semen. Fertil Steril. 1995;63(6):1143–57.
31. Plante M, de Lamirande E, Gagnon C. Reactive oxygen species released by activated neutrophils, but not by deficient spermatozoa, are sufficient to affect normal sperm motility. Fertil Steril. 1994;62(2):387–93.
32. Potts JM, Pasqualotto FF. Seminal oxidative stress in patients with chronic prostatitis. Andrologia. 2003;35(5):304–8.
33. Babior BM. NADPH oxidase: an update. Blood. 1999;93(5):1464–76.
34. Agarwal A, Rana M, Qiu E, AlBunni H, Bui AD, Henkel R. Role of oxidative stress, infection and inflammation in male infertility. Andrologia. 2018;50(11):e13126.
35. Sabeti P, Pourmasumi S, Rahiminia T, Akyash F, Talebi AR. Etiologies of sperm oxidative stress. Int J Reprod Biomed. 2016;14(4):231–40.
36. Wang K, Gao Y, Wang C, Liang M, Liao Y, Hu K. Role of oxidative stress in varicocele. Front Genet. 2022;13:850114.
37. World Health Organization. WHO laboratory manual for the examination and processing of human semen. 6th ed. Geneva, Switzerland: WHO Press; 2021. Available online: https://www.who.int/publications/i/item/9789240030787
38. Schlegel PN, Sigman M, Collura B, et al. Diagnosis and treatment of infertility in men: AUA/ASRM guideline part I. Fertil Steril. 2021;115(1):54–61.
39. Agarwal A, Finelli R, Selvam MKP, et al. A global survey of reproductive specialists to determine the clinical utility of oxidative stress testing and antioxidant use in male infertility. World J Mens Health. 2021;39(3):470–88.
40. Agarwal A, Roychoudhury S, Sharma R, Gupta S, Majzoub A, Sabanegh E. Diagnostic application of oxidation-reduction potential assay for measurement of oxidative stress: clinical utility in male factor infertility. Reprod Biomed Online. 2017;34(1):48–57.
41. Agarwal A, Panner Selvam MK, Arafa M, et al. Multi-center evaluation of oxidation-reduction potential by the MiOXSYS in males with abnormal semen. Asian J Androl. 2019;21(6):565–9.
42. Finelli R, Leisegang K, Kandil H, Agarwal A. Oxidative stress: a comprehensive review of biochemical, molecular, and genetic aspects in the pathogenesis and management of varicocele. World J Mens Health. 2022;40(1):87–103.
43. Agarwal A, Sharma R, Roychoudhury S, Du Plessis S, Sabanegh E. MiOXSYS: a novel method of measuring oxidation reduction potential in semen and seminal plasma. Fertil Steril. 2016;106(3):566–573.e10.
44. Agarwal A, Bui AD. Oxidation-reduction potential as a new marker for oxidative stress: Correlation to male infertility. Investig Clin Urol. 2017;58(6):385–99.
45. Bergsma AT, Li HT, Eliveld J, Bulthuis MLC, Hoek A, van Goor H, et al. Local and systemic oxidative stress biomarkers for male infertility: the ORION study. Antioxidants (Basel, Switzerland). 2022;11(6):1045.
46. Cannarella R, Condorelli RA, Mongioì LM, Vignera SL, Calogero AE. Molecular biology of spermatogenesis: novel targets of apparently idiopathic male infertility. Int J Mol Sci. 2020;21(5):1728.

47. Krzyściak W, Papież M, Bąk E, et al. Sperm antioxidant biomarkers and their correlation with clinical condition and lifestyle with regard to male reproductive potential. J Clin Med. 2020;9(6):1785.
48. Huang C, Cao X, Pang D, et al. Is male infertility associated with increased oxidative stress in seminal plasma? A-meta analysis. Oncotarget. 2018;9(36):24494–513.
49. Martins AD, Agarwal A. Oxidation reduction potential: a new biomarker of male infertility. Panminerva Med. 2019;61(2):108–17.
50. Aitken RJ, Bromfield EG, Gibb Z. The impact of oxidative stress on reproduction: a focus on gametogenesis and fertilization. Reproduction. 2022;164:F79–94.
51. Majzoub A, Agarwal A. Systematic review of antioxidant types and doses in male infertility: benefits on semen parameters, advanced sperm function, assisted reproduction and live-birth rate. Arab J Urol. 2018;16(1):113–24.
52. de Ligny W, Smits RM, Mackenzie-Proctor R, et al. Antioxidants for male subfertility. Cochrane Database Syst Rev. 2022;5(5):CD007411.
53. Schlegel PN, Sigman M, Collura B, et al. Diagnosis and treatment of infertility in men: AUA/ASRM guideline Part II. J Urol. 2021;205(1):44–51.
54. Gill K, Kups M, Harasny P, et al. The negative impact of varicocele on basic semen parameters, sperm nuclear DNA dispersion and oxidation-reduction potential in semen. Int J Environ Res Public Health. 2021;18(11):5977.
55. Dave P, Farber N, Vij S. Conventional semen analysis and advanced sperm function tests in diagnosis and management of varicocele. Andrologia. 2021;53(2):e13629.
56. Agarwal A, Cannarella R, Saleh R, Boitrelle F, Gül M, Toprak T, Salvio G, Arafa M, Russo GI, Harraz AM, Singh R, Garrido N, Hamoda TAA, Rambhatla A, Kavoussi P, Kuroda S, Çalik G, Saini P, Ceyhan E, Dimitriadis F, Henkel R, Crafa A, Palani A, Duran MB, Maziotis E, Saïs É, Bendayan M, Darbandi M, Le TV, Gunes S, Tsioulou P, Sengupta P, Hazir B, Çeker G, Darbandi S, Durairajanayagam D, Aghamajidi A, Alkhalidi N, Sogutdelen E, Leisegang K, Alarbid A, Ho CCK, Malhotra V, Finocchi F, Crisóstomo L, Kosgi R, ElBardisi H, Zini A, Birowo P, Colpi G, Park HJ, Serefoglu EC, Nguyen Q, Ko E, de la Rosette J, Pinggera GM, Nguyen HVP, Kandil H, Shah R. Impact of varicocele repair on semen parameters in infertile men: a systematic review and meta-analysis. World J Mens Health. 2023;41(2):289–310. https://doi.org/10.5534/wjmh.220142.
57. Cannarella R, Shah R, Hamoda TAA, Boitrelle F, Saleh R, Gul M, Rambhatla A, Kavoussi P, Toprak T, Harraz AM, Ko E, Çeker G, Durairajanayagam D, Alkahidi N, Kuroda S, Crafa A, Henkel R, Salvio G, Hazir B, Darbandi M, Bendayan M, Darbandi S, Falcone M, Garrido N, Kosgi R, Sawaid Kaiyal R, Karna K, Phuoc NHV, Birowo P, Colpi GM, de la Rosette J, Pinggera GM, Nguyen Q, Zini A, Zohdy W, Singh R, Saini P, Glina S, Lin H, Mostafa T, Rojas-Cruz C, Arafa M, Calogero AE, Dimitriadis F, Kothari P, Karthikeyan VS, Okada K, Chiba K, Kadıoglu A, Altay B, Turunc T, Zilaitiene B, Gokalp F, Adamyan A, Katz D, Chung E, Mierzwa TC, Zylbersztejn DS, Paul GM, Sofikitis N, Sokolakis I, Malhotra V, Brodjonegoro SR, Adriansjah R, Tsujimura A, Amano T, Balercia G, Ziouziou I, Deswanto IA, Martinez M, Park HJ, Bakırcıoglu ME, Ceyhan E, Aydos K, Ramsay J, Minhas S, Al Hashimi M, Ghayda RA, Tadros N, Sindhwani P, Ho CCK, Rachman RI, Rodriguez Pena M, Motawi A, Ponnusamy AK, Dipankar S, Amir A, Binsaleh S, Serefoglu EC, Banthia R, Khalafalla K, Basukarno A, Bac NH, Singla K, Ambar RF, Makarounis K, Priyadarshi S, Duarsa GWK, Atmoko W, Jindal S, Arianto E, Akhavizadegan H, El Bardisi H, Shoshany O, Busetto GM, Moussa M, Jamali M, Al-Marhoon MS, Ruzaev M, Farsi HMA, Mutambirwa S, Lee DS, Kulaksiz D, Cheng YS, Bouzouita A, Sarikaya S, Kandil H, Tsampoukas G, Farkouh A, Bowa K, Savira M, Mogharabian N, Le TV, Harjanggi M, Anh DT, Long TQT, Soebadi MA, Hakim L, Tanic M, Ari UC, Parikh FR, Calik G, Kv V, Dorji G, Rezano A, Rajmil O, Tien DMB, Yuan Y, Lizarraga-Salas JF, Eze B, Ngoo KS, Lee J, Arslan U, Agarwal A, Global Andrology Forum. Does varicocele repair improve conventional semen parameters? A meta-analytic study of before-after data. World J Mens Health. 2024;42(1):92–132. https://doi.org/10.5534/wjmh.230034.

58. Chen SS, Huang WJ, Chang LS, Wei YH. Attenuation of oxidative stress after varicocelectomy in subfertile patients with varicocele. J Urol. 2008;179(2):639–42.
59. Mostafa T, Anis TH, El-Nashar A, Imam H, Othman IA. Varicocelectomy reduces reactive oxygen species levels and increases antioxidant activity of seminal plasma from infertile men with varicocele. Int J Androl. 2001;24(5):261–5.
60. Abdelbaki SA, Sabry JH, Al-Adl AM, Sabry HH. The impact of coexisting sperm DNA fragmentation and seminal oxidative stress on the outcome of varicocelectomy in infertile patients: a prospective controlled study. Arab J Urol. 2017;15(2):131–9.
61. Kavoussi PK, Gilkey MS, Machen GL, Kavoussi SK, Dorsey C. Varicocele repair improves static oxidation reduction potential as a measure of seminal oxidative stress levels in infertile men: a prospective clinical trial using the MiOXSYS system. Urology. 2022;165:193–7. https://doi.org/10.1016/j.urology.2022.04.007.
62. La Vignera S, Vicari E, Condorelli RA, D'Agata R, Calogero AE. Male accessory gland infection and sperm parameters (review). Int J Androl. 2011;34(5 Pt 2):e330–47.
63. Calogero AE, Duca Y, Condorelli RA, La Vignera S. Male accessory gland inflammation, infertility, and sexual dysfunctions: a practical approach to diagnosis and therapy. Andrology. 2017;5(6):1064–72.
64. Haidl G, Haidl F, Allam JP, Schuppe HC. Therapeutic options in male genital tract inflammation. Andrologia. 2019;51(3):e13207.
65. Omolaoye TS, Omolaoye VA, Kandasamy RK, Hachim MY, Du Plessis SS. Omics and male infertility: highlighting the application of transcriptomic data. Life. 2022;12:280. https://doi.org/10.3390/life12020280.
66. Mehrparavar B, Minai-Tehrani A, Arjmand B, Gilany K. Metabolomics of male infertility: a new tool for diagnostic tests. J Reprod Infertil. 2019;20:64–9.
67. Minai-Tehrani A, Jafarzadeh N, Gilany K. Metabolomics: a state-of-the-art technology for better understanding of male infertility. Andrologia. 2016;48:609–16.
68. Walters JLH, Gadella BM, Sutherland JM, Nixon B, Bromfield EG. Male infertility: shining a light on lipids and lipid-modulating enzymes in the male germline. J Clin Med. 2020;9:327.
69. Kołodziejczyk J, Blixt O, Olejnik B, Zimmer M, Ferens-Sieczkowska M. Application of lectin microarrays for the analysis of seminal plasma glycome. Andrologia. 2018;50:e13018.

Chapter 7
Management of Male Oxidative Stress Infertility (MOSI)

Edmund Y. Ko and Vilvapathy S. Karthikeyan

Key Points

- Male infertility is idiopathic in up to 50% of cases and may be due to male oxidative stress.
- Oxidative stress can be attributed to intrinsic or extrinsic causes.
- Reactive oxygen species assays include chemiluminescence, nitroblue tetrazolium (NBT) staining, oxidation-reduction potential (ORP), flow cytometry, Endtz test, malondialdehyde-thiobarbituric acid (MDA-TBA), and total antioxidant capacity (TAC).
- Management strategies for male oxidative stress infertility (MOSI) include empiric medical therapy, antioxidants, weight loss, antibiotics, or varicocele repair, depending on the etiology.

Introduction

The etiology of male infertility is unknown in up to 30–50% of cases and falls under the broad category of idiopathic male infertility (IMI) [1–3]. In the quest of reducing the diagnosis of IMI, oxidative stress (OS) is now increasingly being identified to have an independent role in male infertility. This has led to coining the new terminology of male oxidative stress infertility (MOSI) [1–6]. The reported incidence of seminal reactive oxygen species (ROS) ranges from 30% to 80% [1].

Seminal reactive oxygen species (ROS) are produced by seminal leukocytes. These ROS can also arise from immature sperms and are formed as a result of oxidative metabolic pathways. Though small amounts of ROS are required for normal cellular function in spermatogenesis, sperm capacitation, hyperactivation, acrosome reaction, and sperm-oocyte fusion, it becomes harmful when the proportion of ROS overwhelms the capacity of body's endogenous antioxidants (AOXs) [1, 3, 7–11].

E. Y. Ko (✉)
Department of Urology, Kaiser Permanente, Fontana, CA, USA

V. S. Karthikeyan
Male Infertility & Men's Health and Urologist, Apollo Hospitals, Greams Road, Chennai, Tamil Nadu, India

A. Agarwal et al. (eds.), *Current and Future Advances in Male Infertility*,
https://doi.org/10.1007/978-3-031-62648-7_7

Oxidative stress damages sperm membrane and DNA, causes lipid peroxidation and protein modification, and also affects the potential of the sperm to fertilize the ovum [9, 10]. It has been observed that OS results in mutagenic and genotoxic products, thereby putting the embryo at an increased risk [1]. OS can lead to arrested embryonic development, implantation failure, recurrent pregnancy loss, and even reduced live birth rate [3]. Additionally, OS can result in epigenetic alterations, telomere attrition, and even Y chromosomal microdeletions [4]. Hence, OS assessment may play an important role in the evaluation of male reproductive potential.

Causes of OS and Male Infertility

Oxidative stress is considered as a physiological redox imbalance [4]. The important causes of MOSI may be intrinsic or extrinsic [3].

Intrinsic Causes

Intrinsic causes include sperm abnormalities, varicocele (especially higher grades), obesity, undescended testis, aging, torsion testis, prostatitis (inflammatory), metabolic syndrome, genitourinary or male accessory gland infections, spinal cord injury, strenuous exercise, or psychological stress [1, 4, 9, 12]. Adipose fibroblasts precipitate proinflammatory leukocyte recruitment and increased NADPH oxidase activity [3]. Scrotal heat following varicocele, obesity, tight underwear, hot water bathing for prolonged periods, use of laptop on closed legs, and long-distance cycling can also impede spermatogenesis, resulting in higher quantities of immature spermatozoa, thereby contributing to ROS production [3]. In men with varicoceles, it has been observed that seminal plasma ROS are high coupled with a deficiency in AOX levels and elevated sperm DNA fragmentation [3, 12].

Extrinsic Causes

The important extrinsic causes of OS include exposure to tobacco, alcohol, chemicals such as phthalates, heat, radiation including exposure to mobile phones, environmental pollution, heavy metals, recreational drugs, and some medications [3, 4, 9, 13, 14]. Smoke contains nicotine, tar, heavy metals, and carbon monoxide, which can recruit proinflammatory white blood cells. Seminal OS can also be induced by centrifugation or cryopreservation [3].

Diagnosis of MOSI

Reactive oxygen species are fragments or whole of atoms or molecules resulting from oxygen, nitrogen, organic compounds, copper, or iron, with at least one unpaired electron valency. Direct methods of ROS assays include chemiluminescence, nitroblue tetrazolium stain (NBT), oxidative reduction potential (ORP), and flow cytometry. The indirect methods include Endtz test (myeloperoxidase), malondialdehyde-thiobarbiturate (MDA-TBA), and total antioxidant capacity (TAC) assay [3].

Semen Analysis

Conventional semen analysis (SA) is deemed insufficient to identify the cause of male infertility, especially in IMI. It is because of the well-recognized hitches associated with SA testing, such as subjectivity in assessment and poor reproducibility [1, 15]. Semen analysis can display the source of ROS such as seminal leukocytes, immature sperms with head morphology defects and cytoplasmic retention in the residual body of midpiece of flagellum, and abnormal or deficient sperms [3, 4, 9, 16]. Seminal Sertoli cells also have the ability to produce ROS [9].

Peroxidase-positive white blood cells in semen can produce 1000-fold higher ROS by enhancing NADPH production (nicotinamide-adenine dinucleotide phosphate) [4]. Myeloperoxidase stains these leukocytes brown, indicating that there is excess ROS production [3]. Nitroblue tetrazolium detects ROS production by immature sperms, and the positivity can be measured using a light microscope or by spectrophotometry, changing its color from yellow to blue (due to diformazan). It is a relatively user-friendly technique helping to identify the source of ROS. The intensity of change in color has been correlated with levels of intracellular ROS [3].

ROS Assays

ROS assay is the commonly used direct assay, with most preferred being the chemiluminescence method. It relies upon the reaction between luminol and oxidizing compounds. It measures extracellular and intracellular ROS such as superoxide, hydrogen peroxide, and hydroxyl radicals, with higher sensitivity and specificity [3, 9]. However, it is time consuming and laborious, with the need for costly equipment, and is dependent upon semen characteristics like volume, centrifugation, background activity, temperature, and keeping time [1]. The test results are expressed as relative light units per second per million sperm, with a cutoff of 102.2 RLU/million sperm [9].

The indirect method for ROS estimation is MDA-TBA, measuring the lipid peroxidation by colorimetry or fluoroscopy, due to excessive OS and is performed less commonly than direct assays [1, 9]. The MDA may also be indicative of DNA damage, as it is a mutagenic agent [9].

Total Antioxidant Capacity

The TAC test measures the cumulative AOXs in the semen, which carry the ability to scavenge free radicals. It is a rapid colorimetric method, but does not measure enzymatic AOXs and also requires an expensive setup. The TAC levels can help differentiate good- from poor-quality semen samples [9, 17].

ROS-TAC Score

The ROS-TAC score is a better overall diagnostic test when compared with ROS or TAC alone. Since it does not directly measure ROS, it is more of a prediction of OS and relies upon statistical modeling. ROS and TAC values taken from controls are used to create a reference point. However, it is nonspecific and requires rigorous controls [1].

Oxidative Reduction Potential

Seminal ORP measures all known and unknown AOXs and oxidants. It is affected by semen viscosity but can be done quickly (roughly 4 min) and does not require expertise to conduct the test. It can be measured even in frozen specimens, semen, and seminal plasma [1]. This test was developed because of variability in assessment and bias due to level of expertise required for performing the tests. The ORP (redox potential) measures the relationship between AOXs donating electrons and oxidants acquiring these electrons and is a comprehensive assessment, indicating the balance. The ORP denotes the level of OS and can also aid in the measurement of response to treatment. It also measures known and unknown contributors of OS unlike ROS or TAC measurements [9].

MiOXSYS is a system which measures static ORP by galvanostatic method [10]. It requires a small sample (30 μm) of semen and measures electron activity (mV/million sperm), and the cutoff of 1.34 mV/million sperm is reported to have good sensitivity (98.6%) and positive predictive value (94.7%), reasonable negative predictive value (66.7%), but low specificity (40.6%). Seminal ORP correlates inversely with normal sperm morphology and is elevated in men with oligoasthenoteratozoospermia [9, 10]. Elevated ORP levels also directly correlate with DNA fragmentation [1, 3].

Treatment of Male Oxidative Stress Infertility

Empiric Medical Therapy

Empiric medical therapy (EMT), or medical therapy in the absence of a specific etiology, is utilized widely for male infertility despite the lack of consensus statements or clinical algorithms. Some associations advise against recommending EMT for the treatment of infertility [18]. Regardless, these treatments have been utilized for many decades despite no Food and Drug Administration approval [19]. EMT treatments are utilized in hopes of improving low sperm counts.

A survey of the American Urologic Association urologists treating male infertility revealed that two-thirds of respondents utilized some form of EMT for IMI or unexplained male infertility (UMI) despite the lack of consensus on the optimal medication as well as the perceived impact on semen parameters [19]. The survey was repeated in 2020 and continued to demonstrate similar findings [20]. These findings have also been confirmed by another survey from Saudi Arabia demonstrating 86.5% of respondents utilizing EMT for men with IMI with oligoasthenoteratozoospermia (OAT) [21]. These surveys demonstrate that clinicians are willing to try treatments in hopes of improving male semen parameters and therefore fertility potential to aid couples in conceiving naturally or improving assisted reproduction outcomes. Despite these findings and lack of consensus guidelines, there is still a potential role of using EMT for the treatment of IMI and UMI.

Empiric medical therapies are divided into two general categories: hormonal and nonhormonal agents or AOXs. Hormonal therapies are utilized to modulate the hypothalamic-pituitary-gonadal (HPG) axis. Hormonal therapies can be further divided into androgens, gonadotropins, selective estrogen receptor modulators (SERMs), and antiestrogens [22, 23].

Empiric medical therapy for the treatment of MOSI is utilized by many clinicians worldwide, but its efficacy continues to be debated [24]. The evidence in support of utilizing EMT in male infertility seems promising, but further studies are needed to fully understand the impact not only on semen parameters but also on pregnancy rates.

Antioxidants

In-depth discussion on OS and ROS formation and impact on sperm production and function and ultimately negative impact on male fertility has been provided in a previous chapter. Antioxidants as potential treatments for MOSI have been studied extensively. Antioxidants are chemicals that participate in redox reactions by donating electrons or reducing reactive molecules to less harmful products. Essentially, they are scavengers of ROS and protect against OS and damage caused by ROS [25]. There are two main sources for AOXs: physiologic and dietary [26]. Physiologic AOXs are present within the sperm or seminal plasma, while dietary AOXs are obtained orally from food products or supplements.

Antioxidants are classified as enzymatic or nonenzymatic reducing agents. Enzymatic AOXs in the male reproductive tract include superoxide dismutase (SOD), catalase, and glutathione peroxidase (GPX) [27]. SOD is a scavenger of the superoxide anion and converts it to hydrogen peroxide. Cellularly, it exists in three isoenzymes: mitochondrial manganese SOD, cytoplasmic copper-zinc SOD, and extracellular SOD [28]. SOD in the semen has been demonstrated to function against OS markers, protect against sperm membrane phospholipid peroxidation, and decrease sperm DNA damage [29–31]. Catalase converts hydrogen peroxide, a potent oxidizer, to water and oxygen and protects against oxidative damage [32]. GPX catalyzes hydrogen peroxide and superoxide anion by utilizing an electron donated from glutathione. This enzyme protects against sperm phospholipid peroxidation [31].

Nonenzymatic reducing agents also occur naturally in the male reproductive tract. They can directly protect against the effects of OS or act as cofactors for the enzymatic reducing agents. The main agents in the male reproductive tract include ascorbic acid, glutathione, lycopene, selenium, and tocopherol. Ascorbic acid (vitamin C) neutralizes ROS and protects against OS [33]. Glutathione is available abundantly in the male genital tract and is a free radical scavenger and coenzyme for GPX [34]. Lycopene is the main carotenoid in the testis and is thought to protect against ischemia-reperfusion injury from OS [35]. Selenium is a trace element that is a cofactor to specific isoforms of GPX [36]. Tocopherol (vitamin E) reduces spermatozoa plasma membrane lipid peroxidation [37].

Although there are reducing agents produced within the male reproductive tract, there may not be enough TAC to counter the negative effects of excess ROS and OS from various pathologies. Therein lie the potential benefits of AOX supplementation in MOSI. There are many studies that demonstrate that exogenous administration of AOX mono- or combination therapy may help improve the TAC and reduce the level of OS within the reproductive tract, thereby improving semen parameters and male fertility potential. In 2021, Agarwal and colleagues performed a systematic review and analysis of the evidence on the utility of AOX in male infertility; 1978 articles were reviewed, and 97 were included in the systematic review [38]. The authors concluded that even though there were positive fertility outcomes with AOX utilization, additional well-designed, randomized, double-blinded, placebo-controlled trials were needed and evidence-based clinical guidelines were needed for the treatment community. A 2022 Cochrane Library review including 90 studies looking at AOX for male subfertility suggested positive findings. The authors found that AOX supplementation may increase clinical pregnancy rates (OR 1.89, 95% CI 1.45–2.47, $P < 0.00001$, $I^2 = 3\%$) and live birth rates (OR 1.45, 95% CI 1.07–1.91, $P = 0.02$, $I^2 = 44\%$) [39]. However, the authors cautioned that the overall evidence is inconclusive due to low-certainty evidence as a result of heterogeneous methods of randomization, incomplete reporting of pregnancy and live birth rates, small sample size of many studies, and high attrition rates. They also, like Agarwal and colleagues, called for further large well-designed, randomized, placebo-controlled trials.

The review here will present common AOXs that have been studied extensively and commonly used by the male infertility community (in alphabetic order).

Arginine

Arginine is a precursor of nitric oxide. It has a role in the cellular inflammatory response and protects against oxidative damage [40]. It is a biochemical precursor for putrescine, spermidine, and spermine and is important for sperm motility [41]. Supplementation up to 4 g per day has been demonstrated to improve sperm concentration and motility [42, 43]. Studies from the 1970s including Pryor's double-blind crossover trial of 64 infertile oligozoospermic men treated for 12 weeks have demonstrated no improvement in semen parameters or pregnancy rates [44, 45]. Other studies have demonstrated that excessive arginine can impair sperm function highlighting that oversupplementation can have deleterious paradoxical results [46].

Carnitines

Carnitines are amines synthesized from lysine and methionine. They transport long-chain fatty acids into the mitochondria for intracellular metabolism. Carnitines have a role in sperm metabolism, motility, and sperm maturation as well as an antioxidant role against ROS [47, 48]. L-carnitine (LC) and L-acetylcarnitine (LAC) are the two main forms, both of which are found in the epididymis, seminal plasma, and spermatozoa [49, 50]. Supplementation with carnitine has been demonstrated to improve multiple semen parameters including concentration, motility, morphology, viability, and TAC [51–55]. Pregnancy rates were higher in treatment groups, although not statistically significant. In a study with 170 men treated for 6 months, the authors found that semen carnitine concentration was significantly correlated with sperm concentration, total count, total motility, forward progression, live sperm count, membrane function, and nuclear DNA integrity compared to pretreatment levels [56]. Despite all of these positive results, studies have also shown carnitine supplementation for treating idiopathic asthenozoospermia to be inferior to placebo [57].

Coenzyme Q10

Coenzyme Q10 (CoQ10) aids in transport of electrons in the mitochondrial respiratory chain. Within the sperm, it promotes energy within the sperm midpiece [58]. It also holds an important role in protecting and stabilizing the lipoprotein-rich sperm cell membrane as a lipid-soluble AOX, thereby protecting it from OS [59]. CoQ10 can be measured in the semen and is directly correlated with sperm count and motility, with a 4.5–6% improvement of motility with CoQ10 supplementation [58, 60].

Folic Acid

Folic acid, also known as vitamin B9 or folate, is involved in purine and pyrimidine production and has an important role in DNA synthesis and cell function [61]. It is also a potent free radical scavenger by providing methyl donors methionine and S-adenosylmethionine [62]. Adequate folate intake is important in preventing sperm DNA abnormalities as studies have shown that there is a 30% lower frequency of disomy X and disomy 21, sex nullisomy, and aneuploidy compared to those with inadequate intake [63]. The impact of folate supplementation on male infertility is mixed as some studies have demonstrated a 74% increase in sperm count but concurrently a 4% increase in abnormal sperm morphology with folate and zinc intake [64]. Other studies have failed to find any improvement in any semen or DNA parameters with supplementation [61, 65].

Glutathione

As previously discussed, glutathione is an abundant endogenously produced AOX. It is produced in the liver and synthesized from cysteine, glutamic acid, and glycine and keeps exogenous AOXs like vitamins C and E in their active reduced states [34]. Glutathione supplementation has been shown to improve sperm motility [66, 67]. Studies have shown improved sperm count and decreased DNA fragmentation when used in combination with vitamins C and E, but it is difficult to directly attribute the positive changes to only one supplement [68].

Lycopene

Lycopene is an AOX that plays many roles including cell growth regulation, gap junction communication, gene expression modulation, immune response, and protection of lipid peroxidation [69]. It belongs to the family of carotenoids found in many bright fruits and vegetables that includes alpha-tocopherol, alpha-carotene, beta-cryptoxanthin, beta-carotene, and lutein and is the most effective antioxidant among the carotenoid family [70]. Lycopene is concentrated in the prostate and testes and many other human tissues like adrenal gland, breast, and liver [71]. Lycopene intake with supplements or through dietary intake (i.e., tomato soup) has been demonstrated to have a positive impact on semen parameters including increased sperm concentration, count, motility, morphology, and viability [70, 72]. The current lycopene studies were reviewed and given support from the Italian Society of Andrology and Sexual Medicine in their consensus statement for male infertility treatment [73]. A recent review also found improvement in sperm quality with lycopene supplementation [74].

Selenium

Selenium is a component of GPX and serves as a reduction cofactor of enzymatic AOXs [75]. It has important role in maintaining male fertility functions including testicular development, spermatogenesis, and sperm motility and capacitation [36]. Selenium deficiency leads to decreased motility, sperm midpiece stability, and poor morphology due to abnormal sperm development [76]. Selenium supplementation alone or in combination with other AOXs, such as vitamin E or N-acetylcysteine, has been noted to improve semen parameters, including sperm count, motility, and morphology (Vezina et al. 1996) [77]. A 3-month placebo-controlled study with selenium alone or selenium used in combination with other vitamins demonstrated a 12.9% increase in sperm motility ($P < 0.05$), and 11% in the treatment group achieved pregnancy and none in the placebo group [78]. Interestingly, an uncontrolled selenium-only study did not find any changes in sperm count, motility, or morphology in subfertile men taking the supplement, highlighting that the benefits of selenium may be only realized when taken in conjunction with other vitamins and AOX [79]. Judicious supplementation is important as excess selenium supplementation can also result in sperm abnormalities such as decreased motility and increase in DNA strand breaks [80].

Vitamin A

Carotenoids and retinoids, including vitamin A, are fat-soluble vitamins that play multiple physiologic roles involving mucous membranes, eyes, skin, and gastrointestinal and genitourinary tracts. Vitamin A has a role in preventing oxidation of low-density lipoproteins and may have a role in stabilizing the sperm cell membrane [81]. Animal studies published in the 1920s and 1930s demonstrated that vitamin A deficiency had a negative impact on the epithelium of the epididymis, prostate, and seminal vesicles replacing them with stratified squamous keratinizing epithelium, resulting in the cessation of spermatogenesis. Subsequent vitamin A replacement resulted in reversal of the epithelial changes [82]. Subsequent studies have also demonstrated return of spermatogenesis on correction of vitamin A deficiency [83]. Vitamin A deficiency has been found to also have a negative impact on Sertoli cell tight junction integrity, thereby compromising the blood-testis barrier [84].

Most human studies currently in literature have utilized combination therapy with vitamin A as there are no current studies focused solely on vitamin A. Therapy with a combination of supplements including vitamins A, C, and E and selenium, N-acetylcysteine, and zinc has demonstrated improvements in sperm motility and count [78, 85]. Because vitamin A is a fat-soluble vitamin readily stored in the body, judicious supplementation is important to avoid side effects and toxicity.

Vitamin C

Ascorbic acid, or vitamin C, is a water-soluble vitamin that is an important cofactor for hydroxylation and amidation reactions [86]. It is involved in the physiological processes of collagen synthesis and is part of the components of intercellular matrix and proteoglycans [87]. It is an important AOX that has a role in recycling oxidized vitamin E and also protects sperm and DNA from oxidative damage by counteracting ROS [87, 88]. It is found concentrated in seminal plasma, and decreased levels can have a negative impact on sperm morphology and DNA fragmentation [89, 90].

Vitamin C supplementation has been found to have positive impacts on overall sperm quality, morphology, sperm DNA fragmentation, and viability. Vitamin C alone, or in combination with other AOXs like beta-carotene, vitamin E, or zinc, has also demonstrated synergistic improvements in sperm quality [91, 92]. Improvements appear to be dose dependent as there has been found to be a direct correlation with serum and seminal vitamin C levels and sperm improvements. As such, daily intake between 200 and 1000 mg has been demonstrated to have the most impact with a study on smokers demonstrating 34% viability and count improvements, 5% motility improvement, and 33% morphology improvement over baseline ($P < 0.05$) [93].

Vitamin E

Vitamin E is part of the tocopherol family, with alpha-tocopherol being the most abundant form in nature. It is a potent AOX that inhibits lipid peroxidation, inhibits free radical cell membrane damage, and synergistically improves the activity of other AOXs [94]. Vitamin E supplementation can reduce seminal ROS levels in infertile men [95]. It has also been shown to improve sperm counts and motility when taken alone or with other AOXs [91]. Other studies have also demonstrated decreased lipid peroxidation and sperm DNA fragmentation rates as well as improved pregnancy rates [37, 88].

Despite these benefits, supplementation with vitamin E is not completely safe as doses greater than 400 IU/day can increase the risk of cardiovascular complications [96, 97]. It has also been demonstrated that doses above 800 IU/day increase antiplatelet effects and bleeding risks and can interact with medications like warfarin [98]. Caution is advised especially in patients with bleeding disorders or those requiring antiplatelet or anticoagulation medications. Vitamin E supplementation should therefore be taken with caution, and counseling of the risks and potential side effects is recommended.

Zinc

Zinc is a trace mineral that has antiapoptotic and AOX properties and is important for human immune function [99]. It is an important component in many physiologic processes and serves a necessary role as a cofactor for many enzymes that are involved in DNA transcription and protein synthesis [100]. Zinc is found in high concentrations within the male genitourinary tract, especially in the prostate and seminal plasma. It is involved with many aspects of male reproduction including testicular steroidogenesis, testicular development, sperm oxygen management, nuclear chromatin condensation, sperm chromatin stabilization, acrosome reaction, acrosin activity, testosterone synthesis, and conversion of testosterone to 5a-dihydrotestosterone [61]. Zinc deficiency has been demonstrated to be associated with male infertility due to decreased sperm counts and lower testosterone levels [101–103]. Zinc taken in conjunction with vitamins C and E has been shown to improve sperm motility and AOX-carrying capacity and decrease ROS, sperm apoptosis, and DNA fragmentation [92]. It has also been shown to decrease sperm aneuploidy when taken with folate [63].

Lifestyle and Dietary Modification

Obesity, tobacco and/or drug use, and excessive alcohol have been associated with male infertility. These are modifiable risk factors as changes in diet, exercise, and cessation of usage of substances may result in improvement in fertility status [104].

Obesity

Obesity continues to increase and is a major public health concern [105]. It has been associated with many different aspects of male hormonal abnormalities and male infertility, and the causes are multifactorial [106].

Obese men have been found to have lower serum testosterone and luteinizing hormone levels [107]. This may be due to disruption or suppression of gonadotropin-releasing hormone (GnRH) or the hypothalamic-pituitary-gonadal (HPG) axis [108]. Potential causes include excess conversion of testosterone to estradiol in the excess adipose tissue or increased endorphins suppressing the GnRH production [109].

Sperm quality has also been noted to be impaired in obese men. This may be due to obesity being a proinflammatory state resulting in systemic inflammation [110]. This can increase ROS and result in OS leading to sperm damage and decreased fertility. Lack of exercise and a sedentary lifestyle have also been associated with increased scrotal temperature [111]. Another potential cause is increased testicular temperature from increased leg, abdominal, or scrotal adipose tissue [112, 113].

More contemporary studies have confirmed these earlier findings with increased body mass index (BMI) associated with higher scrotal temperatures and subfertility [102, 114].

Interestingly, the first meta-analysis with 31 studies found no significant association looking at BMI and semen parameters [115]. The authors noted that their main limitation was the inability to aggregate a lot of data to run the meta-analysis. A subsequent meta-analysis in 2013 with 21 included studies found that men with elevated BMI have increased rates of oligozoospermia or azoospermia [116]. Another study looking at BMI and waist circumference on semen quality also found decreasing ejaculate volume and sperm concentration with rising body size [117].

Obese men are also more likely to have insulin resistance and diabetes. A study found that there is increased nuclear and mitochondrial DNA damage in the sperm of these men, thereby impairing their fertility and reproductive health [118]. Another study did not find higher levels of sperm DNA damage in overweight men with BMI >25.0 [119].

With the rising obesity rates and negative impact on fertility, lifestyle and dietary modification are of the utmost importance to reverse the negative effects. Diet and exercise resulting in weight reduction have been demonstrated to improve hormones as well as semen parameters. A study looked at the impact of diet and exercise for 14 weeks in 43 obese men [120]. Men with higher weight loss up to 25.4% had statistically significant improvements in sperm concentration and morphology as well as serum testosterone, testosterone/estradiol ratio, and sex hormone-binding globulin. This study did not find any improvement in the DNA fragmentation index in those men.

Diet can positively impact semen analysis parameters. A meta-analysis has shown that improving diet to healthier patterns, including high consumption of vegetables, fruits, whole grain, olive oil, fish, soy, poultry, and low-fat dairy products, results in higher sperm concentrations compared to poor dietary patterns [121]. The Mediterranean diet has been associated with improved semen quality, including sperm concentration, total sperm count, total motility, progressive motility, and sperm morphology [122]. These findings have been confirmed in a recent review and meta-analysis that men on healthy diet patterns, including the Mediterranean diet, Dietary Approaches to Stop Hypertension (DASH), and prudent diets, had higher sperm concentrations, total sperm count, and progressive sperm motility [123]. Diets containing higher levels of polyunsaturated fatty acids have been demonstrated to reduce oxidative damage [124]. Utilization of artificial sweeteners to avoid unnecessary carbohydrates and calories may have a deleterious effect on fertility demonstrated in rat studies. For example, aspartame has been demonstrated to increase the production of ROS and induce OS [125]. Similarly, Stevia has been shown to lower sperm count and testosterone level [126].

Exercise, or any activity involving bodily movements that are used to maintain or improve physical fitness, has also been shown to improve male fertility. Different types and intensity of exercise will impact fertility differently. Exercise-induced weight loss has been demonstrated to improve testosterone levels and semen parameters [120]. Low- to moderate-intensity aerobic exercise, like swimming, can increase AOX enzymes in testicular tissue [127]. Studies have found that exercise can increase epididymal dehydroepiandrosterone and may reduce damage from OS [128]. Moderate-intensity treadmill training can improve sperm concentration, motility, and morphology as well as increase semen TAC [129].

However, not all types or intensity of exercise may be beneficial. Moderate- and high-intensity endurance athletes have been shown to have decreased free and total serum testosterone compared to sedentary controls [130, 131]. Excessive exercise, including high-intensity and endurance activities, can increase ROS production and decrease AOX activity in the testicular tissue [132]. It can also increase sperm DNA fragmentation and decrease DNA integrity [133, 134].

Fertility changes in men undergoing gastric bypass versus lifestyle modification have also been studied. Weight loss after gastric bypass has been demonstrated to decrease an obesity-induced chronic proinflammatory state and OS [132]. Some studies have demonstrated that despite improvements in testosterone levels with weight loss, there were no improvements in semen parameters [135]. The authors also noted that the semen parameters did not worsen after gastric bypass. Other authors have demonstrated sperm concentration and hormonal improvements after bariatric surgery [136, 137]. Other studies, however, have reported worsening semen parameters after bariatric surgery [138–140]. A recent meta-analysis including 9 studies with 218 patients with follow-up of 24 months found that bariatric surgery does not improve semen quality [141]. With these conflicting findings in bariatric surgery studies, it is important to counsel patients preoperatively that their semen parameters may not change or even potentially worsen after surgery.

Obese men with infertility should be counseled to improve their diet and exercise to lose weight in order to improve their fertility. They should be cautioned about high-intensity exercise as it may have a negative impact on fertility. For those unable to lose weight with diet and exercise and who are considering bariatric surgery, they need to be counseled that the current outcome data are controversial and may negatively impact their fertility.

Antibiotics

Bacterial infection of the male genitourinary (GU) tract, including the testicles, epididymis, and accessory sex glands, can cause impaired sperm production, function, and delivery. Male GU infection and inflammation contribute up to 35% of male infertility cases [142]. Not all infections have to be sexually transmitted as urinary tract infections involving the kidneys, bladder, or urethra can also have a negative impact on fertility. Bacteriospermia, defined as >1000 colony-forming units of bacteria per milliliter of semen, can have a significant negative impact on fertility [143]. It is found in 15% of infertile men [142]. Leukocytospermia (≥10/mL [6]) found on semen analysis may be a result of an infection or environmental or toxic factors [144]. A study looking at 1750 male partners in infertile couples found that increasing leukocyte concentration was associated with decreased sperm concentration and morphology [145]. Leukocytes have been found to be a major producer of ROS and result in OS [146]. This can have a negative impact on sperm count, motility, morphology, as well as the DNA.

Common sexually transmitted infections include *Chlamydia trachomatis* and *Neisseria gonorrhoeae* and can cause urethritis, epididymitis, or orchitis. Other GU bacteria that can be found include *Ureaplasma* species and *Mycoplasma* species [142]. Both may colonize the male GU tract without any symptoms but may result in infertility. *Ureaplasma* infection in the absence of leukocytospermia can also increase seminal ROS and cause sperm DNA fragmentation [147]. A study by Jung and colleagues found that antibiotics can improve overall semen quality by treating the underlying cause of leukocytospermia [148]. They also found that AOXs can potentially be used for leukocytospermia also and may improve sperm function. Up to 60% of men with acute epididymitis have been shown to have temporarily impaired spermatogenesis, and it appears to be reversible after antibiotic therapy [144]. Antibiotics, including doxycycline, erythromycin, levofloxacin, and trimethoprim/sulfamethoxazole, have been demonstrated to improve sperm morphology, motility, and concentration [142]. Therefore, if leukocytospermia is found on semen analysis, additional investigative testing is recommended to rule out infectious etiology, and if found, it should be treated appropriately with antibiotics.

Varicocele Repair

Varicoceles are one of the most common causes for male infertility and found in up to 50% of men with primary and up to 69% of men with secondary infertility [149]. Varicocele is one of the most correctable causes for male infertility, and repair has resulted in improved semen parameters as well as spontaneous pregnancy rates [150].

Many studies have demonstrated increased OS markers in men with varicocele: higher seminal ROS levels and lower TAC, higher nitric oxide and hexanoyl-lysine activity, higher seminal hydrogen peroxide and lower AOX levels (SOD, CAT, GPX, vitamins C and E), and increased seminal malondialdehyde (MDA) [151–154].

Varicocelectomy has been shown to reduce MDA and increase SOD, CAT, GPX, and vitamin C and E levels at 3 and 6 months after surgery [155]. Other studies have also demonstrated decreased seminal ROS levels at 1 and 3 months after varicocele repair [156]. With these studies, the improvements seem to be time dependent, with most clinicians evaluating the impact on OS 6 months after surgery [157]. Conversely, other studies have demonstrated no significant changes in TAC and differences in MDA, SOD, or ROS levels compared to control groups after varicocele repair [158, 159].

Overall, it appears that varicocele repair can decrease OS for infertile men with clinical varicoceles. However, a significant amount of the data available comes from uncontrolled studies with small sample sizes or short follow-up periods. Pregnancy data is also lacking in many of the studies. Therefore, further research is needed in this area.

New Strategies

The future of therapeutics for MOSI will rely on improved testing and diagnosis of infertile males. As the field of -omics (genomics, transcriptomics, proteomics, epigenomics, metagenomics, metabolomics, nutriomics, etc.) continues to grow within male infertility, we anticipate that the treatments for MOSI will evolve and grow beyond the current limited therapies discussed in this chapter. With new larger datasets from infertility testing, it is challenging for scientists and clinicians to analyze and utilize all information gathered for each patient. Artificial intelligence or machine learning enables handling large amounts of data and opens the door to overcome these challenges [160]. Artificial intelligence may help predict the diagnosis, guide treatment, and predict outcomes. This is currently used in some areas like radiology and breast and colorectal cancer screening [161–163]. Research utilizing deep learning to improve computer-assisted sperm analysis has already been started [164]. Continued development of new technologies will enhance the diagnosis, and development of personalized therapies, as well as outcomes of infertile men diagnosed with MOSI.

Summary

MOSI is a major contributing factor in IMI. Although a necessary component to ensure normal sperm development and function, an excess of ROS can result in OS and male infertility. Traditional semen analysis is inadequate to identify and diagnosis MOSI. Therefore, specialized ROS testing must be employed, and most are readily available. Treatment strategies for MOSI include addressing the underlying cause of the OS and include EMT, antioxidants, and lifestyle and dietary modification. The future of MOSI management includes improving diagnostic testing, especially in the field of -omics and artificial intelligence.

References

1. Agarwal A, Parekh N, Panner Selvam MK, Henkel R, Shah R, Homa ST, et al. Male oxidative stress infertility (MOSI): proposed terminology and clinical practice guidelines for management of idiopathic male infertility. World J Mens Health. 2019;37(3):296–312.
2. Chehab M, Madala A, Trussell JC. On-label and off-label drugs used in the treatment of male infertility. Fertil Steril. 2015;103(3):595–604.
3. Takeshima T, Usui K, Mori K, Asai T, Yasuda K, Kuroda S, et al. Oxidative stress and male infertility. Reprod Med Biol. 2020;20(1):41–52.
4. Bui AD, Sharma R, Henkel R, Agarwal A. Reactive oxygen species impact on sperm DNA and its role in male infertility. Andrologia. 2018;50(8):e13012.
5. Aitken RJ, De Iuliis GN, Drevet JR. Role of oxidative stress in the etiology of male infertility and the potential therapeutic value of antioxidants. In: Henkel R, Samanta L, Agarwal

A, editors. Oxidants, antioxidants, and impact of the oxidative status in male reproduction. London: Elsevier/Academic Press; 2018. p. 91–100.
6. Wagner H, Cheng JW, Ko EY. Role of reactive oxygen species in male infertility: an updated review of literature. Arab J Urol. 2017;16(1):35–43.
7. Aitken RJ. Reactive oxygen species as mediators of sperm capacitation and pathological damage. Mol Reprod Dev. 2017;84(10):1039–52.
8. Du Plessis SS, Agarwal A, Halabi J, Tvrda E. Contemporary evidence on the physiological role of reactive oxygen species in human sperm function. J Assist Reprod Genet. 2015;32(4):509–20.
9. Agarwal A, Roychoudhury S, Bjugstad KB, Cho CL. Oxidation-reduction potential of semen: what is its role in the treatment of male infertility? Ther Adv Urol. 2016;8(5):302–18.
10. Agarwal A, Sharma R, Roychoudhury S, Du Plessis S, Sabanegh E. MiOXSYS: a novel method of measuring oxidation reduction potential in semen and seminal plasma. Fertil Steril. 2016;106(3):566–573.e10.
11. Kothari S, Thompson A, Agarwal A, du Plessis SS. Free radicals: their beneficial and detrimental effects on sperm function. Indian J Exp Biol. 2010;48(5):425–35.
12. Shiraishi K, Matsuyama H, Takihara H. Pathophysiology of varicocele in male infertility in the era of assisted reproductive technology. Int J Urol. 2012;19(6):538–50.
13. Ko EY, Sabanegh ES Jr, Agarwal A. Male infertility testing: reactive oxygen species and antioxidant capacity. Fertil Steril. 2014;102(6):1518–27.
14. Lavranos G, Balla M, Tzortzopoulou A, Syriou V, Angelopoulou R. Investigating ROS sources in male infertility: a common end for numerous pathways. Reprod Toxicol. 2012;34(3):298–307.
15. Patel AS, Leong JY, Ramasamy R. Prediction of male infertility by the World Health Organization laboratory manual for assessment of semen analysis: a systematic review. Arab J Urol. 2017;16(1):96–102.
16. Agarwal A, Tvrda E, Sharma R. Relationship amongst teratozoospermia, seminal oxidative stress and male infertility. Reprod Biol Endocrinol. 2014;12:45.
17. Mahfouz R, Sharma R, Sharma D, Sabanegh E, Agarwal A. Diagnostic value of the total antioxidant capacity (TAC) in human seminal plasma. Fertil Steril. 2009;91(3):805–11.
18. Minhas S, Bettocchi C, Boeri L, Capogrosso P, Carvalho J, Cilesiz NC, Cocci A, Corona G, Dimitropoulos K, Gül M, Hatzichristodoulou G, Jones TH, Kadioglu A, Martínez Salamanca JI, Milenkovic U, Modgil V, Russo GI, Serefoglu EC, Tharakan T, Verze P, Salonia A, EAU Working Group on Male Sexual and Reproductive Health. European Association of Urology guidelines on male sexual and reproductive health: 2021 update on male infertility. Eur Urol. 2021;80(5):603–20. https://doi.org/10.1016/j.eururo.2021.08.014.
19. Ko EY, Siddiqi K, Brannigan RE, Sabanegh ES Jr. Empirical medical therapy for idiopathic male infertility: a survey of the American Urological Association. J Urol. 2012;187(3):973–8. https://doi.org/10.1016/j.juro.2011.10.137.
20. Thaker H, Ko EY, Sabanegh ES, Brannigan RE, Alukal JP, Samplaski MK. Empirical medical therapy for idiopathic male infertility. F S Rep. 2020;1(1):15–20. https://doi.org/10.1016/j.xfre.2020.04.003.
21. Al Khayal AM, Balaraj FK, Alferayan TA, Al Sait MA, Abumelha SM, Alrabeeah KA. Empirical therapy for male factor infertility: survey of the current practice. Urol Ann. 2021;13(4):346–50. https://doi.org/10.4103/UA.UA_22_20.
22. Tadros NN, Sabanegh ES. Empiric medical therapy with hormonal agents for idiopathic male infertility. Indian J Urol. 2017;33(3):194–8. https://doi.org/10.4103/iju.IJU_368_16.
23. Garg H, Kumar R. Empirical drug therapy for idiopathic male infertility: what is the new evidence? Urology. 2015;86(6):1065–75. https://doi.org/10.1016/j.urology.2015.07.030.
24. Buhling KJ, Chan P, Kathrins M, Showell M, Vij SC, Sigman M. Should empiric therapies be used for male factor infertility? Fertil Steril. 2020;113(6):1121–30. https://doi.org/10.1016/j.fertnstert.2020.04.015.

25. Ross C, Morriss A, Khairy M, Khalaf Y, Braude P, Coomarasamy A, El-Toukhy T. A systematic review of the effect of oral antioxidants on male infertility. Reprod Biomed Online. 2010;20(6):711–23. https://doi.org/10.1016/j.rbmo.2010.03.008.
26. Tremellen K. Oxidative stress and male infertility—a clinical perspective. Hum Reprod Update. 2008;14(3):243–58. https://doi.org/10.1093/humupd/dmn004.
27. Makker K, Agarwal A, Sharma R. Oxidative stress & male infertility. Indian J Med Res. 2009;129(4):357–67.
28. Peeker R, Abramsson L, Marklund SL. Superoxide dismutase isoenzymes in human seminal plasma and spermatozoa. Mol Hum Reprod. 1997;3(12):1061–6. https://doi.org/10.1093/molehr/3.12.1061.
29. Kobayashi T, Miyazaki T, Natori M, Nozawa S. Protective role of superoxide dismutase in human sperm motility: superoxide dismutase activity and lipid peroxide in human seminal plasma and spermatozoa. Hum Reprod. 1991;6(7):987–91. https://doi.org/10.1093/oxfordjournals.humrep.a137474.
30. Chen H, Chow PH, Cheng SK, Cheung AL, Cheng LY, O WS. Male genital tract antioxidant enzymes: their source, function in the female, and ability to preserve sperm DNA integrity in the golden hamster. J Androl. 2003;24(5):704–11. https://doi.org/10.1002/j.1939-4640.2003.tb02730.x.
31. Tavilani H, Goodarzi MT, Doosti M, Vaisi-Raygani A, Hassanzadeh T, Salimi S, Joshaghani HR. Relationship between seminal antioxidant enzymes and the phospholipid and fatty acid composition of spermatozoa. Reprod Biomed Online. 2008;16(5):649–56. https://doi.org/10.1016/s1472-6483(10)60478-6.
32. Jeulin C, Soufir JC, Weber P, Laval-Martin D, Calvayrac R. Catalase activity in human spermatozoa and seminal plasma. Gamete Res. 1989;24(2):185–96. https://doi.org/10.1002/mrd.1120240206.
33. Fraga CG, Motchnik PA, Shigenaga MK, Helbock HJ, Jacob RA, Ames BN. Ascorbic acid protects against endogenous oxidative DNA damage in human sperm. Proc Natl Acad Sci U S A. 1991;88(24):11003–6. https://doi.org/10.1073/pnas.88.24.11003.
34. Irvine DS. Glutathione as a treatment for male infertility. Rev Reprod. 1996;1(1):6–12. https://doi.org/10.1530/ror.0.0010006.
35. Hekimoglu A, Kurcer Z, Aral F, Baba F, Sahna E, Atessahin A. Lycopene, an antioxidant carotenoid, attenuates testicular injury caused by ischemia/reperfusion in rats. Tohoku J Exp Med. 2009;218(2):141–7. https://doi.org/10.1620/tjem.218.141.
36. Ursini F, Heim S, Kiess M, Maiorino M, Roveri A, Wissing J, Flohé L. Dual function of the selenoprotein PHGPx during sperm maturation. Science. 1999;285(5432):1393–6. https://doi.org/10.1126/science.285.5432.1393.
37. Suleiman SA, Ali ME, Zaki ZM, el-Malik EM, Nasr MA. Lipid peroxidation and human sperm motility: protective role of vitamin E. J Androl. 1996;17(5):530–7.
38. Agarwal A, Leisegang K, Majzoub A, Henkel R, Finelli R, Panner Selvam MK, Tadros N, Parekh N, Ko EY, Cho CL, Arafa M, Alves MG, Oliveira PF, Alvarez JG, Shah R. Utility of antioxidants in the treatment of male infertility: clinical guidelines based on a systematic review and analysis of evidence. World J Mens Health. 2021;39(2):233–90. https://doi.org/10.5534/wjmh.200196.
39. de Ligny W, Smits RM, Mackenzie-Proctor R, Jordan V, Fleischer K, de Bruin JP, Showell MG. Antioxidants for male subfertility. Cochrane Database Syst Rev. 2022;5(5):CD007411. https://doi.org/10.1002/14651858.CD007411.pub5.
40. Appleton J. Arginine: clinical potential of a semi-essential amino acid. Altern Med Rev. 2002;7(6):512–22.
41. Sinclair S. Male infertility: nutritional and environmental considerations. Altern Med Rev. 2000;5(1):28–38.
42. Schachter A, Friedman S, Goldman JA, Eckerling B. Treatment of oligospermia with the amino acid arginine. Int J Gynaecol Obstet. 1973;11(5):206–9.

43. De Aloysio D, Mantuano R, Mauloni M, Nicoletti G. The clinical use of arginine aspartate in male infertility. Acta Eur Fertil. 1982;13(3):133–67.
44. Miroueh A. Effect of arginine on oligospermia. Fertil Steril. 1970;21(3):217–9.
45. Pryor JP, Blandy JP, Evans P, Chaput De Saintonge DM, Usherwood M. Controlled clinical trial of arginine for infertile men with oligozoospermia. Br J Urol. 1978;50(1):47–50. https://doi.org/10.1111/j.1464-410x.1978.tb02765.x.
46. Srivastava S, Agarwal A. Effect of anion channel blockers on L-arginine action in spermatozoa from asthenospermic men. Andrologia. 2010;42(2):76–82. https://doi.org/10.1111/j.1439-0272.2009.00959.x.
47. Palmero S, Bottazzi C, Costa M, Leone M, Fugassa E. Metabolic effects of L-carnitine on prepubertal rat Sertoli cells. Horm Metab Res. 2000;32(3):87–90. https://doi.org/10.1055/s-2007-978596.
48. Vicari E, La Vignera S, Calogero AE. Antioxidant treatment with carnitines is effective in infertile patients with prostatovesiculoepididymitis and elevated seminal leukocyte concentrations after treatment with nonsteroidal anti-inflammatory compounds. Fertil Steril. 2002;78(6):1203–8. https://doi.org/10.1016/s0015-0282(02)04350-9.
49. Agarwal A, Nallella KP, Allamaneni SS, Said TM. Role of antioxidants in treatment of male infertility: an overview of the literature. Reprod Biomed Online. 2004;8(6):616–27.
50. Bøhmer T, Hoel P, Purvis K, Hansson V. Carnitine levels in human accessory sex organs. Arch Androl. 1978;1(1):53–9. https://doi.org/10.3109/01485017808988318.
51. Moncada ML, Vicari E, Cimino C, Calogero AE, Mongioì A, D'Agata R. Effect of acetylcarnitine treatment in oligoasthenospermic patients. Acta Eur Fertil. 1992;23(5):221–4.
52. Costa M, Canale D, Filicori M, D'lddio S, Lenzi A. L-carnitine in idiopathic asthenozoospermia: a multicenter study. Italian Study Group on Carnitine and Male Infertility. Andrologia. 1994;26(3):155–9.
53. Lenzi A, Sgrò P, Salacone P, Paoli D, Gilio B, Lombardo F, Santulli M, Agarwal A, Gandini L. A placebo-controlled double-blind randomized trial of the use of combined l-carnitine and l-acetyl-carnitine treatment in men with asthenozoospermia. Fertil Steril. 2004;81(6):1578–84. https://doi.org/10.1016/j.fertnstert.2003.10.034.
54. Balercia G, Regoli F, Armeni T, Koverech A, Mantero F, Boscaro M. Placebo-controlled double-blind randomized trial on the use of L-carnitine, L-acetylcarnitine, or combined L-carnitine and L-acetylcarnitine in men with idiopathic asthenozoospermia. Fertil Steril. 2005;84(3):662–71. https://doi.org/10.1016/j.fertnstert.2005.03.064.
55. Zhou X, Liu F, Zhai S. Effect of L-carnitine and/or L-acetyl-carnitine in nutrition treatment for male infertility: a systematic review. Asia Pac J Clin Nutr. 2007;16(Suppl. 1):383–90.
56. De Rosa M, Boggia B, Amalfi B, Zarrilli S, Vita A, Colao A, Lombardi G. Correlation between seminal carnitine and functional spermatozoal characteristics in men with semen dysfunction of various origins. Drugs R D. 2005;6(1):1–9. https://doi.org/10.2165/00126839-200506010-00001.
57. Sigman M, Glass S, Campagnone J, Pryor JL. Carnitine for the treatment of idiopathic asthenospermia: a randomized, double-blind, placebo-controlled trial. Fertil Steril. 2006;85(5):1409–14. https://doi.org/10.1016/j.fertnstert.2005.10.055.
58. Littarru GP, Tiano L. Clinical aspects of coenzyme Q10: an update. Nutrition. 2010;26(3):250–4. https://doi.org/10.1016/j.nut.2009.08.008.
59. Bentinger M, Tekle M, Dallner G. Coenzyme Q-biosynthesis and functions. Biochem Biophys Res Commun. 2010;396(1):74–9. https://doi.org/10.1016/j.bbrc.2010.02.147.
60. Mancini A, De Marinis L, Oradei A, Hallgass ME, Conte G, Pozza D, Littarru GP. Coenzyme Q10 concentrations in normal and pathological human seminal fluid. J Androl. 1994;15(6):591–4.
61. Ebisch IM, Thomas CM, Peters WH, Braat DD, Steegers-Theunissen RP. The importance of folate, zinc and antioxidants in the pathogenesis and prevention of subfertility. Hum Reprod Update. 2007;13(2):163–74. https://doi.org/10.1093/humupd/dml054.

62. Joshi R, Adhikari S, Patro BS, Chattopadhyay S, Mukherjee T. Free radical scavenging behavior of folic acid: evidence for possible antioxidant activity. Free Radic Biol Med. 2001;30(12):1390–9. https://doi.org/10.1016/s0891-5849(01)00543-3.
63. Young SS, Eskenazi B, Marchetti FM, Block G, Wyrobek AJ. The association of folate, zinc and antioxidant intake with sperm aneuploidy in healthy non-smoking men. Hum Reprod. 2008;23(5):1014–22. https://doi.org/10.1093/humrep/den036.
64. Wong WY, Merkus HM, Thomas CM, Menkveld R, Zielhuis GA, Steegers-Theunissen RP. Effects of folic acid and zinc sulfate on male factor subfertility: a double-blind, randomized, placebo-controlled trial. Fertil Steril. 2002;77(3):491–8. https://doi.org/10.1016/s0015-0282(01)03229-0.
65. Landau B, Singer R, Klein T, Segenreich E. Folic acid levels in blood and seminal plasma of normo- and oligospermic patients prior and following folic acid treatment. Experientia. 1978;34(10):1301–2. https://doi.org/10.1007/BF01981432.
66. Lenzi A, Lombardo F, Gandini L, Culasso F, Dondero F. Glutathione therapy for male infertility. Arch Androl. 1992;29(1):65–8. https://doi.org/10.3109/01485019208987710.
67. Lenzi A, Picardo M, Gandini L, Lombardo F, Terminali O, Passi S, Dondero F. Glutathione treatment of dyspermia: effect on the lipoperoxidation process. Hum Reprod. 1994;9(11):2044–50. https://doi.org/10.1093/oxfordjournals.humrep.a138391.
68. Kodama H, Yamaguchi R, Fukuda J, Kasai H, Tanaka T. Increased oxidative deoxyribonucleic acid damage in the spermatozoa of infertile male patients. Fertil Steril. 1997;68(3):519–24. https://doi.org/10.1016/s0015-0282(97)00236-7.
69. Rao AV, Ray MR, Rao LG. Lycopene. Adv Food Nutr Res. 2006;51:99–164. https://doi.org/10.1016/S1043-4526(06)51002-2.
70. Durairajanayagam D, Agarwal A, Ong C, Prashast P. Lycopene and male infertility. Asian J Androl. 2014;16(3):420–5. https://doi.org/10.4103/1008-682X.126384.
71. Rao AV, Rao LG. Carotenoids and human health. Pharmacol Res. 2007;55(3):207–16. https://doi.org/10.1016/j.phrs.2007.01.012.
72. Goyal A, Chopra M, Lwaleed BA, Birch B, Cooper AJ. The effects of dietary lycopene supplementation on human seminal plasma. BJU Int. 2007;99(6):1456–60. https://doi.org/10.1111/j.1464-410X.2007.06804.x.
73. Calogero AE, Aversa A, La Vignera S, Corona G, Ferlin A. The use of nutraceuticals in male sexual and reproductive disturbances: position statement from the Italian Society of Andrology and Sexual Medicine (SIAMS). J Endocrinol Investig. 2017;40(12):1389–97. https://doi.org/10.1007/s40618-017-0699-6.
74. Cannarella R, Calogero AE, Condorelli RA, Giacone F, Mongioi' LM, La Vignera S. Non-hormonal treatment for male infertility: the potential role of Serenoa repens, selenium and lycopene. Eur Rev Med Pharmacol Sci. 2019;23(7):3112–20. https://doi.org/10.26355/eurrev_201904_17595.
75. Brown KM, Arthur JR. Selenium, selenoproteins and human health: a review. Public Health Nutr. 2001;4(2B):593–9. https://doi.org/10.1079/phn2001143.
76. Watanabe T, Endo A. Effects of selenium deficiency on sperm morphology and spermatocyte chromosomes in mice. Mutat Res. 1991;262(2):93–9. https://doi.org/10.1016/0165-7992(91)90113-i.
77. Safarinejad MR, Safarinejad S. Efficacy of selenium and/or N-acetyl-cysteine for improving semen parameters in infertile men: a double-blind, placebo controlled, randomized study. J Urol. 2009;181(2):741–51. https://doi.org/10.1016/j.juro.2008.10.015.
78. Scott R, MacPherson A, Yates RW, Hussain B, Dixon J. The effect of oral selenium supplementation on human sperm motility. Br J Urol. 1998;82(1):76–80. https://doi.org/10.1046/j.1464-410x.1998.00683.x.
79. Iwanier K, Zachara BA. Selenium supplementation enhances the element concentration in blood and seminal fluid but does not change the spermatozoal quality characteristics in subfertile men. J Androl. 1995;16(5):441–7.

80. Shalini S, Bansal MP. Dietary selenium deficiency as well as excess supplementation induces multiple defects in mouse epididymal spermatozoa: understanding the role of selenium in male fertility. Int J Androl. 2008;31(4):438–49. https://doi.org/10.1111/j.1365-2605.2007.00789.x.
81. Esterbauer H, Striegl G, Puhl H, Oberreither S, Rotheneder M, el-Saadani M, Jürgens G. The role of vitamin E and carotenoids in preventing oxidation of low density lipoproteins. Ann N Y Acad Sci. 1989;570:254–67. https://doi.org/10.1111/j.1749-6632.1989.tb14925.x.
82. Wolbach SB, Howe PR. Tissue changes following deprivation of fat-soluble a vitamin. J Exp Med. 1925;42(6):753–77.
83. Van Pelt AM, De Rooij DG. The origin of the synchronization of the seminiferous epithelium in vitamin A-deficient rats after vitamin A replacement. Biol Reprod. 1990;42(4):677–82. https://doi.org/10.1095/biolreprod42.4.677.
84. Morales A, Cavicchia JC. Spermatogenesis and blood-testis barrier in rats after long-term vitamin A deprivation. Tissue Cell. 2002;34(5):349–55. https://doi.org/10.1016/s0040816602000356.
85. Paradiso Galatioto G, Gravina GL, Angelozzi G, et al. May antioxidant therapy improve sperm parameters of men with persistent oligospermia after retrograde embolization for varicocele? World J Urol. 2008;26(1):97–102.
86. Linster CL, Van Schaftingen E, Vitamin C. Biosynthesis, recycling and degradation in mammals. FEBS J. 2007;274(1):1–22.
87. Kefer JC, Agarwal A, Sabanegh E. Role of antioxidants in the treatment of male infertility. Int J Urol. 2009;16(5):449–57. https://doi.org/10.1111/j.1442-2042.2009.02280.x.
88. Greco E, Iacobelli M, Rienzi L, Ubaldi F, Ferrero S, Tesarik J. Reduction of the incidence of sperm DNA fragmentation by oral antioxidant treatment. J Androl. 2005;26(3):349–53. https://doi.org/10.2164/jandrol.04146.
89. Dawson EB, Harris WA, Rankin WE, Charpentier LA, McGanity WJ. Effect of ascorbic acid on male fertility. Ann N Y Acad Sci. 1987;498:312–23. https://doi.org/10.1111/j.1749-6632.1987.tb23770.x.
90. Colagar AH, Marzony ET. Ascorbic acid in human seminal plasma: determination and its relationship to sperm quality. J Clin Biochem Nutr. 2009;45(2):144–9. https://doi.org/10.3164/jcbn.08-251.
91. Eskenazi B, Kidd SA, Marks AR, Sloter E, Block G, Wyrobek AJ. Antioxidant intake is associated with semen quality in healthy men. Hum Reprod. 2005;20(4):1006–12. https://doi.org/10.1093/humrep/deh725.
92. Omu AE, Al-Azemi MK, Kehinde EO, Anim JT, Oriowo MA, Mathew TC. Indications of the mechanisms involved in improved sperm parameters by zinc therapy. Med Princ Pract. 2008;17(2):108–16. https://doi.org/10.1159/000112963.
93. Dawson EB, Harris WA, Teter MC, Powell LC. Effect of ascorbic acid supplementation on the sperm quality of smokers. Fertil Steril. 1992;58(5):1034–9.
94. Brigelius-Flohé R, Traber MG. Vitamin E: function and metabolism. FASEB J. 1999;13(10):1145–55.
95. Kessopoulou E, Powers HJ, Sharma KK, Pearson MJ, Russell JM, Cooke ID, Barratt CL. A double-blind randomized placebo cross-over controlled trial using the antioxidant vitamin E to treat reactive oxygen species associated male infertility. Fertil Steril. 1995;64(4):825–31. https://doi.org/10.1016/s0015-0282(16)57861-3.
96. Lonn E, Bosch J, Yusuf S, Sheridan P, Pogue J, Arnold JM, Ross C, Arnold A, Sleight P, Probstfield J, Dagenais GR, HOPE and HOPE-TOO Trial Investigators. Effects of long-term vitamin E supplementation on cardiovascular events and cancer: a randomized controlled trial. JAMA. 2005;293(11):1338–47. https://doi.org/10.1001/jama.293.11.1338.
97. Miller ER 3rd, Pastor-Barriuso R, Dalal D, Riemersma RA, Appel LJ, Guallar E. Meta-analysis: high-dosage vitamin E supplementation may increase all-cause mortality. Ann Intern Med. 2005;142(1):37–46. https://doi.org/10.7326/0003-4819-142-1-200501040-00110.

98. Mousa SA. Antithrombotic effects of naturally derived products on coagulation and platelet function. Methods Mol Biol. 2010;663:229–40. https://doi.org/10.1007/978-1-60761-803-4_9.
99. Zago MP, Oteiza PI. The antioxidant properties of zinc: interactions with iron and antioxidants. Free Radic Biol Med. 2001;31(2):266–74. https://doi.org/10.1016/s0891-5849(01)00583-4.
100. Maret W, Sandstead HH. Zinc requirements and the risks and benefits of zinc supplementation. J Trace Elem Med Biol. 2006;20(1):3–18. https://doi.org/10.1016/j.jtemb.2006.01.006.
101. Colagar AH, Marzony ET, Chaichi MJ. Zinc levels in seminal plasma are associated with sperm quality in fertile and infertile men. Nutr Res. 2009;29(2):82–8. https://doi.org/10.1016/j.nutres.2008.11.007.
102. Marmar JL, Katz S, Praiss DE, DeBenedictis TJ. Semen zinc levels in infertile and postvasectomy patients and patients with prostatitis. Fertil Steril. 1975;26(11):1057–63. https://doi.org/10.1016/s0015-0282(16)41470-6.
103. Saaranen M, Suistomaa U, Kantola M, Saarikoski S, Vanha-Perttula T. Lead, magnesium, selenium and zinc in human seminal fluid: comparison with semen parameters and fertility. Hum Reprod. 1987;2(6):475–9. https://doi.org/10.1093/oxfordjournals.humrep.a136573.
104. Yao DF, Mills JN. Male infertility: lifestyle factors and holistic, complementary, and alternative therapies. Asian J Androl. 2016;18(3):410–8. https://doi.org/10.4103/1008-682X.175779.
105. Ogden CL, Carroll MD, Curtin LR, McDowell MA, Tabak CJ, Flegal KM. Prevalence of overweight and obesity in the United States, 1999–2004. JAMA. 2006;295(13):1549–55. https://doi.org/10.1001/jama.295.13.1549.
106. Du Plessis SS, Cabler S, McAlister DA, Sabanegh E, Agarwal A. The effect of obesity on sperm disorders and male infertility. Nat Rev Urol. 2010;7(3):153–61. https://doi.org/10.1038/nrurol.2010.6.
107. Al-Ali BM, Gutschi T, Pummer K, Zigeuner R, Brookman-May S, Wieland WF, Fritsche HM, Aziz A. Body mass index has no impact on sperm quality but on reproductive hormones levels. Andrologia. 2014;46(2):106–11. https://doi.org/10.1111/and.12051.
108. Michalakis K, Mintziori G, Kaprara A, Tarlatzis BC, Goulis DG. The complex interaction between obesity, metabolic syndrome and reproductive axis: a narrative review. Metabolism. 2013;62(4):457–78. https://doi.org/10.1016/j.metabol.2012.08.012. Epub 2012 Sep 20
109. Blank DM, Clark RV, Heymsfield SB, Rudman DR, Blank MS. Endogenous opioids and hypogonadism in human obesity. Brain Res Bull. 1994;34(6):571–4. https://doi.org/10.1016/0361-9230(94)90142-2.
110. Tsatsanis C, Dermitzaki E, Avgoustinaki P, Malliaraki N, Mytaras V, Margioris AN. The impact of adipose tissue-derived factors on the hypothalamic-pituitary-gonadal (HPG) axis. Hormones (Athens). 2015;14(4):549–62. https://doi.org/10.14310/horm.2002.1649.
111. Hjollund NH, Storgaard L, Ernst E, Bonde JP, Olsen J. The relation between daily activities and scrotal temperature. Reprod Toxicol. 2002;16(3):209–14. https://doi.org/10.1016/s0890-6238(02)00026-6.
112. Mieusset R, Bujan L, Mondinat C, Mansat A, Pontonnier F, Grandjean H. Association of scrotal hyperthermia with impaired spermatogenesis in infertile men. Fertil Steril. 1987;48(6):1006–11. https://doi.org/10.1016/s0015-0282(16)59600-9.
113. Shafik A, Olfat S. Scrotal lipomatosis. Br J Urol. 1981;53(1):50–4. https://doi.org/10.1111/j.1464-410x.1981.tb03128.x.
114. Jo J, Kim H. The relationship between body mass index and scrotal temperature among male partners of subfertile couples. J Therm Biol. 2016;56:55–8. https://doi.org/10.1016/j.jtherbio.2016.01.003.
115. MacDonald AA, Herbison GP, Showell M, Farquhar CM. The impact of body mass index on semen parameters and reproductive hormones in human males: a systematic review with meta-analysis. Hum Reprod Update. 2010;16(3):293–311. https://doi.org/10.1093/humupd/dmp047.
116. Sermondade N, Faure C, Fezeu L, Shayeb AG, Bonde JP, Jensen TK, Van Wely M, Cao J, Martini AC, Eskandar M, Chavarro JE, Koloszar S, Twigt JM, Ramlau-Hansen CH, Borges E Jr, Lotti F, Steegers-Theunissen RP, Zorn B, Polotsky AJ, La Vignera S, Eskenazi B,

Tremellen K, Magnusdottir EV, Fejes I, Hercberg S, Lévy R, Czernichow S. BMI in relation to sperm count: an updated systematic review and collaborative meta-analysis. Hum Reprod Update. 2013;19(3):221–31. https://doi.org/10.1093/humupd/dms050.

117. Eisenberg ML, Kim S, Chen Z, Sundaram R, Schisterman EF, Buck Louis GM. The relationship between male BMI and waist circumference on semen quality: data from the LIFE study. Hum Reprod. 2014;29(2):193–200. https://doi.org/10.1093/humrep/det428. Epub 2013 Dec 4. Erratum in: Hum Reprod 2015 Feb;30(2):493–4. Erratum in: Hum Reprod. 2015 Feb;30(2):493–4. PMID: 24306102; PMCID: PMC3896223
118. Agbaje IM, Rogers DA, McVicar CM, McClure N, Atkinson AB, Mallidis C, Lewis SE. Insulin dependant diabetes mellitus: implications for male reproductive function. Hum Reprod. 2007;22(7):1871–7. https://doi.org/10.1093/humrep/dem077.
119. Bandel I, Bungum M, Richtoff J, Malm J, Axelsson J, Pedersen HS, Ludwicki JK, Czaja K, Hernik A, Toft G, Bonde JP, Spanò M, Malm G, Haugen TB, Giwercman A. No association between body mass index and sperm DNA integrity. Hum Reprod. 2015;30(7):1704–13. https://doi.org/10.1093/humrep/dev111.
120. Hakonsen LB, Thulstrup AM, Aggerholm AS, Olsen J, Bonde JP, Andersen CY, Bungum M, Ernst EH, Hansen ML, Ernst EH, Ramlau-Hansen CH. Does weight loss improve semen quality and reproductive hormones? Results from a cohort of severely obese men. Reprod Health. 2011;8:24. https://doi.org/10.1186/1742-4755-8-24.
121. Arab A, Rafie N, Mansourian M, Miraghajani M, Hajianfar H. Dietary patterns and semen quality: a systematic review and meta-analysis of observational studies. Andrology. 2018;6(1):20–8. https://doi.org/10.1111/andr.12430. Epub 2017 Oct 12
122. Karayiannis D, Kontogianni MD, Mendorou C, Douka L, Mastrominas M, Yiannakouris N. Association between adherence to the Mediterranean diet and semen quality parameters in male partners of couples attempting fertility. Hum Reprod. 2017;32(1):215–22. https://doi.org/10.1093/humrep/dew288.
123. Cao LL, Chang JJ, Wang SJ, Li YH, Yuan MY, Wang GF, Su PY. The effect of healthy dietary patterns on male semen quality: a systematic review and meta-analysis. Asian J Androl. 2022;24(5):549–57. https://doi.org/10.4103/aja202252. Epub ahead of print
124. Ferramosca A, Zara V. Diet and male fertility: the impact of nutrients and antioxidants on sperm energetic metabolism. Int J Mol Sci. 2022;23(5):2542. https://doi.org/10.3390/ijms23052542.
125. Anbara H, Sheibani MT, Razi M. Long-term effect of aspartame on male reproductive system: evidence for testicular histomorphometrics, Hsp70-2 protein expression and biochemical status. Int J Fertil Steril. 2020;14(2):91–101. https://doi.org/10.22074/ijfs.2020.6065.
126. Melis MS. Effects of chronic administration of Stevia rebaudiana on fertility in rats. J Ethnopharmacol. 1999;67(2):157–61. https://doi.org/10.1016/s0378-8741(99)00081-1.
127. Zhao X, Bian Y, Sun Y, Li L, Wang L, Zhao C, Shen Y, Song Q, Qu Y, Niu S, Wu W, Gao F. Effects of moderate exercise over different phases on age-related physiological dysfunction in testes of SAMP8 mice. Exp Gerontol. 2013;48(9):869–80. https://doi.org/10.1016/j.exger.2013.05.063.
128. Tatara K, Sato K. Aerobic exercise training and dehydroepiandrosterone administration increase testicular sex steroid hormones and enhance reproductive function in high-sucrose-induced obese rats. J Steroid Biochem Mol Biol. 2019;190:37–43. https://doi.org/10.1016/j.jsbmb.2019.03.019.
129. Rosety-Rodriguez M, Rosety JM, Fornieles G, Rosety MA, Diaz AJ, Rosety I, Rodríguez-Pareja A, Rosety M, Ordonez FJ, Elosegui S. Home-based treadmill training improved seminal quality in adults with type 2 diabetes. Actas Urol Esp. 2014;38(9):589–93. https://doi.org/10.1016/j.acuro.2013.10.013.
130. De Souza MJ, Arce JC, Pescatello LS, Scherzer HS, Luciano AA. Gonadal hormones and semen quality in male runners. A volume threshold effect of endurance training. Int J Sports Med. 1994;15(7):383–91. https://doi.org/10.1055/s-2007-1021075.

131. Safarinejad MR, Azma K, Kolahi AA. The effects of intensive, long-term treadmill running on reproductive hormones, hypothalamus-pituitary-testis axis, and semen quality: a randomized controlled study. J Endocrinol. 2009;200(3):259–71. https://doi.org/10.1677/JOE-08-0477.
132. Minas A, Fernandes ACC, Maciel Júnior VL, Adami L, Intasqui P, Bertolla RP. Influence of physical activity on male fertility. Andrologia. 2022;54(7):e14433. https://doi.org/10.1111/and.14433. Epub 2022 Apr 12
133. Vaamonde D, Algar-Santacruz C, Abbasi A, García-Manso JM. Sperm DNA fragmentation as a result of ultra-endurance exercise training in male athletes. Andrologia. 2018;50(1):e12793. https://doi.org/10.1111/and.12793.
134. Min T, Prior SL, Dunseath G, Churm R, Barry JD, Stephens JW. Temporal effects of bariatric surgery on adipokines, inflammation and oxidative stress in subjects with impaired glucose homeostasis at 4 years of follow-up. Obes Surg. 2020;30(5):1712–8. https://doi.org/10.1007/s11695-019-04377-3.
135. Reis LO, Zani EL, Saad RD, Chaim EA, de Oliveira LC, Fregonesi A. Bariatric surgery does not interfere with sperm quality—a preliminary long-term study. Reprod Sci. 2012;19(10):1057–62. https://doi.org/10.1177/1933719112440747.
136. El Bardisi H, Majzoub A, Arafa M, AlMalki A, Al Said S, Khalafalla K, Jabbour G, Basha M, Al Ansari A, Sabanegh E Jr. Effect of bariatric surgery on semen parameters and sex hormone concentrations: a prospective study. Reprod Biomed Online. 2016;33(5):606–11. https://doi.org/10.1016/j.rbmo.2016.08.008.
137. Samavat J, Cantini G, Lotti F, Di Franco A, Tamburrino L, Degl'Innocenti S, Maseroli E, Filimberti E, Facchiano E, Lucchese M, Muratori M, Forti G, Baldi E, Maggi M, Luconi M. Massive weight loss obtained by bariatric surgery affects semen quality in morbid male obesity: a preliminary prospective double-armed study. Obes Surg. 2018;28(1):69–76. https://doi.org/10.1007/s11695-017-2802-7.
138. Magalhaes DP, Mahalingaiah S, Perry MJ. Exploring the causes of semen quality changes post-bariatric surgery: a focus on endocrine-disrupting chemicals. Hum Reprod. 2022;37(5):902–21. https://doi.org/10.1093/humrep/deac039.
139. Razzaq A, Soomro FH, Siddiq G, Khizar S, Ali KM. Decrease in sperm count after bariatric surgery: case reports. Cureus. 2021;13(12):e20388. https://doi.org/10.7759/cureus.20388.
140. Sermondade N, Massin N, Boitrelle F, Pfeffer J, Eustache F, Sifer C, Czernichow S, Lévy R. Sperm parameters and male fertility after bariatric surgery: three case series. Reprod Biomed Online. 2012;24(2):206–10. https://doi.org/10.1016/j.rbmo.2011.10.014.
141. Gao Z, Liang Y, Yang S, Zhang T, Gong Z, Li M, Yang J. Bariatric surgery does not improve semen quality: evidence from a meta-analysis. Obes Surg. 2022;32(4):1341–50. https://doi.org/10.1007/s11695-022-05901-8. Epub 2022 Feb 10. Erratum in: Obes Surg 2022 Feb 22
142. Das S, Roychoudhury S, Roychoudhury S, Agarwal A, Henkel R. Role of infection and leukocytes in male infertility. Adv Exp Med Biol. 2022;1358:115–40. https://doi.org/10.1007/978-3-030-89340-8_6.
143. Ruggeri M, Cannas S, Cubeddu M, Molicotti P, Piras GL, Dessole S, Zanetti S. Bacterial agents as a cause of infertility in humans. New Microbiol. 2016;39(3):206–9.
144. Keck C, Gerber-Schäfer C, Clad A, Wilhelm C, Breckwoldt M. Seminal tract infections: impact on male fertility and treatment options. Hum Reprod Update. 1998;4(6):891–903. https://doi.org/10.1093/humupd/4.6.891.
145. Yanushpolsky EH, Politch JA, Hill JA, Anderson DJ. Is leukocytospermia clinically relevant? Fertil Steril. 1996;66(5):822–5.
146. Henkel RR. Leukocytes and oxidative stress: dilemma for sperm function and male fertility. Asian J Androl. 2011;13(1):43–52. https://doi.org/10.1038/aja.2010.76.
147. Potts JM, Sharma R, Pasqualotto F, Nelson D, Hall G, Agarwal A. Association of ureaplasma urealyticum with abnormal reactive oxygen species levels and absence of leukocytospermia. J Urol. 2000;163(6):1775–8.

148. Jung JH, Kim MH, Kim J, Baik SK, Koh SB, Park HJ, Seo JT. Treatment of leukocytospermia in male infertility: a systematic review. World J Mens Health. 2016;34(3):165–72. https://doi.org/10.5534/wjmh.2016.34.3.165.
149. Witt MA, Lipshultz LI. Varicocele: a progressive or static lesion? Urology. 1993;42(5):541–3. https://doi.org/10.1016/0090-4295(93)90268-f.
150. Schauer I, Madersbacher S, Jost R, Hübner WA, Imhof M. The impact of varicocelectomy on sperm parameters: a meta-analysis. J Urol. 2012;187(5):1540–7. https://doi.org/10.1016/j.juro.2011.12.084.
151. Hendin BN, Kolettis PN, Sharma RK, Thomas AJ Jr, Agarwal A. Varicocele is associated with elevated spermatozoal reactive oxygen species production and diminished seminal plasma antioxidant capacity. J Urol. 1999;161(6):1831–4.
152. Sakamoto Y, Ishikawa T, Kondo Y, Yamaguchi K, Fujisawa M. The assessment of oxidative stress in infertile patients with varicocele. BJU Int. 2008;101(12):1547–52. https://doi.org/10.1111/j.1464-410X.2008.07517.x.
153. Mostafa T, Anis T, Imam H, El-Nashar AR, Osman IA. Seminal reactive oxygen species-antioxidant relationship in fertile males with and without varicocele. Andrologia. 2009;41(2):125–9. https://doi.org/10.1111/j.1439-0272.2008.00900.x.
154. Ni K, Steger K, Yang H, Wang H, Hu K, Zhang T, Chen B. A comprehensive investigation of sperm DNA damage and oxidative stress injury in infertile patients with subclinical, normozoospermic, and astheno/oligozoospermic clinical varicocoele. Andrology. 2016;4(5):816–24. https://doi.org/10.1111/andr.12210.
155. Mostafa T, Anis TH, El-Nashar A, Imam H, Othman IA. Varicocelectomy reduces reactive oxygen species levels and increases antioxidant activity of seminal plasma from infertile men with varicocele. Int J Androl. 2001;24(5):261–5. https://doi.org/10.1046/j.1365-2605.2001.00296.x.
156. Dada R, Shamsi MB, Venkatesh S, Gupta NP, Kumar R. Attenuation of oxidative stress & DNA damage in varicocelectomy: implications in infertility management. Indian J Med Res. 2010;132(6):728–30.
157. Lai TC, Roychoudhury S, Cho CL. Oxidative stress and varicocele-associated male infertility. Adv Exp Med Biol. 2022;1358:205–35. https://doi.org/10.1007/978-3-030-89340-8_10.
158. Mancini A, Meucci E, Milardi D, Giacchi E, Bianchi A, Pantano AL, Mordente A, Martorana GE, de Marinis L. Seminal antioxidant capacity in pre- and postoperative varicocele. J Androl. 2004;25(1):44–9. https://doi.org/10.1002/j.1939-4640.2004.tb02757.x.
159. Yeşilli C, Mungan G, Seçkiner I, Akduman B, Açikgöz S, Altan K, Mungan A. Effect of varicocelectomy on sperm creatine kinase, HspA2 chaperone protein (creatine kinase-M type), LDH, LDH-X, and lipid peroxidation product levels in infertile men with varicocele. Urology. 2005;66(3):610–5. https://doi.org/10.1016/j.urology.2005.03.078.
160. Botezatu A, Vladoiu S, Fudulu A, Albulescu A, Plesa A, Muresan A, Stancu C, Iancu IV, Diaconu CC, Velicu A, Popa OM, Badiu C, Dinu-Draganescu D. Advanced molecular approaches in male infertility diagnosis. Biol Reprod. 2022;107(3):684–704. https://doi.org/10.1093/biolre/ioac105.
161. Wu N, Phang J, Park J, Shen Y, Huang Z, Zorin M, Jastrzebski S, Fevry T, Katsnelson J, Kim E, Wolfson S, Parikh U, Gaddam S, Lin LLY, Ho K, Weinstein JD, Reig B, Gao Y, Toth H, Pysarenko K, Lewin A, Lee J, Airola K, Mema E, Chung S, Hwang E, Samreen N, Kim SG, Heacock L, Moy L, Cho K, Geras KJ. Deep neural networks improve radiologists' performance in breast cancer screening. IEEE Trans Med Imaging. 2020;39(4):1184–94. https://doi.org/10.1109/TMI.2019.2945514.
162. McKinney SM, Sieniek M, Godbole V, Godwin J, Antropova N, Ashrafian H, Back T, Chesus M, Corrado GS, Darzi A, Etemadi M, Garcia-Vicente F, Gilbert FJ, Halling-Brown M, Hassabis D, Jansen S, Karthikesalingam A, Kelly CJ, King D, Ledsam JR, Melnick D, Mostofi H, Peng L, Reicher JJ, Romera-Paredes B, Sidebottom R, Suleyman M, Tse D, Young KC, De Fauw J, Shetty S. International evaluation of an AI system for breast cancer screen-

ing. Nature. 2020;577(7788):89–94. https://doi.org/10.1038/s41586-019-1799-6. Epub 2020 Jan 1. Erratum in: Nature. 2020 Oct;586(7829):E19

163. Gong D, Wu L, Zhang J, Mu G, Shen L, Liu J, Wang Z, Zhou W, An P, Huang X, Jiang X, Li Y, Wan X, Hu S, Chen Y, Hu X, Xu Y, Zhu X, Li S, Yao L, He X, Chen D, Huang L, Wei X, Wang X, Yu H. Detection of colorectal adenomas with a real-time computer-aided system (ENDOANGEL): a randomised controlled study. Lancet Gastroenterol Hepatol. 2020;5(4):352–61. https://doi.org/10.1016/S2468-1253(19)30413-3. Epub 2020 Jan 22. Erratum in: Lancet Gastroenterol Hepatol. 2020 Apr;5(4):e3
164. Marín R, Chang V. Impact of transfer learning for human sperm segmentation using deep learning. Comput Biol Med. 2021;136:104687. https://doi.org/10.1016/j.compbiomed.2021.104687.

Part IV
Genetics and Epigenetics of Male Infertility

Chapter 8
Advances in Genetics of Male Infertility

Taymour Mostafa, Khalid A. Fakhro, and Mohamed Arafa

Key Points

- Male infertility is a multifactorial disorder, whereas some genetic factors are comparatively present. Males with azoospermic are at increased risk to carry genetic anomalies, but such occurrence decreases with increased sperm production.
- Karyotype and Y chromosome microdeletion analyses are indicated in men having severe oligozoospermia or azoospermia.
- AZF deletion test is of diagnostic as well as prognostic importance in men with azoospermia.
- New genetic tests (next-generation DNA sequencing and whole-exome sequencing) are important in discovering single genetic defects causing male infertility.
- Gene therapy for male infertility is still experimental but will play a major role in male fertility management in cases with severe affection of spermatogenesis.

T. Mostafa (✉)
Department of Andrology, Sexology & STIs, Faculty of Medicine, Cairo University, Cairo, Egypt

K. A. Fakhro
Department of Human Genetics, Sidra Medical and Research Center, Doha, Qatar

Department of Genetic Medicine, Weill Cornell Medical College, Doha, Qatar
e-mail: kfakhro@sidra.org

M. Arafa
Department of Andrology, Sexology & STIs, Faculty of Medicine, Cairo University, Cairo, Egypt

Department of Urology, Hamad Medical Corporation, Doha, Qatar

Department of Urology, Weill Cornell Medical-Qatar, Doha, Qatar

A. Agarwal et al. (eds.), *Current and Future Advances in Male Infertility*,
https://doi.org/10.1007/978-3-031-62648-7_8

Introduction

Male infertility has many causes and risk factors that might play a role in its causation, including lifestyle factors, metabolic conditions, genital trauma, varicocele, genitourinary infections, cryptorchidism, and iatrogenic causes [1]. During the previous decades, the management of infertility has rapidly evolved. Nevertheless, a lot is yet to be discovered including the physiopathology of altered spermatogenesis and its genetic origin. Also, little is known about the genetic and epigenetic consequences for the gamete that may affect the course of conception [2].

It was estimated that about 15% of male infertility cases are attributed to the various genetic defects, which can be broadly categorized into pretesticular causes (disorders of the hypothalamic-pituitary axis), testicular causes, and seminal ductal obstruction or dysfunction [3]. Diagnosis of genetic causes of infertility has significant prognostic value in the management of the patient and has great implications on the well-being of his offspring [4].

Research has shown great advances in recent years with the emergence of several techniques for genetic analysis, such as exome sequencing, whole-genome association studies, and next-generation sequencing leading to the discovery of a panel of candidate genes (Fig. 8.1). However, these technologies are not yet established in clinical practice and are still limited to research purposes.

Chromosomal Alterations

Chromosomal alterations are prevalent in about 13–16% of infertile men, leading to different semen parameter changes [5, 6]. The most common are listed below:

- *Klinefelter syndrome (KS)*

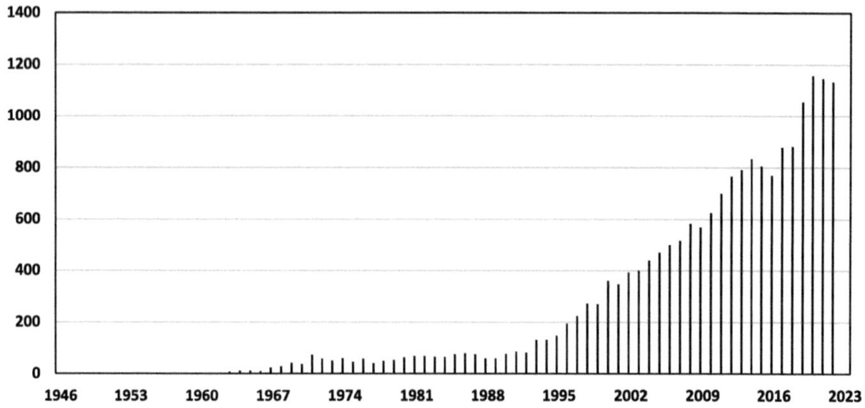

Fig. 8.1 Studies related to genetics and male infertility

- KS is a famous chromosomal abnormality linked to male infertility affecting up to 3% of infertile males, 5% of males with severe oligozoospermia, and 11% of males with azoospermia [7]. It is characterized by the occurrence of an extra X chromosome in a phenotypical male. The common form is 47,XXY and comprises about 80% of KS cases. Other forms include 48,XXXY, 48,XXYY, or structurally abnormal X chromosome [8]. KS may show a mosaic form 46,XY/47,XXY with different percentages of affected cells or may be nonmosaic [9]. KS is caused by nondisjunction from paternal or maternal origin [10].
- Clinically, men with KS are characterized by hypogonadal features, tall stature, defective bone mineralization, gynecomastia, and small firm testes and may be associated with cardiovascular disease and cognitive deficits. Patients have hypergonadotropic hypogonadism with spermatogenic failure resulting in nonobstructive azoospermia or severe oligozoospermia in a few cases [11]. After the introduction of ICSI and surgical sperm retrieval, males with KS may have the chance to father their own biological children. The surgical sperm retrieval rate in these patients ranges from 30% to 70% [12].
- *47,XYY male:*
- 47,XYY syndrome occurs in approximately 1/1000 live male births. Diagnosis of 47,XYY syndrome is problematic and often delayed due to diversity and lack of symptoms, which are usually related to cognitive functions, e.g., delayed speech development with learning difficulties and greater risk of behavioral problems [13]. Most cases are diagnosed later in life with infertility problems. Semen analysis in these cases varies from azoospermia to normal parameters [14].
- *46,XX testicular disorder of sex development (DSD)*
- DSD occurs in about 1:20,000 males [15]. Patients have male phenotype but exhibit female 46,XX karyotype. The male phenotype is maintained due to translocation of the sex-determining region Y (SRY) gene to another chromosome in approximately 80% of patients or due to hidden mosaicism for the SRY gene in SRY-negative cases [16].
- Patients may present at puberty with ambiguous genitalia, micropenis, hypospadias, and undescended testes or may present with infertility later in life [17]. In these cases, there is complete absence of spermatogenic cells owing to lack of the azoospermia factor (AZF) region, and testicular histopathology usually shows Sertoli cell only [18].
- *Chromosomal translocations:*
- These are structural chromosomal rearrangements that are prevalent in 2–8% of infertile men and can be one of the two types, reciprocal or nonreciprocal, or Robertsonian translocations [19]. Reciprocal translocation occurs when chromosomal material is exchanged between the arms of two heterologous chromosomes. This will result in changing the order of the genetic material [20]. The commonest chromosome in reciprocal translocations is chromosomes 12, 22, and Y although any chromosome can be affected [21]. On the other hand, Robertsonian translocations result from the centromeric fusion of acrocentric

chromosomes (13, 14, 15, 21, and 22). This results in the presence of the translocated chromosome made up of the long arms of two acrocentric chromosomes and loss of the chromosome made of the fused short arms. Therefore, the karyotype has only 45 chromosomes [20].

- Clinically, patients with either type of translocation will show normal phenotype, but the translocation may lead to spermatogenic defects leading to semen defects—either oligozoospermia or azoospermia. Both types are at high risk of creating unstable karyotypes in the offspring resulting in repeated miscarriages [22].
- *Chromosomal inversions:*
- A common chromosomal structural defect where a part of the chromosome breaks off rotates 180° and reattaches to the same chromosome [23] and may be one of the two types: pericentric inversion including the centromere and break happens in the chromosome arms, and paracentric inversion does not include the centromere, but the break occurs in the distal part of one arm of a chromosome [24]. Chromosome 9 inversion including inv9(p11q13) or inv9(p12q13) is the common pericentric inversion observed in 1–3.57% of the general population [25]. While it used to be considered a normal variant, recently chromosome 9 inversion has been linked to male infertility [26].
- *Y chromosome microdeletions (YCMDs)*
- YCMDs are deletions in the euchromatic part of the long arm of the Y chromosome, including AZF regions leading to different grades of spermatogenic failure. AZF is divided into AZFa, AZFb, and AZFc [27]. YCMDs are common genetic abnormalities in male infertility occurring in about 13–100% of cases of oligozoospermia and azoospermia, respectively [27].
- The most common YCMD is AZFc, probably because it has the largest size. It has the best prognosis among other types of YCMD as one-third of cases with this defect show moderate to severe oligozoospermia, while the rest show nonobstructive azoospermia with varying degrees of spermatogenic failure, but sperms can be surgically retrieved in approximately 50% of cases [28]. AZFa region deletions are the most severe leading to Sertoli cell only [29]. Microdeletions of AZFb show a large pattern of spermatogenic affection ranging from SCO syndrome to hypospermatogenesis but most commonly primary spermatocyte arrest [30].

Epigenetic Factors

Epigenetic factors play important roles in sperm function as well as fertilization. Regulation of these mechanisms, such as chromatin remodeling, DNA methylation, histone tail modifications, and ncRNAs throughout spermatogenesis, is crucial for both sperm outcome and utility [31].

- *DNA methylation*
- Process of DNA methylation shifts a methyl group (-CH3) from S-adenosyl methionine to the fifth carbon of cytosine ring in different methylated regions (DMRs) by DNA methyltransferases (DNMTs). Methylation of cytosine at DMRs leads to transcriptional inactivation by hindering TF's binding to the gene regulatory regions. Inversely, hypomethylation of the regulatory areas is linked with heightened gene expression. DNMT1 enzyme is elaborated in maintaining DNA methylation throughout DNA replication, whereas its absence could lead to defects in spermatogenesis genes [32].
- In this context, methylation of repetitive elements, genome-wide DNA methylation, and imprinted and non-imprinted genes are the critical DNA methylation steps. While imprinted genes are biallelic, their expression is monoallelic, depending on being transmitted from either parent. This process lasts with type I spermatocyte remethylation and spermatogonia transmitting the father's signature to the sperms [33].
- *Igf2/Dlk-Gtl2*, *Rasgrfl*, *H19*, and *Zdbf2* are paternally imprinted/methylated genes in the sperms. Hypomethylation of *H19* gene has been recognized in males with oligozoospermia and azoospermia, whereas hypermethylation of *SNRPN* gene is observed in men with azoospermia and teratozoospermia compared with normozoospermic men [34]. In their study, Darbandi et al. correlated significantly between ROS levels and H19-Igf2 gene methylation and sperm indices [35]. Besides, Santi et al. found that mesoderm-specific transcript (MEST) methylation levels were greater in idiopathic infertile men in comparison with fertile males [36]. Precisely, the inappropriate DNA methylation at MEST has been (i) related to reduced sperm count, motility, and normal sperm morphology in infertile men [37]; (ii) present in primary spermatocytes of azoospermia men with complete/incomplete maturation arrest; (iii) linked with small testis volume and elevated serum FSH levels [38]; and (iv) linked to abnormal protamine ratio in men with oligozoospermia [39].
- *Chromatin reorganization/remodeling*
- This essential process permits sperms to pack DNA into the nucleus. Protamines are minute proteins, whereas their transition from histones lets sperm DNA occupy less space in the nucleus with tight condensation, thus enhancing sperm motility and protecting against oxidative stress in the female genital tract [40]. Replacement of histones by protamines encompasses hyperacetylation of histone tails, which leads to chromatin loosening and stimulation of DNA strand breaks by topoisomerase. At first, histones are substituted by transition proteins, then TP1 and TP2 fasten to DNA, and lastly, transition proteins are substituted by protamines [41].
- *Histone modifications*
- Histone modifications stimulate the binding of regulatory factors to DNA inducing decreased/increased gene activity as well as expression. Precise amendments as acetylation of H3 and H4, methylation of H3K4, and ubiquitination of H2B

lead to amplified gene expression in the testis. Contrariwise, ubiquitination of H2A and methylation of H3K9 and H3K27 lead to gene expression silencing [42]. In their study, la Spina et al. showed partial heterogeneous adjustments of histones and existence of H3K79Me2, H3K4Me1, H3K9Me2, H3K4Me3, and H3K36Me3 marks in normal sperms, but it increases in semen samples with poor sperm motility [43]. Besides, Vieweg et al. [44] addressed that abnormal histone acetylation of H4K12 in the promoters of imperative genes indicates poor compacted sperm chromatin. Lately, Schon et al. [45] observed important histone posttranslational amendment in abnormal sperm samples compared with normal sperms suggesting their importance in normal sperm function.

- *Noncoding RNAs*
- Noncoding RNAs (ncRNAs) are classified into two groups related to its length. Short ncRNAs are grouped into three main classes: miRNAs, siRNAs, and piRNAs, which regulate gene expression after transcription. miRNAs and siRNAs are expressed copiously in male germ cells during spermatogenesis process, but piRNAs are expressed merely in spermatocytes and round spermatids at the pachytene stage [46].
- *Posttranslational modifications (PTMs)*
- PTMs are important variations essential for protein regulation. Such modifications are essential to control protein function as sperms are transcriptionally and translationally inactive. Seminal proteins are classified into energy-producing proteins, structural proteins, and proteins influencing sperm maturation and coordinating capacitation, acrosome reaction, and zona pellucida binding in the female reproductive tract [47].
- *S-nitrosylation and tyrosine nitration*
- ROS exert a twofold effect on sperms, whereas at low levels play a part in sperm physiology linked to sperm motility and capacitation, and at elevated levels, they cause OS. Sperms produce NO due to the action of NO synthase acting by forming cGMP from sGC leading to tyrosine phosphorylation. Also, NO induces protein S-nitrosylation acting on the mobilization of stored calcium ion synergistically to progesterone by moderating flagellum [48].
- It was observed that 240 proteins were nitrosylated in normozoospermic men in the presence of NO donors involved in energy generation and signal translation [49]. Important proteins are S-nitrosylated, as heat shock proteins, ryanodine receptors, A-kinase anchoring proteins 3 and 4, and glycolytic enzymes, as GAPDHs [50].
- *Glycosylation*
- Glycosylation includes covalent addition of glycans or sugars to proteins. N-glycosylation is the commonest PTM, playing a significant role in cell-cell, cell-matrix, and protein folding interactions [51].
- Glycodelin, which is elaborated in modulating sperm functions through the female genital tract, has four isoforms differing in their glycosylation patterns: [52] glycodelin-S inhibits capacitation; glycodelin-A and glycodelin-F take part in inhibiting sperm-oocyte binding; glycodelin-F inhibits acrosome reaction; and glycodelin-C stimulates sperm binding to zona pellucida [53].

- Sialylation took place as a final step of glycosylation with the transferring of sialic acid to the glycan structure. Collectively, 6069 sites are recognized as acknowledged PTM sites; 543 were N-glycosylated in the sperm head (especially in the acrosome) and are elaborated in weakened fertilization [54].
- *SUMOylation*
- Small ubiquitin-related modifier (SUMO) is a reversible PTM that has several actions when targeted. SUMO proteins are covalently linked to other proteins by conjugating, activating, and binding enzymes [55]. Though protein SUMOylation is a significant PTM during spermatogenesis, many SUMO-1-conjugated proteins have been reported in ejaculated sperms. SUMO-1 positivity in sperms was inversely correlated to active sperm motility [56]. These investigators pointed out that SUMO-1 confined principally to the sperm nucleus and in the midpiece, demonstrating that SUMOylation of dynamin-related protein 1 (DRP1) is a probable reason of low sperm motility being linked to mitochondrial alterations.
- Vigodner et al. [55] characterized SUMO 1 as well as SUMO 2/3, primarily in the sperm neck, but also in the sperm head and flagella. Defective sperms discovered elevated levels of SUMOylation. Marchiani et al. [57] positively correlated between protein SUMOylation and sperm DNA fragmentation. An interaction between SUMOylation and other PTMs was reported in sperms, whereas proteins were concurrently SUMOylated and ubiquitinated [55]. Lately, Kekäläinen et al. [58] indicated that female-induced sperm protein SUMOylation is selective, permitting females to increase sperm motility in some men and decreasing it in others. Therefore, it was suggested that follicular fluid may non-randomly adjust the utility and structure of sperm proteome facilitating gamete-mediated mate choice.
- *Acetylation*
- It involves transferring of an acetylated group to the amino group of the amino-terminal residue or to the amino group of the lysine residues with a vital role in regulating transcription and nuclear homeostasis. Schon et al. showed that abnormal semen samples had a decrease in H4 acetylation [45]. In their studies, Rajabi et al. [59] and Kim et al. [60] addressed negative correlation between sperm motility, sperm DNA fragmentation, morphology, fertilization rate, and H4K12 acetylation.
- Collectively, 1206 acetylation sites were reported in human seminal plasma, consistent with 576 acetylated proteins. Out of them, 9 were connected to the NADH dehydrogenase and ATP synthetase complexes with a pertinent role in manufacturing ATP. It has been reported that acetylated proteins are frequently located in the sperm [61]. Meanwhile, it was verified that asthenozoospermia leads to decreased acetylated α-tubulin expression in the flagella [62].
- *Histone methylation*
- Histone methylation is the addition of a methyl group to a lysine/arginine residue of the histones by direct action of the enzyme histone methyltransferase (HMT). This process could epigenetically turn on/off gene expression [63]. Schon et al. pointed out that semen samples with asthenozoospermia, with/without teratozoospermia, have an aberrant methylation pattern [45]. Therefore, normal his-

tone methylation is significant for the appropriate spermatogenesis, to form heterochromatin, and for DNA replication and its protection.

- *Ubiquitination*
- The ubiquitination-proteasome system plays two roles: acting on histone modification during protamination and eliminating abnormal sperms. Besides, ubiquitination regulates paternal mitochondrial inheritance, and during spermatid differentiation, mitochondria are generally ubiquitinated [64].
- Damaged sperms are ubiquitinated throughout epididymal transit since ubiquitin is expressed by the epididymal epithelium and stored in the apical microvilli [65]. Hosseinpour et al. reported that males with grade III varicocele have a little degree of ubiquitination, suggestive of diminished epididymal function to eliminate defective sperms [66].
- Besides, the presence of ubiquitination marks on sperms was linked to decreased seminal feature, whereas infertile men exhibited higher percentages of sperm head ubiquitination. The location of ubiquitinated proteins differed in normal and abnormal sperm morphology, suggesting dissimilar patterns of ubiquitination in the tail and cytoplasmic residue [66].

Advances in Genetic Testing for Male Infertility

The evaluation of male infertility for genetic factors is increasing in clinical settings, with the recent advances in gene discovery related to spermatogenic abnormalities in humans as well as murine models. Depending on the underlying condition, most clinicians would request that chromosomal abnormality testing be done as a first-tier test, through either karyotyping or microarrays. Following this, patients that remain negative despite a strong genetic suspicion may be tested for individual genes and/or gene panels known to correlate with their specific clinical presentation. A summary of these strategies appears below.

Chromosomal Alteration Testing

Traditionally, genetic investigation of male infertility was performed using low-resolution approaches (such as karyotyping and FISH) to detect gross chromosomal abnormalities. Karyotyping allows the assessment of the overall structure of all chromosomes in an individual [67]. A karyotype can be assessed using a light microscope and will reveal missing or duplicated chromosomal bands, aneuploidies, chromosomal breaks, and fusions. Some examples of chromosomal abnormalities include Klinefelter and chromosomal translocations.

Next in terms of resolution would be the use of fluorescent in situ hybridization (FISH). This is an approach similar to karyotyping, but able to detect smaller size ranges that could be missed by regular karyotyping, including inversions, translocations, fusions, or copy number variants, usually affecting critical genes and causing disease. However, unlike karyotyping which looks at all chromosomes, FISH requires the use of a specific probe to bind target DNA sequences, which could be challenging to know beforehand. However, over the years, the availability of fluorescent probes has increased dramatically, making FISH capable of screening tens of loci at once.

Although these tests are commonly used to investigate male infertility, they are increasingly being replaced with single-gene testing at the point of care, improving diagnosis and treatment in the future [68].

Gene Panel Testing and Next-Generation Sequencing Approaches

The search for single-gene defects is constantly evolving in male infertility. While some initial successes were achieved from re-sequencing known genes from mouse and other organisms, recent advances in unbiased, genome-wide sequencing technologies have enabled the identification of novel variants related to infertility, influencing known pathways such as hormonal control and spermatogenesis. Spermatogenesis, in particular, involves coordinated interaction of hundreds of genes in complex pathways, each contributing different roles of varying criticality to normal sperm formation. Mutations in these genes may influence count, motility, morphology, and/or ability to achieve successful fusion and fertilization. Depending on the number of patients and their clinical presentations, screening for these genes separately may be unnecessarily laborious for clinical labs to undertake, prompting the use of higher throughput approaches, such as gene panels and exome sequencing [69].

Such efforts have led to the identification of a number of genes that are strongly related to male infertility. These include AR, CCDC155, DNAH6, MCM8, MEIOB, NANOS2, NPAS2, SPINK2, SPO11, SYCE1, TAF4B, TDRD9, TEX14, TEX15, WNK3, and ZMYND15. Functional studies and animal models have now shown that many of these genes play important roles in the fertility pathway, including in meiosis, acrosome biogenesis, DNA replication checkpoints, etc. Moreover, in some instances, these genes are observed to act in a dose-dependent manner, where homozygous mutations may for example cause azoospermia, while heterozygous mutations cause oligospermia [70]. However, the rarity of these mutations in individual patients makes it difficult to find multiple individuals sharing mutations in the same gene, motivating the creation of large-scale global consortia for data sharing and analysis in infertility. These global consortia leverage cohort size and high-throughput technologies to screen many genes at the same time in a very large number of patients (and fertile control), to establish strong statistical evidence for the association of genetic variants in a given gene and a particular infertility subtype.

The most well-studied male infertility subtype using NGS is quantitative abnormalities, i.e., nonobstructive azoospermia and oligozoospermia. To date, many genes have been discovered in these patients using NGS approaches [71]. In a seminal study in 2013, a group of 520 NOA and 477 controls were studied using next-gen approaches, and variants in SIRPA and RISPG were identified and replicated in another cohort [72]. This was followed by other gene panel studies performed either in cases vs. controls or in families where a genetic etiology was suspected, which led to the identification of several genes, including TAF4B and ZMYND15, SYCE1, TEX15, NPAS2, MEIOB and DNAH6, SPINK2, MAGEB4, TDRD9, CFTR and SYCP3, and ADGRG2 [73]. In all cases, the mutations segregated with the affected members within each family and were rare in control databases, making them prime candidates for causing infertility. In 2018, the use of whole-exome sequencing for idiopathic azoospermia directly at the point of care was demonstrated, leading to the discovery of novel pathogenic variants in five genes (CCDC155, NANOS2, SPO11, TEX14, and WNK3) affecting fertility in eight multiplex families [73]. Those examples were followed later by numerous studies that led to the identification of hundreds of genes now related to male infertility.

In addition to identifying single genes with mutation in infertile men, next-generation sequencing allows the detection of copy number and structural variants in patients. Akin to a high-resolution microarray, NGS can detect deletions and duplications that are as small as 50 base pairs, and this high resolution opens a window of discovery in the sub-250 kb range that was previously difficult to detect with traditional microarrays. As these technologies become more routine, it is expected that a growing number of microdeletions and microduplication will be observed in infertile men, and understanding their impact and heritability, as well as the pathways they disrupt, will enhance our understanding of this complex condition.

As a final point, it is important to reiterate the value of knowing the exact genetic mutation in individual patients. First, knowledge of genetic etiology in a given patient allows for screening of other male first-degree relatives to rule in/out infertility. Second, advances in IVF can help screen for embryos free of these single-gene mutations to limit vertical transmission of genetic abnormalities to future males in the family. Finally, knowledge of these genes and how they correlate with clinical presentation provides valuable information on the pathways regulating spermatogenesis in humans, which could potentially be targeted by therapy or pharmacologic intervention.

Impact of Genetic Mutations on Male Infertility Management

Congenital Hypogonadotropic Hypogonadism (cHH)

Since in most of cHH patients spermatogenesis can be prompted by the intake of gonadotrophins, gene mutations can be transmitted naturally or by ART, but it is difficult to calculate the health costs to the offspring. Therefore, PGD should be accessible to the couples [74].

Congenital Absent Vas Deferens (CAVD)

Screening for defects in the cystic fibrosis transmembrane regulator (CFTR) gene is recommended in patients with CAVD, agenesis of the seminal vesicles, and epididymal malformations [75]. There are five classes of CFTR mutations: protein production, protein processing, gating, conduction, and insufficient protein. Based on CFTR mutations alone, 92.4% of non-Hispanic white patients, 69.7% of Black/African American patients, 75.6% of Hispanic patients, and 80.5% of other race patients are eligible for CFTR modulators. For each CFTR modulator, Black/African American patients were least likely to have eligible mutations, and non-Hispanic white patients were most likely [76]. Conception of a biological child is likely in these cases via ICSI using sperm aspirated from the epididymis or testis since they have normal spermatogenesis. In the Caucasian ethnicity, the carrier frequency of CFTR mutations is high (1:25); thus, the CFTR screening of the partners is mandatory. The risk of an offspring with CF is high if major mutations are identified in both partners and PGD is needed in these couples [77].

A recent candidate gene was recognized in CBAVD, the adhesion G protein-coupled receptor G2 (ADGRG2) gene, located on chromosome Xp22.13 with five pathogenic reported variants, accounting for 11–15% of CFTR-negative CBAVD patients. Therefore, ADGRG2 testing should be done on CFTR-negative patients to exclude X-linked transmission [78].

Teratozoospermia and Asthenozoospermia

- *Macrozoospermia (sperm macrocephalia)*
- AURKC gene mutations are encoded for a part crucial for right meiotic chromosomal segregation and cytokinesis. The commonest mutation is the deletion of a cytosine in the exon 3 (c.144delC), reported in >85% of these patients being somewhat common in heterozygosis in the Maghrebians (1/50 men), whereas in Europeans, a mutation in exon 6 (p.Y248*) was identified [78]. AURKC mutation

screening is limited to males with macrocephalic sperms. Homozygous or compound heterozygous mutation carriers present sperms with polyploidy; thus, ICSI is not recommended [79].
- *Globozoospermia*
- This is usually associated with mutations of DPY19L2 gene (most frequently complete deletion of this gene (80.4%)). Since DPY19L2 deletions are not extraordinarily rare, screening in the female partners of male carriers is recommended before ICSI. In male cases with 100% globozoospermia, only ICSI can be performed. However, the lack of acrosome phospholipase C zeta hinders oocyte activation, thus leading to fertilization failure [80].
- *Acephalic sperms*
- The phenotype of the SUN5-mutated cases possesses acephalic sperms with a low proportion of abnormal head-tail junctions and tailless heads. Also, mutations at two candidate genes (BRDT and TSGA10) were described. These cases should be screened for SUN5 mutations. ICSI is their only hope for paternity via the selection of tailless sperm heads [81].
- *Sperm tail abnormalities:*
- These may be due to dysplasia of fibrous sheath in sperm flagellum. Screening for DNAH1 mutations is advised in cases with severe or complete asthenozoospermia due to sperm flagellar variations. However, Wambergue et al. [82] showed that some men with these mutations exhibited normal sperm chromatin with low aneuploidy and DNA fragmentation rates.
- *Primary ciliary dyskinesia (PCD)*
- DNAI1 and DNAH5 gene mutations account for about 30% of such cases. ICSI is an effective modality, but fertility of these cases is not equivalent to the normal population. Wife testing before ICSI procedure is advisable, and in the case of a heterozygous father, PGD can be suggested lest for transmitting the entire symptoms if the partner is a heterozygous carrier of a pathogenic mutation of the same gene [83].

Impaired Sperm Capacitation and Fertilizing Capacity

The cation channel of sperm (CATSPER)-related asthenozoospermia possesses the incapacity of sperms to undergo hyperactivated motility during capacitation. In humans, CATSPER-related infertility was associated with mutations in CATSPER1 as well as CATSPER2. The advised ART is ICSI. Since the carrier frequency of CATSPER2-STRC deletions is somewhat high in the population (heterozygous carriers 1.09%), screening in the wives before ICSI should be advised [84].

Quantitative Spermatogenic Disturbances

- *Klinefelter syndrome (KS)*
- Early diagnosis is pertinent for conserving fertility since germ cell loss is progressive with age and mTESE has a good recovery rate in cases <30 years [85].
- *46,XX male (de la Chapelle syndrome)*
- This disorder is not compatible with spermatogenesis due to lack of AZF regions. Careful endocrine checkup with a follow-up is recommended as these cases may present hypoandrogenism [15].
- *47,XYY male*
- These patients may range from severe oligozoospermia to normozoospermia. Normozoospermia phenotype raised the question about the pathogenic role of this karyotype anomaly in compromised sperm output. Sperm electron microscopy of 47,XYY carriers showed distorted sex vesicle formation [86].
- *Chromosomal structural anomalies*
- Cases having Y chromosomal structural anomalies are not linked with an increased risk for hypoandrogenism, and TESE can be tried according to the presence/absence of variable AZF regions. Evaluation of 45,X cell percentage is important since mosaicism represents a poor prognosis for TESE. In cases undergoing ART, PGD is advised lest increasing the risk of aneuploidy and uniparental disomies in the fetus [87].
- Testing for AZF deletions in men with azoospermia has both a diagnostic and a prognostic value for TESE. TESE procedure could be carried out in men with azoospermia carrying AZFc microdeletion due to the presence of a good chance (~50%) of sperm retrieval. On the other hand, in cases with complete deletion of AZFa and b, surgical sperm retrieval rate is nil, and these cases should be counseled against undergoing SSR [88]. However, oligozoospermic AZFc deletion carriers should carry out sperm cryoconservation in a younger age as a progressive decline in sperm output was described [89].
- The occurrence of 46,XY/45, X0 mosaicism deliberates a poor prognostic TESE value in those cases [89]. “gr/gr” deletion carrier should know that this deletion adds to the etiopathogenesis of impaired spermatozoa output. Therefore, the partners should be alert that such deletion would be transmitted to the male offspring and it might develop a complete AZFc deletion [90].

Gene Therapy

This approach is the treatment of a disorder via transmitting genetic material into cells of the patient. This technique comprises addition of a "normal" gene to a patient's genome, eliminating or mutating an "abnormal" gene permitting it to function properly [91].

There are two approaches of gene transfer to the testis, in vivo and ex vivo. In vivo method is easier and more practical for clinical application. Adenoviral or baculoviral mediated gene transfer may be valuable to transfect testicular Sertoli cells, somatic cells, or Leydig cells, since there is introduction of exogenous genes into germ cells [92].

Intratubular injection is a valuable approach to introduce genes into Sertoli cells, whereas intratesticular injection may be beneficial for Leydig cells. Two techniques are available for intratubular injection, antegrade and retrograde approach. In retrograde injection, the micropipette is introduced into the rete testis through the efferent duct to permit direct injection into the seminiferous tubules. In intratesticular injection, DNA solution is injected straight in the testis letting DNA spread through the interstitial space [93].

Kojima et al. injected DNA into the mouse testes in vivo using three approaches, liposome, electroporation, and adenovirus vector using the same exogenous DNA to identify the most suitable method [94]. Although electroporation and liposome methods were simple, they had short physiological effect and high spermatogenic damage that depend on DNA concentration, liposomes, and electric conditions used throughout electroporation compared with adenovirus-mediated gene transfer [95].

Adenovirus is an effective vector for gene therapy because of its capability to infect postmitotic cells, high effectiveness of cell transduction, and low pathogenicity. Intratesticular injection of the adenoviral vector causes strong transgene expression in the interstitial cells. Conversely, intratubular injection results in transgene expression along the seminiferous tubules with robust expression in Sertoli cells [96]. It has been demonstrated that fetuses and offspring produced by mating with males several days after adenovirus-mediated gene transfer to the testis were normal and not significantly different from the controls [97]. Ex vivo gene transfer to the testis is another method. Advances in spermatogonial stem cell transplantation have provided an entrance to the cell and the chance to modify the male germ line [98].

There are numerous candidate genes of future gene therapy for male infertility. Marker genes of Sertoli cells include anti-Müllerian hormone, aromatase, cytokeratin-18, GATA1, laminin 5, M2A antigen, p27kip1, vimentin, connexin 26, connexin 43, inhibin, sulfated glycoprotein 2, androgen receptor, and WT-1. Transcription factors include Pem (Rhox5), CREB, Sox3, and DAX1 that are essential for spermatogenesis and are expressed in Sertoli cells. Additionally, Leydig cells may also be target cells in KS having insufficiency and distressed apoptosis regulation [99]. Marker genes, including P450 steroid hydroxylase, 3-HSD, androgen receptor, LHR, and Ad4BP/SF-1, are expressed in Leydig cells and are concerned in steroidogenesis as well as spermatogenesis [100].

Establishment of approaches for further efficient and safer gene transfer should be encouraged and could provide great benefit to male infertility patients. However, in comparison with other organs, testicular gene transfer needs caution and careful consideration of the biological and ethical issues involved.

Conclusion

Although genetic abnormalities play a major role in male infertility, this field is not yet fully explored. Several genetic defects related to male infertility are already known, and their presence affects the management of male infertility and may necessitate special considerations during IVF treatment. Advances in genetic studies, with the emergence of whole-exome sequencing, have led to the discovery of new candidate genes that are related to different semen abnormalities. Both mouse studies and emerging human sequencing studies support the role played by single genes in male infertility. As more advanced technologies come closer to the bedside, this should increase new gene discovery as well as translational outcomes for patients with male infertility in the future.

References

1. Tournaye H, Krausz C, Oates RD. Novel concepts in the aetiology of male reproductive impairment. Lancet Diabetes Endocrinol. 2017;5:544–53.
2. Ferlin A, Dipresa S, Delbarba A, Maffezzoni F, Porcelli T, Cappelli C, Foresta C. Contemporary genetics-based diagnostics of male infertility. Expert Rev Mol Diagn. 2019;19(7):623–33.
3. Cioppi F, Rosta V, Krausz C. Genetics of Azoospermia. Int J Mol Sci. 2021;22(6):3264.
4. Krausz C, Riera-Escamilla A. Genetics of male infertility. Nat Rev Urol. 2018;15:369–84.
5. Radojcić Badovinac A, Buretić-Tomljanović A, Starcević N, Kapović M, Vlastelić I, Randić L. Chromosome studies in patients with defective reproductive success. Am J Reprod Immunol. 2000;44(5):279–83.
6. Butnariu L, Covic M, Onofriescu M, Grămescu M, Bujoran C, Caba L, Gorduza EV. Chromosomal evaluation in couples with reproductive disorders - retrospective study of a selected group of 266 couples. Rev Med Chir Soc Med Nat Iasi. 2010;114(4):1107–13.
7. Van Assche E, Bonduelle M, Tournaye H, Joris H, Verheyen G, Devroey P, Van Steirteghem A, Liebaers I. Cytogenetics of infertile men. Hum Reprod. 1996;11(Suppl. 4):1–24.
8. Bojesen A, Juul S, Gravholt CH. Prenatal and postnatal prevalence of Klinefelter syndrome: a national registry study. J Clin Endocrinol Metab. 2003;88(2):622–6.
9. Foresta C, Galeazzi C, Bettella A, Stella M, Scandellari C. High incidence of sperm sex chromosomes aneuploidies in two patients with Klinefelter's syndrome. J Clin Endocrinol Metab. 1998;83:203–5.
10. Thomas NS, Hassold TJ. Aberrant recombination and the origin of Klinefelter syndrome. Human Reprod Update. 2003;9(4):309–17.
11. Groth KA, Skakkebæk A, Høst C, Gravholt CH, Bojesen A. Clinical review: Klinefelter syndrome—a clinical update. J Clin Endocrinol Metab. 2013;98(1):20–30.

12. Majzoub A, Arafa M, Al Said S, Agarwal A, Seif A, Al Naimi A, El Bardisi H. Outcome of testicular sperm extraction in nonmosaic Klinefelter syndrome patients: what is the best approach? Andrologia. 2016;48(2):171–6.
13. Jo WH, Jung MK, Kim KE, Chae HW, Kim DH, Kwon AR, Kim HS. XYY syndrome: a 13-year-old boy with tall stature. Ann Pediatr Endocrinol Metab. 2015;20(3):170–3.
14. Abdel-Razic MM, Abdel-Hamid LA, Elsobky ES. Nonmosaic 47, XYY syndrome presenting with male infertility: case series. Andrologia. 2012;44:200–4.
15. de La Chapelle A. Etiology of maleness in XX men. Hum Genet. 1981;58:105.
16. Rajender S, Rajani V, Gupta NJ, Chakravarty B, Singh L, Thangaraj K. SRY-negative 46,XX male with normal genitals, complete masculinization and infertility. Mol Hum Reprod. 2006;12(5):341–6.
17. Tan TT, Khalid BA. Primary infertility in a phenotypic male with 46XX chromosomal constitution. Postgrad Med. 1983;69(810):315–7.
18. Majzoub A, Arafa M, Starks C, Elbardisi H, Al Said S, Sabanegh E. 46 XX karyotype during male fertility evaluation; case series and literature review. Asian J Androl. 2017;19(2):168–72.
19. Ferlin A, Raicu F, Gatta V, Zuccarello D, Palka G, Foresta C. Male infertility: role of genetic background. Reprod Biomed Online. 2007;14(6):734–45.
20. Vozdova M, Oracova E, Kasikova K, Prinosilova P, Rybar R, Horinova V, Gaillyova R, Rubes J. Balanced chromosomal translocations in men: relationships among semen parameters, chromatin integrity, sperm meiotic segregation and aneuploidy. J Assist Reprod Genet. 2013;30(3):391–405.
21. Hsu LY. Phenotype/karyotype correlations of Y chromosome aneuploidy with emphasis on structural aberrations in postnatally diagnosed cases. Am J Med Genetics. 1994;53(2):108–40.
22. Chen X, Zhou C. Reciprocal translocation and Robertsonian translocation in relation to semen parameters: a retrospective study and systematic review. Andrologia. 2022;54(1):e14262.
23. Gardner RM, Sutherland GR, Shaffer LG. Chromosome abnormalities and genetic counseling. OUP USA; 2011.
24. Madan K. Paracentric inversions: a review. Hum Genet. 1995;96(5):503–15.
25. Kosyakova N, Grigorian A, Liehr T, Manvelyan M, Simonyan I, Mkrtchyan H, Aroutiounian R, Polityko AD, Kulpanovich AI, Egorova T, Jaroshevich E, Frolova A, Shorokh N, Naumchik IV, Volleth M, Schreyer I, Nelle H, Stumm M, Wegner RD, Reising-Ackermann G, Merkas M, Brecevic L, Martin T, Rodríguez L, Bhatt S, Ziegler M, Kreskowski K, Weise A, Sazci A, Vorsanova S, Cioffi Mde B, Ergul E. Heteromorphic variants of chromosome 9. Mol Cytogenet. 2013;6(1):14.
26. Xie X, Li F, Tan W, Tang J. Analysis of the clinical features of pericentric inversion of chromosome 9. J Int Med Res. 2020;48(9):300060520957820.
27. Yuen W, Golin AP, Flannigan R, Schlegel PN. Histology and sperm retrieval among men with Y chromosome microdeletions. Transl Androl Urol. 2021;10(3):1442–56.
28. Navarro-Costa P, Goncalves J, Plancha CE. The AZFc region of the Y chromosome: at the crossroads between genetic diversity and male infertility. Hum Reprod Update. 2010;16:525–42.
29. Krausz C, Quintana-Murci L, McElreavey K. Prognostic value of Y deletion analysis: what is the clinical prognostic value of Y chromosome microdeletion analysis? Hum Reprod. 2000;15:1431–4.
30. Brandell RA, Mielnik A, Liotta D, Ye Z, Veeck LL, Palermo GD, Schlegel PN. AZFb deletions predict the absence of spermatozoa with testicular sperm extraction: preliminary report of a prognostic genetic test. Hum Reprod. 1998;13(1O):2812–5.
31. Gunes S, Arslan MA, Hekim GNT, Asci R. The role of epigenetics in idiopathic male infertility. J Ass Reprod Genet. 2016;33:553–69.
32. Gunes S, Esteves SC. Role of genetics and epigenetics in male infertility. Andrologia. 2021;53(1):e13586.
33. Boissonnas CC, Jouannet P, Jammes H. Epigenetic disorders and male subfertility. Fertil Steril. 2013;99:624–31.

34. Dong H, Wang Y, Zou Z, Chen L, Shen C, Xu S, Zhang J, Zhao F, Ge S, Gao Q, Hu H, Song M, Wang W. Abnormal methylation of imprinted genes and cigarette smoking: assessment of their association with the risk of male infertility. Reprod Sci. 2017;4:114–23.
35. Darbandi M, Darbandi S, Agarwal A, Baskaran S, Dutta S, Sengupta P, Khorshid HRK, Esteves S, Gilany K, Hedayati M, Nobakht F, Akhondi MM, Lakpour N, Sadeghi MR. Reactive oxygen species-induced alterations in H19-Igf2 methylation patterns, seminal plasma metabolites, and semen quality. J Assist Reprod Genet. 2019;36:241–53.
36. Santi D, de Vincentis S, Magnani E, Spaggiari G. Impairment of sperm DNA methylation in male infertility: a meta-analytic study. Andrology. 2017;5:695–703.
37. Kläver R, Gromoll J. Bringing epigenetics into the diagnostics of the andrology laboratory: challenges and perspectives. Asian J Androl. 2014;16:669–74.
38. Marques PI, Fernandes S, Carvalho F, Barros A, Sousa M, Marques CJ. DNA methylation imprinting errors in spermatogenic cells from maturation arrest azoospermic patients. Andrology. 2017;5(3):451–9.
39. Hammoud SS, Purwar J, Pflueger C, Cairns BR, Carrell DT. Alterations in sperm DNA methylation patterns at imprinted loci in two classes of infertility. Fertil Steril. 2010;94:1728–33.
40. Esteves SC, Santi D, Simoni M. An update on clinical and surgical interventions to reduce sperm DNA fragmentation in infertile men. Andrology. 2020;8(1):53–81.
41. Moritz L, Hammoud SS. The art of packaging the sperm genome: molecular and structural basis of the histone-to-protamine exchange. Front Endocrinol. 2022;13:895502.
42. Werner M, Ruthenburg AJ. The United States of histone ubiquitylation and methylation. Mol Cell. 2011;43:5–7.
43. la Spina FA, Romanato M, Brugo-Olmedo S, de Vincentiis S, Julianelli V, Rivera RM, Buffone MG. Heterogeneous distribution of histone methylation in mature human sperm. J Assist Reprod Genet. 2014;31:45–9.
44. Vieweg M, Dvorakova-Hortova K, Dudkova B, Waliszewski P, Otte M, Oels B, Hajimohammad A, Turley H, Schorsch M, Schuppe HC, Weidner W, Steger K, Paradowska-Dogan A. Methylation analysis of histone H4K12ac-associated promoters in sperm of healthy donors and subfertile patients. Clin Epigenetics. 2015;7:31.
45. Schon SB, Luense LJ, Wang X, Bartolomei MS, Coutifaris C, Garcia BA, Berger SL. Histone modification signatures in human sperm distinguish clinical abnormalities. J Assist Reprod Genet. 2019;36:267–75.
46. Song R, Hennig GW, Wu Q, Jose C, Zheng H, Yan W. Male germ cells express abundant endogenous siRNAs. Proc Natl Acad Sci U S A. 2011;108(32):13159–64.
47. Maciel VL Jr, Tamashiro LK, Bertolla RP. Post-translational modifications of seminal proteins and their importance in male fertility potential. Expert Rev Proteomics. 2019;16(11-12):941–50.
48. Foster MW, Stamler JS. New insights into protein S-Nitrosylation: mitochondria as a model system. J Biol Chem. 2004;279:25891–7.
49. Machado-Oliveira G, Lefièvre L, Ford C, Herrero MB, Barratt C, Connolly TJ, Nash K, Morales-Garcia A, Kirkman-Brown J, Publicover S. Mobilisation of Ca^{2+} stores and flagellar regulation in human sperm by S-nitrosylation: a role for NO synthesised in the female reproductive tract. Development. 2008;135(22):3677–86.
50. Morielli T, O'Flaherty C. Oxidative stress impairs function and increases redox protein modifications in human spermatozoa. Reproduction. 2015;149:113–23.
51. Yang X, Liu F, Yan Y, Zhou T, Guo Y, Sun G, Zhou Z, Zhang W, Guo X, Sha J. Proteomic analysis of N-glycosylation of human seminal plasma. Proteomics. 2015;15(7):1255–8.
52. Olejnik B, Kratz EM, Zimmer M, Ferens-Sieczkowska M. Glycoprotein fucosylation is increased in seminal plasma of subfertile men. Asian J Androl. 2015;17:274–80.
53. Seppälä M, Koistinen H, Koistinen R, Chiu PCN, Yeung WSB. Glycosylation related actions of glycodelin: gamete, cumulus cell, immune cell and clinical associations. Hum Reprod Update. 2007;13:275–87.

54. Wang Y, Wan J, Ling X, Liu M, Zhou T. The human sperm proteome 2.0: an integrated resource for studying sperm functions at the level of posttranslational modification. Proteomics. 2016;16:2597–601.
55. Vigodner M, Shrivastava V, Gutstein LE, Schneider J, Nieves E, Goldstein M, Feliciano M, Callaway M. Localization and identification of sumoylated proteins in human sperm: excessive sumoylation is a marker of defective spermatozoa. Hum Reprod. 2013;28:210–23.
56. Marchiani S, Tamburrino L, Giuliano L, Nosi D, Sarli V, Gandini L, Piomboni P, Belmonte G, Forti G, Baldi E, Muratori M. Sumo1-ylation of human spermatozoa and its relationship with semen quality. Int J Androl. 2011;34:581–93.
57. Marchiani S, Tamburrino L, Ricci B, Nosi D, Cambi M, Piomboni P, Belmonte G, Forti G, Muratori M, Baldi E. SUMO1 in human sperm: new targets, role in motility and morphology and relationship with DNA damage. Reproduction. 2014;148:453–67.
58. Kekäläinen J, Hiltunen J, Jokiniemi A, Kuusipalo L, Heikura M, Leppänen J, Malinen M. Female-induced selective modification of sperm protein SUMOylation-potential mechanistic insights into the non-random fertilization in humans. J Evol Biol. 2022;35(2):254–64.
59. Rajabi H, Mohseni-Kouchesfehani H, Eslami-Arshaghi T, Salehi M. Sperm DNA fragmentation affects epigenetic feature in human male pronucleus. Andrologia. 2018;50:e12800.
60. Kim JH, Jee BC, Lee JM, Suh CS, Kim SH. Histone acetylation level and histone acetyltransferase/deacetylase activity in ejaculated sperm from normozoospermic men. Yonsei Med J. 2014;55:1333–40.
61. Sun G, Jiang M, Zhou T, Guo Y, Cui Y, Guo X, Sha J. Insights into the lysine acetylproteome of human sperm. J Proteome. 2014;109:199–211.
62. Yu H, Diao H, Wang C, Lin Y, Yu F, Lu H, Xu W, Li Z, Shi H, Zhao S, Zhou Y, Zhang Y. Acetylproteomic analysis reveals functional implications of lysine acetylation in human spermatozoa (sperm). Mol Cell Proteomics. 2015;14:1009–23.
63. Krejčí J, Stixová L, Pagáčová E, Legartová S, Kozubek S, Lochmanová G, Zdráhal Z, Sehnalová P, Dabravolski S, Hejátko J, Bártová E. Post-translational modifications of histones in human sperm. J Cell Biochem. 2015;116:2195–209.
64. Samanta L, Swain N, Ayaz A, Venugopal V, Agarwal A. Post-translational modifications in sperm proteome: the chemistry of proteome diversifications in the pathophysiology of male factor infertility. Biochim Biophys Acta. 2016;1860:1450–65.
65. Sutovsky P, Terada Y, Schatten G. Ubiquitin-based sperm assay for the diagnosis of male factor infertility. Hum Reprod. 2001;16:250–8.
66. Hosseinpour E, Shahverdi A, Parivar K, Sedighi Gilani MA, Nasr-Esfahani MH, Salman Yazdi R, Sharbatoghli M, Tavalaee M, Chehrazi M. Sperm ubiquitination and DNA fragmentation in men with occupational exposure and varicocele. Andrologia. 2014;46:423–9.
67. White MJD. The chromosomes. 6th ed. London: Chapman & Hall; 1973. p. 45.
68. Okutman O, Rhouma MB, Benkhalifa M, Muller J, Viville S. Genetic evaluation of patients with non-syndromic male infertility. J Assist Reprod Genet. 2018;35:1939–51.
69. Mitchell MJ, Metzler-Guillemain C, Toure A, Coutton C, Arnoult C, Ray PF. Single gene defects leading to sperm quantitative anomalies. Clin Genet. 2017;91:208–16.
70. Consortium GT. The genotype-tissue expression (GTEx) project. Nat Genet. 2013;45:580–5.
71. Fakhro KA, Elbardisi H, Arafa M, Robay A, Rodriguez-Flores JL, Al-Shakaki A, Syed N, Mezey JG, Abi Khalil C, Malek JA, Al-Ansari A, Al Said S, Crystal RG. Point-of-care whole-exome sequencing of idiopathic male infertility. Genet Med. 2018;20:1365–73.
72. Lu C, Xu M, Wang R, Qin Y, Wang Y, Wu W, Song L, Wang S, Shen H, Sha J, Miao D, Hu Z, Xia Y, Wang X. Pathogenic variants screening in five non-obstructive azoospermia-associated genes. Mol Hum Reprod. 2014;20:178–83.
73. Okutman O, Muller J, Skory V, Garnier JM, Gaucherot A, Baert Y, Lamour V, Serdarogullari M, Gultomruk M, Röpke A, Kliesch S, Herbepin V, Aknin I, Benkhalifa M, Teletin M, Bakircioglu E, Goossens E, Charlet-Berguerand N, Bahceci M, Tüttelmann F, Viville S. A no-stop mutation in MAGEB4 is a possible cause of rare X-linked azoospermia and oligozoospermia in a consanguineous Turkish family. J Assist Reprod Genet. 2017;34:683–94.

74. Dwyer AA, Raivio T, Pitteloud N. Reversible hypogonadotropic hypogonadism. Eur J Endocrinol. 2016;174:R267–74.
75. Bieth E, Hamdi SM, Mieusset R. Genetics of the congenital absence of the vas deferens. Hum Genet. 2021;140(1):59–76.
76. McGarry ME, McColley SA. Cystic fibrosis patients of minority race and ethnicity less likely eligible for CFTR modulators based on CFTR genotype. Pediatr Pulmonol. 2021;56(6):1496–503.
77. Cuppens H, Cassiman JJ. CFTR mutations and polymorphisms in male infertility. Int J Androl. 2004;27:251–6.
78. Pagin A, Bergougnoux A, Girodon E, Reboul MP, Willoquaux C, Kesteloot M, Raynal C, Bienvenu T, Humbert M, Lalau G, Bieth E. Novel ADGRG2 truncating variants in patients with X-linked congenital absence of vas deferens. Andrology. 2020;8(3):618–24.
79. Coutton C, Escoffier J, Martinez G, Arnoult C, Ray PF. Teratozoospermia: spotlight on the main genetic actors in the human. Hum Reprod Update. 2015;21:455–85.
80. Alimohammadi F, Ebrahimi Nasab M, Rafaee A, Hashemi M, Totonchi M, Mohseni Meybodi A, Sadighi Gilani MA, Sabbaghian M. Deletion of dpy-19 like 2 (DPY19L2) gene is associated with total but not partial globozoospermia. Reprod Fertil Dev. 2020;32(8):727–37.
81. Sha YW, Sha YK, Ji ZY, Mei LB, Ding L, Zhang Q, Qiu PP, Lin SB, Wang X, Li P, Xu X, Li L. TSGA10 is a novel candidate gene associated with acephalic spermatozoa. Clin Genet. 2018;93(4):776–83.
82. Wambergue C, Zouari R, Fourati Ben Mustapha S, Martinez G, Devillard F, Hennebicq S, Satre V, Brouillet S, Halouani L, Marrakchi O, Makni M, Latrous H, Kharouf M, Amblard F, Arnoult C, Ray PF, Coutton C. Patients with multiple morphological abnormalities of the sperm flagella due to DNAH1 mutations have a good prognosis following intracytoplasmic sperm injection. Hum Reprod. 2016;31:1164–72.
83. Jayasena CN, Sironen A. Diagnostics and management of male infertility in primary ciliary dyskinesia. Diagnostics (Basel). 2021;11(9):1550.
84. Hoppman N, Aypar U, Brodersen P, Brown N, Wilson J, Babovic-Vuksanovic D. Genetic testing for hearing loss in the United States should include deletion/duplication analysis for the deafness/infertility locus at 15q15.3. Mol Cytogenet. 2013;6:19.
85. Corona G, Pizzocaro A, Lanfranco F, Garolla A, Pelliccione F, Vignozzi L, Ferlin A, Foresta C, Jannini EA, Maggi M, Lenzi A, Pasquali D, Francavilla S, Klinefelter ItaliaN Group (KING). Sperm recovery and ICSI outcomes in Klinefelter syndrome: a systematic review and meta-analysis. Hum Reprod Update. 2017;23:1–11.
86. Bardsly MZ, Kowal K, Levy C, Gosek A, Ayari N, Tartaglia N, Lahlou N, Winder B, Grimes S, Ross JL. 47,XYY syndrome: clinical phenotype and timing of ascertainment. J Pediatr. 2013;163(4):1085–94.
87. Lange J, Skaletsky H, van Daalen SK, Embry SL, Korver CM, Brown LG, Oates RD, Silber S, Repping S, Page D. Isodicentric Y chromosomes and sex disorders as byproducts of homologous recombination that maintains palindromes. Cell. 2009;138:855–69.
88. Mao JM, Zhao LM, Liu DF, Lin HC, Yang YZ, Zhang HT, Hong K, Li R, Jiang H. Analysis of clinical outcome of synchronous micro-dissection testicular sperm extraction and intracytoplasmic sperm injection in male infertility with Y chromosome azoospermia factor C region deletion. Beijing Da Xue Xue Bao. 2022;54(4):652–7.
89. Krausz C, Hoefsloot L, Simoni M, Tüttelmann F, European Academy of Andrology, European Molecular Genetics Quality Network. EAA/EMQN best practice guidelines for molecular diagnosis of Y-chromosomal microdeletions: state-of-the-art 2013. Andrology. 2014;2:5–19.
90. Lu C, Zhang J, Li Y, Xia Y, Zhang F, Wu B, Wu W, Ji G, Gu A, Wang S, Jin L, Wang X. The b2/b3 subdeletion shows higher risk of spermatogenic failure and higher frequency of complete AZFc deletion than the gr/gr subdeletion in a Chinese population. Hum Mol Genet. 2009;18:1122–30.
91. Tang R, Xu Z. Gene therapy: a double-edged sword with great powers. Mol Cell Biochem. 2020;474(1-2):73–81.

92. Kojima Y, Sasaki S, Hayashi Y, Umemoto Y, Morohashi K, Kohri K. Role of transcription factors Ad4BP/SF-1 and DAX-1 in steroidogenesis and spermatogenesis in human testicular development and idiopathic azoospermia. Int J Urol. 2006;13:785–93.
93. Watanabe S, Kanatsu-Shinohara M, Ogonuki N, Matoba S, Ogura A, Shinohara T. In vivo genetic manipulation of spermatogonial stem cells and their microenvironment by adeno-associated viruses. Stem Cell Rep. 2018;10(5):1551–64.
94. Kojima Y, Sasaki S, Umemoto Y, Hashimoto Y, Hayashi Y, Kohri K. Comparison of characteristics of several vectors to testicular gene transfer system. J Urol. 2005;173:407–8.
95. Schellander K, Berm G. The direct gene transfer through mammal spermatozoa. In: Houdebine LM, editor. Transgenic animal: generation and use. Amsterdam: Harwood Academic Publishers; 1997. p. 41–4.
96. Blanchard KT, Boekelheide K. Adenovirus-mediated gene transfer to rat testis in vivo. Biol Reprod. 1997;56:495–500.
97. Kojima Y, Hayashi Y, Kurokawa S, Mizuno K, Sasaki S, Kohri K. No evidence of germline transmission by adenovirus-mediated gene transfer to mouse testes. Fertil Steril. 2008;89(Suppl. 5):1448–54.
98. Gul M, Hildorf S, Dong L, Thorup J, Hoffmann ER, Jensen CFS, Sønksen J, Cortes D, Fedder J, Andersen CY, Goossens E. Review of injection techniques for spermatogonial stem cell transplantation. Hum Reprod Update. 2020;26(3):368–91.
99. Aksglaede L, Wikström AM, Rajpert-De Meyts E, Dunkel L, Skakkebaek NE, Juul A. Natural history of seminiferous tubule degeneration in Klinefelter syndrome. Hum Reprod Update. 2006;12:39–48.
100. Parrington J, Coward K, Gadea J. Sperm and testis mediated DNA transfer as a means of gene therapy. Syst Biol Reprod Med. 2011;57(1-2):35–42.

Chapter 9
Epigenetic Alterations in Male Infertility

A. Navarro-Gomezlechon and N. Garrido

Key Points

- Spermatozoa are extremely specialized cells which undergo several epigenetic changes during differentiation to become a mature and functional entity with a unique epigenome.
- Spermatozoa epigenome is changed during spermatogenesis where epigenetic modifications such as protamination take place, which are susceptible to be altered by several factors resulting in adverse conditions affecting phenotype and potentially being transmitted to offspring.
- Epigenetic alterations in spermatozoa could be associated with impaired semen parameters, ART outcomes and, more importantly, offspring's health.
- In the near future, with improvements in NGS technologies, we will improve our understanding of sperm epigenetics leading to the discovery of epigenetic biomarkers, which could be used for diagnosis and targeted therapies, overall improving fertility care.

A. Navarro-Gomezlechon · N. Garrido (✉)
IVIRMA Global Research Alliance, IVI Foundation, Instituto de Investigación Sanitaria La Fe (IIS La Fe), Valencia, Spain
e-mail: ana.navarro@ivirma.com; nicolas.garrido@ivirma.com

A. Agarwal et al. (eds.), *Current and Future Advances in Male Infertility*,
https://doi.org/10.1007/978-3-031-62648-7_9

Narrative Review

Introduction

Infertility is defined as the inability to conceive after 1 year of regular unprotected sexual intercourse, and this condition affects approximately 15% of couples in reproductive age. Moreover, a male factor can be attributed in about half of the cases of infertility either solely or combined with female factors [1–9].

Male infertility is a multifactorial pathological condition [8], reflected by either absolute inability to produce spermatozoa, presentation of lower counts or being physiologically incompetent (unable to perform their task) or lack of functionality and completeness of the genital tract. These may occur due to hormonal or physiologic alterations and blockage or absence of pathways to let spermatozoa pass through the tract, among others. The explicative causes can be genetic, environmental or a mixture of both existing in a certain genetic predisposition that acts together with the influence of environmental factors that originate the infertile phenotype in an unknown proportion [3–5, 9–11].

Spermatozoa are extremely specialized cells which transmit to the offspring the genetic material and also cytoplasmic components as RNAs, proteins and gene expression regulatory information, leading to competent embryo formation [2, 3, 12]. Spermatogenesis involves the interplay of a lot of genes, and during this process, spermatozoa undergo multiple variations in their genetic, cellular and chromatin structures, which permit gene expression and function control that may result in fertility/infertility condition [3].

Epigenetics is defined as the study of changes in gene expression and function due to modifications in DNA and histone structure without altering the DNA sequence [3, 5, 10, 13–15], while epigenomics is the study of the epigenetics of the whole genome [3]. Epigenetic information will result in the specific phenotype of an individual [3, 16]. Epigenetic changes are very important for development, differentiation and normal physiological processes within the cell [13]. However, epigenetic states can be altered by certain internal and external factors, and these epigenetic changes can be associated with the development of disease [13–15].

The mechanisms of epigenetic regulation include histone modifications, DNA methylation, chromatin remodelling and small non-coding RNAs (Fig. 9.1). Several studies have demonstrated an association of the epigenetic mechanisms with male infertility/subfertility condition [3–5, 10, 17, 18]. The genome, epigenome, transcriptome and proteome are essential for complete functionality of spermatozoa; therefore, research has been done to study the epigenetic modifications involved in male infertility [3, 4].

In this chapter, we will provide an overview of the current knowledge regarding the epigenetic alterations involved in male infertility along with essential information of the epigenetics in spermatozoa and the association with reproductive outcomes, offspring health and risks as well as future directions in this research field.

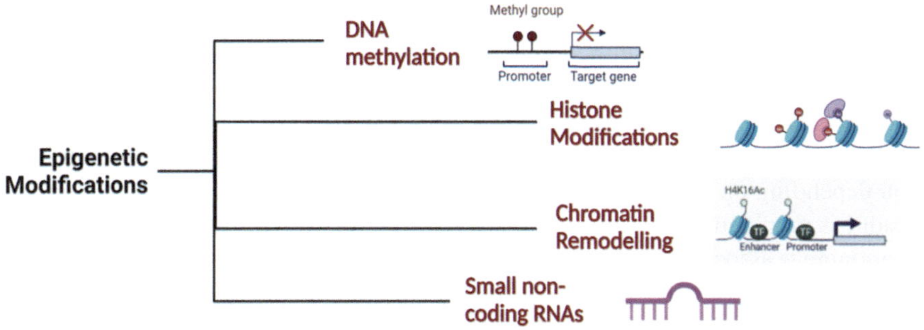

Fig. 9.1 The mechanisms of epigenetic regulation: DNA methylation, histone modifications, chromatin remodelling and small non-coding RNAs. (Created with BioRender.com)

Epigenetic Mechanisms

DNA Methylation (CpG Sites)

DNA methylation consisting of the addition of a methyl group (-CH_3) by DNA methyltransferases [19], mainly at cytosine-guanine (CpG) dinucleotides, occurs in almost all vertebrates, many invertebrates and many plant species [20]. In mammals, on the one hand, the maintenance of methylation patterns is ensured by the enzyme DNA methyltransferase (DNMT1), which methylates new daughter DNA strands on replication based on the parental strand. On the other hand, de novo methylation of unmethylated sites is mainly ensured by DNA methylation enzymes DNMT3A and DNMT3B [15, 20, 21].

Normally, DNA methylation at the promoter region has been implicated in transcriptional repression, inhibiting gene transcription, through the alteration of the conformation of DNA preventing the adequate binding of regulatory proteins [15, 19, 22]. DNA methylation is important in imprinting, X-chromosome inactivation, genome stability and developmental gene regulation [20–22]. In fact, abnormal DNA methylation could be potentially responsible for certain diseases, such as cancer [22].

Histone Modification

Chromatin is formed by a mixture of genomic DNA and proteins into the nucleus, and its fundamental unit is the nucleosome formed of an octamer of histones (containing two units of each histone H2A, H2B, H3 and H4) bound to DNA [15, 21, 23]. Histones are alkaline proteins containing a negatively charged N-terminus, which can be chemically modified causing a change in chromatin structure (alteration in their binding to DNA and the accessibility of other proteins), which can have an influence in gene expression [19, 24].

Histone modifications carried out by enzymes include methylation, acetylation, phosphorylation and ubiquitination. Histone acetylation targets lysine residues, and it activates gene expression by promoting an open chromatin structure. Histone phosphorylation involves serine residues, and it is also associated with the activation of gene expression. Histone methylation can either activate or repress transcription depending on the residues targeted (arginine or lysine) and to what extent the residue is modified (mono-, di- or trimethylation); for example, histone methylation of arginine is associated with gene activation. Ubiquitination targets lysine residues, and it can activate or inhibit gene expression depending on specific cell conditions [15, 19, 21, 25]. Moreover, specific and related modifications may cause certain genomic states, such as gene activation, repression and DNA repair [25]. Histone modifications regulate many different physiological mechanisms, and, as in the case of DNA methylation, its deregulation is involved in various diseases, such as cancer [26].

Chromatin Remodelling

The basic unit of chromatin is the nucleosome, and nucleosomes are linked by linker DNA. Chromatin can condensate in a polynucleosome fibre formed by histone H1, nucleosomes and linker DNA [23], and its structure can affect gene expression, DNA replication, DNA repair and recombination [21, 23].

In chromatin, DNA is not very accessible, so remodelling makes DNA sequences accessible to interacting proteins or promotes packing. Remodelling enzymes may make accessible DNA segments by nucleosome disassembly, change nucleosome composition regarding histones and alter nucleosomal fibre folding [27]. Chromatin remodelling causes chromatin assembly and disassembly [21], which is very important for the regulation of gene expression [23], and this process needs the utilization of energy from ATP hydrolysis [19, 27]. Some ATP-dependent chromatin remodelling complexes are the SWI/SNF and ISWI families [21]. Defects in chromatin remodelling can be linked to several human diseases [23, 27].

Additionally, chromatin remodelling can be coupled with other epigenetic mechanisms to produce stable epigenetic patterns [27].

Small Non-coding RNAs

Non-coding RNAs are a type of RNAs that are not translated into proteins and that regulate gene expression. In this group, regulatory non-coding RNAs that have a regulatory role are divided into short non-coding RNAs (small interfering RNAs (siRNAs), microRNAs (miRNAs), and Piwi-interacting RNAs (piRNAs)) and long non-coding RNA (lncRNAs). These non-coding RNAs have an important role in epigenetic regulation and can control gene and chromosome expression. In this regard, siRNAs can produce transcriptional and post-transcriptional gene silencing in cells, and their pathway may be involved in the maintenance and regulation of the epigenome. Moreover, miRNAs also mediate transcriptional gene silencing and may participate in epigenetic regulation. piRNAs bind to Piwi proteins, and they may have an important role in epigenetic regulation (DNA methylation). Regarding lncRNAs, they can be divided into sense, antisense, bidirectional, intronic and intergenic, and they may play a role in the regulation of gene expression (*H19* in genomic imprinting and *Xist* in X chromosome inactivation) [28–30].

Epigenetics and Sperm

Epigenetics in Spermatogenesis

Epigenetic reprograming or erasure of epigenetic marks takes place in male mammals during germ cell development and early embryogenesis, and epigenetic marks in male germ cells are established during foetal development. Alterations in this process have clinical relevance [15, 20].

Spermatogenesis is a complex process regulated by epigenetic modifications, and sperm cells undergo several epigenetic changes during differentiation to become mature to ensure the delivery of adequate DNA to the future embryo [3]. Epigenetic modifications are regulators of spermatogenesis, and these include chromatin remodelling, DNA methylation and histone modifications [31]. It is very important to have an appropriate paternal epigenome in order to have an adequate sperm function and embryo development [3, 19], as paternal epigenome can have an effect on them and offspring traits and health [4, 5, 19].

Human spermatozoa have a unique and elegant epigenome. In human sperm, there are several types of epigenetic modifications that can modulate gene transcription: chromatin structure modifications due to the replacement of histones with protamines during spermiogenesis, chemical modifications of retained histones, methylation of sperm DNA (mainly hypomethylation) and non-coding RNAs found in mature sperm. All these changes are necessary to accomplish natural sperm functions [3, 24].

Protamination is an epigenetic modification exclusive of sperm that increases packaging of sperm DNA that results in a high level of compaction of the nucleus ceasing transcriptional activity. Protamination is a multistep process: (1) replacement of histones with histone variants that are expressed during spermatogenesis, (2) increase of acetylation of other histones, (3) replacement by transition proteins and (4) replacement of transition proteins by protamines (protamines 1 and 2). The most frequent histone variant found in spermatozoa is testis-specific histone 2B [24, 31, 32]. However, approximately 5–10% of DNA remains bound to histones. These retained histones suffer modifications and are part of the epigenetic status of sperm; they account for the past spermatogenesis and the future embryo development [3, 5, 18, 19, 24, 31]. Moreover, in mature sperm cells, promoters of developmental genes and genes encoding signalling factors are hypomethylated [31, 33].

Interestingly, according to a study from Camprubí et al., spermatozoa methylome is homogeneous and mainly hypomethylated, and genes with hypomethylated promoters are associated with spermatogenesis and embryogenesis functions [12].

Factors Contributing to Epigenetic Changes in Sperm

Sperm epigenetic states can be altered by several factors including smoke, lifestyle, diet, physical activity, alcohol, endocrine disruptors, stress and environment affecting male fertility, and this characteristic can be transmitted to offspring [4, 5, 19]. Altered sperm epigenetics, mainly DNA methylation, can be associated with adverse reproductive conditions [18, 19, 34].

In this regard, Schuller et al. investigated the epigenetic impact of paternal exposure to simulated wildfire smoke in $Apoe^{-/-}$ mouse model demonstrating that 40 days of exposure altered sperm DNA methylation in adult mice. DNA methylation varied significantly in 3353 differentially methylated regions (mainly hypermethylated), which were annotated to 2117 genes [35]. Similarly, Liu et al. found that normozoospermic heavy tobacco smokers had significantly higher levels of global sperm DNA methylation and that they had a significantly higher methylation level in the cg11193865 site in the *DLK1* gene (paternally imprinted gene) [36]. Likewise, Laqqan et al. assessed the impact of tobacco heavy smoking on sperm DNA methylation patterns finding a significant variation between heavy smokers and non-smokers in the methylation level at all CpGs within the *PRICKLE2* and *ALS2CR12* gene amplicon, at 9 CpGs within the *ALDH3B2* gene amplicon and at 18 CpGs within the *PTGIR* gene amplicon [37].

Another study evaluated the effect of nut consumption on sperm DNA methylation patterns in healthy individuals consuming a regular Western-style diet and identified in the nut group 36 genomic regions that were significantly differentially methylated (mainly hypermethylated) in sperm between the start and the end of the trial demonstrating that there are some regions of the sperm epigenome that could respond to diet [38]. The exposure to PM_{10}, an air pollutant, was found to be positively associated with 5-hydroxymethylcytosine levels, and PM_{10} exposure decreased sperm DNA methylation [39].

Furthermore, Zhao et al. identified differentially methylated regions in the whole genome of sperm APA mice and suggested that this may lead to risks for the offspring, such as aberrant glucose metabolism and development of autism spectrum disorder (ASD) behaviours [40]. Therefore, evidence supports that certain factors can lead to an alteration in sperm epigenetic states.

Techniques to Assess Sperm Epigenetics

Technological evolution has allowed significant developments in the way scientific research is done and understood. Advances in molecular technologies as well as reproductive technologies have the potential to identify genetic variants associated with male infertility [4, 6, 15]. Since the development of microarrays, next-generation sequencing (NGS), genome-wide association studies and related technologies, an increasing number of genetic abnormalities have been related to male infertility. NGS provides more powerful tools to study the epigenome and allows the investigation of the underlying causes of male infertility [3, 4, 6, 13, 14].

A gold standard technology used for the detection of DNA methylation is bisulfite genomic sequencing based on bisulfite conversion of DNA using sodium bisulfite, which converts unmethylated cytosines to uracil and leaves methylated cytosines unchanged. This is followed by a PCR amplification, and then either direct sequencing of PCR products (Fig. 9.2) or cloning of PCR products and sequencing can be done [41]. Bisulfite genomic sequencing has been widely used in

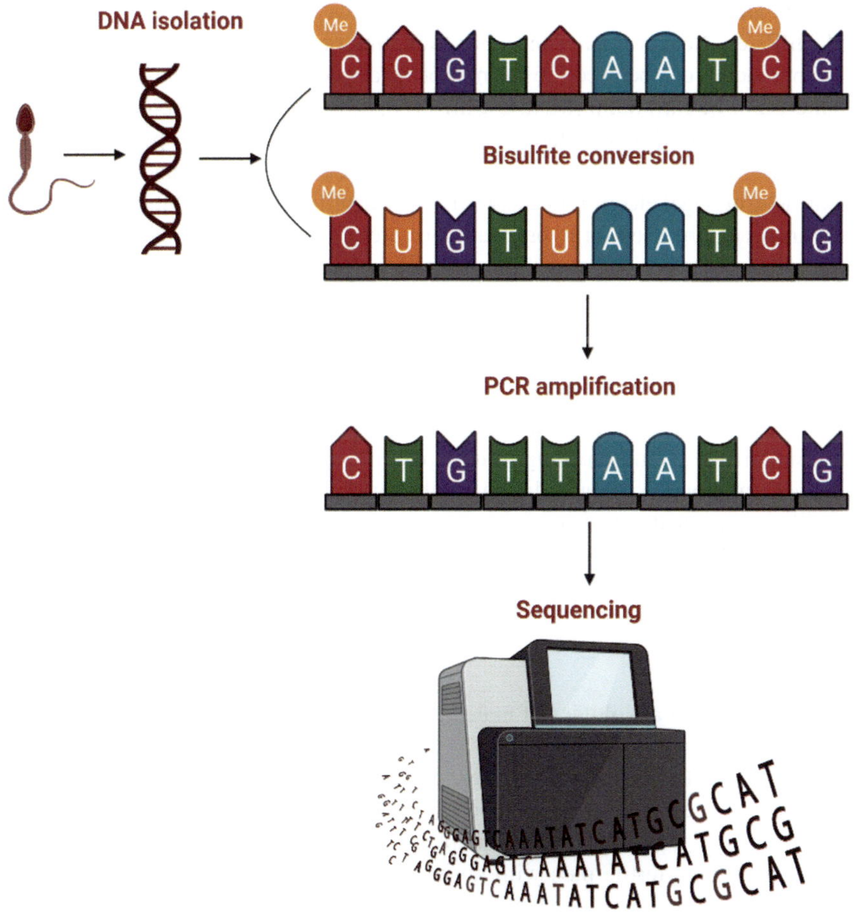

Fig. 9.2 Flow chart with the main steps of the bisulfite genomic sequencing technology consisting of DNA isolation (in this case from a sperm cell), bisulfite conversion, PCR amplification and sequencing. (Created with BioRender.com)

several studies for sperm DNA methylation [22, 35, 42–45]. Interestingly, bisulfite conversion can also be used with array-based techniques, so bisulfite-converted DNA is then hybridized to a methylation array [12, 17, 36, 38]. For example, the Human Methylation 450 Infinium Bead Chip array [12, 17, 46], Infinium Methylation EPIC Bead Chip microarray [38] or Infinium Human Methylation 27 Bead Chip [47] has been used in several studies.

Furthermore, other techniques can also be used to assess sperm epigenetics. In this regard, Cheng et al. used MethylFlash Global DNA Methylation ELISA Easy Kit and MethylFlash Global DNA Hydroxymethylation ELISA Easy Kit to measure the genomic levels of 5-methylcytosine (5mC) and 5-hydroxymethylcytosine in sperm DNA [39]. For the detection of histone modification patterns, chromatin immunoprecipitation (ChIP) can be used where antibodies specific for each histone modification are used for immunoprecipitation of chromatin with the specific modification. This technique has genome-wide applications: ChIP-chip (microarrays) and ChIP-seq (Solexa sequencing). For validation of histone codes, mass spectrometry approaches can be used [26]. A micrococcal nuclease step allows analysing the smallest unit of chromatin (MNase-ChIP) [26, 45]. Also high-throughput sequencing can be done [45]. For protamine studies, a protocol followed is sperm protamine extraction and quantification consisting of extraction of sperm nuclear proteins, acetic acid-urea gel electrophoresis for P1/P2 quantification and quality control [48, 49]. Arrays can be used for hybridization of protamine-associated DNA [45].

Epigenetic Alterations in Male Infertility

Evidence has demonstrated an association of epigenetic signatures with male infertility/subfertility condition, suggesting a possible association of altered sperm epigenetics, mainly DNA methylation, with gene regulation in unexplained male infertility, abnormal semen parameters, pregnancy rate in ART, male subfertility and progeny health [3–5, 10, 17–19, 34].

Impact on Fertility

There are different aetiologies of male infertility that have been found to be associated with epigenetic alterations.

In 30–40% of male infertility cases, the aetiology remains unknown, and these cases are classified as 'unexplained' or 'idiopathic' infertility [3–6, 9–11]. Urdinguio et al. performed a study including couples with unexplained infertility comparing normozoospermic fertile men with normozoospermic infertile men and identified 2752 differentially methylated CpGs (1447 hypermethylated and 1305 hypomethylated), 54 CpG sites associated with 48 imprinted genes aberrantly methylated and significantly lower methylation levels of Alu Yb8 (repetitive sequences) in infertile individuals. These results suggest that aberrant sperm DNA methylation might contribute to infertility in couples with unexplained infertility [46]. A study considering in vitro fertilization (IVF) cycles with donor oocytes and normozoospermic men investigated unexplained male factor infertility identifying 1634 CpG sites at retained histones that had significantly different sperm DNA methylation between the group of good and poor blastocyst development and that ten sperm miRNAs were significantly altered, which may contribute to the poor blastocyst development [50].

Altered methylation has been found in the imprinted genes of men with oligozoospermia, obstructive azoospermia undergoing testicular sperm aspiration, known defects of protamination and idiopathic infertility [24]. *H19* and *MEST* are imprinted genes whose methylation patterns were studied in human testicular spermatozoa from patients with anejaculation, secondary obstructive azoospermia, primary obstructive azoospermia or secretory azoospermia due to hypospermatogenesis, finding that *H19* complete methylation was statistically significantly reduced in secretory azoospermia patients with hypospermatogenesis (affecting the CTCF-binding site 6) and that for *MEST* gene all patients presented complete unmethylation being statistically significantly reduced in the anejaculation group [44]. In 2012, Camprubí et al. analysed sperm DNA methylation profile of *H19*-ICR, KvDMR, *SNRPN*-ICR, *IG*-DMR and *MEG3*-DMR finding more spermatozoa with abnormal DNA methylation in regions regulated by genetic imprinting in infertile individuals compared to controls, but these methylation anomalies did not influence ART outcomes [51].

Moreover, a study considering abnormal protamine patients, oligozoospermic patients and fertile donors examined CpG methylation patterns at seven imprinted loci (*LIT1, MEST, SNRPN, PLAGL1, PEG3, H19* and *IGF2*) finding that at six of the imprinted genes, the overall DNA methylation patterns at their differentially methylated regions were significantly altered in both infertile patient populations, specifically *LIT1, SNRPN, MEST, PLAGL1* and *PEG3* that were hypermethylated and *H19* that was hypomethylated. These results suggested a significant association between altered sperm DNA methylation at imprinted loci and male factor infertility [42]. In contrast, no significant differences in the distribution of *MTHFR* rs1801133 polymorphism genotypes and no associations between the genotypes and the characteristics of semen analysis or the presence of an abnormal sperm DNA hypomethylation pattern in paternally methylated H19-ICR or IG-DMR were found in a study comparing fertile and infertile individuals. In addition, frameshift, nonsense or missense mutations of the *CTCFL* gene were not identified, and *CTCFL* mutations were not associated with the pattern of sperm hypomethylation at the paternally imprinting loci [52].

Furthermore, 696 differentially methylated CpGs (184 hypomethylated and 512 hypermethylated) associated with 501 genes and 17 differentially methylated genes (*ATXN7L1, APCS, PATE4, PRDM1, ANK2, RPS6KA2, RHOBTB1, C6orf118, ANKRD53, LOC100271702/LINC00940, EIF2AK3, JAM3, NCAPD3, TEX261, CACNA2D4, FOXK1 and FOXK2*) were identified in a study comparing infertile and fertile individuals. Interestingly, a significant association was found between *JAM3/NCAPD3* hypermethylation and altered FISH pattern, *RPS6KA2* hypermethylation and advanced age, *ANK2* hypermethylation and lower pregnancy rate, and *APCS* hypermethylation and oligozoospermia [53]. Another study analysed DNA methylation profiles in peripheral blood leukocytes from fertile and infertile individuals identifying 471 significantly differentially methylated CpG loci corresponding to 287 genes with enrichment of the functions of piRNA binding (*PIWIL1* and *PIWIL2* genes, allele-specific methylation) and MHC class II receptor activity (*HLA-DRB1, HLA-DQB1* and *HLA-DQA1* genes), whose genes can be associated with disorders of spermatogenesis. 445 of 471 differentially methylated CpGs were associated with SNPs [54]. Additionally, infertility patients have shown impaired H4 hyperacetylation [32].

Incorrect processing of the protamine transcripts, as well as altered P1/P2 ratio, has been associated with subfertility [24]. Aoki et al. identified a significantly increased proportion of infertile males within their low and high P1/P2 ratio groups and a significantly higher proportion of fertile males in their normal P1/P2 ratio group, with this aberrant P1/P2 ratios arising from an abnormal concentration of P1 and/or P2, associated with male infertility [48].

Impact on Semen Parameters

Abnormal semen parameters have shown to be associated with epigenetic alterations, including oligozoospermia and asthenozoospermia. In this regard, Sujit et al. highlighted the association between methylation changes and loss of fertility using sperm DNA from oligozoospermic/oligoasthenozoospermic infertile patients and normozoospermic fertile men and found 1680 differentially methylated CpGs (1436 hypermethylated and 244 hypomethylated in the infertile group) across 1052 genes, such as *HOXB1, EBF3, ANK2, PRDM1, TP73, GATA3, VAX2, MLPH, SMC1B, KCNJ5, ASB4, BCAN, CTNNA3, DLGAP2, MAGI2, SPATA5, SPATA7, SPATA16, SPATA22, TET2, KDM4C, TCERG1L, JMJD1C, HDAC4, SMYD3, HLA-C, HLA-DRB6, HLA-DQA1, CRISPLD1, LPHN3* and *CPEB2* [33]. Laqqan et al. found that tobacco heavy smoking can impact spermatozoa DNA methylation patterns and that alterations in the methylation level for certain CpGs can be correlated with several semen parameters causing a negative impact on semen parameters and spermatozoa quality. In this respect, they found a significant negative association between the methylation levels at CpG within the *ALDH3B2* gene amplicon and normal form of spermatozoa, total motility of spermatozoa, progressive motility, non-progressive motility, vitality level and sperm count; within the *PTGIR* gene amplicon and sperm non-progressive motility; within the *PRICKLE2* gene amplicon and total motility of spermatozoa, non-progressive motility and normal form of spermatozoa; and within the *ALS2CR12* gene amplicon and the sperm non-motile, normal form of spermatozoa and vitality test [37]. Abnormal protamine replacement of histones and abnormal protamine expression have been associated with decreased semen quality [24]. In addition, Houshdaran et al. found that sperm DNA methylation at numerous sequences was increased in poor-quality semen (concentration, motility and morphology) and suggested that it could be due to improper erasure of DNA methylation during epigenetic reprogramming of the male germ line [3, 18, 55].

Asthenozoospermia is mainly characterized by low sperm motility. A study investigated DNA methylation differences at CpGs in promoter regions between high and low motile sperm cells from normozoospermic and asthenozoospermic individuals finding that there were no statistically significant differences in the global DNA methylation profiles between sperm from men with normozoospermia or asthenozoospermia. However, in terms of DNA methylation rates at CpGs, they identified 134 differentially methylated CpGs (corresponding to 127 genes), 50 hypermethylated and 84 hypomethylated in group low-motile sperm cells from asthenozoospermic patients compared to group high-motile sperm cells from normozoospermic controls, 41 differentially methylated regions and 134 differentially variable CpGs [56]. Another study found that 9189 CpGs had significantly altered methylation associated with motility, 1827 hypermethylated and 7362 hypomethylated in the low-motility samples; 194 CpGs associated with imprinted genes (corresponding to 92 genes) had significant associations with motility, 92 hypermethylated (predominantly paternally expressed) and 102 hypomethylated (predominantly maternally expressed) in the low-motility samples; 58 CpGs associated with genes involved in spermatogenesis were significantly altered in low-motility sperm, 41 hypomethylated and 17 hypermethylated in low-motility samples; and 13 CpG loci associated with epigenetic regulatory genes had significantly altered methylation in low-motility sperm samples, 8 hypomethylated and 5 hypermethylated [47].

Oligozoospermia is an alteration related to sperm count. Sperm DNA methylation has been analysed in oligozoospermic and normospermic individuals finding hypomethylation of at least one CpG island of the *H19*-DMR in men with mild oligozoospermia and with severe oligozoospermia; 20% of oligozoospermia cases showed methylation errors in *H19*-DMR and hypermethylation in at least one CpG island of *PEG1/MEST*-DMR in men with mild oligozoospermia and severe oligozoospermic, and 3% of oligozoospermia cases showed methylation errors in *PEG1/MEST*-DMR. Interestingly, the study found no association between epimutations and genetic variants or ART outcome [43]. Comparison of oligospermic infertile and normospermic fertile individuals found significant differences between methylation level of *H19* gene being hypomethylated in oligospermic cases, which was related to an up-regulation of gene expression level for the *H19* gene in oligospermic group, which can inhibit spermiogenesis resulting in defects in semen quality. The study suggested that *H19* hypomethylation could serve as epigenomic biomarkers for the assessment of oligospermia infertility in men with multiple sperm defects. Other studies have also found that aberrant DNA methylation of the paternally imprinted gene *H19* is significantly associated with decreased sperm count [57]. Also, semen quality parameters have been found to be diminished in patients with abnormal (low or high) P1/P2 ratios [49].

Aberrant DNA methylation in some imprinted genes has been identified to be associated with non-obstructive azoospermia, oligozoospermia and other abnormal semen parameters [56]. Santi et al.'s meta-analysis found an association between male infertility and reduced sperm *H19* methylation and increased *MEST* and

SNRPN methylation, and no differences for *LINE-1* methylation levels in sperm DNA methylation considering studies of men with oligozoospermia, oligoasthenoteratozoospermia or idiopathic infertility and fertile controls [4, 19, 34].

Impact on ART Outcomes

Sperm DNA methylation is proposed to be crucial for fertilization and early embryogenesis [33]. Abnormal protamine replacement of histones or altered protamine expression has been associated with diminished IVF embryo quality and pregnancy rates [24]. Alterations in the protamine ratio are implicated in infertility and fertilization failure. Moreover, sperm epigenetics could possibly impact embryo development, and epigenetic alterations could be implicated in pregnancy loss [19]. A study conducted by Aoki et al. evaluated aberrant sperm P1/P2 ratios and ART (IVF or intracytoplasmic sperm injection (ICSI)) outcomes finding that standard IVF fertilization rates were significantly reduced in patients with low and high P1/P2 ratios compared to those with normal ratios, chemical pregnancy rates were reduced in patients with low ratios compared to those with normal and high ratios, and clinical pregnancy rates were significantly decreased in patients with a low ratio compared to those with normal and high ratios. However, overall fertilization rate, ICSI fertilization rate, IVF embryo quality and spontaneous abortion rates were similar between the groups [49]. Another study from the same author found that overall fertilization rate (IVF and ICSI) was significantly decreased in patients with low P1/P2 ratio compared with patients with normal and elevated P1/P2 [48].

Montjean et al. did not find any difference in the pregnancy rate of oligozoospermic patients with altered methylation profiles when compared to oligozoospermic patients with normal methylation profiles, independent of the ART used [43]. Another study identified two genomic regions (*HSPA1L* and *HSPA1B*) where significantly decreased methylation appeared to be associated with decreased pregnancy rates and three genomic regions (*USP6NL, SPON2* and *PTPRN2*) where significantly increased methylation appeared to be associated with pregnancy outcome, suggesting that decreased fecundity could be associated with alterations in DNA methylation at specific genomic loci [4, 17].

Recurrent pregnancy loss (RPL) is defined as the loss of two or more pregnancies. Comparison of sperm DNA methylation in RPL couples with no identifiable cause and fertile couples found a significant decrease in sperm global 5mC levels in the RPL group; a significant hypomethylation in the RPL group at specific CpG sites at *LINE1* promoter, *IGF2-H19* DMR and *IG*-DMR; no significant differences between the groups for total methylation in the *LINE1* promoter, *IGF2-H19* DMR and *IG*-DMR; a significant hypermethylation of differentially methylated regions of the maternally imprinted genes (commonly unmethylated in the sperm) *MEST, ZAC, KvDMR, PEG10, PEG3,* except for *SNRPN*; and a significant increase in the total methylation of *MEST, ZAC, KvDMR, PEG10* and *PEG3* in the RPL group, except for *SNRPN*, suggesting that aberrations in sperm DNA methylation of several imprinted genes are associated with RPL [58]. Rotondo et al. found that *MTHFR* promoter hypermethylation was more frequent in recurrent spontaneous abortion (RSA) couples than in no history of RSA (NRSA) couples and fertile men. They found that the methylated *MTHFR* epigenotype (including samples where it coexisted with unmethylated epigenotypes) was in 75% of semen samples from RSA men, 54% from NRSA men and 15% from fertile controls; *MTHFR* methylation was in the whole sperm population in semen samples from 55% of RSA men, 8% in NRSA men and 0% in fertile men; and CpG islands within the *MTHFR* promoter region were 100% methylated (hypermethylation of *MTHFR* gene promoter) [59].

A systematic review reported a significant *H19* hypomethylation in patients with idiopathic recurrent pregnancy loss compared to fertile controls, while altered methylation of other paternally expressed imprinted genes was not associated with recurrent pregnancy loss. They also reported no significant differences in ART outcomes (pregnancy, live birth rate, fertilization rate or good-quality embryos) in patients with aberrant and normal methylation for *H19, GLT2, LIT1, SNRPN, KCNQ1OT1, PEG1/MEST, PEG3 and NESPAS.* In contrast, they reported a study that showed an association between altered *GTL2* methylation and poorer ART results [60]. ALU hypomethylation is associated with male infertility, poor sperm quality and poor ART outcome (pregnancy, abortion and live birth). This was concluded by el Hajj et al., who analysed germline differentially methylated regions of *H19* and *GTL2* (paternally imprinted genes) and *LIT1, MEST, NESPAS, PEG3* and *SNRPN* (maternally imprinted genes), and ALU and LINE1 repetitive elements in semen samples from men with normal and abnormal semen analyses finding also that *GTL2* and *SNRPN* showed significant methylation differences between infertile and fertile individuals and that aberrant methylation imprints occurred significantly more frequently in infertile males (abnormal semen parameters), but did not seem to influence ART outcomes [61].

Epigenetic Inheritance and Impact on Offspring Health

Epigenetic reprogramming is the major barrier for epigenetic inheritance [16, 62], as during this process, DNA methylation, histone modification and small RNAs are reset. Imprinted loci (at imprinted genes), as well as other non-imprinted sequences (at non-imprinted genes), can resist demethylation after fertilization and inherit methylation from parental gametes [16, 63]. This shows that some sequences may escape reprogramming events, and this failure to erase epigenetic marks can contribute to epigenetic inheritance [15, 62].

Parental environmental epigenetic marks can be transmitted to the offspring through gamete epigenomes and influence their phenotype. DNA methylation, chromatin proteins and non-coding RNA can produce stable epigenetic effects that are transmitted from parents to offspring. In this regard, DNA methylation is a heritable epigenetic marker implicated in epigenetic inheritance, so environmentally induced sperm DNA methylation alterations can be potentially transmitted to the offspring. Non-coding RNAs in gametes including miRNAs, siRNAs and piRNAs are involved in environmental epigenetic inheritance. Regarding chromatin proteins, certain genes could maintain their histone marks at their promoters possibly carrying epigenetic information between generations and participating in transgenerational epigenetic inheritance [16, 62].

Epigenetic inheritance is the concept used to define that the father had certain preconception environmental exposures and these exposures modify offspring's epigenetics [19]. Transgenerational epigenetic inheritance describes the epigenetic effects, which can be inherited from one generation to the next [16]. Several studies have demonstrated that sperm epigenetic reprogramming can be altered by certain factors affecting male fertility, and this trait can be transmitted to offspring [36, 40]. Therefore, paternal epigenome can impact early embryo development and possibly even overall offspring's health [4, 5, 19]. The disruption of epigenetic inheritance could affect embryonic development, as this process is important for appropriate fertilization and embryo viability [63]. In this regard, studies have been done to investigate a possible association between altered paternal epigenome and the development of certain diseases in offspring.

Parental lifestyle can change the development of disease in the offspring [19]. Epigenetics is the mechanism to justify how the experiences from a father can affect the development of its offspring, as epigenetic marks are relatively stable and can be transmitted transgenerationally through the germline. Paternal factors before conception could play a significant role in offspring's health. For example, psychological, metabolic and environmental factors can alter offspring's neurodevelopment and endocrine and metabolic functions. Paternal malnutrition can affect the epigenome from spermatozoa and therefore foetal development and affect offspring's health by causing an increased risk of metabolic diseases and breast cancer in adulthood. However, paternal consumption of certain food compounds can be beneficial for the health of the father and the offspring [64]. Therefore, nutritional factors' exposure before offspring conception can affect its metabolism [19].

Similarly, paternal obesity and diabetes have also been associated with epigenetic inheritance, as both obesity and diabetes change DNA and histone methylation, histone acetylation and non-coding RNAs in sperm [65]. Chang et al. found an association between paternal preconception smoking and a significant increased risk of acute myeloid leukaemia and a non-significant increased risk of acute lymphoblastic leukaemia [66], and although other reasons could be responsible for this, probably epigenetics is also involved [19].

Alterations in sperm epigenome have been associated with the development of certain neuropsychiatric diseases in offspring. Kimura et al. suggested that one of the causes that can explain the increased risk of ASD due to paternal ageing is age-related alteration in sperm DNA methylation [67]. A recent study from Garrido et al. found 805 differential DNA methylation regions in paternal sperm, 303 with increase and 502 with decrease in DNA methylation in the autistic compared to the non-autistic male children group, showing a highly significant set of differential DNA methylated regions that could act as a biomarker to identify paternal offspring autism susceptibility [68].

Another study conducted by Feinberg et al. identified 193 differentially methylated regions in paternal sperm from an ASD-enriched risk cohort associated with

12-month ASD-related phenotypes in offspring and top ten differentially methylated regions corresponding to the following genes: *SNORD115-15, SNORD115-11, SNORD115-17, SMYD3, MUC17, RBM19, FAM13A, GPR125* and *WDR1*. Some differentially methylated regions showed enrichment for genes involved in cellular movement, neurogenesis and neuronal development. They suggested that epigenetic differences in paternal sperm may contribute to offspring's autism risk [69]. Jenkins et al. identified 139 regions significantly hypomethylated with age (112 associated with a gene) and 8 regions significantly hypermethylated with age (7 associated with a gene) in sperm DNA and 4 diseases most commonly associated with the 117 genes, specifically diabetes mellitus, hypertension, bipolar disorder and schizophrenia. Interestingly, bipolar disorder and schizophrenia appeared to be more frequently associated with the identified set of genes, raising the possibility of an increased risk of these diseases in the offspring of older fathers due to sperm DNA methylation alterations associated with age [70].

In summary, evidence points towards an association between altered epigenetics, which in some cases even involves imprinted loci, and male infertility conditions, semen parameters, ART outcomes and offspring's health (Fig. 9.3). However, it must be noticed that not all studies done until now have found such associations. Further studies are needed to acquire a better understanding of these differences and identify possible biomarkers that can be used for diagnosis and for targeted therapy, and this will help in improving counselling and fertility care of couples reaching an ART clinic.

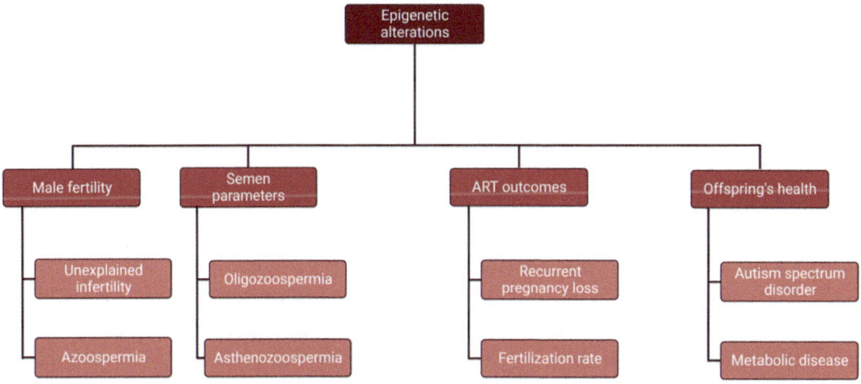

Fig. 9.3 Schematic and brief representation of the male infertility conditions, semen parameters, ART outcomes and offspring's health that can be affected by alterations in epigenetic signatures. (Created with BioRender.com)

Insights into the Future Research of Epigenetic Alterations in Male Infertility

SWOT (Strengths, Weaknesses, Opportunities and Threats) Analysis of the Current Research on Epigenetics

Spermatozoa undergo several epigenetic changes during differentiation, and they have a unique epigenome [5, 24]. Scientific research has supported the association between sperm epigenome and male infertility, semen parameters, ART outcomes and, more importantly, offspring's health. This not only gives rise to the possibility of considering these epigenetic marks as potential targets for the development of biomarkers to improve diagnosis in male infertility and for the development of therapeutic options, but also allows the early detection, prediction of susceptibility and prevention of transmission of epigenetic marks linked to offspring's non-genetic disease and assessing offspring's health risks. Nevertheless, there is still much to be done, and additional investigations are needed to elucidate the role and biological implication of epigenetic mechanisms in sperm and translate all this knowledge into the clinical practice [4, 10, 16, 17, 19, 34, 55, 68]. To this end, NGS has enabled the analysis of the different epigenetic modifications [30], and its application will help unravel these possible associations and overall will permit an improvement of reproductive counselling of couples reaching infertility clinics.

Prospects for Future Research on Epigenetics

Histone codes could be used as prognostic markers and in therapy discerning altered histone codes in various diseases and then restoring the altered histone codes in disease by therapeutically targeting the corresponding epigenetic regulatory enzymes. HDACs have been considered in epigenetic therapy, and histone deacetylase inhibitor (HDACi) could be used for the treatment of some diseases, such as cancer [26], but there is still a need of acquiring more knowledge of these molecules. For example, for the treatment of acute promyelocytic leukaemia, a combined treatment of retinoic acid with histone deacetylase/histone methyltransferase (HDAC/HMT) inhibitors could be used [23].

Our goal should be to identify the mechanisms of regulation by epigenetic markers and their interactions with normal and disease states [28]. In addition, evaluating the effect of environmental risk factors on sperm epigenetics and sperm epigenetic markers, as well as offspring's heritability of the epigenetic modifications and phenotypes, is also necessary to prevent the transmission of non-genetic disease [16, 24]. Moreover, the identification of methylation markers that could be used for the development of methylation screening panels of infertility holds a great promise in the future [33]. Further basic science studies, as well as translational studies, are needed [24], and high-throughput technologies should be applied. In upcoming years, with the improvement in epigenetic testing and the better understanding of sperm epigenomics and its relation with disease states, we would be able to improve diagnosis, prediction, prevention, management, counselling, therapeutics, treatment and overall infertility care.

Summary

Epigenetics is the study of changes in gene expression and function without altering the DNA sequence. During spermatogenesis, spermatozoa undergo several epigenetic modifications, such as protamination, resulting in the formation of spermatozoa with a unique epigenome, which could later on be altered by several factors, such as diet or smoke. Paternal epigenome is very important for sperm function, fertilization, embryo development and offspring's health. Altered epigenetic states could be associated with male infertility (unexplained infertility), semen parameters (asthenozoospermia or oligozoospermia) and ART outcomes (pregnancy or fertilization rate). Aberrant methylation in imprinted genes such as *H19* or *MEST* could be associated with male factor infertility. More importantly, altered sperm epigenetics can have an effect on offspring's health leading to the development of disease (autism spectrum disorder) due to epigenetic inheritance where paternal epigenetic marks can be transmitted to the offspring through sperm and influence their phenotype. This brings up the possibility of identifying new candidates as epigenetic biomarkers for improvement in diagnosis, development of targeted therapies and allowing an early detection of susceptibility of transmission of non-genetic disease to offspring. Still there is much to be done in this intriguing field of epigenetics, and further basic and translational studies are necessary. In the near future, with improvements in high-throughput technologies and its application in the study of epigenomes, we would be able to increase our understanding in the underlying mechanisms and open up new possibilities where specialists can participate to improve fertility care.FundingAna Navarro-Gomezlechon is granted by the Ministerio de Ciencia, Innovación y Universidades para la Formación de Profesorado Universitario (FPU19/06126), Spain.

References

1. Stouffs K, Seneca S, Lissens W. Genetic causes of male infertility. Ann Endocrinol (Paris). 2014;75(2):109–11.
2. Garrido N, Hervás I. Personalized medicine in infertile men. Urol Clin North Am. 2020;47(2):245–55.
3. Sinha A, Singh V, Yadav S. Multi-omics and male infertility: status, integration and future prospects. Front Biosci (Schol Ed). 2017;9(3):375–94.
4. Krzastek SC, Smith RP, Kovac JR. Future diagnostics in male infertility: genomics, epigenetics, metabolomics and proteomics. Transl Androl Urol. 2020;9(7):S195–205.

5. Halder A, Kumar P, Jain M, Kalsi AK. Genomics: tool to predict and prevent male infertility. Front Biosci (Schol Ed). 2017;9(4):448–508.
6. Alhathal N, Maddirevula S, Coskun S, Alali H, Assoum M, Morris T, et al. A genomics approach to male infertility. Genet Med [Internet]. 2020;22(12):1967–75. Available from: https://doi.org/10.1038/s41436-020-0916-0
7. Hu Z, Xia Y, Guo X, Dai J, Li H, Hu H, et al. A genome-wide association study in Chinese men identifies three risk loci for non-obstructive azoospermia. Nat Genet. 2012;44(2):183–6.
8. Shiraishi K. Genome medicine in male infertility: from karyotyping to single-cell analysis. J Obstet Gynaecol Res. 2021;47(8):2586–96.
9. Robay A, Abbasi S, Akil A, El-Bardisi H, Arafa M, Crystal RG, et al. A systematic review on the genetics of male infertility in the era of next-generation sequencing. Arab J Urol. 2018;16(1):53–64.
10. Pelzman DL, Hwang K. Genetic testing for men with infertility: techniques and indications. Transl Androl Urol. 2021;10(3):1354–64.
11. Oud MS, Smits RM, Smith HE, Mastrorosa FK, Holt GS, Houston BJ, et al. A de novo paradigm for male infertility. Nat Commun. 2022;13(1):154.
12. Camprubí C, Cigliano RA, Salas-Huetos A, Garrido N, Blanco J. What the human sperm methylome tells us. Epigenomics. 2017;9(10):1299–315.
13. Philip C. Introduction. Epigenetics: nature insigth. 2007;447(7143):395.
14. Berger SL, Kouzarides T, Shiekhattar R, Shilatifard A. An operational definition of epigenetics. Genes Dev. 2009;23(7):781–3.
15. Dupont C, Armant DR, Brenner CA. Epigenetics: definition, mechanisms and clinical perspective. Semin Reprod Med. 2009;27(5):351–7.
16. Wei Y, Schatten H, Sun Q. Environmental epigenetic inheritance through gametes and implications for human reproduction. Hum Reprod Update. 2015;21(2):194–208.
17. Jenkins TG, Aston KI, Meyer TD, Hotaling JM, Shamsi MB, Johnstone EB, et al. Decreased fecundity and sperm DNA methylation patterns. Fertil Steril. 2016;105(1):51–57.e3.
18. Marzouni ET, Ilkhani H, Harchegani AB, Shafaghatian H, Layali I, Shahriary A. Epigenetic modifications, a new approach to male infertility etiology: a review. Int J Fertil Steril. 2022;16(1):1–9.
19. Ibrahim Y, Hotaling J. Sperm epigenetics and its impact on male fertility, pregnancy loss, and somatic health of future offsprings. Semin Reprod Med. 2018;36(3–4):233–9.
20. Reik W, Dean W. DNA methylation and mammalian epigenetics. Electrophoresis. 2001;22(14):2838–43.
21. Nakao M. Epigenetics: interaction of DNA methylation and chromatin. Gene. 2001;278:25–31.
22. Jones PA, Takai D, Jones PA, Takai D. The role of DNA methylation in mammalian epigenetics. 2001;2013(1068):1068–70.
23. Quina AS, Buschbeck M, Di CL. Chromatin structure and epigenetics. Biochem Pharmacol. 2006;72:1563–9.
24. Carrell DT, Ph D. Epigenetics of the male gamete. Fertil Steril [Internet]. 2012;97(2):267–74. https://doi.org/10.1016/j.fertnstert.2011.12.036.
25. Berger SL. Histone modifications in transcriptional regulation. Curr Opin Genet Dev. 2002;12(2):142–8.
26. Lennartsson A, Ekwall K. Histone modi fi cation patterns and epigenetic codes. Biochim Biophy Acta. 2009;1790:863–8.
27. Becker PB, Workman JL. Nucleosome remodeling and epigenetics. 2013;5(9):a017905.
28. Wei J, Huang KAI, Yang C, Kang C. Non-coding RNAs as regulators in epigenetics (Review). Oncol Rep. 2017;37(1):3–9.
29. Kaikkonen MU, Lam MTY, Glass CK. Non-coding RNAs as regulators of gene expression and epigenetics. Cardiovasc Res. 2011;90(3):430–40.
30. Collins LJ, Schönfeld B, Chen XS. Chapter 4—The epigenetics of non-coding RNA. In: TBT T, editor. Handbook of epigenetics. San Diego: Academic Press; 2011. p. 49–61. Available from: https://www.sciencedirect.com/science/article/pii/B9780123757098000046.

31. Güneş S, Kulaç T. The role of epigenetics in spermatogenesis. Turk J Urol. 2013;39(3):181–7.
32. Oliva R. Protamines and male infertility. Hum Reprod Update. 2006;12(4):417–35.
33. Sujit KM, Sarkar S, Singh V, Pandey R, Agrawal NK, Trivedi S, et al. Genome-wide differential methylation analyses identi fi es methylation signatures of male infertility. Hum Reprod Update. 2018;33(12):2256–67.
34. Santi D, De Vincentis S, Magnani E, Spaggiari G. Impairment of sperm DNA methylation in male infertility: a meta-analytic study. Andrology. 2017;5(4):695–703.
35. Schuller A, Bellini C, Jenkins TG, Eden M, Matz J, Oakes J, et al. Simulated wildfire smoke significantly alters sperm DNA methylation patterns in a murine model. Toxics. 2021;9(9):1–10.
36. Liu Y, Chen S, Pang D, Zhou J, Xu X, Yang S, et al. Effects of paternal exposure to cigarette smoke on sperm DNA methylation and long-term metabolic syndrome in offspring. Epigenet Chromatin [Internet]. 2022;1–12. Available from: https://doi.org/10.1186/s13072-022-00437-8.
37. Laqqan MM, Yassin MM. Cigarette heavy smoking alters DNA methylation patterns and gene transcription levels in humans spermatozoa. Environ Sci Pollut Res [Internet]. 2022;26835–49. Available from: https://doi.org/10.1007/s11356-021-17786-8.
38. Salas-huetos A, James ER, Salas-salvadó J, Bulló M, Aston KI, Carrell DT, et al. Sperm DNA methylation changes after short-term nut supplementation in healthy men consuming a Western-style diet. Andrology. 2021;9:260–8.
39. Cheng Y, Tang Q, Lu Y, Li M, Zhou Y, Wu P, et al. Semen quality and sperm DNA methylation in relation to long-term exposure to air pollution in fertile men: a cross-sectional study. Environ Pollut [Internet]. 2022;300:118994. https://doi.org/10.1016/j.envpol.2022.118994.
40. Zhao W, Gu N, Li Z, Wang G, Cheng CY. Autism-like behaviors and abnormality of glucose metabolism in offspring derived from aging males with epigenetically modified sperm. Aging (Albany NY). 2020;12(19):19766–84.
41. Li Y, Tollefsbol TO. DNA methylation detection: bisulfite genomic sequencing analysis. Methods Mol Biol. 2011;791:11–21.
42. Hammoud SS, Purwar J, Pflueger C, Cairns BR, Ph D. Alterations in sperm DNA methylation patterns at imprinted loci in two classes of infertility. Fertil Steril [Internet]. 2010;94(5):1728–33. https://doi.org/10.1016/j.fertnstert.2009.09.010.
43. Montjean D, Ravel C, Benkhalifa M, Cohen-Bacrie P, Berthaut I, Bashamboo A, et al. Methylation changes in mature sperm deoxyribonucleic acid from oligozoospermic men: assessment of genetic variants and assisted reproductive technology outcome. Fertil Steril. 2013;100(5):1241–7.
44. Marques CJ, Francisco T, Sousa S, Carvalho F, Barros A, Sousa M. Methylation defects of imprinted genes in human testicular spermatozoa. Fertil Steril. 2010;94(2):585–94.
45. Hammoud SS, Nix DA, Hammoud AO, Gibson M, Cairns BR, Carrell DT. Genome-wide analysis identifies changes in histone retention and epigenetic modifications at developmental and imprinted gene loci in the sperm of infertile men. Hum Reprod. 2011;26(9):2558–69.
46. Urdinguio RG, Bayón GF, Dmitrijeva M, Toraño EG, Bravo C, Fraga MF, et al. Aberrant DNA methylation patterns of spermatozoa in men with unexplained infertility. Hum Reprod. 2015;30(5):1014–28.
47. Pacheco SE, Houseman EA, Christensen BC, Marsit CJ, Kelsey KT, Sigman M, et al. Integrative DNA methylation and gene expression analyses identify DNA packaging and epigenetic regulatory genes associated with low motility sperm. PLoS One. 2011;6(6):1–10.
48. Aoki VW, Liu L, Carrell DT. Identification and evaluation of a novel sperm protamine abnormality in a population of infertile males. Hum Rerod. 2005;20(5):1298–306.
49. Aoki VW, Liu L, Jones KP, Hatasaka HH. Sperm protamine 1 / protamine 2 ratios are related to in vitro fertilization pregnancy rates and predictive of fertilization ability. Fertil Steril. 2006;86(5):1408–15.
50. Denomme MM, Mccallie BR, Parks JC, Schoolcraft WB, Katz-jaffe MG. Alterations in the sperm histone- retained epigenome are associated with unexplained male factor infertility and poor blastocyst development in donor oocyte IVF cycles. Hum Reprod. 2017;32(12):2443–55.

51. Camprubí C, Pladevall M, Grossmann M, Garrido N, Pons MC, Blanco J. Semen samples showing an increased rate of spermatozoa with imprinting errors have a negligible effect in the outcome of assisted reproduction techniques. Epigenetics. 2012;7(10):1115–24.
52. Camprubí C, Pladevall M, Grossmann M, Garrido N, Pons MC, Blanco J. Lack of association of MTHFR rs1801133 polymorphism and CTCFL mutations with sperm methylation errors in infertile patients. J Assist Reprod Genet. 2013;30(9):1125–31.
53. Camprubí C, Salas-Huetos A, Aiese-Cigliano R, Godo A, Pons MC, Castellano G, et al. Spermatozoa from infertile patients exhibit differences of DNA methylation associated with spermatogenesis-related processes: an array-based analysis. Reprod Biomed Online [Internet]. 2016;33(6):709–19. https://doi.org/10.1016/j.rbmo.2016.09.001.
54. Friemel C, Ammerpohl O, Gutwein J, Schmutzler AG, Siebert R, Caliebe A, et al. Array-based DNA methylation profiling in male infertility reveals allele-specific DNA methylation in PIWIL1 and PIWIL2. Fertil Steril. 2014;101(4):1097–1103.e1.
55. Houshdaran S, Cortessis VK, Siegmund K, Yang A, Laird PW, Sokol RZ. Widespread epigenetic abnormalities suggest a broad DNA methylation erasure defect in abnormal human sperm. PLoS One. 2007;2(12):e1289.
56. Du Y, Li M, Chen J, Duan Y, Wang X, Qiu Y, et al. Promoter targeted bisulfite sequencing reveals DNA methylation profiles associated with low sperm motility in asthenozoospermia. Hum Reprod. 2016;31(1):24–33.
57. Al-qazzaz HK, Al-awadi SJ. Gene reports epigenetic alteration in DNA methylation pattern and gene expression level using H19 on oligospermia patients in Iraqi men. Gene Rep [Internet]. 2020;20(June):100780. https://doi.org/10.1016/j.genrep.2020.100780.
58. Khambata K, Raut S, Deshpande S, Mohan S, Sonawane S, Gaonkar R, et al. DNA methylation defects in spermatozoa of male partners from couples experiencing recurrent pregnancy loss. Hum Reprod. 2021;36(1):48–60.
59. Rotondo JC, Bosi S, Bazzan E, Di DM, De MM, Selvatici R, et al. Methylenetetrahydrofolate reductase gene promoter hypermethylation in semen samples of infertile couples correlates with recurrent spontaneous abortion. Hum Reprod. 2012;27(12):3632–8.
60. Cannarella R, Crafa A, Condorelli RA, Mongioì LM, La VS, Calogero AE, et al. Systems Biology in Reproductive Medicine Relevance of sperm imprinted gene methylation on assisted reproductive technique outcomes and pregnancy loss: a systematic review technique outcomes and pregnancy loss: a systematic review. Syst Biol Reprod Med. 2021;67(4):251–9. https://doi.org/10.1080/19396368.2021.1909667.
61. El Hajj N, Zechner U, Schneider E, Tresch A, Gromoll J, Hahn T, et al. Methylation status of imprinted genes and repetitive elements in sperm DNA from infertile males. Sex Dev. 2011;5(2):60–9.
62. Xavier MJ, Roman SD, Aitken RJ, Nixon B. Transgenerational inheritance: how impacts to the epigenetic and genetic information of parents affect offspring health. Hum Reprod Update. 2019;25(5):518–40.
63. Denomme MM, Ph D, Mccallie BR, Sc B, Parks JC, Sc B, et al. Inheritance of epigenetic dysregulation from male factor infertility has a direct impact on reproductive potential. Fertil Steril [Internet]. 2018;110(3):419–428.e1. https://doi.org/10.1016/j.fertnstert.2018.04.004.
64. De FG, Pascoal L, Geraldi MV, Mar R, Ong TP. Effect of paternal diet on spermatogenesis and offspring health: focus on epigenetics and interventions with food bioactive compounds. Nutrients. 2022;14(10):2150.
65. Ou X-H, Zhu C-C, Sun S-C. Effects of obesity and diabetes on the epigenetic modification of mammalian gametes. J Cell Physiol. 2019;234(6):7847–55.
66. Chang JS, Selvin S, Metayer C, Crouse V, Golembesky A, Buffler PA. Parental smoking and the risk of childhood leukemia. Am J Epidemiol. 2006;163(12):1091–100.
67. Kimura R, Yoshizaki K, Osumi N. Risk of neurodevelopmental disease by paternal aging: a possible influence of epigenetic alteration in sperm. Adv Exp Med Biol. 2018;1012:75–81.

68. Garrido N, Cruz F, Egea RR, Simon C, Sadler-Riggleman I, Beck D, et al. Sperm DNA methylation epimutation biomarker for paternal offspring autism susceptibility. Clin Epigenet [Internet]. 2021;13(1) https://doi.org/10.1186/s13148-020-00995-2.
69. Feinberg JI, Bakulski KM, Jaffe AE, Tryggvadottir R, Brown SC, Goldman LR, et al. Paternal sperm DNA methylation associated with early signs of autism risk in an autism-enriched cohort. Int J Epidemiol. 2015;44(4):1199–210.
70. Jenkins TG, Aston KI, Pflueger C, Cairns BR, Carrell DT. Age-associated sperm DNA methylation alterations: possible implications in offspring disease susceptibility. PLoS Genet. 2014;10(7):e1004458.

Part V
Varicocele Revisited

Chapter 10
New Insights into the Pathophysiology of Varicocele in Male Infertility

Parviz K. Kavoussi and Ioannis Sokolakis

Key Points

- Although some fertile and some infertile men with varicoceles may have similar conventional semen parameters, many have diminished parameters which improve with varicocele repair, and there is a significant association between varicocele and male infertility.
- Of the available sperm function tests, sperm DNA fragmentation assays and assays measuring seminal oxidative stress have been deemed clinically useful as these processes are associated with male infertility and spermatogenic dysfunction.
- Oxidative stress levels are significantly higher in varicocele patients and significantly reduced following varicocele repair.
- Elevated sperm DNA fragmentation levels correlate with poor semen quality, impaired preimplantation development, and increased spontaneous pregnancy loss rates.

Introduction

Varicocele is defined as an abnormal dilation and tortuosity of the veins of the pampiniform plexus (Fig. 10.1) with the presence of malfunctioning valves and is the most common correctable cause of male infertility [1]. Varicocele affects nearly 15% of men in the general population and is diagnosed in up to 41% of men with primary infertility and 80% secondary infertility cases [2]. The venous drainage from the testis forms multiple anastomoses at the mediastinum of the testis, which is known as the pampiniform plexus. The pampiniform plexus is created by three groups of veins: the anterior, middle, and posterior veins. The anterior spermatic

P. K. Kavoussi (✉)
Department of Reproductive Urology, Austin Fertility & Reproductive Medicine/Westlake IVF, Austin, TX, USA

I. Sokolakis
Department of Urology, Medical School, Aristotle University of Thessaloniki, Thessaloniki, Greece

A. Agarwal et al. (eds.), *Current and Future Advances in Male Infertility*, https://doi.org/10.1007/978-3-031-62648-7_10

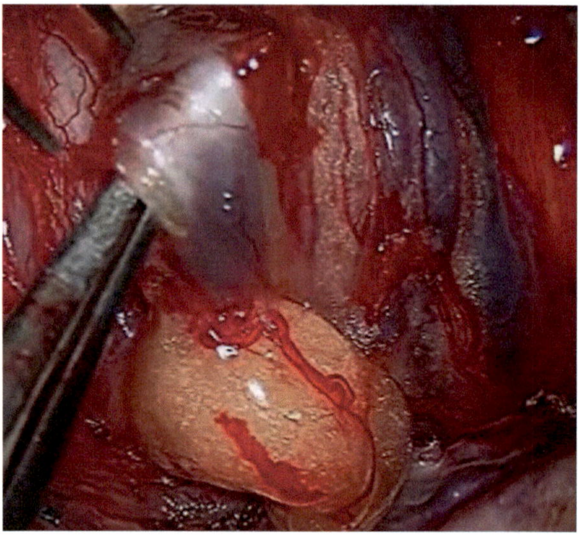

Fig. 10.1 Microsurgical view of the spermatic cord demonstrating abnormal dilation of the veins of the pampiniform plexus in a patient undergoing varicocele repair

veins course alongside the internal spermatic artery and coalesce into three or four veins traveling into the pelvis at the level of the superficial inguinal ring. These veins eventually combine to form a single internal spermatic vein at the level of the internal inguinal ring before draining into the inferior vena cava on the right and the renal vein on the left. The middle deferential veins travel alongside the vas deferens and drain via the internal iliac vein. The posterior spermatic veins course alongside the spermatic cord and drain into the external pudendal and cremasteric veins. The order of significance of venous drainage ranks internal spermatic vein first, followed by the external pudendal vein, the deferential vein, and then the cremasteric veins [3]. The objective of this chapter is to review and comprehensively discuss the pathophysiology of varicocele and its role in male infertility.

Animal Models to Study the Pathophysiology of Varicoceles

A significant amount of research is currently ongoing in order to elucidate the pathophysiology of varicocele. However, due to the fact that varicocele is virtually exclusively seen in humans (probably because of our upright position), basic science research opportunities are challenging. To address this issue, numerous animal models have been developed, but the most popular one includes the partial closure of the left renal vein just medial to the insertion of the internal spermatic vein in dogs or rodents, and most frequently in rats [4]. Because of the increased pressure in the internal spermatic vein caused by the partial closure, this surgical approach can produce a varicocele model. The left internal spermatic vein and the pampiniform venous plexus enlarge as a result of the elevated venous pressure [5]. The varicocele model with this technique can cause an increase in testicular blood flow, an increase in intratesticular temperature, a decrease in sperm concentration and motility, and a decrease in intratesticular testosterone levels. While some studies have had success using this model to replicate the effects of varicocele, other researchers have had varying degrees of success [6].

In rats, partial blockage of the left renal vein does not always result in a successful varicocele model (the most effective series had a success rate of about 90%) [7]. The variable venous architecture of the rat testis is probably to blame for these erratic outcomes. Two distinct left gonadal veins have been identified by some researchers, one emptying into the left renal vein and the other into the left common iliac vein. In comparison to the left gonadal vein emptying into the left renal vein, the left gonadal vein typically has a sixfold bigger diameter [8]. Failure to recognize supplementary gonadal veins may result in a failed varicocele formation. The significance of locating and ligating the second left gonadal vein, which empties into the left common iliac vein, is obvious. Utilizing a microsurgical technique, ligation of the gonadal vein draining into the common iliac vein and partial occlusion of the left renal vein produced a more effective varicocele model in rats compared to partial occlusion alone [9].

For the partial occlusion of the left renal vein, several techniques have been described. Usually, a 4-0 silk suture is used to partially occlude the vein. In order to create a consistent model, the suture is tied down around the vein and an interposed metal wire or needle of 0.8 mm diameter. After the suture has been tied, the metal wire is removed and the vessel will expand as much as the suture will allow [7]. Recently, a study has described the partial occlusion of left renal vein using a clip with 0.7 mm gap width instead of suture ligature placed at the same point on the renal vein [10].

Laboratory Finding Associated with the Pathophysiology of Varicoceles

A major question regarding the pathophysiology of varicocele-induced male infertility is why does a unilateral left varicocele cause bilateral effect. To explain the pathogenesis of varicoceles, numerous researchers recently published brand-new molecular results. The first researchers to specifically note that elevated levels of reactive oxygen species (ROS) and nitrous oxide (N_2O) were seen bilaterally in cases with a unilateral varicocele were Santoro and Romeo [11]. Additionally, Mostafa et al. evaluated the ROS levels in men with varicoceles and found a correlation between the ROS levels and the grade of the varicocele [12]. Furthermore, Deepinder et al. highlighted that the diagnostic and prognostic capabilities of seminal oxidative stress measurement can exceed the capabilities of conventional sperm quality tests [13].

Additionally, investigations on infertile men with varicoceles have produced additional supportive laboratory evidence and offered novel methods of testing for this population. According to Zini et al., men with varicoceles were more likely to experience sperm DNA damage, which was reversed by having the varicoceles repaired [14]. Furthermore, Finelli et al. carried out proteomic analyses on infertile men with varicoceles and identified mitochondrial aconitate hydratase (ACO2) and fatty acid synthase (FASN) as possible proteins involved in DNA repair, whose altered expression may contribute to DNA damage in varicocele pathophysiology [15]. Esteves et al. point out that the understanding of the role of sperm DNA fragmentation in male infertility requires an in-depth analysis of the multifactorial pathophysiological processes and the theories involved [16]. These findings indicate that additional laboratory studies may be considered for the basic workup of patients with varicoceles.

Some other novel laboratory findings regarding the pathophysiology of varicocele include the presence of heat shock proteins which may identify heat-sensitive men with varicoceles [17]. In other studies, varicocele seemed to affect the Leydig cells of some men, which may affect the production of testosterone. Lately, with an arising interest in investigating the role of microRNAs in the control of Sertoli cells, spermatogenesis and male fertility have emerged [18, 19]. MicroRNA testing could help us understand the pathophysiology of varicocele-induced infertility in the future.

Anatomic Hypotheses of Origin of Varicoceles

The anatomic hypothesis of varicocele formation is likely multifactorial. It is mainly based on the fact that the right internal spermatic vein empties directly into the inferior vena cava, while the left internal spermatic vein into the left renal vein lateral to the vertebral column [20]. Due to this modification, three anatomic hypotheses of varicocele origin have been developed: the hydrostatic pressure hypothesis, the valvular dysfunction hypothesis, and the nutcracker phenomenon hypothesis. All three hypotheses are anchored on the fact that patients present, in most cases, with unilateral left-sided varicocele.

1. ***Hydrostatic pressure hypothesis:*** The left internal spermatic vein is about 8–10 cm longer compared to the right internal spermatic vein. The increased length of the left internal spermatic vein leads to a greater venous pressure in the left venous drainage system, resulting in dilation of the pampiniform plexus. Additionally, the left spermatic vein terminates into the left renal vein at an angle of 90°, whereas the right spermatic vein terminates more obliquely. This "twist" of the left internal spermatic vein seems to increase the hydrostatic venous pressure in the left venous drainage system, resulting in dilation of the pampiniform plexus [21]. Another theory that supports the hydrostatic pressure hypothesis is that the blood flow in the inferior vena cava is higher compared to the left renal vein, leading to increased venous flow from the right internal spermatic vein into the inferior vena cava based on the principles of the Venturi effect [22].

2. ***Valvular dysfunction hypothesis:*** This hypothesis is based on the fact that spermatic veins might have dysfunctional valves or even no valves which cause varicocele in line with the pathophysiological mechanism leading to venous insufficiency [23]. Observational data support that an association between varicose veins of the lower extremities and varicocele might exist [24]. Still, the hypothesis of valvular dysfunction is controversial since it does not explain why varicocele manifests more often on the left side. Importantly, autopsy findings have demonstrated that the absence of valves can also occur in men without varicocele [25]. Therefore, the valvular dysfunction hypothesis is reserved only for some cases of varicocele.
3. ***Nutcracker phenomenon hypothesis:*** The nutcracker phenomenon or the left renal vein entrapment syndrome is the compression of the left renal vein between the abdominal aorta and the superior mesenteric artery. This leads to stasis in the left renal vein, causing, in turn, dilatation of the pampiniform plexus [21]. Even though the nutcracker phenomenon manifests only in rare cases of varicocele, it can be easily diagnosed with ultrasound through estimation of the left renal vein diameter and through measurement of the left renal vein peak velocity [26]. It is also a rare cause of varicocele.

Scrotal Hyperthermia

Even though the cause of varicocele seems to be anatomic, the cause of varicocele-related male infertility seems to be multifactorial. A principal factor contributing to abnormal sperm physiology might be the scrotal hyperthermia. Physiologically, the scrotal temperature is about 1° lower compared to the core body temperature for optimal testicular function and spermatogenesis [27]. This temperature regulation is also supported by the pampiniform plexus. In particular, the inflowing arterial blood is cooled by the outflowing venous blood of the pampiniform plexus. Still, in patients with varicocele, the dilatation of the pampiniform plexus leads to venous and, in turn, to testicular hyperthermia [28]. Testicular hyperthermia leads to dysfunction of a plethora of enzymes involved in DNA synthesis, such as topoisomerase 1 and DNA polymerase, which normally exhibit optimal activity at a lower temperature [29]. Accordingly, it has been postulated that gene expression and protein synthesis might also be negatively affected by testicular hyperthermia [30].

However, human studies report controversial findings. More specifically, some studies have demonstrated increased scrotal temperatures in infertile men with varicocele compared to normal controls [31], while other studies did not find a direct association between varicocele and elevated scrotal temperature [32]. Therefore, it seems that a clear relation between scrotal hyperthermia leading to infertility in patients with varicocele does not exist, but animal and human studies suggest that the elevation of testicular temperatures might be caused by varicocele, leading to dysregulation of the spermatogenesis in some cases [33].

Hormonal Disturbances

It has been postulated that male infertility in men with varicocele might be attributed to hormonal disturbances. In these patients, dysfunction of Leydig cells leads to decreased intratesticular testosterone levels and, in turn, to the development of male infertility [34]. This postulation has been concurred by a plethora of studies suggesting a decrease in serum and intratesticular testosterone levels due to varicocele. The mechanism leading to reduction of intratesticular and serum testosterone levels seems to be explained by an attenuated response to human chorionic gonadotrophin stimulation or by a decreased binding of human chorionic gonadotrophin hormone to Leydig cells [34]. On the other hand, several studies suggest no difference in the concentrations of FSH, LH, testosterone, and estradiol in both peripheral and testicular blood in men with and without varicocele [35]. Similarly, other studies indicate no difference in testosterone concentration before and after varicocele repair [36]. It seems that the decrease in testosterone levels occurring in some patients with varicocele is compensated through some degree of Leydig cell hyperplasia [37]. Thus, men with varicocele and abnormal Leydig cell function might benefit the most from varicocelectomy.

Hypoperfusion of the Testis

The hypoperfusion of the testis might also contribute to male infertility. An increase of the testicular venous pressure caused by the varicocele may lead to vasoconstriction of the precapillary arterioles, hypoperfusion of the testis, and, in turn, disturbance of the normal spermatogenesis [38]. Moreover, the increased testicular venous pressure may change the paracrine environment of the hormones involved in spermatogenesis and negatively affect fluid exchange. Although this hypothesis has been formulated based on findings from animal models, studies on human subjects have demonstrated that the majority of patients with varicocele and increased testicular venous pressure have normal semen parameters, questioning whether there is a direct association between increased testicular venous pressure and impaired spermatogenesis [39]. Nevertheless, correction of varicocele in patients with abnormal semen parameters results in improved semen parameters and pregnancy rates. Of note, it has been suggested that the greater improvement in sperm parameters has been observed in patients who had a decrease in venous pressure postoperatively [40].

Metabolic Reflux to the Testis

Venous reflux is a common feature in early venography studies on men with varicocele [41]. According to this hypothesis, the reflux of toxic metabolites from the kidney and adrenal gland, including urea, prostaglandins, and adrenaline, can contribute to chronic vasoconstriction, endothelial cell failure, and hypoperfusion/hypoxia of the testicles. These substances are also known to encourage cellular oxidative stress in numerous in vitro human cell cultures [42]. However, research investigating this hypothesis has produced conflicting findings. For example, in contrast to levels found in the peripheral circulation, MacLeod et al. reported a threefold rise in the mean catecholamines content from testicular venous blood taken during varicocelectomy [43]. However, investigations comparing the levels of additional adrenal metabolites, such as dehydroepiandrosterone and cortisol, in the peripheral circulation and testicular venous blood of infertile men with varicocele did not discover any statistically significant variations [44].

Another interesting study found higher PGE and PGF levels in the spermatic venous blood of varicocele patients. However, they failed to detect a rise in cortisol levels, assuming that adrenal metabolites do not reflux in contrast to renal metabolites [45]. Others, however, disagreed, finding no rise in the renin concentration in the spermatic venous blood of varicocele males, which should have been elevated if renal blood flow was refluxing down the spermatic veins [46]. Additionally, another study also disregarded retrograde flow of renal/adrenal metabolites after performing adrenalectomy on varicocelized Wistar rats and found no reversal of the pathologic changes caused by varicocele, including increased testicular temperature, decreased sperm count and motility, and decreased testicular weight [47]. Another animal investigation that added to the evidence disputing the metabolic reflux idea involved tagged microspheres infused into the left renal vein that did not show up in either testis of animals with induced left varicocele [48]. Therefore, the theory of metabolic reflux to the testis could not be supported by robust evidence.

Genetics of Varicocele Pathophysiology

Over 15% of infertile men and 2–8% of men with unexplained infertility and azoospermia or oligozoospermia have genetic disorders, which significantly contributes to spermatogenesis failures [49]. The structural and numerical chromosomal abnormalities, gene mutations, polymorphisms, and copy number variations were emphasized among the genetic abnormalities linked to varicocele formation [50].

1. ***Somatic Chromosomal Alterations:*** The prevalence of chromosomal abnormalities in men with varicocele varies greatly and may be influenced by a number of variables, especially those related to spermatic abnormalities. In contrast to males who experienced idiopathic infertility, individuals with varicocele had greater incidences of chromosomal abnormalities. They included inversions on

chromosomes 9 and 2, translocations between chromosomes 4 and 15, deletions on chromosome 4, and insertions onto chromosome 9. On chromosomes 21 and 22, additional genetic material was also seen to have been added. Additionally, several patients with varicocele and chromosomal issues also exhibited microdeletions in the Y chromosome's NS153, SI158, and SI254 regions [51]. The association between deletions in various AZF areas and the varicocele phenotype has been examined in several studies [52]. It is crucial to know whether the genetic changes linked to varicocele are somatic or germline based in order to better understand the etiology and guide treatment decisions for these individuals, which should include genetic counseling to avoid potentially unfavorable surgical outcomes [53].

2. ***Genetic Mutations and Polymorphisms*:** The effects of various single nucleotide polymorphisms (SNPs) on the infertility phenotypes in males with varicocele have been the subject of several research. The glutathione S-transferase (GST) gene polymorphism, which is connected to oxidative stress and antioxidant capability, is one of the most researched polymorphisms in men with varicocele [54]. Additionally, men with varicoceles are more likely to have the Cys/Cys null genotype of the human 8-oxoguanine DNA glycosylase 1 (hOGG1) gene polymorphism [55]. 8-Hydroxydeoxyguanosine is a sensitive indicator of the oxidative DNA damage brought on by reactive oxygen species (ROS) in human sperm cells [56]. Moreover, men with varicocele and the Cys/Cys null genotype have the poorest semen analysis outcomes, which are not seen in individuals with subclinical varicocele [55]. The transition nuclear protein (TNP) gene is another site of a different mutation that has been observed in men with varicocele. DNA damage is connected to single nucleotide polymorphisms (SNPs) in the TNP genes [57]. Several other mutations and polymorphisms have been connected to male infertility, but future studies are needed to prove the etiological connection to varicocele-induced infertility.
3. ***Epigenetic Mechanisms*:** Histone modifications, DNA methylation, and noncoding RNA (ncRNA) expression are examples of epigenetic mechanisms. The sperm cells of males with varicocele have lower levels of global DNA methylation than those of fertile people, according to Bahreinian et al. This study also demonstrated a negative correlation between methylation and DNA fragmentation, suggesting that the sperm cells of people with varicocele were more vulnerable to DNA damage when the DNA was hypomethylated [58]. In another study, the analysis of the expression of miRNA-122, miRNA-181a, and miRNA-34c5 in the sperm cells of varicocele-affected men revealed decreased levels of these miRNAs in the presence of varicocele and oligoasthenoteratozoospermia, suggesting that these miRNAs may be connected to semen quality in varicocele-affected men. These miRNAs also connected negatively with oxidative stress and apoptotic indicators, the grade of the varicocele, and the side on which it developed [59].
4. ***Gene Expression*:** Since varicocele produces heat and oxidative stress, which may affect DNA and RNA integrity and the Sertoli cells' ability to function, it may change the expression patterns of numerous genes [60].

Independently to the degree of varicocele, genetic and epigenetic variables are linked to low sperm quality and production in males with varicocele and, as a result, to the loss of fertility. The variety of phenotypes seen points to a multifactorial disorder, in which the anatomical changes associated with it can change the environment of the testis and perhaps have an impact on spermatogenesis. No precise biomarkers could be found for varicocele because of its multifactorial and diverse character; nonetheless, a number of modifications, including chromosomal alterations, gene polymorphisms, mutations, SNPs, changes in DNA methylation, and epigenetic mutations, are frequently seen in patients with varicocele. However, identifying the key processes and associated genetic and epigenetic abnormalities in varicocele would help us better understand the condition. Additionally, in particular for people who are infertile, they may aid in varicocele prevention and help guide patient care and prognosis.

Sperm Proteomics

The understanding of structural and functional sperm proteins is advancing the molecular field of sperm biology. Cellular and molecular pathways are dysregulated in the spermatozoa of infertile men and particularly in those with varicoceles [61]. Altered expression of sperm proteins and metabolites in infertile men suggests compromised spermatogenesis or defects in crucial sperm functions such as capacitation, hyperactivation, and acrosome reaction, all of which are necessary for the fertilization process. There is a paucity of data in the medical literature on sperm proteomics and specifically in men with varicoceles. Protein profiling was performed in normozoospermic men without varicocele and oligospermic men with varicocele, but as the technique had inferior sensitivity, only 15 differential enrichment analyses of proteomic data (DEPs) were identified. Molecular pathways involving mitochondrial proteins, heat shock protein, and cytoskeleton proteins were affected in varicocele patients [30]. It has also been demonstrated that the expression of sperm proteins, mitochondrial expression protein (ATP5D), antioxidant protein (SOD1), and heat shock protein (HSPA5), was significantly increased following varicocele repair in comparison to preoperatively when varicocele was intact [62]. A high state of oxidative stress (OS) secondary to varicoceles induces mitochondrial dysfunction, and expression of mitochondrial proteins has been shown to be altered in men with varicoceles [63, 64]. Altered expression of sperm proteins impacts molecular pathways, posttranslational modification, free radical scavenging, protein ubiquitination, and mitochondrial dysregulation, which can negatively impact the normal physiological function of the spermatozoa. Twenty-nine proteins associated with sperm maturation, motility, hyperactivation, capacitation, and acrosome reaction were shown to be altered in spermatozoa in men with varicoceles [65].

Effect of Varicocele on Testicular Function

It has been well established that varicoceles may have an adverse impact on testicular function. There are a number of theories of mechanisms by which this may occur. The majority of the data indicate that varicoceles impact testicular function by elevating intratesticular temperatures secondary to the interruption of the countercurrent heat exchange in the pampiniform plexus with opposing flows in a central arterial system [28, 31, 66]. In men without varicoceles, the countercurrent provided by the venous plexus in the spermatic cords allows the testicles to remain at a temperature of 1–2 °C below core body temperature [27]. Proposed potential mechanisms of cellular damage due to varicoceles include sperm DNA fragmentation (SDF), apoptosis, increasing reactive oxygen species (ROS) through OS, intracellular ionic and metabolic changes, predisposition to sperm aneuploidy, and molecular pathways and altered sperm protein expression [61, 63, 67–81]. A rat animal model study supports the theory of retrograde flow of adrenal and renal metabolites increasing the severity of varicocele-induced testicular damage [82]. Another study found adrenal and renal metabolites within the venous plexus of the testicles, suggesting valvular incompetence resulting in reflux of blood, which can further contribute to venous dilation and hemostasis [83].

Varicocele and Conventional Semen Analysis

The conventional semen analysis remains as the cornerstone of the laboratory evaluation of the infertile male and the most globally used biomarker to estimate male fertility potential [84]. Some data have revealed that fertile and infertile men with varicoceles have similar semen parameters to those without varicoceles [85]. This indicates that varicocele affects semen quality and fertility in some but not all men with varicoceles. Current data demonstrate a significant association between varicocele and male infertility, indicated by the reduction of testicular volume on the ipsilateral side of the testis in many men with varicoceles [86]. Varicoceles can impact all semen parameters including sperm concentration, motility, and morphology [87, 88]. Men with varicoceles were shown to have significant decreases in the mean total sperm count, percent motility, and percent with normal morphology in comparison to controls without varicoceles in a study including 9034 men performed by the World Health Organization [89]. A meta-analysis evaluating ten studies on conventional semen parameters in men with varicoceles revealed a significantly reduced sperm count, motility, and morphology, but not semen volume in men with varicoceles [87]. Varicocele has been shown to negatively impact semen parameter values, and varicocele grade has an inverse association with sperm concentration, motility, and morphology [89]. The most appreciable difference is noted in men with grade 3 varicoceles [90]. In men with grade 3 varicoceles, the sperm concentration is typically less than half of that in men without a varicocele [89].

It has been indicated that varicocele repair significantly improves the fertility profile; however; there have been conflicting data in the medical literature as well [91–93]. Varicocele repair in randomized clinical trials resulted in significant improvement in conventional semen parameters with a sperm concentration improvement by 75%, motility improvement by 5.2%, and morphology improvement by 8% [94]. Other studies showed that regardless of the surgical technique, there were significant improvements in sperm count and motility with varicocele repair [85, 95]. Varicocele repair improves sperm concentration and motility in all varicocele grades, but most significantly among grade 3 varicoceles, and it may take 6 months to demonstrate this rather than 3 months postoperatively [90].

Varicocele and Oxidative Stress

A physiological level of ROS is necessary for sperm capacitation regulation and enzymatic and nonenzymatic antioxidant scavenging systems' ability to maintain a balanced cellular environment [96–98]. ROS are highly reactive molecules which are unstable and increase cell membrane peroxidation of polyunsaturated fatty acids. This results in adverse effects on the sperm head structure and the midpiece membrane, resulting in suboptimal motility and fertilization [99]. OS has been demonstrated to be a major factor in varicocele-associated infertility. Higher levels of OS and lipid peroxidation have been found in infertile men with varicoceles in comparison to infertile men without varicoceles. Even fertile men with varicoceles were found to have higher levels of OS than those without varicoceles [100]. Scrotal temperature elevation caused by varicoceles increases ROS production from mitochondria, plasma membrane, cytoplasm, and peroxisome due to heat stress [99]. ROS are a known cause of SDF by damaging mitochondrial and sperm nuclear DNA. Varicocele is associated with SDF as fertile and infertile men with varicoceles have been shown to have higher SDF than those without varicoceles. ROS can also induce apoptosis in spermatozoa [100]. A direct relationship has been demonstrated between seminal ROS levels and the grade of the varicocele [101].

Varicocele repair can decrease seminal OS levels but may take up to 6 months to do so [102–104]. A rapid decline in high levels of seminal ROS free radicals has also been demonstrated as early as 1 month post-varicocele repair [104, 105]. A prospective clinical trial by Kavoussi et al. demonstrated that varicocele repair improved static oxidation reduction potential as a measure of seminal OS levels in infertile men [106].

Varicocele and Antisperm Antibodies

Disruption of the blood-testis barrier may result in the production of antisperm antibodies (ASAs) as a result of a man's immune system identifying haploid sperm cells. ASAs can interfere with fertilization by affecting sperm agglutination (Fig. 10.2), cervical mucus penetration, and sperm-oocyte interaction. ASAs may also negatively impact sperm differentiation, capacitation, acrosome reaction, zona binding and penetration, and sperm-oocyte membrane interaction [107, 108]. ASAs were only detected in approximately 30% of men with clinical varicoceles [109]. The impact of varicocele repair on ASAs is controversial. One study revealed a nearly 50% reduction of ASA titers following varicocele repair, most notably in men with high-grade varicoceles, and pregnancy within a year post-varicocele repair was 2.8 times more likely in ASA-negative than ASA-positive men following varicocele repair [110]. Another study revealed that decreasing ASA titers did not predict improvement in semen parameter values [109]. With the lack of clarity, with the current level of data, ASA testing in response to the presence of a varicocele remains controversial.

Varicocele and Sperm Vitality

Vitality testing is recommended when there is low sperm motility and sperm have lost their flagellation and have metabolic dysfunction or axonemal defects, in cases of necrozoospermia. Vitality can be assessed through hypo-osmotic swelling test, eosin test, or eosin-nigrosin test [111]. Varicoceles have been implicated in altering sperm membrane function, but there is a paucity of data on varicocele repair impact on sperm vitality [112].

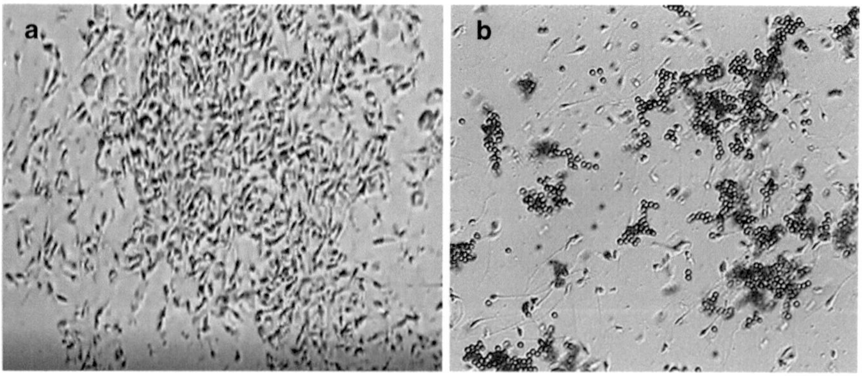

Fig. 10.2 (**a**) Microscopic view of agglutinated sperm. (**b**) Microscopic view of immunobead assay for antisperm antibodies

Varicocele and Sperm Capacitation

Sperm capacitation is a reversible process, which is time dependent, where extrinsic protein loss, such as acrosome-stabilizing factors and membrane cholesterols, occurs. This makes for a more pliable, fluid sperm membrane which facilitates acrosome reaction and sperm hyperactivation [113]. A prospective study revealed that sperm from men with grade 2 and grade 3 varicoceles had severe impairment in the ability to develop hyperactive motility in comparison to normozoospermic men. There was a significantly lower incidence of sperm with phosphotyrosine immunoreactive tails among varicocele patients. The normozoospermic cells had significantly more fluid membranes in comparison to the lower membrane fluidity in spermatozoa from varicocele patients [114]. Men with varicoceles have spermatozoa with impairment in their ability to have capacitation-associated changes such as protein tyrosine phosphorylation, which may contribute to the lower membrane fluidity due to higher levels of peroxidative damage to the membrane.

Varicocele and Sperm Binding to Zona Pellucida

The zona pellucida is critical for fertilization as it induces acrosome reaction [84, 115]. Abnormal sperm-zona pellucida interaction results in unsuccessful fertilization. Sperm binding to the zona may be assessed by two assays: competitive intact zona binding assay and the hemizona assay [84, 115]. Although the negative effects of varicoceles on sperm fusion and penetration of the zona pellucida have been reported, the use of these assays in predicting which men would benefit from varicocele repair from a sperm binding to zona pellucida aspect remains controversial. Sperm binding to zona pellucida only improved in varicocele patients whose partners achieved pregnancy [116, 117]. Hemizona assay results had a positive correlation with pregnancy following varicocele repair. The hemizona assay improved after varicocele repair in patients who achieved an early pregnancy [116]. Due to a lack of large-scale studies confirming its utility, the use of this assay to predict who would benefit from varicocele repair remains controversial.

Varicocele and Sperm DNA Fragmentation

High levels of sperm DNA damage in the form of DNA fragmentation have been associated with poor semen quality, impaired preimplantation embryonic development, and increased spontaneous pregnancy loss [108, 118–120]. In men with varicoceles, OS has been directly correlated with increased SDF levels [121]. ROS can damage nuclear and mitochondrial DNA, resulting in base modification, DNA strand breaks, and chromatin cross-links and apoptosis-like process, which can impact sperm maturation and nuclear protamination [121, 122]. Men with varicoceles with high levels of SDF have been shown to have detrimental effects on spontaneous fertility as well as assisted fertility [118]. Assays for SDF assess for single- and/or double-strand DNA breaks. There are multiple assays for SDF including direct methods to detect breaks such as the comet assay and terminal deoxynucleotidyl transference-mediated deoxyuridine triphosphate (dUTP) nick end labeling (TUNEL) assay or indirect methods using sperm chromatin structure assay (SCSA) and sperm chromatin dispersion assay (SCDA) (Fig. 10.3) [108, 118]. Varicocele is associated with increased levels of SDF, with a 9.84% higher SDF level in men with varicoceles in comparison to controls, and elevated SDF levels may be detected in men with varicoceles with normal semen parameter values [14, 123–125]. In one study, varicocele repair decreased SDF by a mean of 3.37% in comparison with no treatment and was associated with improved pregnancy rates, but was only effective in clinical varicoceles, not subclinical ones [126, 127]. A separate prospective clinical trial revealed a mean decrease in SDF by 14% 3 months following varicocele repair [106]. Elevation of abnormal chromatin packaging has also been identified in the semen of men with varicoceles, which adversely impacts the process of fertilization [128–130]. Following varicocele repair, the rate of chromatin condensation has been shown to improve, along with decreasing free radical levels 1 month post-repair and decreasing SDF 3–6 months post-repair [128]. A publication endorsed by the Society of Translational Medicine, with guidelines on

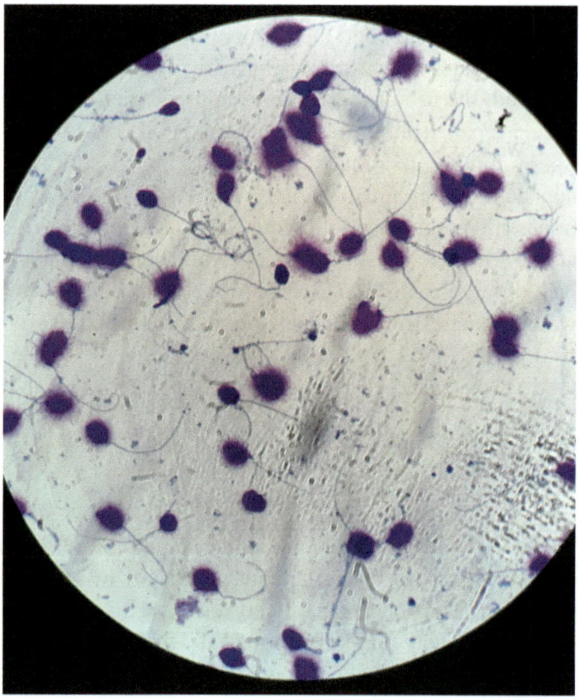

Fig. 10.3 Microscopic view of sperm DNA fragmentation assay using the sperm chromatin dispersion assay

the utility of SDF in clinical practice, recommends SDF testing in varicocele patients to help select candidates for varicocele repair [131]. This recommendation was also published in a clinician guideline study on SDF for clinicians [132].

Summary

There is a great deal of data in the medical literature suggesting that varicoceles have a pathological effect on the testes and their function. There are numerous mechanisms by which varicoceles result in this testicular insult. Although a number of men with varicoceles are capable of spontaneous conception or may have normal conventional semen parameters, in many men, the primary culprit affecting their fertility potential is a clinical varicocele. Specialized sperm function tests are gaining more acceptance for utility in the evaluation of the infertile male with a varicocele, and varicocele repair has been shown to improve semen parameters, sperm function tests, and clinical outcomes for many men. Large-scale, controlled, well-designed studies are needed to identify which infertile men with varicoceles will benefit from repair.

References

1. Su JS, Farber NJ, Vij SC. Pathophysiology and treatment options of varicocele: an overview. Andrologia. 2021;53(1):e13576.
2. Alsaikhan B, Alrabeeah K, Delouya G, Zini A. Epidemiology of varicocele. Asian J Androl. 2016;18(2):179–81.
3. Wishahi MM. Anatomy of the spermatic venous plexus (pampiniform plexus) in men with and without varicocele: intraoperative venographic study. J Urol. 1992;147(5):1285–9.
4. Katz MJ, Najari BB, Li PS, Goldstein M. The role of animal models in the study of varicocele. Transl Androl Urol. 2014;3(1):59.
5. Saypol DC, Howards SS, Turner TT, Miller E. Influence of surgically induced varicocele on testicular blood flow, temperature, and histology in adult rats and dogs. J Clin Invest. 1981;68(1):39–45.
6. Li H, Dubocq F, Jiang Y, Tiguert R, Gheiler EL, Dhabuwala C. Effect of surgically induced varicocele on testicular blood flow and Sertoli cell function. Urology. 1999;53(6):1258–62.
7. Turner T. The study of varicocele through the use of animal models. Hum Reprod Update. 2001;7(1):78–84.
8. Pascual JA, Lemmi C, Rajfer J. Variability of venous anatomy of rat testis: application to experimental testicular surgery. Microsurgery. 1992;13(6):335–7.
9. Najari BB, Li PS, Ramasamy R, Katz M, Sheth S, Robinson B, et al. Microsurgical rat varicocele model. J Urol. 2014;191(2):548–53.
10. Guo W-b, Yang C, Bian J, Xia H, Yang J-k, Q-z Z, et al. With a new clip technique surgically inducing varicocele in Sprague-Dawley rats. BMC Urol. 2018;18(1):1–6.
11. Santoro G, Romeo C. Normal and varicocele testis in adolescents. Asian J Androl. 2001;3(4):259–62.
12. Mostafa T, Anis T, El Nashar A, Imam H, Osman I. Seminal plasma reactive oxygen species–antioxidants relationship with varicocele grade. Andrologia. 2012;44(1):66–9.

13. Deepinder F, Cocuzza M, Agarwal A. Should seminal oxidative stress measurement be offered routinely to men presenting for infertility evaluation? Endocr Pract. 2008;14(4):484–91.
14. Zini A, Azhar R, Baazeem A, Gabriel M. Effect of microsurgical varicocelectomy on human sperm chromatin and DNA integrity: a prospective trial. Int J Androl. 2011;34(1):14–9.
15. Finelli R, Darbandi S, Pushparaj PN, Henkel R, Ko E, Agarwal A. In silico sperm proteome analysis to investigate DNA repair mechanisms in varicocele patients. Front Endocrinol. 2021;12:757592.
16. Esteves SC, Agarwal A, Cho C-L, Majzoub A. A Strengths-Weaknesses-Opportunities-Threats (SWOT) analysis on the clinical utility of sperm DNA fragmentation testing in specific male infertility scenarios. Transl Androl Urol. 2017;6(Suppl 4):S734.
17. Ferlin A, Speltra E, Patassini C, Pati MA, Garolla A, Caretta N, et al. Heat shock protein and heat shock factor expression in sperm: relation to oligozoospermia and varicocele. J Urol. 2010;183(3):1248–52.
18. Gholami D, Amirmahani F, Yazdi RS, Hasheminia T, Teimori H. MiR-182-5p, MiR-192-5p, and MiR-493-5p constitute a regulatory network with CRISP3 in seminal plasma fluid of teratozoospermia patients. Reprod Sci. 2021;28(7):2060–9.
19. Procópio MS, de Avelar GF, Costa GM, Lacerda S, Resende RR, de França LR. MicroRNAs in Sertoli cells: implications for spermatogenesis and fertility. Cell Tissue Res. 2017;370(3):335–46.
20. Lechter A, Lopez G, Martinez C, Camacho J. Anatomy of the gonadal veins: a reappraisal. Surgery. 1991;109(6):735–9.
21. Coolsaet B. The varicocele syndrome: venography determining the optimal level for surgical management. J Urol. 1980;124(6):833–8.
22. Shafik A, Moftah A, Olfat S, Mohi-el-Din M, El-Sayed A. Testicular veins: anatomy and role in varicocelo genesis and other pathologic conditions. Urology. 1990;35(2):175–82.
23. Mohseni MJ, Nazari H, Amini E, Javan-Farazmand N, Baghayee A, Farzi H, et al. Shunt-type and stop-type varicocele in adolescents: prognostic value of these two different hemodynamic patterns. Fertil Steril. 2011;96(5):1091–6.
24. Yasim A, Resim S, Sahinkanat T, Eroglu E, Ari M, Efe E. Clinical and subclinical varicocele incidence in patients with primary varicose veins requiring surgery. Ann Vasc Surg. 2013;27(6):758–61.
25. Ahlberg N, Bartley O, Chidekel N. Right and left gonadal veins: an anatomical and statistical study. Acta Radiol Diagn. 1966;4(6):593–601.
26. Takebayashi S, Ueki T, Ikeda N, Fujikawa A. Diagnosis of the nutcracker syndrome with color Doppler sonography: correlation with flow patterns on retrograde left renal venography. J Urol. 1999;162(1):274–5.
27. Dahl EV, Herrick JF. A vascular mechanism for maintaining testicular temperature by counter-current exchange. Surg Gynecol Obstet. 1959;108(6):697–705.
28. Zorgniotti AW, Macleod J. Studies in temperature, human semen quality, and varicocele. Fertil Steril. 1973;24(11):854–63.
29. Fujisawa M, Yoshida S, Matsumoto O, Kojima K, Kamidono S. Deoxyribonucleic acid polymerase activity in the testes of infertile men with varicocele. Fertil Steril. 1988;50(5):795–800.
30. Hosseinifar H, Gourabi H, Salekdeh GH, Alikhani M, Mirshahvaladi S, Sabbaghian M, et al. Study of sperm protein profile in men with and without varicocele using two-dimensional gel electrophoresis. Urology. 2013;81(2):293–300.
31. Goldstein M, Eid J-F. Elevation of intratesticular and scrotal skin surface temperature in men with varicocele. J Urol. 1989;142(3):743–5.
32. Lund L, Nielsen K. Varicocele testis and testicular temperature. Br J Urol. 1996;78(1):113–5.
33. Green KF, Turner TT, Howards SS. Varicocele: reversal of the testicular blood flow and temperature effects by varicocele repair. J Urol. 1984;131(6):1208–11.
34. Organization WH. The influence of varicocele on parameters of fertility in a large group of men presenting to infertility clinics. Fertil Steril. 1992;57(6):1289–93.

35. Swerdloff RS, Walsh PC. Pituitary and gonadal hormones in patients with varicocele. Fertil Steril. 1975;26(10):1006–12.
36. Hudson RW, Perez-Marrero RA, Crawford VA, McKay DE. Hormonal parameters of men with varicoceles before and after varicocelectomy. Fertil Steril. 1985;43(6):905–10.
37. Sirvent J, Bernat R, Navarro M, Tolra JR, Guspi R, Bosch R. Leydig cell in idiopathic varicocele. Eur Urol. 1990;17:257–61.
38. Sweeney TE, Rozum JS, Gore RW. Alteration of testicular microvascular pressures during venous pressure elevation. Am J Phys Heart Circ Phys. 1995;269(1):H37–45.
39. Kantartzi P, Goulis CD, Goulis G, Papadimas I. Male infertility and varicocele: myths and reality. Hippokratia. 2007;11(3):99.
40. Shafik A. Venous tension patterns in cord veins. II. After varicocele correction. J Urol. 1983;129(4):749–51.
41. Comhaire F, Kunnen M. Selective retrograde venography of the internal spermatic vein: a conclusive approach to the diagnosis of varicocele. Andrologia. 1976;8(1):11–24.
42. Zhang Z, Dmitrieva NI, Park J-H, Levine RL, Burg MB. High urea and NaCl carbonylate proteins in renal cells in culture and in vivo, and high urea causes 8-oxoguanine lesions in their DNA. Proc Natl Acad Sci. 2004;101(25):9491–6.
43. Macleod J. Seminal cytology in the presence of varicocele. Fertil Steril. 1965;16(6):735–57.
44. Steeno O, Koumans J, De Moor P. Adrenal cortical hormones in the spermatic vein of 95 patients with left varicocele. Andrologia. 1976;8(2):101–4.
45. Ito H, Fuse H, Minagawa H, Kawamura K, Murakami M, Shimazaki J. Internal spermatic vein prostaglandins in varicocele patients. Fertil Steril. 1982;37(2):218–22.
46. Lindholmer C, Thulin L, Eliasson R. Concentrations of cortisol and renin in the internal spermatic vein of men with varicocele. Andrologie. 1973;5(1):21–2.
47. Sofikitis N, Miyagawa I. Bilateral effect of unilateral varicocele on testicular metabolism in the rabbit. Int J Fertil Menopausal Stud. 1994;39(4):239–47.
48. Turner T, Lopez T. Testicular blood flow in peripubertal and older rats with unilateral experimental varicocele and investigation into the mechanism of the bilateral response to the unilateral lesion. J Urol. 1990;144(4):1018–21.
49. Foresta C, Ferlin A, Gianaroli L, Dallapiccola B. Guidelines for the appropriate use of genetic tests in infertile couples. Eur J Hum Genet. 2002;10(5):303–12.
50. Finelli R, Leisegang K, Kandil H, Agarwal A. Oxidative stress: a comprehensive review of biochemical, molecular, and genetic aspects in the pathogenesis and management of varicocele. World J Men's Health. 2022;40(1):87.
51. Rao L, Babu A, Kanakavalli M, Padmalatha V, Singh A, Singh PK, et al. Chromosomal abnormalities and y chromosome microdeletions in infertile men with varicocele and idiopathic infertility of South Indian origin. J Androl. 2004;25(1):147–53.
52. de Sousa FE, Christofolini D, Barbosa C, Glina S, Bianco B. Y chromosome microdeletions and varicocele as aetiological factors of male infertility: a cross-sectional study. Andrologia. 2018;50(3):e12938.
53. Cayan S, Lee D, Black LD, Pera RAR, Turek PJ. Response to varicocelectomy in oligospermic men with and without defined genetic infertility. Urology. 2001;57(3):530–5.
54. Wu Q, Xing J, Xue W, Sun J, Wang X, Jin X. Influence of polymorphism of glutathione S-transferase T1 on Chinese infertile patients with varicocele. Fertil Steril. 2009;91(3):960–2.
55. Chen SS, Chiu LP. The hOGG1 Ser326Cys polymorphism and male subfertility in Taiwanese patients with varicocele. Andrologia. 2018;50(5):e13007.
56. Shen H-M, Ong C-N. Detection of oxidative DNA damage in human sperm and its association with sperm function and male infertility. Free Radic Biol Med. 2000;28(4):529–36.
57. Miyagawa Y, Nishimura H, Tsujimura A, Matsuoka Y, Matsumiya K, Okuyama A, et al. Single-nucleotide polymorphisms and mutation analyses of the TNP1 and TNP2 genes of fertile and infertile human male populations. J Androl. 2005;26(6):779–86.

58. Bahreinian M, Tavalaee M, Abbasi H, Kiani-Esfahani A, Shiravi AH, Nasr-Esfahani MH. DNA hypomethylation predisposes sperm to DNA damage in individuals with varicocele. Syst Biol Reprod Med. 2015;61(4):179–86.
59. Mostafa T, Rashed LA, Nabil NI, Osman I, Mostafa R, Farag M. Seminal miRNA relationship with apoptotic markers and oxidative stress in infertile men with varicocele. Biomed Res Int. 2016;2016
60. Naugton D, Nangia A, Agarwal A. Varicocele and male infertility: Part II. Pathophysiology of varicoceles in male infertility. Hum Reprod Update. 2001;7:473–81.
61. du Plessis SS, Kashou AH, Benjamin DJ, Yadav SP, Agarwal A. Proteomics: a subcellular look at spermatozoa. Reprod Biol Endocrinol. 2011;9:36.
62. Hosseinifar H, Sabbaghian M, Nasrabadi D, Modarresi T, Dizaj AV, Gourabi H, et al. Study of the effect of varicocelectomy on sperm proteins expression in patients with varicocele and poor sperm quality by using two-dimensional gel electrophoresis. J Assist Reprod Genet. 2014;31(6):725–9.
63. Smith R, Kaune H, Parodi D, Madariaga M, Rios R, Morales I, et al. Increased sperm DNA damage in patients with varicocele: relationship with seminal oxidative stress. Hum Reprod. 2006;21(4):986–93.
64. Samanta L, Agarwal A, Swain N, Sharma R, Gopalan B, Esteves SC, et al. Proteomic signatures of sperm mitochondria in varicocele: clinical use as biomarkers of varicocele associated infertility. J Urol. 2018;200(2):414–22.
65. Agarwal A, Sharma R, Durairajanayagam D, Ayaz A, Cui Z, Willard B, et al. Major protein alterations in spermatozoa from infertile men with unilateral varicocele. Reprod Biol Endocrinol. 2015;13:8.
66. Masson P, Brannigan RE. The varicocele. Urol Clin North Am. 2014;41(1):129–44.
67. Benoff SH, Millan C, Hurley IR, Napolitano B, Marmar JL. Bilateral increased apoptosis and bilateral accumulation of cadmium in infertile men with left varicocele. Hum Reprod. 2004;19(3):616–27.
68. Baccetti BM, Bruni E, Capitani S, Collodel G, Mancini S, Piomboni P, et al. Studies on varicocele III: ultrastructural sperm evaluation and 18, X and Y aneuploidies. J Androl. 2006;27(1):94–101.
69. Bertolla RP, Cedenho AP, Hassun Filho PA, Lima SB, Ortiz V, Srougi M. Sperm nuclear DNA fragmentation in adolescents with varicocele. Fertil Steril. 2006;85(3):625–8.
70. Enciso M, Muriel L, Fernandez JL, Goyanes V, Segrelles E, Marcos M, et al. Infertile men with varicocele show a high relative proportion of sperm cells with intense nuclear damage level, evidenced by the sperm chromatin dispersion test. J Androl. 2006;27(1):106–11.
71. Lima SB, Cenedeze MA, Bertolla RP, Filho PA, Oehninger S, Cedenho AP. Expression of the HSPA2 gene in ejaculated spermatozoa from adolescents with and without varicocele. Fertil Steril. 2006;86(6):1659–63.
72. Zeh JA, Bonilla MM, Adrian AJ, Mesfin S, Zeh DW. From father to son: transgenerational effect of tetracycline on sperm viability. Sci Rep. 2012;2:375.
73. Shiraishi K, Naito K. Effects of 4-hydroxy-2-nonenal, a marker of oxidative stress, on spermatogenesis and expression of p53 protein in male infertility. J Urol. 2007;178(3 Pt 1):1012–7. discussion 1017
74. Agarwal A, Makker K, Sharma R. Clinical relevance of oxidative stress in male factor infertility: an update. Am J Reprod Immunol. 2008;59(1):2–11.
75. Blumer CG, Fariello RM, Restelli AE, Spaine DM, Bertolla RP, Cedenho AP. Sperm nuclear DNA fragmentation and mitochondrial activity in men with varicocele. Fertil Steril. 2008;90(5):1716–22.
76. Pasqualotto FF, Sundaram A, Sharma RK, Borges E Jr, Pasqualotto EB, Agarwal A. Semen quality and oxidative stress scores in fertile and infertile patients with varicocele. Fertil Steril. 2008;89(3):602–7.
77. Ghabili K, Shoja MM, Agutter PS, Agarwal A. Hypothesis: intracellular acidification contributes to infertility in varicocele. Fertil Steril. 2009;92(1):399–401.

78. Wu GJ, Chang FW, Lee SS, Cheng YY, Chen CH, Chen IC. Apoptosis-related phenotype of ejaculated spermatozoa in patients with varicocele. Fertil Steril. 2009;91(3):831–7.
79. Abd-Elmoaty MA, Saleh R, Sharma R, Agarwal A. Increased levels of oxidants and reduced antioxidants in semen of infertile men with varicocele. Fertil Steril. 2010;94(4):1531–4.
80. El-Domyati MM, Al-Din AB, Barakat MT, El-Fakahany HM, Honig S, Xu J, et al. The expression and distribution of deoxyribonucleic acid repair and apoptosis markers in testicular germ cells of infertile varicocele patients resembles that of old fertile men. Fertil Steril. 2010;93(3):795–801.
81. Hassan A, el-Nashar EM, Mostafa T. Programmed cell death in varicocele-bearing testes. Andrologia. 2009;41(1):39–45.
82. Camoglio FS, Zampieri N, Corroppolo M, Chironi C, Dipaola G, Giacomello L, et al. Varicocele and retrograde adrenal metabolites flow. An experimental study on rats. Urol Int. 2004;73(4):337–42.
83. Ozbek E, Yurekli M, Soylu A, Davarci M, Balbay MD. The role of adrenomedullin in varicocele and impotence. BJU Int. 2000;86(6):694–8.
84. Franken DR, Oehninger S. Semen analysis and sperm function testing. Asian J Androl. 2012;14(1):6–13.
85. Fuse H, Akashi T, Fujishiro Y, Kazama T, Katayama T. Effect of varicocele on fertility potential: comparison between impregnating and nonimpregnating groups. Arch Androl. 1995;35(2):143–8.
86. Gorelick JI, Goldstein M. Loss of fertility in men with varicocele. Fertil Steril. 1993;59(3):613–6.
87. Agarwal A, Sharma R, Harlev A, Esteves SC. Effect of varicocele on semen characteristics according to the new 2010 World Health Organization criteria: a systematic review and meta-analysis. Asian J Androl. 2016;18(2):163–70.
88. Agarwal A, Sharma RK, Sharma R, Assidi M, Abuzenadah AM, Alshahrani S, et al. Characterizing semen parameters and their association with reactive oxygen species in infertile men. Reprod Biol Endocrinol. 2014;12:33.
89. The influence of varicocele on parameters of fertility in a large group of men presenting to infertility clinics. World Health Organization. Fertil Steril. 1992;57(6):1289–93.
90. Vahidi S, Moein M, Nabi A, Narimani N. Effects of microsurgical varicocelectomy on semen analysis and sperm function tests in patients with different grades of varicocele: role of sperm functional tests in evaluation of treatments outcome. Andrologia. 2018;50(8):e13069.
91. Krause W, Muller HH, Schafer H, Weidner W. Does treatment of varicocele improve male fertility? results of the 'Deutsche Varikozelenstudie', a multicentre study of 14 collaborating centres. Andrologia. 2002;34(3):164–71.
92. Johnson D, Sandlow J. Treatment of varicoceles: techniques and outcomes. Fertil Steril. 2017;108(3):378–84.
93. Schlesinger MH, Wilets IF, Nagler HM. Treatment outcome after varicocelectomy. A critical analysis. Urol Clin North Am. 1994;21(3):517–29.
94. Agarwal A, Deepinder F, Cocuzza M, Agarwal R, Short RA, Sabanegh E, et al. Efficacy of varicocelectomy in improving semen parameters: new meta-analytical approach. Urology. 2007;70(3):532–8.
95. Baazeem A, Belzile E, Ciampi A, Dohle G, Jarvi K, Salonia A, et al. Varicocele and male factor infertility treatment: a new meta-analysis and review of the role of varicocele repair. Eur Urol. 2011;60(4):796–808.
96. Aitken J, Fisher H. Reactive oxygen species generation and human spermatozoa: the balance of benefit and risk. BioEssays. 1994;16(4):259–67.
97. Aitken RJ. The role of free oxygen radicals and sperm function. Int J Androl. 1989;12(2):95–7.
98. Mancini A, Milardi D, Conte G, Festa R, De Marinis L, Littarru GP. Seminal antioxidants in humans: preoperative and postoperative evaluation of coenzyme Q10 in varicocele patients. Horm Metab Res. 2005;37(7):428–32.

99. Cho CL, Esteves SC, Agarwal A. Novel insights into the pathophysiology of varicocele and its association with reactive oxygen species and sperm DNA fragmentation. Asian J Androl. 2016;18(2):186–93.
100. Hendin BN, Kolettis PN, Sharma RK, Thomas AJ Jr, Agarwal A. Varicocele is associated with elevated spermatozoal reactive oxygen species production and diminished seminal plasma antioxidant capacity. J Urol. 1999;161(6):1831–4.
101. Agarwal A, Prabakaran S, Allamaneni SS. Relationship between oxidative stress, varicocele and infertility: a meta-analysis. Reprod Biomed Online. 2006;12(5):630–3.
102. Chen SS, Huang WJ, Chang LS, Wei YH. Attenuation of oxidative stress after varicocelectomy in subfertile patients with varicocele. J Urol. 2008;179(2):639–42.
103. Dada R, Shamsi MB, Venkatesh S, Gupta NP, Kumar R. Attenuation of oxidative stress & DNA damage in varicocelectomy: implications in infertility management. Indian J Med Res. 2010;132:728–30.
104. Hurtado de Catalfo GE, Ranieri-Casilla A, Marra FA, de Alaniz MJ, Marra CA. Oxidative stress biomarkers and hormonal profile in human patients undergoing varicocelectomy. Int J Androl. 2007;30(6):519–30.
105. Mostafa T, Anis TH, El-Nashar A, Imam H, Othman IA. Varicocelectomy reduces reactive oxygen species levels and increases antioxidant activity of seminal plasma from infertile men with varicocele. Int J Androl. 2001;24(5):261–5.
106. Kavoussi PK, Gilkey MS, Machen GL, Kavoussi SK, Dorsey C. Varicocele repair improves static oxidation reduction potential as a measure of seminal oxidative stress levels in infertile men: a prospective clinical trial using the MiOXSYS system. Urology. 2022;165:193–7.
107. Majzoub A, Esteves SC, Gosalvez J, Agarwal A. Specialized sperm function tests in varicocele and the future of andrology laboratory. Asian J Androl. 2016;18(2):205–12.
108. Samplaski MK, Agarwal A, Sharma R, Sabanegh E. New generation of diagnostic tests for infertility: review of specialized semen tests. Int J Urol. 2010;17(10):839–47.
109. Djaladat H, Mehrsai A, Rezazade M, Djaladat Y, Pourmand G. Varicocele and antisperm antibody: fact or fiction? South Med J. 2006;99(1):44–7.
110. Bozhedomov VA, Lipatova NA, Alexeev RA, Alexandrova LM, Nikolaeva MA, Sukhikh GT. The role of the antisperm antibodies in male infertility assessment after microsurgical varicocelectomy. Andrology. 2014;2(6):847–55.
111. Bjorndahl L, Soderlund I, Kvist U. Evaluation of the one-step eosin-nigrosin staining technique for human sperm vitality assessment. Hum Reprod. 2003;18(4):813–6.
112. Fuse H, Kazama T, Katayama T. Hypoosmotic swelling test in patients with varicocele. Arch Androl. 1991;27(3):149–54.
113. Bailey JL. Factors regulating sperm capacitation. Syst Biol Reprod Med. 2010;56(5):334–48.
114. Buffone MG, Calamera JC, Verstraeten SV, Doncel GF. Capacitation-associated protein tyrosine phosphorylation and membrane fluidity changes are impaired in the spermatozoa of asthenozoospermic patients. Reproduction. 2005;129(6):697–705.
115. Oehninger S, Franken D, Alexander N, Hodgen GD. Hemizona assay and its impact on the identification and treatment of human sperm dysfunctions. Andrologia. 1992;24(6):307–21.
116. Hauser R, Yogev L, Greif M, Hirshenbein A, Botchan A, Gamzu R, et al. Sperm binding and ultrasound changes after operative repair of varicocele: correlation with fecundity. Andrologia. 1997;29(3):145–7.
117. Plymate SR, Nagao RR, Muller CH, Paulsen CA. The use of sperm penetration assay in evaluation of men with varicocele. Fertil Steril. 1987;47(4):680–3.
118. Bungum M, Humaidan P, Axmon A, Spano M, Bungum L, Erenpreiss J, et al. Sperm DNA integrity assessment in prediction of assisted reproduction technology outcome. Hum Reprod. 2007;22(1):174–9.
119. Duran HE, Morshedi M, Kruger T, Oehninger S. Intrauterine insemination: a systematic review on determinants of success. Hum Reprod Update. 2002;8(4):373–84.
120. Irvine DS, Twigg JP, Gordon EL, Fulton N, Milne PA, Aitken RJ. DNA integrity in human spermatozoa: relationships with semen quality. J Androl. 2000;21(1):33–44.

121. Dieamant F, Petersen CG, Mauri AL, Conmar V, Mattila M, Vagnini LD, et al. Semen parameters in men with varicocele: DNA fragmentation, chromatin packaging, mitochondrial membrane potential, and apoptosis. JBRA Assist Reprod. 2017;21(4):295–301.
122. Sakkas D, Alvarez JG. Sperm DNA fragmentation: mechanisms of origin, impact on reproductive outcome, and analysis. Fertil Steril. 2010;93(4):1027–36.
123. Ozturk MI, Koca O, Keles MO, Yilmaz S, Karaman MI. Increased sperm DNA damage in experimental rat varicocele model and the beneficial effect of varicocelectomy. Int J Fertil Steril. 2012;6(2):95–100.
124. Li F, Yamaguchi K, Okada K, Matsushita K, Ando M, Chiba K, et al. Significant improvement of sperm DNA quality after microsurgical repair of varicocele. Syst Biol Reprod Med. 2012;58(5):274–7.
125. Wang YJ, Zhang RQ, Lin YJ, Zhang RG, Zhang WL. Relationship between varicocele and sperm DNA damage and the effect of varicocele repair: a meta-analysis. Reprod Biomed Online. 2012;25(3):307–14.
126. Smit M, Romijn JC, Wildhagen MF, Veldhoven JL, Weber RF, Dohle GR. Decreased sperm DNA fragmentation after surgical varicocelectomy is associated with increased pregnancy rate. J Urol. 2010;183(1):270–4.
127. Lacerda JI, Del Giudice PT, da Silva BF, Nichi M, Fariello RM, Fraietta R, et al. Adolescent varicocele: improved sperm function after varicocelectomy. Fertil Steril. 2011;95(3):994–9.
128. Sadek A, Almohamdy AS, Zaki A, Aref M, Ibrahim SM, Mostafa T. Sperm chromatin condensation in infertile men with varicocele before and after surgical repair. Fertil Steril. 2011;95(5):1705–8.
129. Talebi AR, Moein MR, Tabibnejad N, Ghasemzadeh J. Effect of varicocele on chromatin condensation and DNA integrity of ejaculated spermatozoa using cytochemical tests. Andrologia. 2008;40(4):245–51.
130. Evenson DP, Wixon R. Data analysis of two in vivo fertility studies using Sperm Chromatin Structure Assay-derived DNA fragmentation index vs. pregnancy outcome. Fertil Steril. 2008;90(4):1229–31.
131. Agarwal A, Cho CL, Majzoub A, Esteves SC. The Society for Translational Medicine: clinical practice guidelines for sperm DNA fragmentation testing in male infertility. Transl Androl Urol. 2017;6(Suppl 4):S720–33.
132. Agarwal A, Majzoub A, Baskaran S, Panner Selvam MK, Cho CL, Henkel R, et al. Sperm DNA fragmentation: a new guideline for clinicians. World J Mens Health. 2020;38(4):412–71.

Chapter 11
Clinical Dilemmas and Controversies in Varicocele Management

Taha Abo-Almagd Abdel-Meguid Hamoda and Hussein Kandil

Key Points

- Diagnosis of varicocele relies mainly on clinical evaluation except in special clinical contexts where sonographic study is needed.
- The mere presence of varicocele does not indicate a necessity for repair, and an erroneous tendency toward varicocele repair may impose needless overtreatment of a common non-life-threatening condition. On the other hand, avoiding a needed repair may imperil a man's fertility.
- AUA/ASRM and EAU have recommended varicocele repair (VR) in men with clinical varicoceles, infertility, and abnormal sperm parameters.
- Other controversial indications for VR include elevated sperm DNA fragmentation (SDF) prior to ART, nonobstructive azoospermia (NOA) prior to sperm retrieval, and hypogonadism.
- The subinguinal microsurgical varicocelectomy has been identified as the gold standard with the highest efficacy, least morbidity, and lowest recurrence rates, compared to retroperitoneal and non-magnification techniques.
- Studies have demonstrated the superiority of bilateral repair, with better improvement in semen parameters and spontaneous pregnancy rates.
- VR is not recommended for subclinical varicocele.

Controversies in Diagnosis

Varicocele is one of the most common clinical disorders causing male reproductive dysfunction. The prevalence of varicocele, as found in a study on 7035 subjects with median age of 19 years from six European countries, was 15.7% [1]. Yet, its diagnosis remains controversial, with heterogeneous data and no universal diagnostic

T. A.-A. A.-M. Hamoda (✉)
Department of Urology, King Abdulaziz University, Jeddah, Saudi Arabia

Department of Urology, Faculty of Medicine, Minia University, Minia, Egypt

H. Kandil
FAKIH IVF Fertility Center, Abu Dhabi, UAE

A. Agarwal et al. (eds.), *Current and Future Advances in Male Infertility*,
https://doi.org/10.1007/978-3-031-62648-7_11

consensus. In this section, we discuss the diagnosis of varicocele using recommendations from important clinical studies and professional society guidelines.

Clinical Versus Ultrasonographic Diagnosis and Grading

Clinical examination of varicocele requires a comfortable warm environment, to enable scrotal skin relaxation and to facilitate easy venous palpation. The physical examination is routinely performed in both standing and supine positions, with and without Valsalva's maneuver. Clinically palpable varicoceles are graded according to Dubin and Amelar grading system which was developed in the 1970s. Clinical grading of varicocele is described according to the severity as grade I which is palpable only with Valsalva's maneuver, grade II which is palpable without Valsalva, and grade III which is visible without Valsalva [2, 3]. The subclinical entity of varicocele is non-palpable and only diagnosed through imaging studies such as ultrasonography. Despite this standardized approach, there appears to be about 16% inter-observer errors in varicocele evaluation and testicular volume assessment [4]. Nevertheless, clinical examination showed a sensitivity of 71% and specificity of 69% when compared to venography [5].

Ultrasonography is commonly used to diagnose varicoceles, and advanced high-frequency probes have a high sensitivity (97%) and specificity (94%), when compared to venography [4, 5]. As with physical examination, the evaluation in both supine and upright positions, as well as using Valsalva's maneuver, is critical in the assessment of varicocele using ultrasonography [6]. Varicoceles appear as anechoic, dilated, and tortuous vascular channels extending proximal to the upper pole of the testis, although there is no consistent standardization governing the degree of dilation [4]. An additional benefit to using ultrasonography is that testicular parenchymal echotexture is concomitantly assessed, and hence any associated calcifications or presence of atypical lesions can be identified [7].

The indications for using ultrasonography to diagnose varicocele are inconsistent [8], and the examination techniques lack standardization as well [9]. Thus, the examination methods rely on the expertise and protocols adopted by the clinicians [9], and different classifications do exist for ultrasonographic varicocele grading [10–12]. For instance, a grading method relies on the duration of reflux assessed while undergoing Valsalva maneuver in the standing position. Yet, others perform the measurements in the supine position or combine the supine and upright positions. The ESUR-SPIWG Guidelines have shown that using the venous diameter of 3 mm or more being measured in the upright position and under Valsalva maneuver is supported by a level 2 evidence and grade B recommendation [10]. Despite the advanced diagnostic capability of ultrasonography, there seems to be significant variations when it comes to institutional parameters; hence, the role of physical evaluation remains crucial [4].

Guidelines for Varicocele Diagnosis

According to the EAU guidelines, ultrasonography is indicated in the evaluation of varicocele only if physical evaluation is inconclusive or in the context of abnormal semen parameters following varicocele repair suggesting recurrent or persistent varicocele [8]. On the other hand, AUA/ASRM guidelines recommend against the routine use of ultrasonography to detect subclinical varicocele, since repair of subclinical varicocele has not proved beneficial [13]. Additionally, routine abdominal imaging for every isolated mild or moderate right-sided varicocele is not recommended. However, right-sided varicocele may warrant further abdominal imaging when being of new onset or being large and irreducible [13]. In the context of isolated clinical right-sided varicocele, EAU guidelines recommend further evaluation for a possible association with congenital, abdominal, or retroperitoneal pathologies [8]. Nevertheless, a study on 4060 male patients, out of which 8.3% had isolated right-sided varicoceles, has failed to report increased cancer-related diagnoses compared to left-sided varicoceles [14].

In a recent survey by Shah et al., 60 urologists/andrologists from 23 countries have responded to questionnaire aiming to describe the different global practices regarding the management of varicocele. Results of this survey showed that many practitioners rely on ultrasonography to confirm varicocele diagnosis, and surprisingly, 11.2% reported using 2 mm venous diameter as a cutoff value for diagnosing varicocele despite the fact that there is no data supporting this assumption [15]. According to the EAU, a venous diameter above 3 mm in the upright position is the cutoff to diagnose clinically significant varicocele and during Valsalva maneuver in addition to a venous reflux time of more than 2 s [8]. The venous diameter seems to pose a conflicting argument between clinicians; however, in a study on 217 males, it was shown that during rest, a venous diameter of 2.45 mm had a varicocele diagnostic sensitivity and specificity of 84% and 81%, respectively, compared to 84% sensitivity and specificity for a diameter of 2.95 mm during Valsalva [16]. According to the AUA/ASRM guidelines, a venous diameter above 3 mm is considered diagnostic for varicocele under the effect of Valsalva maneuver [13].

In a systematic review released by the ESUR-SPIWG on US utilization for varicocele, the variability in current practices was significant. Additionally, there is absence of a universally standardized system used for varicocele classification (LoR: 3, GoE: C). Furthermore, technically, it is believed that reflux duration assessment is critical in the evaluation (LoR: 3, GoE: C), and an extended abdominal imaging is warranted in cases of acute onset in patients under 9 years (LoE 2, GoR B) [10].

Controversies in Counseling

Evaluating the Real Impact of Varicocele on Male Fertility

Being the most common reversible cause of male infertility, varicocele is present in 15% and 40% of the normal and infertile male populations, respectively [17]. Varicocele is diagnosed in 35% and 81% of males with primary and secondary, respectively [18]. Varicocele-induced male infertility is multifactorial [19] and involves numerous molecular attributes, which result in increased apoptosis [20]. Oxidative stress is believed to be the cornerstone behind varicocele-induced male infertility [21], which is demonstrated by the presence of excessive ROS infiltration, lowered antioxidant capacity, and elevated SDF rates among patients with varicocele and normal semen parameters (DFI = 20.7 ± 4.0) or with abnormal semen parameters (DFI, 35.5 ± 9.0) compared to controls (DFI, 7.1 ± 0.9) [22]. Other changes may include the presence of anti-sperm antibodies [23], testosterone-related abnormalities [24], and abnormal testicular cytokine production [25]. A meta-analysis by Wang et al. noted that in comparison to controls, SDF is reduced by 3.37% following varicocele repair [26].

Clinical Varicocele in the Context of Normal Conventional Semen Parameters

Abnormal semen parameters are present in 25.4% vs. 11.7% in the infertile compared to normal male population [27]. In a study on adolescent population, it was shown that elevation in SDF was confirmed among the varicocele group even though they had normal semen parameters compared to controls [28]. SDF could be used to assess the patients presenting with normal conventional semen parameters and clinical varicocele [29, 30]. Agarwal et al. recommend that SDF be implemented when clinical varicocele is associated with normal conventional semen analysis to help in determining the subset of patients who may benefit from varicocele repair [31].

Role of Varicocele Repair (VR) in the Context of ART

In the context of ART, the role of varicocele repair is currently being studied; however, it is suggested that ART outcome is expected to improve following VR [32]. A study by Daitch et al. demonstrated that compared to those who were left untreated, IUI-related pregnancy rate (11.8% versus 6.3%, $P = 0.04$) and live birth rate (11.8% versus 1.6%, $P = 0.007$) were significantly higher [33]. Furthermore, in patients undergoing ICSI, VR prior to ICSI was associated with increased live birth rates and decline in miscarriage compared to untreated controls as noted by Esteves et al., who analyzed the data obtained from 80 men who had VR and demonstrated that varicocele repair was associated with favorable outcome with evidence of increase in clinical pregnancy rate (60.0% vs. 45.0%, $P = 0.04$) and concomitant increase in live birth rate (46.2% vs. 31.4%, $P = 0.03$), in addition to reduced pregnancy loss (OR: 0.433, 95% CI: 0.22–0.84) [34]. A meta-analysis consisting of 870 ICSI cycles noted similar results confirming the positive impact of VR on pregnancy and live birth rate (OR: 1.59, 95% CI: 1.19–2.12, I2 = 25%; OR: 2.17, 95% CI: 1.55–3.06, I2 = 0%, respectively) [29]. Gokce et al. compared the outcome from 168 patients who had varicocele repair prior to ICSI to 138 untreated patients and noted an increase in pregnancy rate (62.5 vs. 47.1%, $P = 0.001$) and live birth rate (47.6 vs. 29.0%, $P = 0.0002$) in the varicocele-treated arm compared to their untreated counterpart [35].

Varicocele and Hypogonadism

Varicocele has been linked to Leydig cell dysfunction and hence abnormalities in testosterone hormone production [36]. It was shown that hyperthermia induced by varicocele may negatively affect 17,20-lyase enzymes, which are involved in cholesterol biosynthesis with resultant testosterone deficiency [37, 38]. Hsiao et al. demonstrated, in a study on 78 patients, rise in testosterone levels in most subjects ($n = 65$, 83%) following varicocele repair, regardless of the grade with a mean follow-up period of 7 months and mean increase in serum testosterone reaching 109.1 ± 12.8 ng/dL [39]. In a meta-analysis including nine studies, data from a total of 814 post-varicocele repair patients demonstrated an increase in mean serum testosterone by 97.48 ng/dl (95% confidence interval 43.73–151.22, $P = 0.0004$) [37].

Varicocele and NOA

In a systematic review and meta-analysis by Esteves et al., sperm retrieval rate increased following VR in NOA patients compared to those left untreated (OR: 2.65; 95% CI: 1.69–4.14; $P < 0.001$) [40]. In another systematic review on 16 articles, Jensen et al. demonstrated that the average sperm retrieval rate for NOA patients undergoing varicocele reached 27.3% and successful sperm retrieval during micro-TESE following VR reached 48.9% compared to 32.1% among the control group [41]. Elbardisi et al. reported that the presence of sperm in the ejaculate was 26.2% among NOA patients following VR in a follow-up period that reached 6.7 months and that histological subtype was a predictive factor, with hypospermatogenesis being the most favorable among their studied cohort [42].

Varicocele in Adolescence

Dealing with varicocele in the adolescent population is more challenging, knowing that the role of repair lacks some clarity and is still controversial in the prepubertal patients [43]. Varicocele in the adolescent population is commonly discovered incidentally, as it is commonly asymptomatic, yet it is a common cause for testicular hypotrophy [43, 44]. Varicocele in this population could present at various stages of development [45]. Caution is warranted in the context of isolated varicocele on the right side, especially if it is irreducible, which is a condition that raises the suspicion for retroperitoneal mass [46, 47]. When done, semen analysis could be associated with abnormal semen parameters [48]. One of the features associated with varicocele in the adolescent population is testicular growth abnormalities, which is a hallmark for the resulting damage and is noted in 77% of such population [18, 49]. Varicocele repair in a prophylactic fashion is not warranted as it may only be of benefit to 15% of patients, yet it is however advised in patients with testicular size reduction of 2 SD below the designated growth curve or when the difference in size between both sides exceeds 2 ml. Repair is also considered in patients with high-grade varicocele and associated abnormal semen parameters, in those presenting with concomitant pain, and in the presence of bilateral varicocele [50].

Varicocele and Scrotal Pain

Varicocele is commonly asymptomatic, yet approximately 10% of patients may present with variable degrees of scrotal pain [51], which usually presents as a sense of heaviness that increases in intensity following long duration of standing [52]. Pain could result from venous mediated nerve compression, venous congestion, testicular hypoxia, and reflux of adrenal/renal toxic byproducts [19, 53]. Managing chronic orchialgia in the context of varicocele is controversial, as while varicocele repair can be associated with symptomatic improvement in selected patients [53], others may not. Conservative treatment could be initially considered consisting of scrotal elevation, anti-inflammatories (NSAIDs), and reduced physical activity [53]. Surgical treatment is considered after failure of conservative management, consisting of the microsurgical approach, which is the gold standard treatment option [51].

Controversies in Therapy

Although the association between varicocele and male infertility has been almost universally accepted, and the positive impact of varicocele repair on semen quality and human reproductive outcomes has been described in the literature for several decades, many issues related to varicocele treatment are still not well defined. The following section will depict some common varicocele treatment controversies.

Indications for Intervention

Varicocele is a common condition affecting 15% of the general male population [17]; meanwhile, the condition is not life-threatening, and the majority of varicocele men are fertile. On the other hand, conversely, varicocele may jeopardize the fertility potential of a man as evidenced by the strong association between varicocele and male infertility [19] and by reporting varicocele in 35% and 81% of primary and secondary infertility men, respectively [18]. Thus, the mere presence of varicocele does not indicate a necessity for repair, and an erroneous tendency toward varicocele repair may impose needless overtreatment of a common non-life-threatening condition. On the other hand, declining a needed repair may imperil a man's fertility. To further cloud the scene, there is no known effective medical treatment for varicocele, and repair is the only available option when therapy is needed [15]. Given the aforementioned discussion, identifying and selecting the proper patient who needs and may benefit from varicocele repair are still controversial despite many decades of research on varicocelectomies. A well-balanced selection and identifying the proper indications for repair are of utmost importance, although challenging.

The most recent [13] guidelines of the American Urological Association and the American Society for Reproductive Medicine (AUA/ASRM) have recommended VR in men with clinical varicoceles, infertility, and abnormal sperm parameters (but no azoospermia) (moderate recommendation; moderate evidence level). Similarly [54], the European Association of Urology (EAU) guidelines have also recommended VR in men with infertility, clinical varicocele, and abnormal semen parameters (and no other causes of male infertility) (strong recommendation; high evidence level). Nevertheless, the term "abnormal sperm parameters" is not defined in both guidelines.

Other Indications

Several other more controversial indications for VR have emerged during the last few years and are expanding. Notable controversial examples include the need for repair in infertile men having clinical varicocele and one or more of the following:

- Elevated sperm DNA fragmentation (SDF)
- Prior to ART
- Nonobstructive azoospermia (NOA), and prior to sperm retrieval
- Hypogonadism

Elevated SDF

Since varicocele is associated with increased oxidative stress and elevated SDF [55], repair of varicocele may be required to revert this process. Several studies have noted the beneficial effect of VR on SDF, with two recent meta-analyses having, respectively, revealed decreased SDF by 6.14% and 7.23% in men with clinical varicocele [56, 57]. However, in currently existing guidelines, there is no explicit recommendation on the management of couples with clinical varicocele, normal semen parameters, and elevated SDF. Only the EAU has specifically recommended (weak recommendation) varicocele repair in men with elevated SDF and otherwise unexplained infertility or who have failed ART including repeated pregnancy loss (RPL), failed embryogenesis, and failed implantation.

Prior to ART

Repair of clinical varicocele has been reported to improve ART pregnancy rates, probably due to lowering of SDF levels [56, 57]. A meta-analysis was conducted on non-azoospermic infertile men with clinical varicocele who underwent either varicocelectomy prior to ICSI or ICSI without varicocelectomy, to compare their ICSI outcomes [29]. The analysis included 4 studies with a total of 870 ICSI cycles and reported significantly improved clinical pregnancy rates (OR = 1.59) and live birth rates (OR = 2.17) among men who underwent prior repair as compared to those without repair. However, recommending repair prior to ART is a considerable decision since it imposes a 3–6-month delay of ART for an unpredictable benefit [15].

NOA and Prior to Sperm Retrieval

A controversy exists over the role of repair of clinical varicocele in men with NOA, with limited supporting evidence based on observational studies. According to the EAU guidelines [54], repair of clinical varicocele in men with NOA may result in the recovery of ejaculate sperm in 20.8–55% of cases. Nevertheless, if sperm is recovered in the ejaculate, sperm cryopreservation should be considered since recovery could be transient and relapse of azoospermia may ensue [58]. Testicular histopathology was found to be a predictor of ejaculate sperm recovery in NOA after VR, as men having hypospermatogenesis or late maturation arrest have better chances to recover sperm [58].

Additional support for varicocele repair in NOA is derived from studies showing improved sperm retrieval during micro-TESE when a prior varicocele repair has been performed [59, 60]. The EAU guidelines [54] reported improved surgical sperm retrieval rates (OR, 2.65; 95% CI, 1.69–4.14), while a meta-analysis [61] demonstrated higher live birth rates following varicocele repair (OR, 2.208; $P = 0.052$).

Of note, patients with NOA are very heterogeneous with variable testicular sizes, testicular histology, hormonal profiles, varicocele grades, genetic makeup, and association of other underlying etiologies. Hence, the decision to preform repair of varicocele for NOA (usually with large varicoceles, non-atrophied testes, no genetic or known cause for testicular failure) is at the clinician's and patient's discretion after a thorough discussion with the patient or couple [15].

Hypogonadism

Varicocele has been traditionally hypothesized to insult germ and Sertoli cells. In more recent years, the hypothesis has been expanded as a pantesticular insult to involve the Leydig cells as well. Evidence indicates that VR can reverse hypogonadism among infertile men. Post-varicocelectomy improvements in serum testosterone levels inversely correlate to baseline levels, as hypogonadal men demonstrate better improvements than eugonadal men [36, 37, 62]. Notably, most studies investigating the effects of varicocelectomy on hypogonadism have mainly addressed infertile men. Therefore, suggesting varicocelectomy to treat hypogonadism among fertile men is still lacking evidence and not supported by practice guidelines.

Intervention: Which Technique to Select?

Like the controversy on the indications of varicocelectomy, still there is discordance on the techniques of VR. The goal of varicocele treatment is to improve the reproduction potential and alleviate any associated symptoms, with the least morbidity and shortest recovery. The main general technical principle of VR is to occlude the dilated varicose veins, with preservation of the testicular arteries, lymphatics, and vas deferens. However, since the spermatic veins extend from the scrotum up to the retroperitoneum proximally, there is a divergence on the site and technique to occlude the veins, with a myriad of surgical and interventional radiological techniques to repair varicoceles. The surgical techniques vastly dominate the repair procedures and include the subinguinal, inguinal, and retroperitoneal (open or laparoscopic) approaches [63]. The selection of the technique usually depends on the surgeon's expertise, patients' characteristics, and availability of instrumentation and equipment [15].

The subinguinal and inguinal routes are the most popular approaches and generally require some sort of magnification, using surgical magnifying loupes or preferably surgical microscope. The subinguinal approach entails direct access to the spermatic cord distal to the external inguinal ring with no muscle cutting and is, thus, associated with less postoperative pain and faster recovery. The subinguinal approach also facilitates cord delivery in obese patients and in men with previous inguinal surgery. Nevertheless, a subinguinal surgery drawback is being technically challenging, as the proper magnification might require microsurgical expertise. At the subinguinal level, there are numerous veins, and magnification can help identify and ligate all veins and identify and spare the spermatic arteries and lymphatics to avoid recurrence, testicular atrophy, and hydrocele formation.

The inguinal approach requires opening the inguinal canal by incising the external oblique aponeurosis between the external and internal inguinal rings and delivering the spermatic cord at this level. Otherwise, the inguinal approach has similar technicality and outcomes to the subinguinal approach. However, since the inguinal technique involves muscle cutting and closure, it leads to more postoperative pain and more prolonged recovery compared to the subinguinal approach. The inguinal approach is more useful in patients with previous subinguinal surgery and in men with high testicle or short spermatic cord when the distance between external inguinal ring and testis is short.

The traditional open retroperitoneal approach (abdominal; high approach of Palomo) is another muscle-cutting procedure to identify and occlude the spermatic veins proximally at the retroperitoneum near their insertions. The laparoscopic approach was introduced in the early 1990s to replicate the retroperitoneal technique with few minimal incisions to avoid muscle cuttings and to enhance recovery. However, the retroperitoneal approaches to control the veins may overlook several distal collaterals and have several disadvantages and complications including significantly higher recurrence rates and hydrocele formation as compared to microscopic subinguinal surgical treatment [63]. Additionally, the laparoscopic route attains potential complications of significant vascular and gastrointestinal injuries [63] and, although remains popular among pediatric surgeons, is nowadays seldom used in routine varicocele surgeries among urologists and andrologists.

The interventional radiological percutaneous embolization of varicocele was introduced as an alternative to surgical techniques and was claimed to be a less invasive technique of repair with satisfactory outcomes [64]. Generally, via percutaneous angiographic access of the femoral vein, the internal spermatic vein is retrogradely approached and is occluded using a balloon and/or coil. An obvious advantage of the percutaneous approach is the sparing of the testicular artery and lymphatics. Nevertheless, percutaneous embolization harbors several disadvantages and drawbacks. Difficult retrograde access to the spermatic vein can hinder the troublesome procedure. Local complications of femoral vein cannulation may include infection, thrombophlebitis, bleeding, arterial injury, and pseudoaneurysm formation. Proximal coil migration to the renal vein is uncommon but a significant complication. Injection of contrast material may expose the patient to allergic reactions and other contrast problems such as contrast nephropathy. Importantly, fluoroscopy is an integral part of the procedure, thus exposing a mostly subfertile patient to significant radiation and questionable further fertility harm. Further, many patients may sustain post-procedure scrotal "lump" of thrombosed varicose veins, which usually presents as a firm-to-hard indurated irregular scrotal mass above the testis and is associated with a firm indurated thickened cord that may persist for several months, causing significant patients' anxiety (author's observation). Percutaneous embolization should be reserved for men with recurrent or persistent varicoceles after other surgical techniques, and upon referral from urologist or andrologist.

Reference Technique (Subinguinal Microsurgical Varicocelectomy)

Despite necessitating a longer operative time compared to other open non-magnified surgical procedures and laparoscopic technique, the subinguinal microsurgical varicocelectomy has been identified as the reference technique and gold standard to achieve the ultimate goals of repair with the highest efficacy, least morbidity, and lowest recurrence rates, compared to retroperitoneal and non-magnification techniques [65]. A Cochrane meta-analysis of the efficacy and safety of varicocele treatments has shown some evidence that microsurgical procedures, particularly the subinguinal procedure, demonstrate less postoperative complications, rapid recovery, minimal recurrence rates, as well as highest improvements of semen parameters and pregnancy rates, when compared to other surgical and interventional therapies [63].

Subclinical Varicocele: To Treat or Not to Treat?

The management of infertile men with subclinical varicocele represents another dilemma, as there is limited information on long-term outcome of subclinical varicoceles, and its significance remains unclear. A meta-analysis of randomized controlled trials has assessed the impact of varicocele treatment versus no treatment on semen parameters and pregnancy rates in men with subclinical varicocele [66]. Although surgical repair has yielded statistically significant improvements on forward progressive sperm motility (MD 3.94, 95% CI 1.24–6.65), there was no statistically significant difference in pregnancy rate (OR 1.29, 95% CI 0.99–1.67). Nevertheless, the quality of included studies was very low, and thus the evidence is not adequate to provide a definite conclusion [66]. There is currently no consensus on the management of subclinical varicocele with variable practice patterns [15], although the practice guidelines [54, 67] clearly recommend against the interventional treatment.

Bilateral Versus Unilateral VR

In the setting of left clinical varicocele, an associated right subclinical varicocele is a frequent finding among infertile men. In this context, a controversial question arises whether to perform a bilateral or a unilateral repair. However, several original and meta-analysis studies have demonstrated the superiority of bilateral repair, with better improvement in semen parameters and spontaneous pregnancy rates [68–70].

Age of the Couple

The age of both partners is a significant controversial factor when managing an infertile male with varicocele. The AUA/ASRM guidelines [67] indicate that "maternal age is the strongest predictor of fertility outcome." Thus, when the age of the female partner is >35 years, an ART is advisable to avoid the delay associated with varicocelectomy [15].

Similarly, considerable disagreement exists as to whether varicocele repair is effective in older infertile men, possibly due to irreversible varicocele-induced testicular injury with diminished potential recovery. However, Hsiao et al. reported that microsurgical varicocelectomy resulted in significant improvement in sperm parameters and serum testosterone in men of all ages, including the fifth and sixth decades of life [71]. Fırat and Erdemir further evaluated outcomes after VR in 293 couples of different age groups, to report that total motile sperm count has significantly increased in all ages. These findings suggest that age need not be an exclusion criterion and advanced male age is not a deterrent to varicocelectomy, as couples with both partners >35 years old have a reasonable chance of natural pregnancy after varicocelectomy [72].

Role of Medical and AOX-Based Therapy

In infertile men, no medical therapies for varicoceles have been yet proved effective. Although some evidence endorses using dietary supplements and antioxidants to lower the levels of inflammatory markers [73], the effect of antioxidant therapy on fertility is still unknown. A recent meta-analysis suggested that while antioxidants did not significantly improve the pregnancy rates in varicocele men who underwent repair, antioxidants may benefit men with unrepaired varicoceles [74]. However, several methodological concerns regarding the included studies are raised, and, hence, no definitive conclusions about the efficacy of antioxidants in this context can be provided.

Controversies in Posttreatment Evaluation

Role of Ultrasound in Post-VR Evaluation

Doppler scrotal ultrasonography can help confirm the presence of no residual varicocele and preserved integrity of the artery after repair. Also, thickening of the spermatic cord due to thrombosed veins after repair may render clinical examination inconclusive, and, thus, Doppler ultrasonography can detect whether there is significant reflux in the thickened cord. Nevertheless, apart from the required additional cost and time, the test has several disadvantages. Often, the test may detect a varicocele that is not clinically significant and may cause a management dilemma. Additionally, detection of residual "subclinical" varicocele can lead to unjustified patient disappointment, anxiety, and false impression of failed surgery. In a Turkish small study [75] of men after varicocele repair, as high as 60% recurrence rate was reported using Doppler ultrasonography, suggesting that the examination may overestimate the recurrence.

The AUA/ASRM [67] and the EAU [54] guidelines have provided separate recommendations in this regard. While the AUA/ASRM advise against the routine use of scrotal ultrasonography to monitor for recurrent or residual varicocele after repair, the EAU recommends scrotal Doppler ultrasonography in patients demonstrating no improvement in semen parameters after repair. In the huge worldwide survey conducted by the Global Andrology Forum (GAF) to assess the real-world practice [15], there was considerable diversity of 521 practitioners' opinions on follow-up after varicocele repair. While 14.8% request scrotal ultrasonography routinely for all patients, 21.7% never advise for ultrasonography, and the remaining majority ask for ultrasonography conditionally for reasons such as persistence of clinical residual varicocele, no improvement of semen parameters, or unresolved pain.

Optimal Duration to Assess Post-VR Changes in Semen Parameters

Following VR, the expected duration to show maximum semen improvement has clinical implications. Lacking such improvement by that time interval would indicate failure to benefit from VR and the need to proceed with further management to avoid unnecessary delay. Evidence from a few studies [76, 77] suggests that when semen parameter improvement occurs, it will mostly ensue after the first 3 months following repair, which obviously parallels the spermatogenesis cycle. However, patients with severe oligospermia may require up to 6 months for maximal improvement [78]. If by 12 months post-VR no improvement in semen parameters is observed, then it is unlikely to ensue. Contrarily, testing the semen earlier than 3 months after repair may erroneously assess the outcomes. Both AUA/ASRM and

EAU guidelines [54, 67] recommend semen examination within 3–6 months after VR (which corresponds with 1–2 spermatogenic cycles) and every 3 months thereafter for up to 1 year.

Managing Recurrent and Persistent Varicocele

Varicocele recurrence is disturbing to both surgeon and patient. The reported incidence of varicocele recurrence varies widely based on the surgical approach, technique, and duration and method of follow-up [79]. Missing spermatic vein tributaries during repair are the primary source of recurrence, while the role of cremasteric and gubernacular veins is still debated. As discussed in previous sections, microsurgical VR has the lowest recurrence rate since small tributaries can be identified and ligated.

The role of intervention for recurrent varicocele is still undefined, and the clinical guidelines provide no comment on the likelihood of benefit from VR for recurrent varicoceles [54, 67]. However, intervention for recurrent varicocele may be considered but with a cautionary note about chances of semen parameter improvement [15]. To avoid technical difficulties, an alternative approach, another to the previously used one, is advisable. For instance, if the primary surgery was by a retroperitoneal approach, then the redo surgery should be at a subinguinal or inguinal level. If the previous surgery was subinguinal, then a redo intervention by inguinal approach or venographic occlusion could be considered.

Future Perspectives

Semen analysis is pivotal in the evaluation of male infertility, including the varicocele men. Since 1980, the WHO has published several editions of laboratory manuals dedicated to standardizing the methodology of human semen processing. The latest sixth edition was recently published in July 2021 [80]. Certain tests such as SDF have been classified in the "extended examination" section of the sixth edition of the WHO manual. Yet, the WHO manual does not provide reference values for SDF, and further future research is still needed in this area. In the advanced section (research), the WHO manual lists a number of tests to assess seminal oxidative stress. To complete the etiological evaluation of the causes of infertility and varicocele, whole-genome, epigenetic, and proteomic biomarkers are heavily studied, and they are strongly believed to resolve much of the current uncertainty when predicting outcomes of VR. The introduction of artificial intelligence (AI) and robots is also emerging in the management of varicoceles.

Clinical Case Scenario

- A 28-year-old male patient presenting with 2-year history of primary infertility. His wife is otherwise healthy, and his laboratory testing revealed normal endocrine evaluation and semen parameters. His physical evaluation revealed a left-sided palpable grade II varicocele. The patient has been advised by another healthcare provider to pursue ART; however, the couple was reluctant and opted for a second opinion managing their case.

Answer

The presence of clinical varicocele in the context of normal conventional semen is not uncommon with an incidence of 11.7% [81]. This clinical scenario warrants investigating for a possible impact from varicocele despite normal semen parameters, which includes assessing oxidative stress level and sperm DNA integrity [82]. It has been shown that clinical varicocele can be associated with extensive influx of ROS, resulting in significant SDF and decline in sperm-fertilizing capability [83]. With that being said, managing varicocele should be considered as a management option, even though the common practice abiding with the current guidelines does not indicate varicocele repair in the context of normal semen parameters [8]. It was also shown that patients with normal conventional semen analysis can still harbor elevated SDF levels and oxidative stress [84, 85]. Furthermore, seminal ROS was positively correlated between varicocele grades [86]. In 2012, a Cochrane review suggested a role for varicocele repair, which was associated with improved spontaneous pregnancy in couples with unexplained infertility [87].

Clinical Case Scenario 2

- A 33-year-old otherwise healthy gentleman presented with primary infertility for 5 years. He has tried several courses of empirical antioxidants with no success. His clinical examination was unremarkable with normal genitalia. His previous semen analyses have repeatedly demonstrated oligospermia with sperm count ranging between 8 and 13 million/ml. The hormonal profile was normal, but the scrotal ultrasound examination has demonstrated bilateral subclinical varicocele. His wife was 30 years old and has shown unremarkable reproductive evaluation. The couple was anxious, and the husband inquired about the role of VR.

Answer

There is no current consensus on the role of repair of subclinical varicocele. A meta-analysis of randomized controlled trials assessing the impact of varicocele treatment versus no treatment on semen parameters and pregnancy rates in men with subclinical varicocele has shown no statistically significant difference in pregnancy rates [66]. Additionally, the practice guidelines [54, 67] clearly recommend against the interventional treatment for subclinical varicocele. The couple was thus counseled on the role of ART, rather than considering VR, to help solve their infertility problem.

Summary

In conclusion, this chapter has clearly demonstrated the deleterious impact of varicocele on male reproductive function. Moreover, the state of an overwhelming ambiguity, related to the lack of consensus on the diagnosis and management of this disorder, transcended a state of confusion among healthcare providers. It is mandatory that clinicians spend enough time counseling their patients, expounding on the impact of varicocele on the patient's current and future fertility potential. Furthermore, this chapter demonstrates that the clinical controversies and dilemmas are still significantly persisting, despite the advent of the many recent publications and emergence of guidelines that studied and analyzed varicocele management in all its details, from diagnosis to repair.

References

1. Damsgaard J, Joensen UN, Carlsen E, et al. Varicocele is associated with impaired semen quality and reproductive hormone levels: a study of 7035 healthy young men from six European countries. Eur Urol. 2016;70(6):1019–29. https://doi.org/10.1016/j.eururo.2016.06.044.
2. Dubin L, Amelar RD. Varicocele size and results of varicocelectomy in selected subfertile men with varicocele*. Fertil Steril. 1970;21(8):606–9. https://doi.org/10.1016/S0015-0282(16)37684-1.
3. Macey MR, Owen RC, Ross SS, Coward RM. Best practice in the diagnosis and treatment of varicocele in children and adolescents. Ther Adv Urol. 2018;10(9):273–82. https://doi.org/10.1177/1756287218783900.
4. Belay R, Huang G, Shen JC, Ko EK. Diagnosis of clinical and subclinical varicocele: how has it evolved? Asian J Androl. 2016;18(2):182. https://doi.org/10.4103/1008-682X.169991.
5. Trum JW, Gubler FM, Laan R, van der Veen F. The value of palpation, varicoscreen contact thermography and colour Doppler ultrasound in the diagnosis of varicocele. Hum Reprod. 1996;11(6):1232–5. https://doi.org/10.1093/oxfordjournals.humrep.a019362.
6. Kim YS, Kim SK, Cho IC, Min SK. Efficacy of scrotal Doppler ultrasonography with the Valsalva maneuver, standing position, and resting-Valsalva ratio for varicocele diagnosis. Korean J Urol. 2015;56(2):144. https://doi.org/10.4111/kju.2015.56.2.144.

7. Sharlip ID, Jarow JP, Belker AM, et al. Best practice policies for male infertility. Fertil Steril. 2002;77(5):873–82. https://doi.org/10.1016/S0015-0282(02)03105-9.
8. Salonia A, Bettocchi C, Carvalho J, et al. EAU Guidelines on Sexual and Reproductive Health. Edn presented at the EAU Annual Congress Amsterdam 2022. Published online 2022.
9. Lotti F, Maggi M. Ultrasound of the male genital tract in relation to male reproductive health. Hum Reprod Update. 2015;21(1):56–83. https://doi.org/10.1093/humupd/dmu042.
10. Bertolotto M, Freeman S, Richenberg J, et al. Ultrasound evaluation of varicoceles: systematic literature review and rationale of the ESUR-SPIWG Guidelines and Recommendations. J Ultrasound. 2020;23(4):487–507. https://doi.org/10.1007/s40477-020-00509-z.
11. Dhabuwala CB, Kumar AB, Kerkar PD, Bhutawala A, Pierce J. Patterns of Doppler recordings and its relationship to varicocele in infertile men. Int J Androl. 1989;12(6):430–8. https://doi.org/10.1111/j.1365-2605.1989.tb01333.x.
12. Patil V, Shetty SMC, Das SK. Redefining the criteria for grading varicoceles based on reflux times. Ultrasound Q. 2016;32(1):82–5. https://doi.org/10.1097/RUQ.0000000000000168.
13. Schlegel PN, Sigman M, Collura B, et al. Diagnosis and treatment of infertility in men: AUA/ASRM guideline Part I. J Urol. 2021;205(1):36–43. https://doi.org/10.1097/JU.0000000000001521.
14. Elmer DeWitt M, Greene DJ, Gill B, Nyame Y, Haywood S, Sabanegh E. Isolated right varicocele and incidence of associated cancer. Urology. 2018;117:82–5. https://doi.org/10.1016/j.urology.2018.03.047.
15. Shah R, Agarwal A, Kavoussi P, et al. Consensus and diversity in the management of varicocele for male infertility: results of a global practice survey and comparison with guidelines and recommendations. World J Mens Health. 2022;40 https://doi.org/10.5534/wjmh.220048.
16. Pilatz A, Altinkilic B, Köhler E, Marconi M, Weidner W. Color Doppler ultrasound imaging in varicoceles: is the venous diameter sufficient for predicting clinical and subclinical varicocele? World J Urol. 2011;29(5):645–50. https://doi.org/10.1007/s00345-011-0701-4.
17. Kupis Ł, Artur Dobronski P, Radziszewski P. Varicocele as a source of male infertility—current treatment techniques. Cent European J Urol. 2015;68(3) https://doi.org/10.5173/ceju.2015.642.
18. Gorelick JI, Goldstein M. Loss of fertility in men with varicocele. Fertil Steril. 1993;59(3):613–6.
19. Eisenberg M, Lipshultz L. Varicocele-induced infertility: newer insights into its pathophysiology. Indian J Urol. 2011;27(1):58. https://doi.org/10.4103/0970-1591.78428.
20. Hosseini M, Shaygannia E, Rahmani M, et al. Endoplasmic reticulum stress (ER Stress) and unfolded protein response (UPR) occur in a rat varicocele testis model. Oxidative Med Cell Longev. 2020;2020:1–11. https://doi.org/10.1155/2020/5909306.
21. Agarwal A, Sharma RK, Desai NR, Prabakaran S, Tavares A, Sabanegh E. Role of oxidative stress in pathogenesis of varicocele and infertility. Urology. 2009;73(3):461–9. https://doi.org/10.1016/j.urology.2008.07.053.
22. Smith R, Kaune H, Parodi D, et al. Increased sperm DNA damage in patients with varicocele: relationship with seminal oxidative stress. Hum Reprod. 2006;21(4):986–93. https://doi.org/10.1093/humrep/dei429.
23. Tchiokadze S, Galdava G. Humoral immunity status if infertile men antisperm antibodies and various pathologies of reproductive organs. Georgian Med News. 2015;241:58 62.
24. Oh YS, Jo NH, Park JK, Gye MC. Changes in inflammatory cytokines accompany deregulation of claudin-11, resulting in inter-Sertoli tight junctions in varicocele rat testes. J Urol. 2016;196(4):1303–12. https://doi.org/10.1016/j.juro.2016.05.004.
25. Finelli R, Pallotti F, Cargnelutti F, et al. Sperm DNA damage and cytokines in varicocele: a case-control study. Andrologia. 2021;53(5) https://doi.org/10.1111/and.14023.
26. Wang YJ, Zhang RQ, Lin YJ, Zhang RG, Zhang WL. Relationship between varicocele and sperm DNA damage and the effect of varicocele repair: a meta-analysis. Reprod Biomed Online. 2012;25(3):307–14. https://doi.org/10.1016/j.rbmo.2012.05.002.
27. Kruger T. Critical appraisal of conventional semen analysis in the context of varicocele. Asian J Androl. 2016;18(2):202. https://doi.org/10.4103/1008-682X.168691.

28. Bertolla RP, Cedenho AP, Filho PAH, Lima SB, Ortiz V, Srougi M. Sperm nuclear DNA fragmentation in adolescents with varicocele. Fertil Steril. 2006;85(3):625–8. https://doi.org/10.1016/j.fertnstert.2005.08.032.
29. Esteves S, Roque M, Agarwal A. Outcome of assisted reproductive technology in men with treated and untreated varicocele: systematic review and meta-analysis. Asian J Androl. 2016;18(2):254. https://doi.org/10.4103/1008-682X.163269.
30. Kandil H, Shah R. Grades 2/3 varicocele and normal conventional semen analysis. In: Varicocele and male infertility. Springer: Cham; 2019. p. 537–43. https://doi.org/10.1007/978-3-319-79102-9_49.
31. Agarwal A, Majzoub A, Esteves SC, Ko E, Ramasamy R, Zini A. Clinical utility of sperm DNA fragmentation testing: practice recommendations based on clinical scenarios. Transl Androl Urol. 2016;5(6):935–50. https://doi.org/10.21037/tau.2016.10.03.
32. Sönmez MG, Haliloğlu AH. Role of varicocele treatment in assisted reproductive technologies. Arab J Urol. 2018;16(1):188–96. https://doi.org/10.1016/j.aju.2018.01.002.
33. Daitch JA, Bedaiwy MA, Pasqualotto EB, et al. Varicocelectomy improves intrauterine insemination success rates in men with varicocele. J Urol. 2001;165(5):1510–3.
34. Esteves SC, Oliveira F v, Bertolla RP. Clinical outcome of intracytoplasmic sperm injection in infertile men with treated and untreated clinical varicocele. J Urol. 2010;184(4):1442–6. https://doi.org/10.1016/j.juro.2010.06.004.
35. Gokce MI, Gülpınar Ö, Süer E, Mermerkaya M, Aydos K, Yaman Ö. Effect of performing varicocelectomy before intracytoplasmic sperm injection on clinical outcomes in non-azoospermic males. Int Urol Nephrol. 2013;45(2):367–72. https://doi.org/10.1007/s11255-013-0394-2.
36. Çayan S, Akbay E, Saylam B, Kadıoğlu A. Effect of varicocele and its treatment on testosterone in hypogonadal men with varicocele: review of the literature. Balkan Med J. 2020;37(3):121–4. https://doi.org/10.4274/balkanmedj.galenos.2020.2020.1.85.
37. Li F, Yue H, Yamaguchi K, et al. Effect of surgical repair on testosterone production in infertile men with varicocele: a meta-analysis. Int J Urol. 2012;19(2):149–54. https://doi.org/10.1111/j.1442-2042.2011.02890.x.
38. Andò S, Giacchetto C, Colpi G, et al. Physiopathologic aspects of Leydig cell function in varicocele patients. J Androl. 1984;5(3):163–9. https://doi.org/10.1002/j.1939-4640.1984.tb02388.x.
39. Hsiao W, Rosoff JS, Pale JR, Powell JL, Goldstein M. Varicocelectomy is associated with increases in serum testosterone independent of clinical grade. Urology. 2013;81(6):1213–8. https://doi.org/10.1016/j.urology.2013.01.060.
40. Esteves SC, Miyaoka R, Roque M, Agarwal A. Outcome of varicocele repair in men with nonobstructive azoospermia: systematic review and meta-analysis. Asian J Androl. 2016;18(2):246. https://doi.org/10.4103/1008-682X.169562.
41. Jensen S, Ko EY. Varicocele treatment in non-obstructive azoospermia: a systematic review. Arab J Urol. 2021;19(3):221–6. https://doi.org/10.1080/2090598X.2021.1956838.
42. Elbardisi H, el Ansari W, Majzoub A, Arafa M. Does varicocelectomy improve semen in men with azoospermia and clinically palpable varicocele? Andrologia. 2020;52(2):e13486. https://doi.org/10.1111/and.13486.
43. Chung JM, Lee SD. Current issues in adolescent varicocele: pediatric urological perspectives. World J Mens Health. 2018;36(2):123. https://doi.org/10.5534/wjmh.170053.
44. Sayfan J, Siplovich L, Koltun L, Benyamin N. Varicocele treatment in pubertal boys prevents testicular growth arrest. J Urol. 1997;157(4):1456–7.
45. Glassberg KI, Korets R. Update on the management of adolescent varicocele. F1000 Med Rep. 2010;2 https://doi.org/10.3410/M2-25.
46. Ates N, Yüksel M, Yılmaz S, Habibi M, Ipekci T. Retroperitoneal paraganglioma presenting as right-sided varicocele: case report. Ann Saudi Med. 2016;36(2):148–51. https://doi.org/10.5144/0256-4947.2016.21.3.1135.

47. Masson P, Brannigan RE. The varicocele. Urol Clin N Am. 2014;41(1):129–44. https://doi.org/10.1016/j.ucl.2013.08.001.
48. Paduch DA, Niedzielski J. Semen analysis in young men with varicocele. J Urol. 1996:788–90. https://doi.org/10.1097/00005392-199608001-00063. Published online August.
49. Lyon RP, Marshall S, Scott MP. Varicocele in childhood and adolescence: implication in adulthood infertility? Urology. 1982;19(6):641–4. https://doi.org/10.1016/0090-4295(82)90019-X.
50. Paduch DA, Skoog SJ. Current management of adolescent varicocele. Rev Urol. 2001;3(3):120–33.
51. Owen RC, McCormick BJ, Figler BD, Coward RM. A review of varicocele repair for pain. Transl Androl Urol. 2017;6(S1):S20–9. https://doi.org/10.21037/tau.2017.03.36.
52. Lundy SD, Sabanegh ES. Varicocele management for infertility and pain: a systematic review. Arab J Urol. 2018;16(1):157–70. https://doi.org/10.1016/j.aju.2017.11.003.
53. Paick S, Choi WS. Varicocele and testicular pain: a review. World J Mens Health. 2019;37(1):4. https://doi.org/10.5534/wjmh.170010.
54. Minhas S, Bettocchi C, Boeri L, et al. European Association of Urology guidelines on male sexual and reproductive health: 2021 update on male infertility. Eur Urol. 2021;80(5):603–20. https://doi.org/10.1016/j.eururo.2021.08.014.
55. Jeremias JT, Belardin LB, Okada FK, et al. Oxidative origin of sperm DNA fragmentation in the adult varicocele. Int Braz J Urol. 2021;47(2):275–83. https://doi.org/10.1590/S1677-5538.IBJU.2019.0827.
56. Qiu D, Shi Q, Pan L. Efficacy of varicocelectomy for sperm DNA integrity improvement: a meta-analysis. Andrologia. 2021;53(1):e13885. https://doi.org/10.1111/and.13885.
57. Lira Neto FT, Roque M, Esteves SC. Effect of varicocelectomy on sperm deoxyribonucleic acid fragmentation rates in infertile men with clinical varicocele: a systematic review and meta-analysis. Fertil Steril. 2021;116(3):696–712. https://doi.org/10.1016/j.fertnstert.2021.04.003.
58. Abdel-Meguid TA. Predictors of sperm recovery and azoospermia relapse in men with non-obstructive azoospermia after varicocele repair. J Urol. 2012;187(1):222–6. https://doi.org/10.1016/j.juro.2011.09.047.
59. Inci K, Hascicek M, Kara O, Dikmen AV, Gürgan T, Ergen A. Sperm retrieval and intracytoplasmic sperm injection in men with nonobstructive azoospermia, and treated and untreated varicocele. J Urol. 2009;182(4):1500–5. https://doi.org/10.1016/j.juro.2009.06.028.
60. Haydardedeoglu B, Turunc T, Kilicdag EB, Gul U, Bagis T. The effect of prior varicocelectomy in patients with nonobstructive azoospermia on intracytoplasmic sperm injection outcomes: a retrospective pilot study. Urology. 2010;75(1):83–6. https://doi.org/10.1016/j.urology.2009.09.023.
61. Kirby EW, Wiener LE, Rajanahally S, Crowell K, Coward RM. Undergoing varicocele repair before assisted reproduction improves pregnancy rate and live birth rate in azoospermic and oligospermic men with a varicocele: a systematic review and meta-analysis. Fertil Steril. 2016;106(6):1338–43. https://doi.org/10.1016/j.fertnstert.2016.07.1093.
62. Abdel-Meguid TA, Farsi HM, Al-Sayyad A, Tayib A, Mosli HA, Halawani AH. Effects of varicocele on serum testosterone and changes of testosterone after varicocelectomy: a prospective controlled study. Urology. 2014;84(5):1081–7. https://doi.org/10.1016/j.urology.2014.05.029.
63. Persad E, O'Loughlin CA, Kaur S, et al. Surgical or radiological treatment for varicoceles in subfertile men. Cochrane Database Syst Rev. 2021;4(4):CD000479. https://doi.org/10.1002/14651858.CD000479.pub6.
64. Methorst C, Akakpo W, Graziana JP, et al. Recommandations du Comité d'Andrologie et de Médecine Sexuelle de l'AFU concernant la prise en charge de la Varicocèle. Prog Urol. 2021;31(3):119–30. https://doi.org/10.1016/j.purol.2020.11.006.
65. Yuan R, Zhuo H, Cao D, Wei Q. Efficacy and safety of varicocelectomies: a meta-analysis. Syst Biol Reprod Med. 2017;63(2):120–9. https://doi.org/10.1080/19396368.2016.1265161.

66. Kim HJ, Seo JT, Kim KJ, et al. Clinical significance of subclinical varicocelectomy in male infertility: systematic review and meta-analysis. Andrologia. 2016;48(6):654–61. https://doi.org/10.1111/and.12495.
67. Schlegel PN, Sigman M, Collura B, et al. Diagnosis and treatment of infertility in men: AUA/ASRM guideline PART II. J Urol. 2021;205(1):44–51. https://doi.org/10.1097/JU.0000000000001520.
68. Lei SX, Lin WJ, Peng PY, et al. Bilateral is superior to unilateral varicocelectomy in infertile males with left clinical and right subclinical varicocele: a prospective randomized controlled study. Int Urol Nephrol. 2018;50(2):205–10. https://doi.org/10.1007/s11255-017-1749-x.
69. Niu Y, Wang D, Chen Y, et al. Comparison of clinical outcome of bilateral and unilateral varicocelectomy in infertile males with left clinical and right subclinical varicocele: a meta-analysis of randomised controlled trials. Andrologia. 2018;50(9):e13078. https://doi.org/10.1111/and.13078.
70. Ou N, Zhu J, Zhang W, et al. Bilateral is superior to unilateral varicocelectomy in infertile men with bilateral varicocele: systematic review and meta-analysis. Andrologia. 2019;51(11) https://doi.org/10.1111/and.13462.
71. Hsiao W, Rosoff JS, Pale JR, Greenwood EA, Goldstein M. Older age is associated with similar improvements in semen parameters and testosterone after subinguinal microsurgical varicocelectomy. J Urol. 2011;185(2):620–5. https://doi.org/10.1016/j.juro.2010.09.114.
72. Fırat F, Erdemir F. The effect of age on semen quality and spontaneous pregnancy rates in patients who treated with microsurgical inguinal varicocelectomy. Cureus. 2020;12(4):e7744. https://doi.org/10.7759/cureus.7744.
73. Arab D, Doustmohammadi H, Ardestani ZA. Dietary supplements in the management of varicocele-induced infertility: a review of potential mechanisms. Andrologia. 2021;53(1) https://doi.org/10.1111/and.13879.
74. Pyrgidis N, Sokolakis I, Palapelas V, et al. The effect of antioxidant supplementation on operated or non-operated varicocele-associated infertility: a systematic review and meta-analysis. Antioxidants. 2021;10(7):1067. https://doi.org/10.3390/antiox10071067.
75. Akçar Değirmenci N, Turgut M, Ozkan R. Recurrence rate after varicocelectomy in infertile men. Tani Girisim Radyol. 2004;10(2):144–6.
76. Fukuda T, Miyake H, Enatsu N, Matsushita K, Fujisawa M. Assessment of time-dependent changes in semen parameters in infertile men after microsurgical varicocelectomy. Urology. 2015;86(1):48–51. https://doi.org/10.1016/j.urology.2015.04.014.
77. al Bakri A, Lo K, Grober E, Cassidy D, Cardoso JP, Jarvi K. Time for improvement in semen parameters after varicocelectomy. J Urol. 2012;187(1):227–31. https://doi.org/10.1016/j.juro.2011.09.041.
78. Masterson TA, Greer AB, Ramasamy R. Time to improvement in semen parameters after microsurgical varicocelectomy in men with severe oligospermia. Can Urol Assoc J. 2018;13(3) https://doi.org/10.5489/cuaj.5408.
79. Rotker K, Sigman M. Recurrent varicocele. Asian J Androl. 2016;18(2):229. https://doi.org/10.4103/1008-682X.171578.
80. World Health Organization. WHO laboratory manual for the examination and processing of human semen. 6th ed. WHO: Geneva; 2021.
81. World Health Organization. The influence of varicocele on parameters of fertility in a large group of men presenting to infertility clinics. World Health Organization. Fertil Steril. 1992;57(6):1289–93.
82. Takeshima T, Usui K, Mori K, et al. Oxidative stress and male infertility. Reprod Med Biol. 2021;20(1):41–52. https://doi.org/10.1002/rmb2.12353.
83. Shiraishi K, Matsuyama H, Takihara H. Pathophysiology of varicocele in male infertility in the era of assisted reproductive technology. Int J Urol. 2012;19(6):538–50. https://doi.org/10.1111/j.1442-2042.2012.02982.x.

84. Bungum M, Humaidan P, Axmon A, et al. Sperm DNA integrity assessment in prediction of assisted reproduction technology outcome. Hum Reprod. 2007;22(1):174–9. https://doi.org/10.1093/humrep/del326.
85. Kantartzi PD, Goulis CD, Goulis GD, Papadimas I. Male infertility and varicocele: myths and reality. Hippokratia. 2007;11(3):99–104.
86. Cocuzza M, Athayde KS, Alvarenga C, Srougi M, Hallak J. Grade 3 varicocele in fertile men: a different entity. J Urol. 2012;187(4):1363–8. https://doi.org/10.1016/j.juro.2011.11.114.
87. Kroese AC, de Lange NM, Collins J, Evers JL. Surgery or embolization for varicoceles in subfertile men. Cochrane Database Syst Rev. 2012;17 https://doi.org/10.1002/14651858.CD000479.pub5. Published online October.

Part VI
Management of Male Accessory Gland Infection (MAGI)

Chapter 12
Challenges in the Diagnosis and Treatment of Male Accessory Gland Infection (MAGI)

Murat Gül and Gianmaria Salvio

Key Points
- MAGI is a frequent condition in adult males, which has a significant impact on the patient's quality of life.
- The association between MAGI and infertility is frequently observed in clinical practice.
- The outcome of a drug sensitivity test and the clinical characteristics of the patient should guide the selection of a specific antibiotic treatment.

Introduction

The possible role of chronic inflammation of the accessory sex glands on semen abnormalities and, consequently, alterations in spermatozoa functionality has been hypothesized since the 1960s, but initial findings led to conflicting opinions [1]. Only in more recent times, with advances in andrology and the introduction of ultrasound (US) into clinical practice, has the clinical entity defined as male accessory gland inflammation (MAGI), which includes prostatitis, prostate-vesiculitis (PV), and prostate-vesiculo-epididymitis (PVE), been recognized as an important cause of male infertility. In 1993, the World Health Organization (WHO) proposed a series of diagnostic criteria for MAGI, represented by (A) history or signs of genitourinary tract infection (the latter including thickened or tender epididymis, thickened vas deferens, and/or prostate abnormalities found during rectal examination), (B) presence of leukocytes or bacteria in urinary sediment or prostatic fluid after prostate massage, and (C) signs of infection in ejaculate (leukocytospermia, positive culture for pathogenic bacteria, and physicochemical abnormalities of seminal plasma). The diagnosis of MAGI is established if one or more abnormalities of semen analysis (oligo- or astheno- or teratozoospermia) are found in association with one factor A plus one factor B or C, one factor B plus one factor C, or 2 factors

M. Gül (✉)
Department of Urology, Selcuk University School of Medicine, Konya, Turkey

G. Salvio
Department of Endocrinology, Polytechnic University of Marche, Ancona, Italy

A. Agarwal et al. (eds.), *Current and Future Advances in Male Infertility*,
https://doi.org/10.1007/978-3-031-62648-7_12

C [2]. In addition to the classic WHO criteria, US criteria have been recently introduced, and they made the diagnosis of MAGI easier and more accurate (see later). An alternative classification focused on prostatitis has been proposed by the National Institutes of Health (NIH) Chronic Prostatitis Collaborative Research Network, which includes the following categories:

1. Category I: acute bacterial infection of the prostate
2. Category II: chronic bacterial infection of the prostate
3. Category III: chronic nonbacterial prostatitis/chronic pelvic pain syndrome, further divided into inflammatory (IIIA) or noninflammatory (IIIB), depending on the presence or not of leukocytes in the ejaculate
4. Category IV: asymptomatic inflammatory prostatitis, where the only sign is leukocytes in prostate secretion or in prostate tissue [3]

In accordance with both the WHO and NIH definitions, the presence of infection is not strictly necessary for the diagnosis of MAGI, and in the absence of pathogenic bacteria evidenced in seminal culture or prostatic fluid, we speak of abacterial MAGI. In this form, which sometimes follows the successful treatment of a genital infection, inflammation can result in dysfunction of the accessory sex glands, obstruction of the seminal ducts, and dysregulation of spermatogenesis, with consequent adverse effects on male fertility [4].

Since different diagnostic categories of MAGI exist, and the correct application of diagnostic criteria requires both andrological and urological expertise, the impact of MAGI on couple infertility shows a wide variability, ranging from 1.5% to 16% among studies [5].

In order to learn more about this important entity, this chapter provides detailed guidance on the diagnostic pathway to detect MAGI, defines its extent and impact on couple fertility, and discusses current therapeutic indications and future prospects.

Microbiological Investigations in MAGI

There is general agreement that MAGI originates from the spread of an infectious agent from the urethra to the accessory sex glands such as the prostate, seminal vesicles, and epididymis.

According to the WHO definition, the presence of more than 1×10^6 leukocytes/ml is defined as leukocytospermia (or pyospermia), and, together with increased viscosity, they could be associated with infection and poor sperm quality [6]. Although the cutoff of 1×10^6 leukocytes/ml has also been reported in the latest edition of the WHO laboratory manual for the examination and processing of human semen, the clinical significance of leukocytospermia remains controversial. In fact, the presence of leukocytes is not necessarily associated with the presence of active infection, nor does the number of leukocytes reflect their functional status [7]. In addition, a routine assay of peroxidase activity, which is commonly used to identify polymorphonuclear (PMN) leukocytes and distinguish them from multinucleated spermatids, does not detect either PMN leukocytes that have released their granules or other types of leukocytes, including lymphocytes, macrophages, and monocytes, that are all peroxidase-free. Immunochemical staining (CD45) could be useful to identify all classes of leukocytes but is more expensive and time-consuming, and there are currently no evidence-based reference values [6].

Alternatively, the measurement of seminal cytokine and chemokine levels has been proposed as a tool for assessing the inflammatory status of the seminal tract. Cytokines and chemokines are molecules produced by cells of the immune system that play a key role in initiating and maintaining the inflammatory process. For example, semen levels of interleukin (IL)-1 and IL-6 have been reported to be higher in infertile patients, and the latter also negatively correlates with sperm malondialdehyde (MDA) levels, a typical marker of oxidative stress [8]. Among the different molecules proposed over the years by different authors, IL-8 has been recognized by the WHO manual as having the highest accuracy and sensitivity for the diagnosis of chronic urogenital inflammatory diseases, including chronic prostatitis and chronic pelvic syndrome [6]. Indeed, IL-8 levels in the seminal plasma directly correlate with the presence of leukocytospermia, and recent findings support its involvement in inflammation of the prostate, seminal vesicles, and epididymis [9].

According to the 2021 update of the European Association of Urology (EAU) Guidelines on Male Sexual and Reproductive Health, the threshold of 1×10^6 leukocytes/ml should be considered an indicator of inflammation and used to trigger further investigations, including semen culture or polymerase chain reaction (PCR) testing for common urogenital tract pathogens [10].

Sperm culture is a simple and inexpensive test that should be used as a screening for MAGI. The procedure is done by masturbation and requires 3–4 days of sexual abstinence and no prior antibiotic use for at least 1 week. Notably, the patient should be instructed not to contaminate the sample by preceding the collection by accurate hand and external genitalia washing. Urine culture may be an alternate option for patients who refuse to collect semen by masturbation, where the analysis of the first urinary stream may be useful to identify pathogens present in the urethral-prostatic tract, whereas initial and intermediate stream should be used in acute prostatitis [11]. On the other hand, a urine culture test has very low sensitivity for chronic prostatitis (1–10%) [12] and should not be used when this condition is suspected. In such cases, especially when the semen culture provided repeated negative results or when symptoms persist after antibiotic therapy, the Meares-Stamey test could be conducted. It requires three urine samples of 10 ml each, the last one taken after prostate massage. This test is also particularly helpful in discriminating between chronic bacterial prostatitis and complicated lower urinary tract infection (UTI) [11]. Finally, if a sexually transmitted disease is suspected, or if a patient presents signs/symptoms of urethritis, history of phimosis, diabetes mellitus, hypospadias, and persistent UTI, a urethral swab (integrated with a swab from balanopreputial sulcus, if indicated) should be performed [11].

Several microorganisms have been called into question as possible causes of MAGI, although the possibility of specimen contamination must always be considered. For this reason, the involvement of a bacterium should be considered plausible only in the presence of $>10^3$ or $>10^4$ (for pathogenic and nonpathogenic bacteria, respectively) colony-forming unit (CFU) growth in seminal plasma diluted 1:2 with saline solution [8]. Genital ureaplasmas (*Ureaplasma urealyticum, Ureaplasma parvum*) and mycoplasmas (*Mycoplasma hominis, Mycoplasma genitalium*) are frequently found in semen samples of men undergoing evaluation for couple infertility, but a recent meta-analysis confirmed a significant association with male infertility, and a consequent role as etiological agents, only for *U. urealyticum* and *M. hominis* [13]. *Chlamydia trachomatis* is another bacterial species commonly associated with male infertility. According to in vivo and in vitro evidences, the infection of *Chlamydia trachomatis* can affect the canalicular system, causing obstructive azoospermia, or damage spermatogenesis, leading to deterioration of semen quality of varying degrees [14]. Other bacteria for which there is sufficiently strong evidence are *Escherichia coli* and *Staphylococcus aureus*, but several reports on *Enterococcus faecalis, Helicobacter pylori, Streptococcus agalactiae, Gardnerella vaginalis, Anaerococcus, Neisseria gonorrhoeae*, and *Pseudomonas aeruginosa* exist as well [15].

Among other agents, human papillomavirus (HPV) is one of the most common sexually transmitted viruses worldwide. According to the results of a recent meta-analysis, men with HPV infection have a nearly threefold increased risk of being infertile, with HPV DNA prevalence in semen reaching 46.2% and HPV16 being the most common type [16]. In addition, HPV infection is related to a significant decrease in sperm progressive motility and sperm morphology score and leads to an increased risk of miscarriage and lower chances of ongoing patients in men from couple undergoing assisted reproductive technology (ART) [17].

Finally, *Candida albicans* can hamper sperm motility in vitro and reduce the success rate of in vitro fertilization (IVF) [8]. For this reason, its presence should always be ruled out with conventional semen culture, especially in men from couples who are candidates for ART.

Diagnostic Workup of MAGI

According to the WHO definition, clinical criteria suggesting a diagnosis of MAGI are represented by history and physical signs of genitourinary tract infection [2]. Notably, several patients with MAGI may be asymptomatic or falsely asymptomatic. In the latter, minor symptoms may be missed due to a moderate extent of clinical involvement, lack of patient awareness, or inadequacy of investigation modalities. To overcome these limitations, La Vignera proposed an original structured questionnaire (SI-MAGI), with 4 domains (urinary irritative or obstructive symptoms, spontaneous or post-ejaculatory pain or discomfort, sexual dysfunction, quality-of-life impact), with a total of 30 questions scored from 0 to 4 (0 = no symptoms, 4 = worst possible symptoms). Interestingly, the author found a direct correspondence between the severity of symptoms and extension of MAGI (assessed with scrotal and transrectal US), with significantly higher scores in patients with PV and PVE than in those with uncomplicated prostatitis [18]. Additional signs of MAGI include abnormal findings during the examination of the external genitalia (thickening and/or tenderness of the epididymis or vas deferens) or digital rectal exam, and leukocytospermia [2].

The use of US methods in the diagnostic pathway of the infertile male, especially transrectal US, has become popular due to their speed, accuracy, and minimal invasiveness, making them a useful tool in imaging the male genital tract [19]. However, it should be noted that the American Urology Association (AUA) guidelines do not recommend scrotal and transrectal US to be routinely performed in the initial evaluation of infertile men, with the latter being suggested only if ejaculatory duct obstruction is suspected [20]. In selected cases, male genital tract US (MGT-US) not only has the unique capability to discriminate bilateral from unilateral forms of MAGI, but it is also able to define the extent of inflammation and distinguish two variants of MAGI (hypertrophic-congestive or fibro-sclerotic), thus allowing a prognostic judgment to be made and guiding the most appropriate therapeutic choice [5]. The US criteria of MAGI are shown in Table 12.1, whereas the differences between hypertrophic-congestive and fibro-sclerotic MAGI are reported in Table 12.2.

As reported earlier, microbiological investigation is a key element in the diagnostic pathway of MAGI, although it does not always allow the identification of a specific pathogen. According to a practical approach, sperm culture should always be offered in the presence of leukocytospermia and signs of inflammation on objective examination or MGT-US. In addition, molecular detection by PCR on the first-morning molt can be used as a screening method for the detection of pathogenic subspecies of *Chlamydia* and *Mycoplasma* [21]. If the culture test is negative in at least two findings, but a strong suspicion of MAGI persists, the urethral swab (possibly integrated with the swab of the balanopreputial sulcus) or the Meares-Stamey test may be used depending on whether urethritis or bacterial prostatitis is suspected. Identification of a specific agent can then guide antibiotic therapy targeted on the antibiogram, with potential improvement of seminal parameters in MAGI [22].

A diagnostic workup of MAGI is shown in Fig. 12.1. Since the diagnosis can be challenging and cannot be based on the positivity of culture tests alone, it is necessary for the clinician treating male infertility to be familiar with the clinical signs that can be associated with MAGI and to receive adequate training in MGT-US. However, some critical issues persist: the WHO criteria date back to 1993 and did not include the use of the US, while the NIH definition is focused only on prostate inflammation. In addition, the lack of defined guidelines specific to MAGI makes it necessary to raise awareness of this etiologic entity among the major urological and andrological scientific societies.

Table 12.1 Ultrasonographic criteria of MAGI (suspected in the presence of >2 signs) [95]

Prostatitis	• Asymmetry of the gland volume • Areas of low echogenicity • Areas of high echogenicity • Dilatation of periprostatic venous plexus • Single or multiple areas of acinar ectasia • Area/s of moderate increase of vascularity (focal or multiple)
Vesiculitis	• Increased (>14 mm) anteroposterior diameter (mono- or bilateral) • Asymmetry >2.5 mm compared to the contralateral vesicle • Reduced (<7 mm) anteroposterior diameter (mono- or bilateral) • Glandular epithelium thickened and/or calcified • Polycyclic areas separated by hyperechoic septa in one or both vesicles • Fundus/body ratio >2.5 or fundus/body ratio <1 • Anteroposterior diameter unchanged after ejaculation
Epididymitis	• Increase in size of the head (cranio-caudal diameter >12 mm) and/or of the tail (cranio-caudal diameter >6 mm) (mono- or bilateral) • Presence of multiple microcysts in the head and/or tail (mono- or bilateral) • Low echogenicity or high echogenicity (mono- or bilateral) • Large hydrocele mono- or bilateral • Enlargement in superior part of the cephalic tract and superior/inferior part ratio >1 • Unchanged anteroposterior diameter of tail after ejaculation

Table 12.2 Differences between hypertrophic-congestive and fibro-sclerotic variants of MAGI [95]

Hypertrophic-congestive	Prostate: increase of volume, areas of hypoechogenicity, dilatation of periprostatic venous plexus, single or multiple internal similar cystic areas Seminal vesicles: increase of volume, mono- or bilateral increased (>14 mm) anteroposterior diameter, polycyclic areas separated by hyperechoic septa in both vesicles, fundus/body ratio >2.5 Epididymis: increased (>6 mm) tail cranio-caudal diameter, bilateral head and tail areas of hypoechogenicity, unchanged tail anteroposterior diameter just after ejaculation
Fibro-sclerotic	Prostate: areas of hyperechogenicity, asymmetry of the gland volume Seminal vesicles: reduced (<7 mm) mono- or bilateral anteroposterior diameter, thickened and/or calcified glandular epithelium, fundus/body ratio <1 Epididymis: bilateral head and tail areas of hyperechogenicity

MAGI Linked with Sexual Dysfunctions (SDs)

Pathophysiology of SD and MAGI

Dedicated questionnaires identify a high frequency of SD in patients with MAGI. Current scientific evidence demonstrates the connection between prostatitis and SD [23, 24]. It was hypothesized that the etiology could entail multiple linked pathways [25]. These may be precipitated by an initial stimulation, including infection and dysfunctional urine flow under high pressure, trauma, etc., and may result

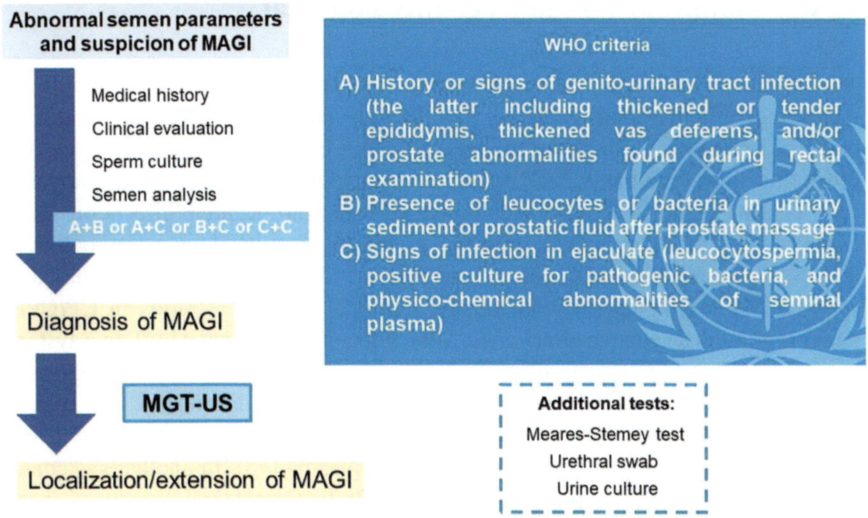

Fig. 12.1 Diagnostic flowchart of MAGI

in a neuropathic state of pelvic nerves and muscles and/or prostatic tissue. Inflammation is initially confined to the prostate and periprostatic region, but due to the persistence of the original component, it might progress and induce a neurogenic reaction, resulting in a state of chronic neuropathy. It has also been discovered that in patients with varicocele, there may be concomitant dilation of the periprostatic venous plexus, which may have implications for persistent deterioration of the seminal viscosity, a parameter associated with chronic inflammation [26]. The neuropathic state is perpetuated by the activation of the pelvic neural circuit. This results in perineal, pelvic, and genital pain; aberrant urine flow parameters; and varying degrees of SD due to the closeness of the structures that regulate the erectile and ejaculatory mechanism [27].

According to some experts, chronic prostatitis and accompanying SDs may have a psychological basis [28–30]. It has been documented that chronic prostatitis reduces sexual activity, that melancholy and psychological disorders are widespread in patients with chronic prostatitis, and that patients with prostatitis tend to be more anxious and fastidious than healthy males [31, 32].

Multiple studies have revealed a higher prevalence of erectile dysfunction (ED) and premature ejaculation (PE) in patients with MAGI than in the general population [33–36]. SDs (ED, PE, and decreased libido) were prevalent in 42% of patients with prostatitis, 52% of patients with prostato-vesiculitis, and 60% of patients with prostato-vesiculo-epididymitis, according to the literature [24, 37–39]. In a recent meta-analysis, the prevalence of SD in men with CP/CPPS was evaluated. It was found that the overall prevalence of SD was 0.62, while the prevalence of ED and PE was 0.29 and 0.40, respectively [36].

MAGI Compromises Male Fertility Potential

According to a meta-analysis, sperm vitality, total sperm motility, and proportion of increasingly motile sperm were all significantly negatively impacted by chronic bacterial prostatitis [40]. Boström and Andersson examined the effects of chronic prostatitis on sperm quality back in 1971 and found no differences in comparison to their control group [41]. Also Weidner et al. found no negative effects on sperm quality [42]. Christiansen et al. produced conflicting results, demonstrating that all three key parameters were drastically decreased [43]. Berg et al. showed increased sperm DNA fragmentation, and mostly abnormal protamine ratios in CP/CPPS patients point to a negative effect on fertility at the molecular level [44]. In a systematic review, reduced semen volume, sperm concentration, and sperm progressive motility all were found to be associated with CP/CPPS. Additionally, they discovered that CP significantly increased the probability of developing ASA and was linked to a lower zinc concentration in seminal plasma [45]. In another systematic review, authors found that patients with CP/CPPS had considerably reduced sperm counts and percentages of morphologically normal sperm and progressively motile sperm [46].

In their studies of patients with acute unilateral epididymitis at 2 weeks, 6 weeks, and 12 weeks ($n = 41$, 32, and 37, respectively), Weidner and colleagues found an improvement in all three fundamental sperm parameters from the first to the last examination. However, 3 months following effective antimicrobial therapy, oligozoospermia occurred in 8/37 patients (22%) and azoospermia in 3/37 patients (8%) [47]. In the follow-up study on epididymitis, semen quality recovered in all published studies within 6 months, but a permanent impairment was found in many patients. Osegbe found the highest rate of poor semen quality, with 10/30 patients (33%) exhibiting oligozoospermia and 8/30 patients (27%) exhibiting azoospermia 2 years later [48].

Although the link between MAGI and infertility is still not clear, obstruction, immunological abnormalities, bacteria, viruses, leukocytes, reactive oxygen species, cytokines, and other substances must be considered as cofactors in the emergence of infertility in patients with MAGI.

Main Mechanisms by which MAGI Impacts Male Infertility

Production of ROS and/or Inflammatory Cytokines

The imbalance between the generation of so-called reactive oxygen species (ROS) and the antioxidant system's protective function, which is responsible for their neutralization and elimination, results in oxidative stress. Due to the high concentration of oxidizable unsaturated fatty acids in spermatozoa's cell membrane and the low concentration of an enzyme that may neutralize ROS in the cytoplasm, spermatozoa are particularly vulnerable to the harmful effects of ROS. The process of lipid oxidation causes structural DNA damage, cell death, a loss of membrane integrity, and an increase in membrane permeability.

Sperm cells are one of the main biological sources of ROS in semen. Male germ cells can create a modest quantity of ROS even in the earliest stages of development [49]. In order to regulate the amount of germ cells by inducing apoptosis or spermatogonia growth, ROS are engaged in the condensation of sperm chromatin [50]. ROS are crucial for capacitation, acrosome reaction, mitochondrial sheath stability, and sperm motility in mature sperm. There are at least two positions and production procedures for them. The first is the membrane NADPH oxidase, an enzyme complex found within the cell membrane. The mitochondria, which leak electrons from the respiratory chain, are the second.

Leukocytes, which create up to 1000 times as much ROS as spermatozoa under normal conditions, are the second source of ROS in the semen [51]. The cellular defense mechanism against infections and inflammation is significantly aided by the increased generation of ROS by leukocytes. In such circumstances, activated leukocytes penetrate the damaged organ and release huge levels of ROS, which causes infectious organisms to be eliminated. Nevertheless, the cells can suffer harm from this oxidant/antioxidant imbalance.

Enzymatic and nonenzymatic components make up the semen's protective antioxidant system. The superoxide dismutase (SOD), catalase, and glutathione peroxidase (GPX) enzyme triad constitutes the primary antioxidant enzyme system in semen. In seminal plasma, SOD exhibits high activity, with 25% of its activity being attributed to SOD-3 and 75% to SOD-1 activity. These two isoenzymes were shown to be most likely originated from the prostate [52]. Nitric oxide-induced sperm cell capacitation is activated by catalase through a complex mechanism including hydrogen peroxide. Many different types of cells have shown their activity in the cytosol, endoplasmic reticulum, mitochondria, and peroxisomes. It was discovered in the sperm cells of rats and humans in semen, as well as in seminal plasma, where the prostate is its source [53]. The GPX enzyme, which is mostly found in the mitochondrial matrix of the cell, is another antioxidant system enzyme in semen. Additionally, GPX has been found in seminal plasma, indicating that it originates from the prostate. The low-molecular-weight, nonenzymatic antioxidants that support enzyme function play a significant part in the antioxidant protection system in addition to the enzymes that neutralize excessive ROS generation [54]. In cases with MAGI, there is increased WBC production of ROS and particular cytokines [interleukin (IL)-1α and IL-8] and their soluble receptor (IL-1 RA) [55].

Impaired Secretory Capacity of the Accessory Glands

Alpha-glucosidase, fructose, prostaglandins, bicarbonate, and citric acid are only a few of the substances secreted by male accessory glands that are essential for sperm physiology. The maturation of sperm is influenced by epididymis secretory factors; the function of the epididymis can be determined by measuring the levels of

L-carnitine, glycerylphosphorylcholine, and alpha-glucosidase in seminal plasma [56]. Fructose, ascorbic acid, ergothioneine, prostaglandins, and bicarbonate are all produced by seminal vesicles. Numerous studies have been conducted on the secretory activity of the prostate gland. Seminal plasma pH, citric acid, gamma-glutamyl transpeptidase, and zinc have been suggested as indicators of its exocrine action [57]. Multiple studies have shown that patients with MAGI had higher pH and decreased a-glucosidase, fructose, zinc, and semen volume levels [58].

Anatomical Obstruction or Sub-obstruction of the Seminal Tract

Infection is typically to blame for unilateral epididymal blockage. On clinical inspection, a swollen epididymis on one side or the lack of one vas can raise suspicions for the diagnosis. In these situations, the ultrasonographic examination might be crucial in making the correct diagnosis [59]. Scrotal ultrasound, in conjunction with color Doppler, offers details on testicle and epididymal morphology, diameters, and condition of the proximal vas deferens. Transrectal ultrasonography (TRUS) can provide crucial information on the size of the prostate gland, the texture of its parenchyma, the existence of tumors or cysts, as well as the condition of the ejaculatory ducts, the distal vas deferens, and the seminal vesicles [37]. According to Garolla et al., patients with oligozoospermia who have normal FSH levels are more likely to have TRUS abnormalities of the prostate, seminal vesicles, or deferent ducts [60]. Obstructive/inflammatory signs at the epididymis, prostate, and seminal vesicles or deferent ducts may be an ultrasound fingerprint of obstructive oligozoospermia and may respond well to the right therapies [61]. In men with obstructive infertility, TRUS has been shown to be a reliable diagnostic method, particularly when paired with seminal analysis [62].

Direct Effect on Spermatozoa

Chlamydia trachomatis

There has been a lot of debate about a potential connection between chlamydia and male infertility because it is linked to infection of the male genital tract. It is extremely debatable whether *C. trachomatis* contributes to male infertility. Serological markers of previous infections and infertility status or semen quality have often been correlated in in vivo studies [63]. Any consequences of prior *C. trachomatis* infections on the male reproductive system are not immediately evident using such methods. The majority of in vitro investigations on *C. trachomatis* infections in males have focused on analyzing the bacterium's direct impact on sperm function in an effort to simulate what may occur should spermatozoa come into contact with the bacteria in the male or female reproductive tracts. The evidence demonstrating that *C. trachomatis* adheres to human spermatozoa is indirect and relies on the visualization of the bacterium next to spermatozoa in fixed preparations using electron microscopy or monoclonal antibodies [64]. At a dosage of 0.1 g/mL, *C. trachomatis* serovar lymphogranuloma venereum lipopolysaccharide was particularly toxic, killing around 65% of spermatozoa after only 60 min [65]. A persistent and/or chronic chlamydial infection in the male genital tract may have a significant impact on fertility and provide some insight into impacts on semen quality [66].

E. coli

E. coli has been demonstrated to quickly and permanently attach to spermatozoa in vitro, leading to agglutination, altered morphology, immobility, and reduced fertilization [67]. Mice can become infertile when exposed to *E. coli* strains that have been found to cause the agglutination of human sperm [68].

Ureaplasma urealyticum

According to in vitro research, the quantity and duration of contact with *U. urealyticum* directly correlated with a considerable loss in sperm membrane integrity [69]. As a result of the *U. urealyticum* infection, oxygen free radicals were released to generate peroxide, which could expose spermatozoa to oxidative assault and cause apoptosis [70].

Staphylococcus aureus

Multiple studies showed a significant decrease in sperm motility caused by *S. aureus* [71, 72]. Majority of the soluble spermicidal components were generated by the bacteria [73].

Mycoplasma genitalium

It has been demonstrated that the spermatozoa's head, midpiece, and tail can be adhered by *Mycoplasma genitalium*. When several *M. genitalium* were adhered, the spermatozoa became immotile [74].

Treatment of MAGI

Importance of the Treatment of MAGI

The goals of treating male genital tract infection/inflammation are to reduce or eliminate pathogenic bacteria from the ejaculate and/or prostate secretions, to normalize inflammatory parameters, to improve aberrant sperm parameters, and ultimately to increase the same. However, accurate patient classification during the diagnostic workup is necessary for effective therapeutic therapy fertility [75]. Distinguishing between ongoing infections and postinfectious or noninfectious inflammatory illness is important. Effective treatment of MAGI is essential not only for the termination of the infective process but also for sexual function and reproduction.

Treatment of Prostatitis

Antimicrobials are advised in both acute bacterial prostatitis (ABP) and chronic bacterial prostatitis (CBP). The best practice is culture-guided antibiotic therapy, although all patients with ABP should also be considered for empirical medicines. High dosages of bactericidal antimicrobials, such as broad-spectrum penicillins, third-generation cephalosporins, or fluoroquinolones, should be administered parenterally while treating ABP [76]. Once infection parameters have returned to normal, oral medication can be substituted and continued for a total of 2–4 weeks. Urethral or suprapubic catheterization can be used to treat urine retention, which affects 10% of men with ABP [77]. Both drainage and conservative treatment options are possible in the case of a prostatic abscess, but aspiration is preferable for abscesses larger than 1 cm [78]. Despite the high rates of uropathogen resistance, fluoroquinolones are advised as first-line medicines in the empirical management of CBP due to their favorable pharmacokinetic characteristics. Doxycycline and azithromycin both work against *C. trachomatis* and genital mycoplasma [79]. Patients with *T. vaginalis* infections should receive treatment with metronidazole [80]. After the initial diagnosis of CBP, antibiotics should be administered for 4–6 weeks. Tetracyclines or macrolides should be administered if intracellular bacteria have been identified [81] (Table 12.3).

Treatment of Vesiculitis

Acute seminal vesiculitis is usually associated with urethritis or epididymitis. The treatment given for these diseases is also sufficient for vesiculitis [82]. Chronic seminal vesiculitis is a rare condition but more challenging to treat. Seminal vesicles have comparatively poor blood circulation, which results in low local drug concentration. Therefore, in case local antibiotherapy application failed, some authors tried seminal vesicle endoscopy to treat refractory seminal vesiculitis with success [83].

Treatment of Epididymitis

Despite rising resistance, fluoroquinolones are still useful for treating enterobacterales orally. Local guidance is advised. Gonorrhea should not be treated with fluoroquinolones. Third-generation cephalosporins administered as a single high parenteral dose are effective against *N. gonorrhoeae*. When administered orally, doxycycline reaches appropriate levels in inflamed male genital tissues and has good clinical and microbiological cure rates in patients with suspected *C. trachomatis* or *M. genitalium* infections [84] (Table 12.4). Epididymitis and orchitis can be treated with antibiotics in addition to analgesics, scrotal elevation, activity restriction, and application of cold packs.

Treatment of Orchitis

Treatment for orchitis is largely supportive and should involve resting in bed and applying hot or cold compresses to relieve pain. The majority of cases of orchitis linked with the mumps recover on their own within 3–10 days, and antibacterial drugs are not recommended for the treatment of viral orchitis. The administration of steroids contributes to the reduction of pain and swelling; however, it does not influence the overall clinical progression of the disease or serve as a preventive measure against future complications [85]. Despite attempting surgical management involving the early incision of the tunica albuginea, the intervention proved unsuccessful in preventing the onset of testicular atrophy [86]. However, the use of interferon-alpha 2B as a systemic treatment demonstrates notable efficacy in preventing

Table 12.3 Antimicrobial therapy for chronic bacterial prostatitis

Antimicrobial	Daily dose	Duration of therapy	Comments
Ciprofloxacin	500 mg b.i.d.	1–3 months	
Levofloxacin	750 mg b.i.d.	1–3 months	
TMP-SMX	400 mg b.i.d.	1–3 months	In fluoroquinolone resistance
Doxycycline	100 mg b.i.d.	10 days	For *C. trachomatis* or mycoplasma infections
Azithromycin	500 mg once daily	3 weeks	For *C. trachomatis* infections
Metronidazole	500 mg t.i.d.	14 days	For *T. vaginalis* infections

Table 12.4 Antimicrobial therapy for epididymitis

Comments	Antimicrobial	Dose	Duration of therapy
Low risk of gonorrhea	Fluoroquinolone active against *C. trachomatis*	Once daily	10–14 days
	Doxycycline + ciprofloxacin	100–500 mg twice daily	10–14 days
Likely gonorrheal	Ceftriaxone + doxycycline	1 g single dose + 100 twice daily	10–14 days
Non-sexually active	Fluoroquinolone	Once or twice daily	10–14 days

sterility and testicular atrophy following bilateral mumps orchitis [87]. Bacterial orchitis requires appropriate antibiotic coverage, as epididymitis [88].

Challenges in the Therapeutic Approaches Towards MAGI

It is often difficult to diagnose MAGI because it is usually asymptomatic and does not meet the diagnostic criteria [27]. Treatment of chronic conditions takes a long time and requires multiple antibiotics. The low eradication rate in patients with chronic bacterial prostatitis is largely due to the inability of antibiotics to penetrate the prostate tissue, altered pharmacokinetics of the inflamed gland, antibiotic resistance of uropathogenic microorganisms, side effects associated with antibiotic treatment, presence of prostate calcification, formation of microcolonies, and biofilm in the ductal and acinar inflamed walls [89].

Insights into the Future Research on MAGI

SWOT (Strengths, Weaknesses, Opportunities and Threats) Analysis of the Current Research on MAGI

Our knowledge of male infertility caused by MAGI has greatly increased over the past 20 years, and inflammation markers and antioxidants have received particular focus [90]. Debatable definitions of prostatitis, particularly chronic prostatitis, have been a topic of discussion for decades because the pathophysiology of the condition is not well understood [91]. According to the most recent NIH consensus categorization, laboratory testing is the primary factor in determining whether a patient has CP/CPPS. However, not all patients with CP/CPPS have laboratory-proven symptoms, and not all laboratory-proven symptoms of CP/CPPS patients are always alleviated by the specific treatment revealed in the laboratory, and vice versa [92]. The classification of prostatitis is intricate, the method of diagnosis is highly debatable, and there are not many trustworthy physical and chemical signs. There is no single accepted standard for clinical diagnosis and assessments of the curative effect, and the cure is typically challenging to evaluate and analyze. Due to the poor efficacy of conventional therapies and recurrence, many patients have turned to alternative therapies.

Prospects for Future Research on MAGI

It is necessary to conduct studies examining the pathogenesis and etiology of MAGI as well as developing innovative treatment methods. There is a need for studies to determine the most appropriate antioxidant treatment and dose [93]. Promising technologies such as nanomaterials could be investigated for chronic diseases [94].

Summary

- MAGI is a prevalent disorder that negatively affects males' sexual function and fertility. MAGI is a hypernym for the clinical conditions of prostatitis, prostate-vesiculitis, prostate-vesiculo-epididymitis, urethritis, and orchitis. The most prevalent infectious agents are *Neisseria gonorrhoeae*, *Chlamydia trachomatis*, and *E. coli* along with enterobacterium and viral infections at a lesser frequency. MAGI is characterized by leukocytospermia, an increased concentration of cytokines, and reactive oxygen species. Treatment of MAGI is usually performed with antibiotics; however, the outcome of a drug sensitivity test and the clinical characteristics of the patient should guide the selection of a specific antibiotic treatment.

References

1. Boström K. Chronic inflammation of human male accessory sex glands and its effect on the morphology of the spermatozoa. Scand J Urol Nephrol. 1971;5(2):133–40.
2. Rowe PJ, Comhaire FH, Hargreave TB, Mellows HJ, World HO. WHO manual for the standardized investigation and diagnosis of the infertile couple/Patrick J. Rowe ... [et al.]. Cambridge, MA: Cambridge University Press; 1993.
3. Nickel JC. Prostatitis: diagnosis and classification. Curr Urol Rep. 2003;4(4):259–60.
4. Grande G, Milardi D, Baroni S, Luca G, Pontecorvi A. Identification of seminal markers of male accessory gland inflammation: from molecules to proteome. Am J Reprod Immunol(New York, NY: 1989). 2018;80(2):e12992.
5. La Vignera S, Vicari E, Condorelli R, D'Agata R, Calogero AE. Hypertrophic-congestive and fibro-sclerotic ultrasound variants of male accessory gland infection have different sperm output. J Endocrinol Investig. 2011;34(10):e330–5.

6. World Health Organization. WHO laboratory manual for the examination and processing of human semen. World Health Organization, 2021.
7. Rusz A, Pilatz A, Wagenlehner F, Linn T, Diemer T, Schuppe HC, et al. Influence of urogenital infections and inflammation on semen quality and male fertility. World J Urol. 2012;30(1):23–30.
8. La Vignera S, Vicari E, Condorelli RA, D'Agata R, Calogero AE. Male accessory gland infection and sperm parameters (review). Int J Androl. 2011;34(5 Pt 2):e330–47.
9. Lotti F, Maggi M. Interleukin 8 and the male genital tract. J Reprod Immunol. 2013;100(1):54–65.
10. Minhas S, Bettocchi C, Boeri L, Capogrosso P, Carvalho J, Cilesiz NC, et al. European association of urology guidelines on male sexual and reproductive health: 2021 update on male infertility. Eur Urol. 2021;80(5):603–20.
11. La Vignera S, Condorelli RA, Vicari E, Salmeri M, Morgia G, Favilla V, et al. Microbiological investigation in male infertility: a practical overview. J Med Microbiol. 2014;63(Pt 1):1–14.
12. Zegarra Montes LZ, Sanchez Mejia AA, Loza Munarriz CA, Gutierrez EC. Semen and urine culture in the diagnosis of chronic bacterial prostatitis. Int Braz J Urol. 2008;34(1):30–7. discussion 38–40.
13. Huang C, Zhu HL, Xu KR, Wang SY, Fan LQ, Zhu WB. Mycoplasma and ureaplasma infection and male infertility: a systematic review and meta-analysis. Andrology. 2015;3(5):809–16.
14. Goulart ACX, Farnezi HCM, França J, Santos AD, Ramos MG, Penna MLF. HIV, HPV and Chlamydia trachomatis: impacts on male fertility. JBRA Assisted Reprod. 2020;24(4):492–7.
15. Farsimadan M, Motamedifar M. Bacterial infection of the male reproductive system causing infertility. J Reprod Immunol. 2020;142:103183.
16. Lyu Z, Feng X, Li N, Zhao W, Wei L, Chen Y, et al. Human papillomavirus in semen and the risk for male infertility: a systematic review and meta-analysis. BMC Infect Dis. 2017;17(1):714.
17. Moreno-Sepulveda J, Rajmil O. Seminal human papillomavirus infection and reproduction: a systematic review and meta-analysis. Andrology. 2021;9(2):478–502.
18. La Vignera S. Male accessory gland infections: anatomical extension of inflammation and severity of symptoms evaluated by an original questionnaire. Andrologia. 2012;44(Suppl 1):739–46.
19. Lotti F, Maggi M. Ultrasound of the male genital tract in relation to male reproductive health. Hum Reprod Update. 2015;21(1):56–83.
20. Schlegel PN, Sigman M, Collura B, et al. Diagnosis and Treatment of Infertility in Men: AUA/ASRM Guideline Part I. J Urol. 2021;205(1):36–43. https://doi.org/10.1097/JU.0000000000001521.
21. López-Corbeto E, González V, Lugo R, Rivaya B, Casabona J, Matas L. Pooling of urine samples for molecular detection of Chlamydia trachomatis, Neisseria gonorrhoeae and Mycoplasma genitalium as a screening strategy among young adults in Catalonia. Enferm Infecc Microbiol Clin (English ed). 2020;38(2):65–71.
22. Krause W. Male accessory gland infection. Andrologia. 2008;40(2):113–6.
23. Evans-Durán B, Tripp DA, Campbell J, Doiron RC, Nickel JC. Chronic prostatitis/chronic pelvic pain syndrome-related pain symptoms and their impact on sexual functioning. Can Urol Assoc J. 2022;16(6):222.
24. La Vignera S, Condorelli R, Vicari E, D'agata R, Calogero A. High frequency of sexual dysfunction in patients with male accessory gland infections. Andrologia. 2012;44:438–46.
25. Nickel JC. Prostatitis and related conditions. In: PC Walsh, AB Retik, ED Vaughan, Wein J, editors. Campbell's urology; Saunders, 2002, p. 603–623.
26. Condorelli RA, Calogero AE, Mongioi L, Vicari E, Russo GI, Lanzafame F, et al. Varicocele and concomitant dilation of the periprostatic venous plexus: effects on semen viscosity sperm parameters. J Endocrinol Investig. 2016;39(5):543–7.
27. Calogero AE, Duca Y, Condorelli RA, La Vignera S. Male accessory gland inflammation, infertility, and sexual dysfunctions: a practical approach to diagnosis and therapy. Andrology. 2017;5(6):1064–72.

28. Keltikangas-Järvinen L, Järvinen H, Lehtonen T. Psychic disturbances in patients with chronic prostatis. Ann Clin Res. 1981;13(1):45–9.
29. Kwon JK, Chang IH. Pain, catastrophizing, and depression in chronic prostatitis/chronic pelvic pain syndrome. Int Neurourol J. 2013;17(2):48–58.
30. Ahn SG, Kim SH, Chung KI, Park KS, Cho SY, Kim HW. Depression, anxiety, stress perception, and coping strategies in Korean military patients with chronic prostatitis/chronic pelvic pain syndrome. Korean J Urol. 2012;53(9):643–8.
31. Mehik A, Hellström P, Sarpola A, Lukkarinen O, Järvelin MR. Fears, sexual disturbances and personality features in men with prostatitis: a population-based cross-sectional study in Finland. BJU Int. 2001;88(1):35–8.
32. Berghuis JP, Heiman JR, Rothman I, Berger RE. Psychological and physical factors involved in chronic idiopathic prostatitis. J Psychosom Res. 1996;41(4):313–25.
33. Screponi E, Carosa E, Di Stasi SM, Pepe M, Carruba G, Jannini EA. Prevalence of chronic prostatitis in men with premature ejaculation. Urology. 2001;58(2):198–202.
34. Liang CZ, Hao ZY, Li HJ, Wang ZP, Xing JP, Hu WL, et al. Prevalence of premature ejaculation and its correlation with chronic prostatitis in Chinese men. Urology. 2010;76(4):962–6.
35. Trinchieri A, Magri V, Cariani L, Bonamore R, Restelli A, Garlaschi MC, et al. Prevalence of sexual dysfunction in men with chronic prostatitis/chronic pelvic pain syndrome. Arch Ital Urol Androl. 2007;79(2):67–70.
36. Li HJ, Kang DY. Prevalence of sexual dysfunction in men with chronic prostatitis/chronic pelvic pain syndrome: a meta-analysis. World J Urol. 2016;34(7):1009–17.
37. La Vignera S, Calogero AE, Condorelli RA, Vicari LO, Catanuso M, D'Agata R, et al. Ultrasonographic evaluation of patients with male accessory gland infection. Andrologia. 2012;44(Suppl 1):26–31.
38. La Vignera S, Condorelli R, D'Agata R, Vicari E, Calogero AE. Semen alterations and flowcitometry evaluation in patients with male accessory gland infections. J Endocrinol Investig. 2012;35(2):219–23.
39. La Vignera S, Condorelli RA, Calogero AE, Bellanca S, Salmeri M, Vicari E. Persistence of ultrasound alterations after antibiotic treatment with levofloxacin in patients with male accessory gland infection. Asian J Androl. 2012;14(6):879–83.
40. Shang Y, Liu C, Cui D, Han G, Yi S. The effect of chronic bacterial prostatitis on semen quality in adult men: a meta-analysis of case-control studies. Sci Rep. 2014;4:7233.
41. Boström K, Andersson L. Creatine phosphokinase relative to acid phosphatase, lactate dehydrogenase, zinc and fructose in human semen with special reference to chronic prostatitis. Scand J Urol Nephrol. 1971;5(2):123–32.
42. Weidner W, Jantos C, Schiefer HG, Haidl G, Friedrich HJ. Semen parameters in men with and without proven chronic prostatitis. Arch Androl. 1991;26(3):173–83.
43. Christiansen E, Tollefsrud A, Purvis K. Sperm quality in men with chronic abacterial prostatovesiculitis verified by rectal ultrasonography. Urology. 1991;38(6):545–9.
44. Berg E, Houska P, Nesheim N, Schuppe HC, Pilatz A, Fijak M, et al. Chronic prostatitis/chronic pelvic pain syndrome leads to impaired semen parameters, increased sperm DNA fragmentation and unfavorable changes of sperm protamine mRNA ratio. Int J Mol Sci. 2021;22(15):7854. https://doi.org/10.3390/ijms22157854.
45. Condorelli RA, Russo GI, Calogero AE, Morgia G, La Vignera S. Chronic prostatitis and its detrimental impact on sperm parameters: a systematic review and meta-analysis. J Endocrinol Investig. 2017;40(11):1209–18.
46. Fu W, Zhou Z, Liu S, Li Q, Yao J, Li W, et al. The effect of chronic prostatitis/chronic pelvic pain syndrome (CP/CPPS) on semen parameters in human males: a systematic review and meta-analysis. PLoS One. 2014;9(4):e94991.
47. Weidner W, Garbe C, Weissbach L, Harbrecht J, Kleinschmidt K, Schiefer HG et al. [Initial therapy of acute unilateral epididymitis using ofloxacin. II. Andrological findings]. Der Urol Ausg A. 1990; 29(5):277–80.

48. Osegbe DN. Testicular function after unilateral bacterial epididymo-orchitis. Eur Urol. 1991;19(3):204–8.
49. Fisher HM, Aitken RJ. Comparative analysis of the ability of precursor germ cells and epididymal spermatozoa to generate reactive oxygen metabolites. J Exp Zool. 1997;277(5):390–400.
50. Aitken RJ. The Amoroso Lecture. The human spermatozoon—a cell in crisis? J Reprod Fertil. 1999;115(1):1–7.
51. Plante M, de Lamirande E, Gagnon C. Reactive oxygen species released by activated neutrophils, but not by deficient spermatozoa, are sufficient to affect normal sperm motility. Fertil Steril. 1994;62(2):387–93.
52. Peeker R, Abramsson L, Marklund SL. Superoxide dismutase isoenzymes in human seminal plasma and spermatozoa. Mol Hum Reprod. 1997;3(12):1061–6.
53. Fraczek M, Kurpisz M. [The redox system in human semen and peroxidative damage of spermatozoa]. Postepy higieny i medycyny doswiadczalnej (Online). 2005;59:523–534.
54. Pasqualotto FF, Sharma RK, Potts JM, Nelson DR, Thomas AJ, Agarwal A. Seminal oxidative stress in patients with chronic prostatitis. Urology. 2000;55(6):881–5.
55. Vicari E. Seminal leukocyte concentration and related specific reactive oxygen species production in patients with male accessory gland infections. Hum Reprod. 1999;14(8):2025–30.
56. Mahmoud AM, Geslevich J, Kint J, Depuydt C, Huysse L, Zalata A, et al. Seminal plasma alpha-glucosidase activity and male infertility. Hum Reprod. 1998;13(3):591–5.
57. Weidner W, Krause W, Ludwig M. Relevance of male accessory gland infection for subsequent fertility with special focus on prostatitis. Hum Reprod Update. 1999;5(5):421–32.
58. Marconi M, Pilatz A, Wagenlehner F, Diemer T, Weidner W. Impact of infection on the secretory capacity of the male accessory glands. Int Braz J Urol. 2009;35(3):299–308. discussion 308-299
59. Armstrong JM, Keihani S, Hotaling JM. Use of ultrasound in male infertility: appropriate selection of men for scrotal ultrasound. Curr Urol Rep. 2018;19(8):58.
60. Garolla A, Grande G, Palego P, Canossa A, Caretta N, Di Nisio A, et al. Central role of ultrasound in the evaluation of testicular function and genital tract obstruction in infertile males. Andrology. 2021;9(5):1490–8.
61. Martin-Du Pan R, Bischof P, de Boccard G, Campana A. Is diclofenac helpful in the diagnosis of partial epididymal obstruction? Hum Reprod. 1997;12(2):396–7.
62. Donkol RH. Imaging in male-factor obstructive infertility. World J Radiol. 2010;2(5):172–9.
63. Krause W, Bohring C. Male infertility and genital chlamydial infection: victim or perpetrator? Andrologia. 2003;35(4):209–16.
64. Wølner-Hanssen P, Mårdh PA. In vitro tests of the adherence of Chlamydia trachomatis to human spermatozoa. Fertil Steril. 1984;42(1):102–7.
65. Hosseinzadeh S, Pacey AA, Eley A. Chlamydia trachomatis-induced death of human spermatozoa is caused primarily by lipopolysaccharide. J Med Microbiol. 2003;52(Pt 3):193–200.
66. Eley A, Pacey AA, Galdiero M, Galdiero M, Galdiero F. Can Chlamydia trachomatis directly damage your sperm? Lancet Infect Dis. 2005;5(1):53–7.
67. Kaur K, Kaur S, Prabha V. Exploitation of sperm-Escherichia coli interaction at the receptor-ligand level for the development of anti-receptor antibodies as the vaginal contraceptive. Andrology. 2015;3(2):385–94.
68. Kaur K, Prabha V. Spermagglutinating Escherichia coli and its role in infertility: in vivo study. Microb Pathog. 2014;69-70:33–8.
69. Núñez-Calonge R, Caballero P, Redondo C, Baquero F, Martínez-Ferrer M, Meseguer MA. Ureaplasma urealyticum reduces motility and induces membrane alterations in human spermatozoa. Hum Reprod. 1998;13(1o):2756–61.
70. Ma XP, Gao XQ. The effect of Ureaplasma urealyticum on the level of P34H expression, the activity of hyaluronidase, and DNA fragmentation in human spermatozoa. Am J Reprod Immunol (New York, NY: 1989). 2017;77(1).
71. Li J, Li B, Song J, Liu H, Bi W, Dong G, et al. Characteristic and mechanism of immobilization effect of Staphylococcus aureus on human spermatozoa. Microb Pathog. 2018;119:28–34.

72. Liu JH, Li HY, Cao ZG, Duan YF, Li Y, Ye ZQ. Influence of several uropathogenic microorganisms on human sperm motility parameters in vitro. Asian J Androl. 2002;4(3):179–82.
73. Paulson JD, Polakoski KL. Isolation of a spermatozoal immobilization factor from Escherichia coli filtrates. Fertil Steril. 1977;28(2):182–5.
74. Svenstrup HF, Fedder J, Abraham-Peskir J, Birkelund S, Christiansen G. Mycoplasma genitalium attaches to human spermatozoa. Hum Reprod. 2003;18(10):2103–9.
75. Haidl G. Advances in the management of male infertility. F1000 Med Rep. 2009;1.
76. Wagenlehner FM, Pilatz A, Bschleipfer T, Diemer T, Linn T, Meinhardt A, et al. Bacterial prostatitis. World J Urol. 2013;31(4):711–6.
77. Hua LX, Zhang JX, Wu HF, Zhang W, Qian LX, Xia GW et al. [The diagnosis and treatment of acute prostatitis: report of 35 cases]. Zhonghua Nan Ke Xue. 2005;11(12):897–9.
78. Chou YH, Tiu CM, Liu JY, Chen JD, Chiou HJ, Chiou SY, et al. Prostatic abscess: transrectal color Doppler ultrasonic diagnosis and minimally invasive therapeutic management. Ultrasound Med Biol. 2004;30(6):719–24.
79. Skerk V, Schönwald S, Krhen I, Banaszak A, Begovac J, Strugar J, et al. Comparative analysis of azithromycin and ciprofloxacin in the treatment of chronic prostatitis caused by Chlamydia trachomatis. Int J Antimicrob Agents. 2003;21(5):457–62.
80. Vickovic N, Skerk V, Granic J, Vargovic M, Pasini M, Turcic P, et al. Metronidazole 1.5 gram dose for 7 or 14 days in the treatment of patients with chronic prostatitis caused by Trichomonas vaginalis: a randomized study. J Chemother (Florence, Italy). 2010;22(5):364–5.
81. Perletti G, Marras E, Wagenlehner FM, Magri V. Antimicrobial therapy for chronic bacterial prostatitis. Cochrane Database Syst Rev. 2013;(8):Cd009071.
82. Furuya R, Takahashi S, Furuya S, Saitoh N, Ogura H, Kurimura Y, et al. Is urethritis accompanied by seminal vesiculitis? Int J Urol. 2009;16(7):628–31.
83. Xu B, Li P, Niu X, Zhang X, Wang Z, Qin C, et al. A new method of chronic and recurrent seminal vesiculitis treatment. J Endourol. 2011;25(11):1815–8.
84. Street E, Joyce A, Wilson J. BASHH UK guideline for the management of epididymo-orchitis, 2010. Int J STD AIDS. 2011;22(7):361–5.
85. Smith IM, Bishir JW. Treatment of mumps orchitis with ACTH and cortisone. N Engl J Med. 1958;258(3):120–4.
86. Nixon N, Lewis DB. Mumps orchitis; surgical treatment. J Urol. 1946;56(5):554–60.
87. Erpenbach KH. Systemic treatment with interferon-alpha 2B: an effective method to prevent sterility after bilateral mumps orchitis. J Urol. 1991;146(1):54–6.
88. Trojian TH, Lishnak TS, Heiman D. Epididymitis and orchitis: an overview. Am Fam Physician. 2009;79(7):583–7.
89. Letkiewicz S, Międzybrodzki R, Kłak M, Jończyk E, Weber-Dąbrowska B, Górski A. The perspectives of the application of phage therapy in chronic bacterial prostatitis. FEMS Immunol Med Microbiol. 2010;60(2):99–112.
90. Chen Q, Feng J, Liu Z, An D, Li Y, Zhou S, et al. Research trends of prostatitis over past 20 years: a bibliometric analysis. Andrologia. 2021;53(10):e14206.
91. Khan FU, Ihsan AU, Khan HU, Jana R, Wazir J, Khongorzul P, et al. Comprehensive overview of prostatitis. Biomed Pharmacother. 2017;94:1064–76.
92. Polackwich AS, Shoskes DA. Chronic prostatitis/chronic pelvic pain syndrome: a review of evaluation and therapy. Prostate Cancer Prostatic Dis. 2016;19(2):132–8.
93. Dutta S, Sengupta P, Roychoudhury S, Chakravarthi S, Wang CW, Slama P. Antioxidant paradox in male infertility: 'a blind eye' on inflammation. Antioxidants (Basel, Switzerland). 2022;11(1).
94. Liu CP, Chen ZD, Ye ZY, He DY, Dang Y, Li ZW, et al. Therapeutic applications of functional nanomaterials for prostatitis. Front Pharmacol. 2021;12:685465.
95. La Vignera S, Crafa A, Condorelli RA, Barbagallo F, Mongioì LM, Cannarella R, et al. Ultrasound evaluation of patients with male accessory gland inflammation: a pictorial review. Andrology. 2021;9(5):1298–305.

Part VII
Sexual Dysfunction in Male Infertility

Chapter 13
Epidemiologic Features and Management of Sexual Dysfunctions in Infertile Men

Eric Huyghe and Peter Ka-Fung Chiu

Key Points
1. Male sexual dysfunction can be associated with male infertility.
2. Erectile dysfunction, ejaculatory dysfunction, and decreased libido are common sexual dysfunctions in infertile men, and they should be treated before assisted reproductive techniques.
3. Multidisciplinary management including a urologist and a specialist in sexual medicine is preferred for infertile men with sexual dysfunction.

Introduction

Currently, in many cultures, fatherhood (as well as motherhood) remains a model of "normality" and self-fulfillment. Sexuality and infertility are linked for several reasons: firstly, sexuality is a fundamental part of the life of the individual and the couple and is particularly sensitive to the crisis of infertility. Secondly, sexual dysfunctions may precede infertility and worsen during the course of management or sometimes even be the cause of infertility. Finally, sexual dysfunctions may be secondary to infertility and its management.

Infertility is a burden for couples who want to have a child that interferes with their sexual life. In this chapter, we will first present the various sexual dysfunctions and anomalies in male and their treatments. In the second part, we will briefly address sexual disorders commonly faced by infertile couples [1].

E. Huyghe
Department of Urology, Toulouse University Hospital, Toulouse, France

P. K.-F. Chiu (✉)
SH Ho Urology Centre, Department of Surgery, The Chinese University of Hong Kong, Hong Kong, China
e-mail: peterchiu@surgery.cuhk.edu.hk

A. Agarwal et al. (eds.), *Current and Future Advances in Male Infertility*,
https://doi.org/10.1007/978-3-031-62648-7_13

Sexual Problems Causing Infertility

Male Problems

Male sexual dysfunction is the cause of infertility in only about 5% of cases [2], but infertility and its management can be associated with the development of male sexual dysfunction.

Congenital Malformations

Micropenis is defined as a stretched penile length below the value corresponding to—2.5 standard deviation of the mean for the age [3]. In adults, a value of 7–7.5 cm on erection corresponds to a micropenis, and this condition may affect the man's ability to penetrate and inseminate. Congenital curvature, due to hypoplasia of one of the two corpora cavernosa or a ventral chord, may make penetration impossible. A recent electronic survey in adults with congenital curvature showed that participants with uncorrected curvature noted more difficulty with intercourse than others because of curvature (4.5 vs. 4.9, $P < 0.001$) [4].

Severe hypospadias (penoscrotal) can compromise semen deposition and procreation. Operated hypospadias with diverticula or urethroplasty-related strictures may also be a cause of ejaculatory dysfunction. Epispadias and complex forms associated with bladder exstrophy are also at risk of infertility. The wish to have their own children is among the main concerns for these patients [5].

Acquired Morphological Anomalies

Curvatures of the erect penis in Peyronie's disease and sequelae of penile trauma can affect a couple's fertility by compromising intromission and deposition of semen.

Erectile Dysfunction

The prevalence of erectile dysfunction (ED) is twice as high in the infertile male population (15–22%) compared to men of the same age category (7–9%) [6]. Severe ED can be a cause of male infertility but is rare in young men and should be managed comprehensively as it may be a sign of paternity denial or severe psychological disorders. Among infertile men, 15–20% show signs of moderate or severe depression [7] and even if infertile men did not report more psychological stress symptoms, they experience more frequent stressful life events than fertile men [8].

The permanence of ED, defined by persistence of the disorder regardless of circumstances and partners, is a sign of severity. In this context, psychogenic factors are to be sought as well as organic factors:

- Individual factors: neurosis, performance anxiety, ignorance of sexuality, depressive syndrome, personality factors, gender identity factors, phobias, and fears. It is also important to do a workup for organic causes of ED including undiagnosed diabetes mellitus, hypertension, hyperlipidemia, and cardiovascular diseases [9].
- Relational factors: conflict between partners, attitude resignation and guilt of one of the partners, aggressive and demanding attitude(s), extramarital relationship(s), and breakup.
- Cultural and social factors: situation(s) or condition(s) of life making the expression of sexuality difficult or fatherhood generating anxiety (unemployment, risk of dishonor, assimilation of fertility with manhood, age difference).

Treatment involves a multipronged approach. Raising awareness of the importance of healthy living, stopping smoking and other addictive substances, and combating sedentary lifestyles are all part of the first level of care and should be advised in all patients with ED [10].

The physician must assess the patient's real goals and take into account the couple as a whole. It is essential to explain the physiology of erection and the mechanism by which performance anxiety can disrupt the erection. The aim is to help the patient understand how to break out of the vicious circle created by low self-esteem and anticipatory stress.

Pharmacologically, there is now a wide range of erectile dysfunction treatments. Selective phosphodiesterase 5 inhibitors (PDE5i) are the first line of treatment [11–13]. In many countries, four molecules are available—sildenafil, tadalafil, vardenafil, and avanafil. Tadalafil differs from the other three molecules in that it has a longer half-life of around 16 h (compared with 3–5 h in the other three drugs), which allows it to be used as a daily treatment [14]. Avanafil has a higher selectivity for PDE5i and less cross-reactivity with other PDE isoenzymes and therefore should result in less side effects like headache, flushing, abnormal vision, and back pain [15]. lodenafil, udenafil, and mirodenafil are the other non-Food and Drug Administration-approved, commercially available drugs [16].

The patient (and possibly his or her partner) should be involved in the choice of treatment as much as possible. It is therefore essential to provide them with detailed information about the methods of taking the treatment, the expected benefits, the possible risks, and the cost of the treatment. Whatever the molecule, efficacy rates are in the order of 65–85%, and the causes of failure are not necessarily organic and may be purely psychogenic (lack of sympathetic inhibition, insufficient excitation). A frequent cause of failure of oral treatment is the absence of explanations at prescription. It is very important to point out that they require sexual stimulation and that the effect may be delayed. There may be improvement over the course of treatment, which is why a minimum of 4–6 attempts is recommended.

Follow-up is essential: The physician should systematically offer the patient a follow-up consultation after 1–2 months to assess his response to the treatment and to ensure that the patient understands how to use the treatment, that it is effective, that there are no side effects, and that he and his partner are satisfied [13].

In case of dissatisfaction or failure of an oral treatment, it is recommended:

- To re-explain the prescription, the objectives, and the mechanism of action of the treatment
- To consider therapeutic adaptations
- To take up the history of the ED and the psychological and relational context
- To look for factors that are not known or that have appeared since the first consultation

If reassessment reveals complex factors (conjugopathy, desire disorder, sexual disharmony, relationship problems), joint management with a sex therapist should be proposed.

Intra-cavernosal injections or intraurethral pellets are second-line treatments that can be prescribed in patients refractory to PDE5i or with an organic component of ED. Vacuum erection devices used alone or in combination with PDE5i have been shown to enable erection in more than 90% men with ED [17]. However, the penile compression ring used with vacuum devices may impede the flow of semen at ejaculation. Low-intensity extracorporeal shockwave therapy (ESWT) used with or without PDE5i was shown in a meta-analysis to improve IIEF-EF score by 2.5 [18]. Penile implants are very rarely necessary except in refractory ED [11].

Ejaculation Disorders

Premature Ejaculation

Premature ejaculation (PE) refers to the triad of (i) a short delay in the onset of ejaculation (that always or nearly always occurs within 1 min of vaginal penetration); (ii) the inability to delay the onset of ejaculation in all or nearly all vaginal penetrations; and (iii) the personal negative consequences (concern and suffering) associated with PE. The most commonly used definitions are those of the International Society of Sexual Medicine (ISSM) [19], the Diagnostic and Statistical Manual of Mental Disorders, 5th revision (DSM-5 [20]), and the 11th revision of the International Classification of Diseases for Mortality and Morbidity Statistics (ICD-11) [21]. They recognize that PE is a multifaceted sexual dysfunction, which may be present from the beginning of sexual life (permanent, primary) or after a period of satisfactory ejaculatory control (acquired). All of the above definitions are limited to intravaginal sex [22]. "Lifelong PE" is characterized by ejaculation that occurs within 1 min of vaginal penetration [23]. In patients with "acquired PE," this latency time may be up to 3 min or less [23].

More recently, the Italian Society of Andrology and Sexual Medicine (SIAMS) has proposed a definition for daily practice that is applicable to other sexual stimuli than intravaginal intercourse, such as masturbation, oral or anal intercourse, as well as nonheterosexual settings [24].

Premature ejaculation does not interfere with fertilization if there is regular penetration and intravaginal ejaculation. However, permanent anteportal ejaculation (ejaculation before intromission) can be a cause of male infertility. While premature ejaculation does not seem to be associated with an increase in overall sexual dysfunction in partners as measured by the Female Sexual Function Index (FSFI) score [25], a correlation between premature ejaculation and female vaginal penetration difficulties has been observed [26]. Moreover, premature ejaculation may impair the quality of the relationship between the two partners and be a sign of suboptimal sexual communication in infertile couples.

Organic causes of PE have been identified as penile hypersensitivity and 5-hydroxytryptamine (5-HT) receptor hypersensitivity; however, psychogenic influences such as anxiety, depression, and stress may further exacerbate PE. Short-acting selective serotonin reuptake inhibitors (SSRIs), like dapoxetine, have been successful in treating PE by activating the 5HT2C receptor and, therefore, readjusting the ejaculatory threshold set point [19]. A meta-analysis on five RCTs on dapoxetine showed the increase in intravaginal ejaculatory latency time (IELT) from about 1 to 3 min (2.5–3.0-fold) vs. 2 min for the placebo [27]. Additionally, several lidocaine-based topical agents are available that aim to treat penile hypersensitivity [28]. It is also important to emphasize the role of sexual therapy, employing cognitive and behavioral techniques, with combination therapy being increasingly considered as the optimal treatment. Involving the partner in the treatment process and encouraging open communication about sexuality are important therapeutic levers.

Anejaculation and Total Retrograde Ejaculation

Psychological anejaculation can be associated with the scheduling of intercourse at the time of ovulation or during the collection of sperm for assisted reproductive technique (ART). In more severe cases, the anejaculation may be directly related to the "child project," either as a refusal of parenthood sometimes justified by a precarious psychological, emotional, social, or financial situation or secondary to the psychological shock linked to the discovery of a male cause of infertility. In some cases, a link with a strict upbringing inhibiting the expression of sexuality has been described. A feeling of fear and/or disgust associated with the act of ejaculation, a rigid personality that tends to rationalize and intellectualize emotions, a feeling of being forbidden to take pleasure, and unacknowledged fantasies that are anxiety-provoking are all possible causes that should be assessed.

Aspermia is the absence of an ejaculation with an orgasm. This may be due to the lack of seminal emission or due to retrograde ejaculation. In both circumstances, the men will have a "dry orgasm" [29]. Retroperitoneal lymph node dissection for testicular cancer is at risk of ejaculatory dysfunction, notably emission failure, due to damage to the sympathetic chains, postganglionic sympathetic nerve fibers, or hypogastric plexus. For this reason, it is important to counsel these men about sperm banking before the surgery.

Retrograde ejaculation can be secondary to medications inhibiting bladder neck closure (i.e., alpha blockers) or due to surgical procedures on the prostate and/or bladder neck, most commonly after endoscopic benign prostatic hyperplasia (BPH) surgery like transurethral resection of prostate (TURP). Other etiologies include various neuropathies affecting bladder neck closure, which can be secondary to diabetes mellitus, spinal cord injury, neurologic disorders, or retroperitoneal lymph node dissection [30]. Antegrade ejaculation may be restored by stopping alpha blocker or improving the control of diabetes. Several drugs (alpha agonists and tricyclic antidepressants such as imipramine) have been tested in this indication with conflicting results [31, 32]. Otherwise, in men with retrograde ejaculation, sperm can be harvested from the urine and used for either intrauterine insemination (IUI) or invitro fertilization (IVF). Conventional protocols involve alkalizing urine for a period of 24 h, followed by a post-orgasm urinalysis. This is essential for ensuring sperm viability so that it can be used effectively for IUI or IVF, depending on the amount and quality of sperm harvested [33]. Endovesical instillation of sterile spermatozoa culture medium before ejaculation may improve spermatozoa quality in patients with retrograde ejaculation [34].

Men with spinal cord injuries may present with aspermia secondary to either the absence of seminal emission or retrograde ejaculation. Many of these men also have anorgasmia, which is the inability to achieve an orgasm. There has been encouraging success with the use of penile vibratory stimulation to enable these patients to reach climax and produce an ejaculate. This is a noninvasive method to help men reach an orgasm and provide sperm for either IUI or IVF. If there is no ejaculate, then the post-orgasm urine can be analyzed to diagnose retrograde ejaculation [35]. If this is ineffective and an ejaculate is desired for fertility purposes, electroejaculation or testicular sperm extraction can be used [36].

Partial retrograde ejaculation is a relatively unknown nosological condition which may reduce the number of fertile spermatozoa in the semen. It may be suspected in cases of hypospermia (decreased ejaculate volume below 1.5 mL). The diagnosis is made by identifying sperm in the urine after orgasm.

Men with ejaculatory duct obstruction may also have absent or significantly reduced seminal emission; these patients may benefit from a transurethral resection or laser incision of the ejaculatory ducts to relieve the obstruction. Additional etiologies for lack of seminal emission can include spinal cord injury, radical prostatectomy, pelvic trauma, diabetes mellitus, multiple sclerosis, and Parkinson's disease. Additionally, patients with ED or ejaculatory dysfunction may want information about sperm banking prior to treatment in the event they cannot produce a semen sample on the day of oocyte retrieval.

Decreased Libido

Men presenting with infertility have concomitant symptomatic hypogonadism (testosterone deficiency) in around 20% of cases [37]. Clinically, testosterone deficiency can be manifested by different symptoms of varying importance and specificity depending on the individual and the extent of the hormonal deficiency. The picture is often dominated by sexual symptoms [38–40], and sexual dysfunction is often the main symptom leading to the diagnosis of testosterone deficiency because testosterone is the main driver of male sexual arousal (stimulating fantasy production, desire, erection, pleasure, and orgasm) [41]. The most suggestive symptoms are decreased sexual desire and loss of early-morning erection. The most suggestive nonsexual symptoms are fatigue and loss of muscle strength. An increase in the body mass index (BMI) is often found. Psychologically, there may be a depressed mood, anxiety, irritability, or simply a decrease in the feeling of well-being. All these symptoms are not necessarily present, and their intensity varies according to the individual.

Correction of testosterone deficiency improves clinical symptoms gradually: In the first 3 months, there is an improvement in sexual desire and general condition. From 3 months onwards, there is an effect on mood, while the effect on fat mass and erectile function is established around 6 months. Bone mineral density is improved from 9 months [42, 43]. Men with complaints related specifically to diminished libido in the setting of hypogonadism may benefit greatly from hormonal therapy [44].

However, in men seeking fertility, exogenous testosterone replacement therapy should be avoided at all costs due to the deleterious effects on spermatogenesis. Exogenous testosterone replacement therapy causes iatrogenic suppression of pituitary gonadotropin secretion, which results in decrease in intratesticular testosterone, and decreased spermatogenesis, often to the point of azoospermia [45]. In young men desiring to father children, hypogonadism can be treated by the use of aromatase inhibitors and "antiestrogens" which will increase serum testosterone level together with intratesticular testosterone levels.

Aromatase inhibitors block the enzyme aromatase, which converts testosterone to estradiol in peripheral tissues [46]. Antiestrogens, also known as selective estrogen receptor modulators (SERMs), such as clomiphene citrate and tamoxifen, inhibit estrogen receptors in the pituitary gland, thereby promoting the secretion of LH and FSH, which will improve testicular function, testosterone production, and spermatogenesis.

Clomiphene citrate may correct sexual dysfunction up to 75% of cases, according to a series of 175 hypogonadal patients [47]. A recent review of literature about clomiphene citrate for the treatment of hypogonadism concluded that consistent literature shows that clomiphene reduces symptoms in hypogonadal men, notably erectile dysfunction and bone mineral density, as well as a reduction in body mass index [48]. Clomiphene is generally considered to be safe and well tolerated despite reports of headache, dizziness, gynecomastia, and exacerbation of psychiatric illnesses. Another possibility to stimulate spermatogenesis together with testosterone secretion is a combined treatment with FSH and hCG. According to EAU guidelines, in order to achieve normal testosterone levels in the blood, a dose of 1500–5000 IU hCG is administered intramuscularly or subcutaneously twice a week, together with an FSH regimen of 150 IU administered intramuscularly or subcutaneously three times a week [49].

The Couple

Sexual Factors in Infertility

Low Sexual Activity

Couples separated for professional reasons may reduce their fertility as they have little sexual intercourse during the fertile period. The frequency of intercourse is a factor in infertility, which may be expressed if there are other infertility cofactors [50]. Other situations may be responsible for a delay or even a temporary cessation of sexual intercourse: bereavement, illness, major surgery, cancer, disabling diseases, onset of disability, etc.

At the Beginning of the Infertility Consultation Process

The impossibility of having a child inevitably causes a narcissistic wound in couples who wish to have children. When a couple comes to the doctor for infertility, they have already been through a long period of waiting, worrying, hoping, and disappointing.

This expectation is all the more difficult to meet, as we live in an era of instant gratification, in a world that advocates the rapid satisfaction of desires and where technical means take center stage. Many couples imagine that they can control conception in the same way that they have been able to control contraception.

During the period when the couple is trying to achieve a pregnancy naturally, but cannot, sex may become less spontaneous. Sexual intercourse is less frequent, with less foreplay, and is preferentially arranged during the ovulatory period [51]. Some patients go so far as to calculate the spacing of intercourse so that the quality of their partner's sperm is optimal during ovulation period.

In the long run, physicians should also pay attention to detrimental life habits in order to optimize the chances of both natural and ART-mediated pregnancy [52]. Sexuality is often dissociated from any sexual desire and reduced to intravaginal ejaculation, which sometimes causes sexual difficulties. Inhibition of sexual desire in couples focused on the desire for pregnancy is a common sexual dysfunction.

During the Infertility Assessment

The medical assessment of infertility in a couple is a moment of profound questioning for the three entities—man, woman, and the couple. The diagnosis of an organic anomaly is a source of narcissistic disturbance and anxiety for young, healthy adults, especially as the diagnosis calls into question the individual's genetic nature and ability to transmit life. Feelings of guilt will almost always be present, and the marital balance may be altered.

A discussion about sexual experience should be opened when the couple is informed about the different examinations that will be prescribed. Details of these examinations must be explained in order to limit their psychological impact and the intrusive nature of the couple's sexual intimacy.

Spermiological examinations (spermogram, semen culture) require masturbation in the laboratory. The experience is extremely variable and may be affected by a man's education, culture, or religion. Semen collection procedures generate a great deal of anxiety because the conditions of intimacy and confidentiality are often absent, and some men are unable to give a semen sample in the clinic. To masturbate in an unfamiliar room that is often uncomfortable, with erotic magazines already used by others, leads to a feeling of mortified sexuality.

On Announcement of Infertility

The announcement of infertility will modify the balance in the couple whether the cause is borne by the man, the woman, or both. Beyond the common project of having a child, it is the individual who may be questioned in his or her normality as a man or woman if the cause of abnormality is genetically related. The man may perceive azoospermia or even asthenozoospermia as a narcissistic wound due to his identity with his spermatozoa or a genetic anomaly as a questioning of his masculinity (Klinefelter) or of his health (CFTR mutation, cystic fibrosis).

Infertility is always a serious illness for the couple, leading at best to a recovery with strengthening of the couple, at worst to a breakup [53]. The sterile subject is doubly affected: by the impossibility of procreating and by the questioning of his person, his power, and his capacity to transmit. Sterility breaks the chain of time that links human beings to those who have preceded them and to those who will succeed them. The life of the sterile couple opens onto nothingness. Even if both partners maintain a good understanding within their couple unit and support each other, a large number of couples experience a reduction in sexual desire [54]. Thus, over time, and with the accumulation of disappointments, a number of couples "fall apart."

Men may experience symptoms of depression, and they may be long-lasting if it is based on a particular psychopathological background. They often feel guilty and look to the past for the reason for the punishment of infertility [55]. A recent case-control study evaluating self-esteem in infertile men concluded that infertility leads to lower self-esteem, sexual performance, and confidence among infertile men as compared to controls and highlighted that increasing duration of infertility, advanced age, diabetes, and higher education were factors significantly lowering the self-esteem scores on univariate analysis [56].

While Undergoing Medically Assisted Reproductive Care

Throughout the ART process, the man may feel excluded, especially as some women transfer to the doctor who is treating them for insemination. The man may be tempted to seek reassurance elsewhere, invest in other areas, or even try to achieve a pregnancy through an extramarital relationship. It is essential to offer the man an equal place in the care of his partner. ART must be at the service of the couple.

The couple may be confronted with the failures of inseminations, IVF, and embryo transfers. Each failure sends both partners back to their identity, to their problems. The couple may not say anything, believing that they are protecting each other. Both may feel guilty and undesirable. These tensions in the couple can lead to a deterioration of the sexual relationship [57].

After the End of Medically Assisted Reproduction

The sexual consequences of infertility seem to depend more on previous sexuality, communication within the couple, and experience of the ART than on its outcome in terms of birth. If the couple had a fragile sexual functionality, infertility may result in a progressive deterioration: decreased desire, pleasure, frequency of intercourse, feelings of estrangement, abandonment, and conflicts may arise. Strengthening of the couple through the ordeal jointly undergone, or the life experience constituted by the experience of couple infertility, reported benefits in almost two-thirds of women and half of men. However, it seems that this marital benefice is not directly correlated with sexual satisfaction parameters. An alteration in the marital relationship is reported by 10% of men and 6% of women, when the infertility problem is kept as a secret from those around them [53].

Conclusion

Sexual disorders are common among men treated for infertility. Sometime, they must be treated prior to the ART procedure. Multidisciplinary management including a urologist and a specialist in sexual medicine is preferred.

In practice, the ART team should:

- Facilitate discussion on sexuality-related issues with the couple.
- Assess the significance and severity of sexual disorders. Establish whether the disorder was preexisting or secondary to male infertility or its treatment. Verify whether the dysfunction is transient or permanent. Search for an organic cause and propose an appropriate treatment.
- Arrange treatment for erectile dysfunction when indicated.
- Assess the psychological consequences of infertility (depression) and its effects on sexuality and quality of life. Search for a primary dysfunction of the couple or

individual that would require treatment (couple therapy, sex therapy, or analytical therapy) prior to ART.
- Help patients to rebuild their sexuality as a source of pleasure after the ART period.

References

1. Greil AL. Infertility and psychological distress: a critical review of the literature. Soc Sci Med 1982. 1997;45(11):1679–704.
2. Rantala ML, Koskimies AI. Sexual behavior of infertile couples. Int J Fertil. 1988;33(1):26–30.
3. Nihal H, Selim K. Micropenis: etiology, diagnosis and treatment approaches. J Clin Res Pediatr Endocrinol. 2013;5(4):217–23.
4. Menon V, Breyer B, Copp HL, Baskin L, Disandro M, Schlomer BJ. Do adult men with untreated ventral penile curvature have adverse outcomes? J Pediatr Urol. 2016;12(1):31.e1–7.
5. Ebert AK, Zwink N, Schwarzer N, Brunner L, Reutter H, Jenetzky E, et al. Needs assessment in care of adults with anorectal malformations and exstrophy-epispadias complex in Germany. Front Pediatr. 2018;6:392.
6. Shindel AW, Nelson CJ, Naughton CK, Ohebshalom M, Mulhall JP. Sexual function and quality of life in the male partner of infertile couples: prevalence and correlates of dysfunction. J Urol. 2008;179(3):1056–9.
7. Nelson CJ, Shindel AW, Naughton CK, Ohebshalom M, Mulhall JP. Prevalence and predictors of sexual problems, relationship stress, and depression in female partners of infertile couples. J Sex Med. 2008;5(8):1907–14.
8. Bräuner EV, Nordkap L, Priskorn L, Hansen ÅM, Bang AK, Holmboe SA, et al. Psychological stress, stressful life events, male factor infertility, and testicular function: a cross-sectional study. Fertil Steril. 2020;113(4):865–75.
9. Skeldon SC, Detsky AS, Goldenberg SL, Law MR. Erectile dysfunction and undiagnosed diabetes, hypertension, and hypercholesterolemia. Ann Fam Med. 2015;13(4):331–5.
10. Duca Y, Calogero AE, Cannarella R, Giacone F, Mongioi LM, Condorelli RA, et al. Erectile dysfunction, physical activity and physical exercise: recommendations for clinical practice. Andrologia. 2019;51(5):e13264.
11. Salonia A, Bettocchi C, Boeri L, Capogrosso P, Carvalho J, Cilesiz NC, et al. European association of urology guidelines on sexual and reproductive health-2021 update: male sexual dysfunction. Eur Urol. 2021;80(3):333–57.
12. Burnett AL, Nehra A, Breau RH, Culkin DJ, Faraday MM, Hakim LS, et al. Erectile dysfunction: AUA guideline. J Urol. 2018;200(3):633–41.
13. Hatzimouratidis K, Salonia A, Adaikan G, Buvat J, Carrier S, El-Meliegy A, et al. Pharmacotherapy for erectile dysfunction: recommendations from the fourth international consultation for sexual medicine (ICSM 2015). J Sex Med. 2016;13(4):465–88.
14. Hong JH, Kwon YS, Kim IY. Pharmacodynamics, pharmacokinetics and clinical efficacy of phosphodiesterase-5 inhibitors. Expert Opin Drug Metab Toxicol. 2017;13(2):183–92.
15. Boeri L, Capogrosso P, Ventimiglia E, Serino A, La Croce G, Russo A, et al. Avanafil—a further step to tailoring patient needs and expectations. Expert Rev Clin Pharmacol. 2016;9(9):1171–81.
16. Dhaliwal A, Gupta M. PDE5 Inhibitors. In: StatPearls [Internet]. Treasure Island: StatPearls Publishing; 2022 [cité 12 févr 2023]. Disponible sur: http://www.ncbi.nlm.nih.gov/books/NBK549843/
17. Beaudreau SA, Van Moorleghem K, Dodd SM, Liou-Johnson V, Suresh M, Gould CE. Satisfaction with a vacuum constriction device for erectile dysfunction among middle-aged and older veterans. Clin Gerontol. 2021;44(3):307–15.

18. Man L, Li G. Low-intensity extracorporeal shock wave therapy for erectile dysfunction: a systematic review and meta-analysis. Urology. 2018;119:97–103.
19. Althof SE, McMahon CG, Waldinger MD, Serefoglu EC, Shindel AW, Ganesan Adaikan P, et al. An update of the international society of sexual medicine's guidelines for the diagnosis and treatment of premature ejaculation (PE). J Sex Med. 2014;11(6):1392–422.
20. Am Psychiatric Assoc. American Psychiatric Association. Diagnostic and statistical manual of mental disorders, fifth edition (DSM-5); 2013.
21. World Health Organization. World Health Organization. International classification of diseases 11th revision for mortality and morbidity statistics (ICD-11-MMS). [Internet]. Geneva; 2018. Disponible sur: https://icd.who.int/browse11/l-m/fr.
22. Serefoglu EC, Yaman O, Cayan S, Asci R, Orhan I, Usta MF, et al. Prevalence of the complaint of ejaculating prematurely and the four premature ejaculation syndromes: results from the Turkish society of andrology sexual health survey. J Sex Med. 2011;8(2):540–8.
23. McMahon CG, Althof SE, Waldinger MD, Porst H, Dean J, Sharlip ID, et al. An evidence-based definition of lifelong premature ejaculation: report of the international society for sexual medicine (ISSM) ad hoc committee for the definition of premature ejaculation. J Sex Med. 2008;5(7):1590–606.
24. Sansone A, Aversa A, Corona G, Fisher AD, Isidori AM, La Vignera S, et al. Management of premature ejaculation: a clinical guideline from the Italian Society of Andrology and Sexual Medicine (SIAMS). J Endocrinol Invest. 2021;44(5):1103–18.
25. Shindel AW, Nelson CJ, Naughton CK, Mulhall JP. Original research—ejaculatory disorders: premature ejaculation in infertile couples: prevalence and correlates. J Sex Med. 2008;5(2):485–91.
26. Bronner G, Kitrey ND, Uziel N, Eli I, Raviv G, Ramon J, et al. Correlation between premature ejaculation and female vaginal penetration difficulties. Int J Impot Res. 2015;27(4):152–6.
27. McMahon CG, Althof SE, Kaufman JM, Buvat J, Levine SB, Aquilina JW, et al. Efficacy and safety of dapoxetine for the treatment of premature ejaculation: integrated analysis of results from five phase 3 trials. J Sex Med. 2011;8(2):524–39.
28. Rowland D, McMahon CG, Abdo C, Chen J, Jannini E, Waldinger MD, et al. Disorders of orgasm and ejaculation in men. J Sex Med. 2010;7(4):1668–86.
29. Sigman M. Introduction. Fertil Steril. 2015;104(5):1049–50.
30. Mehta A, Sigman M. Management of the dry ejaculate: a systematic review of aspermia and retrograde ejaculation. Fertil Steril. 2015;104(5):1074–81.
31. Ochsenkühn R, Kamischke A, Nieschlag E. Imipramine for successful treatment of retrograde ejaculation caused by retroperitoneal surgery. Int J Androl. 1999;22(3):173–7.
32. Proctor KG, Stuart S. The effect of sympathomimetic drugs on post-lymphadenectomy aspermia. J Urol. 1983;129(4):837–8.
33. Gupta S, Sharma R, Agarwal A, Parekh N, Finelli R, Shah R, et al. A comprehensive guide to sperm recovery in infertile men with retrograde ejaculation. World J Mens Health. 2022;40(2):208.
34. Perrin J, Saïas-Magnan J, Lanteaume A, Thiry-Escudié I, Serment G, Bladou F, et al. Résultats préliminaires d'une nouvelle technique de recueil du sperme vésical en présence d'éjaculation rétrograde réfractaire au traitement médical. Prog En Urol. 2011;21(2):134–8.
35. Brackett NL, Ferrell SM, Aballa TC, Amador MJ, Padron OF, Sonksen J, et al. An analysis of 653 trials of penile vibratory stimulation in men with spinal cord injury. J Urol. 1998;159(6):1931–4.
36. Schatte EC, Orejuela FJ, Lipshultz LI, Kim ED, Lamb DJ. Treatment of infertility due to anejaculation in the male with electroejaculation and intracytoplasmic sperm injection. J Urol. 2000;163(6):1717–20.
37. Patel DP, Brant WO, Myers JB, Zhang C, Presson AP, Johnstone EB, et al. Sperm concentration is poorly associated with hypoandrogenism in infertile men. Urology. 2015;85(5):1062–7.

38. Hackett G, Kirby M, Edwards D, Jones TH, Wylie K, Ossei-Gerning N, et al. British society for sexual medicine guidelines on adult testosterone deficiency, with statements for UK practice. J Sex Med. 2017;14(12):1504–23.
39. Khera M, Adaikan G, Buvat J, Carrier S, El-Meliegy A, Hatzimouratidis K, et al. Diagnosis and treatment of testosterone deficiency: recommendations from the fourth international consultation for sexual medicine (ICSM 2015). J Sex Med. 2016;13(12):1787–804.
40. Bhasin S, Brito JP, Cunningham GR, Hayes FJ, Hodis HN, Matsumoto AM, et al. Testosterone therapy in men with hypogonadism: an endocrine society* clinical practice guideline. J Clin Endocrinol Metab. 2018;103(5):1715–44.
41. Buvat J, Maggi M, Guay A, Torres LO. Testosterone deficiency in men: systematic review and standard operating procedures for diagnosis and treatment. J Sex Med. 2013;10(1):245–84.
42. Burte C, Lejeune H, Faix A, Desvaux P, Almont T, Cuzin B, et al. [Practical recommendations for the management of testosterone deficiency]. Progres En Urol J Assoc Francaise Urol Soc Francaise Urol. 2021;31(8–9):458–76.
43. Lunenfeld B, Mskhalaya G, Zitzmann M, Arver S, Kalinchenko S, Tishova Y, et al. Recommendations on the diagnosis, treatment and monitoring of hypogonadism in men. Aging Male. 2015;18(1):5–15.
44. Mulhall JP, Trost LW, Brannigan RE, Kurtz EG, Redmon JB, Chiles KA, et al. Evaluation and management of testosterone deficiency: AUA guideline. J Urol. 2018;200(2):423–32.
45. Patel AS, Leong JY, Ramos L, Ramasamy R. Testosterone is a contraceptive and should not be used in men who desire fertility. World J Mens Health. 2019;37(1):45.
46. de Ronde W, de Jong FH. Aromatase inhibitors in men: effects and therapeutic options. Reprod Biol Endocrinol. 2011;9(1):93.
47. Guay AT, Jacobson J, Perez JB, Hodge MB, Velasquez E. Clomiphene increases free testosterone levels in men with both secondary hypogonadism and erectile dysfunction: who does and does not benefit? Int J Impot Res. 2003;15(3):156–65.
48. Wheeler KM, Sharma D, Kavoussi PK, Smith RP, Costabile R. Clomiphene citrate for the treatment of hypogonadism. Sex Med Rev. 2019;7(2):272–6.
49. Dohle GR, Colpi GM, Hargreave TB, Papp GK, Jungwirth A, Weidner W, et al. EAU guidelines on male infertility. Eur Urol. 2005;48(5):703–11.
50. Kim S, Sundaram R, Buck Louis GM. Joint modeling of intercourse behavior and human fecundability using structural equation models. Biostatistics. 2010;11(3):559–71.
51. Coëffin-Driol C, Giami A. L'impact de l'infertilité et de ses traitements sur la vie sexuelle et la relation de couple: revue de la littérature. Gynécol Obstét Fertil. 2004;32(7–8):624–37.
52. The Annual Capri Workshop Group, Bhattacharya S, JLH E, Gameiro S, Negri E, Somigliana E, et al. Towards a more pragmatic and wiser approach to infertility care. Hum Reprod. 2019;34(7):1165–72.
53. Schmidt L, Holstein B, Christensen U, Boivin J. Does infertility cause marital benefit? Patient Educ Couns. 2005;59(3):244–51.
54. Ohl J, Reder F, Fernandez A, Bettahar-Lebugle K, Rongières C, Nisand I. Impact de l'infertilité et de l'Assistance médicale à la procréation sur la sexualité. Gynécol Obstét Fertil. 2009;37(1):25–32.
55. Sandlow JI. Shattering the myths about male infertility: treatment of male factors may be more successful and cost-effective than you think. Postgrad Med. 2000;107(2):235–45.
56. Jamil S, Shoaib M, Aziz W, Ather MH. Does male factor infertility impact on self-esteem and sexual relationship? Andrologia [Internet]. mars 2020 [cité 11 févr 2023];52(2). Disponible sur: https://onlinelibrary.wiley.com/doi/10.1111/and.13460
57. Schmidt L. Infertility and assisted reproduction in Denmark. Epidemiology and psychosocial consequences. Dan Med Bull. 2006;53(4):390–417.

Part VIII
Current Challenges and Future Perspectives in Male Infertility

Chapter 14
Hypogonadism in Infertile Men: A Clinical Minefield

Amarnath Rambhatla and Widi Atmoko

Key Points

1. Hypogonadism is diagnosed when a patient has signs and symptoms of low testosterone along with biochemical confirmation of low testosterone on two separate morning evaluations.
2. Hypogonadism can be classified as primary (testicular) hypogonadism and secondary (pituitary) hypogonadism.
3. Exogenous testosterone replacement therapy should not be utilized in men with hypogonadism who are interested in fertility.
4. Men who have hypogonadism and are interested in preserving fertility should be treated with selective estrogen receptor modulators (SERMs), aromatase inhibitors (AIs), or human chorionic gonadotropin (hCG).

Introduction

Testosterone plays a vital role in regulating male sexual and reproductive function. During puberty, testosterone determines sexual differentiation and virilization. It also regulates and induces spermatogenesis through several signaling pathways. If there is a defect in the production or function of testosterone, it may cause various clinical features [1, 2]. The term "hypogonadism" only applies if any hypogonadal symptoms accompany a proven low serum testosterone level [3]. It may cause a decrease in quality of life and potentially cause multiple organ problems, including infertility.

Every 10 years, testosterone levels decrease by about 100 ng/dL [4]. A study of 890 men shows that low testosterone level occurs in 20% of men over 60% and 50% of men over 80 years old [5]. Although the exact prevalence of hypogonadism in the

A. Rambhatla (✉)
Department of Urology, Henry Ford Health, Vattikuti Urology Institute, Detroit, MI, USA
e-mail: arambha1@hfhs.org

W. Atmoko
Department of Urology, Faculty of Medicine, Universitas Indonesia, Cipto Mangunkusumo Hospital, Jakarta, Indonesia

A. Agarwal et al. (eds.), *Current and Future Advances in Male Infertility*,
https://doi.org/10.1007/978-3-031-62648-7_14

general population is unknown, it is estimated to be around 25–33% among men who presented to an infertility clinic, and 38% of these men who had a normal semen analysis were found to have hypogonadism [6, 7]. The odds ratio of hypogonadism in subfertile men is ten times higher than in the general population [8]. Therefore, an endocrinology assessment is a crucial part of evaluating male infertility.

The causes of male hypogonadism can be a disturbance at any level of the hypothalamic-pituitary-gonadal axis [9]. A proper diagnosis is needed as it will significantly affect the treatment given. Nevertheless, a large percentage of hypogonadism is currently still undiagnosed and untreated, which should be a warning sign to many physicians. Given the abundance of controversies within the field of hypogonadism in male infertility, it is important to focus on the approach with the most evidence. The aim of this chapter is to provide a comprehensive review of the etiology, pathophysiology, diagnosis, and treatment options of hypogonadism in infertile men.

Etiology of Male Hypogonadism

Physiology of the Hypothalamic-Pituitary-Testis (HPT) Axis

Hypothalamic-pituitary-testis (or gonadal) axis forms an integrated system responsible for maintaining adequate testosterone secretion to ensure normal spermatogenesis. Like any other homeostasis mechanism in our body, the HPT axis also forms a feedback loop for regulating the level of hormones [10].

Pulsatile secretion of gonadotropin-releasing hormone (GnRH) from the mediobasal part of hypothalamus is first stimulated in response to kisspeptin, a neuromodulator that triggers peptide release and activation of the reproductive axis [11]. Production of GnRH begins in early fetal life; however, its production decreases significantly during childhood until after the onset of puberty. In response to GnRH stimulation, the anterior pituitary gland releases LH and FSH, which will subsequently stimulate testicular secretion of testosterone and spermatogenesis. Specifically, LH stimulates testosterone secretion from Leydig cells, whereas FSH stimulates inhibin B secretion from Sertoli cells and spermatogenesis [10].

Testosterone stimulates sperm production and male virilization by acting directly on androgen receptors and being converted into two active metabolites, dihydrotestosterone by the enzyme 5-alpha reductase or estradiol by the enzyme aromatase. The biological effects of testosterone are mediated through androgen receptor activation (AR). At the same time, testosterone and estradiol act as negative feedback on the hypothalamus and pituitary to inhibit the secretion of GnRH, LH, and FSH with the help of inhibin B to inhibit FSH secretion [10]. Interruption within the axis will result in hypogonadism.

Classification of Hypogonadism

With the physiological concept of the HPT axis, it is generally accepted that the problems can originate from the testes (primary hypogonadism) or hypothalamus and pituitary (secondary hypogonadism). In primary hypogonadism, gonadotropin concentration will increase as compensation for low testosterone; hence, it is also called hypergonadotropic hypogonadism. On the contrary, secondary hypogonadism will have a low or inappropriately normal level of gonadotropin hormone despite low level of testosterone; thus, it is called hypogonadotropic hypogonadism [12]. Congenital or acquired problems can cause all types of hypogonadism.

Different classifications of hypogonadism such as "organic" and "functional" can also be used to specify the underlying diseases. Grossman and Matsumoto firstly formalized this term in their article [13]. Organic hypogonadism refers to any specific pathology that may cause disturbance in the HPT axis. Accordingly, it should be treated with conventional medication (i.e., gonadotropins or testosterone therapy). In contrast, functional hypogonadism, characterized by borderline low testosterone, is caused by conditions that physiologically suppress the production or action of gonadotropins or testosterone. However, it is potentially reversible by treating underlying causes and the associated comorbidity. An example of functional hypogonadism is metabolic hypogonadism [13].

Primary Hypogonadism: Definition and Causes

Primary hypogonadism or hypergonadotropic hypogonadism is a classification of hypogonadism that is caused by a primary defect in the testis [12]. Primary testicular failure will result in impaired production of testosterone by the Leydig cells.

Primary Congenital Hypogonadism

Klinefelter's syndrome (KS) is the most frequent congenital cause of primary hypogonadism. Despite its high prevalence which affects 1 in 600–650 men, KS remains highly underdiagnosed because of substantial variation in the clinical presentation [14]. In most cases, KS with 46 XY/47 XXY mosaicism will have milder abnormalities and be more well androgenized [15]. The main features of KS include small testes, gynecomastia, behavioral problems, low IQ, sexual dysfunction, and various degrees of impaired spermatogenesis [14]. Other congenital causes include Noonan syndrome and LH receptor mutations that result in Leydig cell hypoplasia [16, 17].

Congenital structural problems may result from anorchia or cryptorchidism. Uncorrected cryptorchidism predisposes men to germ cell loss and impaired Sertoli and Leydig cell function [18]. Cryptorchidism may present as part of testicular dysgenesis syndrome along with other conditions, such as hypospadias, TGCT (testicular germ cell tumor), and reduced sperm concentration, due to prenatal testicular maldevelopment [19]. To differentiate anorchia and cryptorchidism, HCG administration and measurement of AMH are sometimes essential [20].

Primary Acquired Hypogonadism

Any condition such as trauma, torsion, inflammations/infections, toxins, or other external damages resulting in the testis injury may cause primary hypogonadism [21]. Most orchitis occurs bilaterally and typically develops a few days after the onset of parotitis. Moreover, it can also result in intratesticular atrophy [22]. Another important cause of testicular failure is oncological treatment, including orchiectomy, radiotherapy, or chemotherapy [23]. Several chemotherapeutic agents may cause damage to seminiferous tubules and other testicular cells. Moreover, radiation, especially with a higher dose, may also result in impaired spermatogenesis [24].

Central Hypogonadism: Definition and Causes

Central hypogonadism refers to secondary hypogonadism (hypogonadotropic hypogonadism), which results from any abnormalities in the hypothalamus and/or pituitary gland. GnRH, LH, and/or FSH secretion may be absent or inadequately secreted to stimulate testosterone production [12]. In these cases, FSH and LH concentrations are most likely to be low when tested. Similar to primary hypogonadism, secondary hypogonadism can be caused by congenital and acquired problems.

Secondary Congenital Hypogonadism

One of the most common congenital causes of hypogonadotropic hypogonadism is Kallmann syndrome. It is a heterogeneous clinical and genetic syndrome with the pathognomonic feature of anosmia. Several known genetic mutations for Kallmann syndromes are *KAL1, FGFR1, PROKR2* and *PROK2,* and *FGF8. However, only 30% of the cases have those gene mutations, reflecting that many genetic defects have not been identified yet* [25].

In most cases, Kallmann syndrome results from sporadic cases, whereas in a small subset, it results from familial inheritance (X chromosome-linked recessive, autosomal dominant, or autosomal recessive). The pathophysiology of Kallmann syndrome is hypothesized as early degeneration of olfactory nerve and terminal nerve axons and problems in the embryonic migration of neuroendocrine GnRH cells [25].

The primary differential diagnoses are normosmic idiopathic hypogonadotropic hypogonadism. In idiopathic hypogonadotropic hypogonadism, the etiology is due to a mutation that causes inactivation of GnRH receptors, kisspeptin, or its receptors [26].

Secondary Acquired Hypogonadism

Acquired causes of secondary hypogonadism include inflammatory diseases of the pituitary, pituitary tumors and craniopharyngiomas, hyperprolactinemia, brain injury, and infiltrative/destructive disease, which cause impairment or problems in the production of GnRH from the hypothalamus and FSH/LH from the pituitary [21]. Brain injury, such as after a trauma, can lead to damage and dysfunction of the pituitary. In 25–50% of cases, brain injury results in some degree of hypothalamic-pituitary dysfunction during the first year of brain injury [27]. Inflammation within the hypophysis, tumor, or infiltrative disease can also result in partial hormone deficits, which can be temporary or permanent depending on the disease.

Hyperprolactinemia due to a prolactinoma can result in negative feedback of GnRH as well as gonadotropin secretion. It will result in a suppressed LH and FSH level and, consequently, a low testosterone level. Any medication that increases steroids or glucocorticoids will also disturb the HPG axis [28]. Eating disorders and metabolic syndrome will also negatively impact testosterone levels causing hypogonadism [21]. Similarly, opioids can also suppress testosterone levels [29].

Functional Hypogonadism

Functional hypogonadism is a diagnosis that should be made after excluding other organic causes of hypogonadism. The main purpose of functional hypogonadism is to describe hypogonadism without any structural or specific pathological issue that suppresses the HPT axis such as microprolactinoma and endogenous Cushing syndrome. As opposed to classical hypogonadism, functional hypogonadism typically exhibits more subtle and less specific clinical hypogonadal signs and symptoms. Moreover, in the elderly, the symptoms may also coincide with comorbid illnesses or the aging process [13]. Nevertheless, sexual complaints such as erectile dysfunction are more frequently associated with functional hypogonadism.

Late-onset hypogonadism (LOH) is most frequently experienced by aging men and is accompanied by a decrease in serum testosterone levels. Each year has a 1–2% decrease in testosterone levels [30]. This age-related testosterone decline can also result from comorbidities in older men, including metabolic syndrome [31]. In metabolic hypogonadism, testosterone deficiency is caused by a direct and indirect mechanism. Due to the high adipose tissue, most testosterone is converted into estradiol leading to increased ROS production and disturbing the HPT axis. Hypogonadism also causes an increase in adipose tissue, which will further decrease testosterone levels [32]. The diagnosis of functional hypogonadism should only be made after exclusion of other possible organic causes [33].

Diagnosis of Male Hypogonadism

The diagnosis of male hypogonadism can only be made if there are clinical symptoms and signs that accompany laboratory findings of decreased serum testosterone level. The diagnostic approach is mainly focused on discovering the underlying causes of male hypogonadism and any related comorbidities that may affect the treatment option. To avoid misdiagnosis, male hypogonadism should not be evaluated during the presence of acute or subacute illness [34].

Several international associations, such as the Endocrine Society and the European Association of Urology, are against routine screening of men for hypogonadism in the general population [35, 36]. Instead, it should be done in high-risk patients or those with symptoms indicating a possible hypogonadism diagnosis [35]. Similarly, questionnaires such as ADAM (Androgen Deficiency in the Aging Male), MMAS (the Massachusetts Male Aging Study), and AMS (the Aging Male Symptoms) should not be used to screen all men [35]. Although most of the questionnaires have been validated in many languages worldwide, their use is limited due to low specificity and variable sensitivity [37]. Moreover, its use cannot be a substitute for a comprehensive workup. Instead, screening may be beneficial in academic or research settings.

Similar to other diseases, the approach in male hypogonadism starts with a comprehensive history, physical examination, laboratory test, and other specific tests as needed. Any reversible causes of hypogonadism should be identified and excluded before attempting any further workup or treatment. A complete algorithm of male hypogonadism can be seen in Fig. 14.1.

Patient History

The first and most crucial portion of the hypogonadism workup is a comprehensive history to ascertain the patient's symptoms, general health, and any related disease or behavior that may correlate with low testosterone levels. As the symptoms also largely depend on the onset of hypogonadism, the patient's pubertal and sexual development history is essential to be assessed [2]. Patients with congenital or prepubertal onset of hypogonadism may report small testes and penis, lack of deep voice, minimal body hair, and difficulty gaining muscle mass. In a severe form, the patient may complain of ambiguous genitalia and other specific disease features, such as anosmia in Kallmann syndrome [9]. Any other related congenital deformity and its causes in these subsets of patients should be thoroughly evaluated.

On the other hand, postpubertal hypogonadism will mostly have complaints related to sexual symptoms, including erectile dysfunction, low libido, and orgasmic issues, as well as various degrees of infertility [9]. The patient may also report many nonsexual symptoms, including fatigue, gynecomastia, hot flashes and sweats, depression, mood disturbance, impaired concentration, sleep disturbance, increased

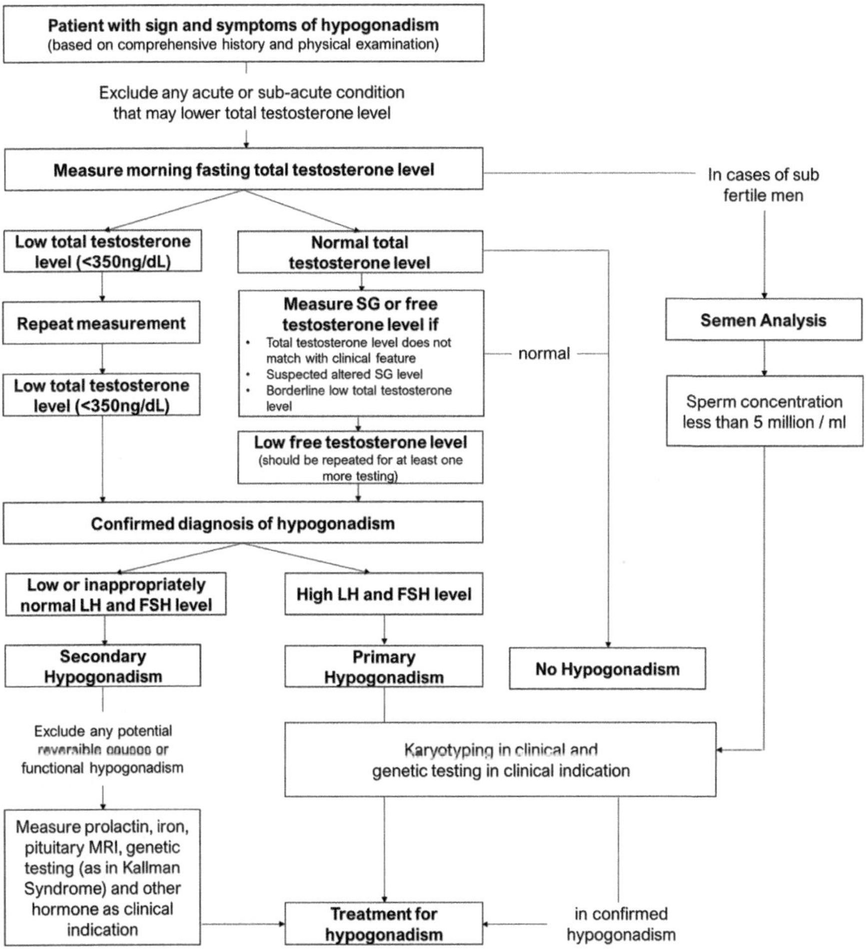

Fig. 14.1 Algorithm of diagnosis for male hypogonadism

body fat, and a general decrease in vitality or quality of life [35]. Depending on the underlying causes, the patient may have other symptoms, such as visual field changes in pituitary tumor patients [9].

Things not to miss out on during the hypogonadism evaluation include looking for a systemic disorder such as metabolic syndrome, obesity, diabetes mellitus, and use of any medications that suppress testosterone production and function such as an anti-androgen, GnRH antagonist, opioid, or even illicit drugs such as marijuana or excessive alcohol intake [21].

In most cases, the probability of male hypogonadism increases in proportion with the number of symptoms. Nevertheless, one symptom is enough to diagnose hypogonadism if there is proof of low testosterone serum. A detailed variety of hypogonadism symptoms has been summarized in Table 14.1. Specific symptoms and signs include incomplete or delayed sexual development, loss of body hair, and small testes [35]. Suggestive symptoms and signs include decreased libido, erectile dysfunction, gynecomastia, eunuchoid body habitus, infertility, low bone mineral density, and hot flushes and sweats [35].

Physical Examination

During the physical examination, it is important to perform a targeted examination for signs of hypogonadism [3]. This should include an assessment of body habitus, virilization and secondary sexual characteristics, dysmorphic features, anthropometry (body mass index and waist circumference), gynecomastia, and genitalia evaluation including testis, scrotum, penis, epididymis, vas deferens, and prostate. Testicular size in an adult normally is greater than 15 ml, and it can be measured using the Prader orchidometer. Penile length should be assessed in a stretched mode. Prostate should be examined, especially in older patients, to find out if any prostate abnormalities are present because testosterone replacement may be contraindicated. The presence of any abnormality should be noted [36].

Congenital cases of hypogonadism, especially due to inadequate stimulation from GnRH during fetal life, will result in various phenotypes of genital ambiguity. If the hypogonadism occurs after gestation, it may cause cryptorchidism or micropenis, whereas if the hypogonadism occurs during prepuberty, it may result in delay of secondary sexual characteristics as well as bone maturation. In postpuberty or adults, however, the signs are often mild, not specific and vague. Hypogonadism can be related to insulin resistance; it may present as acanthosis nigricans. Body mass index and waist circumference are important as hypogonadism can manifest in increased body fat, decreased muscle mass, and accumulation of visceral abdominal fat [3, 9].

Table 14.1 Symptoms of hypogonadism in men [9, 35, 36]

Sexual and reproductive symptoms	Other symptoms
• Delayed or incomplete sexual development • Hypotrophy or atrophy testes • Reduced sexual desire and activity • Erectile dysfunction • Decreased spontaneous erections or nocturnal penile rigidity • Gynecomastia • Loss of body hair • Infertility • Decreased libido	• Lethargic • Mood disturbance • Poor concentration and memory • Sleep disturbances • Anemia • Reduced muscle mass while increase in body fat • Height loss, low-trauma fracture, decreased bone mass density • Hot flushes, sweats • Reduced physical performance

Hormonal Evaluation (Including Stimulation Tests)

Hormonal evaluation is the most crucial workup in the diagnosis of male hypogonadism. There are three forms of testosterone, which include SHBG-bound testosterone (58%), albumin-bound testosterone (40%), and free testosterone (1–2%) [1]. Generally, the first approach in testosterone assessment is measuring total testosterone levels. The most commonly used technique for testosterone is immunoassay and immunometric. However, the accuracy of the test is being questioned nowadays, especially with a very low testosterone level. Thus, the current "gold standard" for measuring testosterone is using liquid chromatography-tandem mass spectrometry (LC-MS/MS). LC-MS/MS has high specificity for measuring testosterone and now is widely available in many countries. The barrier to using LC-MS is the cost, and the technique is rather difficult. In this kind of shortage, a high-quality validated immunoassay can be justified [38].

Due to its pulsatile, circadian, and circannual secretory rhythms, the testosterone level is the highest in the morning, whereas the concentration will lower during the afternoon and evening [39]. Therefore, the most representative testosterone analysis is the one in the morning, preferably between 7 and 11 am [39]. In the older patient, this circadian physiological variation may be blunted, so the use of morning testosterone may not be necessary [40]. One study with more than 300 men with a mean age of 60 shows that only 13% will have a significantly different testosterone level during different time points (before and after 2 pm). However, in healthy elderly males, circadian rhythm is still intact until 70 years old. Glucose consumption can decrease testosterone levels by 15–30%. Thus, it is recommended to measure testosterone in a fasting state [41].

The cutoff used to define low testosterone is varied in the literature. There is no universally accepted threshold below which men will experience symptoms of hypogonadism. The Endocrine Society guideline uses a value of 264 ng/dL as the lower limit of normal in healthy nonobese young men [35]. This corresponds to the 2.5th percentile in cohort studies [42]. The American Urologic Association (AUA) uses a cutoff of 300 ng/dL, and the European Association of Urology (EAU) uses a level of 350 ng/dL below which it is likely that men may experience symptoms of hypogonadism [43, 44]. In certain situations, bioavailable or free testosterone measurements can help guide which patients may benefit from testosterone replacement therapy (TRT).

If the testosterone level is low, a confirmatory test is needed before the diagnosis of hypogonadism can be made as in 30% of the cases the second test can have a normal result [39]. A repeat test should be performed on two separate days/occasions, preferably employing the same laboratory and identical measurement techniques/equipment [35, 36]. Several studies recommend an interval of 2–3 weeks between the two measurements [45].

Total testosterone represents the sum of SHBG-binding testosterone, albumin-binding testosterone, and free testosterone. SHBG has a high affinity; thus, testosterone cannot dissociate to the targeted organ using the usual androgen receptor binding mechanism. On the other hand, albumin has low-affinity binding to testosterone; the process of dissociation can be faster. Based on this physiology, only free testosterone and albumin-binding testosterone are biologically active in the tissue and are known as bioavailable testosterones [1].

Moreover, the concentration of SHBG can be affected by many conditions. Metabolic syndrome, nephrotic syndrome, hypothyroidism, and external steroids may decrease SHBG concentration, while aging, hyperthyroidism, liver cirrhosis, and estrogen can increase SHBG concentration [35]. With this variable concentration, total testosterone will not accurately measure the testosterone level. Therefore, bioavailable and free testosterones generally have better accuracy in the diagnostic workup as it has a better association with clinical and biochemical parameters of androgen deficiency [46, 47]. However, if the SHBG level is normal, the measurement of free testosterone may add little value.

Bioavailable or free testosterone should be considered in cases of borderline range of total testosterone [35, 46]. Additionally, it should also be considered in cases where total testosterone does not match the clinical presentation or is in a condition where SHBG concentration may get affected. The standard for measuring free testosterone and bioavailable testosterone uses equilibrium dialysis and ammonium sulfate precipitation [47]. However, due to its high cost, it is not widely available. On the other hand, immunoassay is widely available, but its reliability has been questioned. The alternative way to calculate free testosterone is using a mathematical calculation based on total testosterone level, SHBG, and albumin level (http://www.issam.ch/freetesto.ht) [36]. The threshold for normal free testosterone is 65 pg/ml (225 pmol/l) or 70 pg/ml (243 pmol/dl) [48].

Once the testosterone level is confirmed to be low in at least two repeated tests, the next step includes central hormonal evaluation, such as LH, FSH, and prolactin. Both LH and FSH concentrations can be used to differentiate primary and secondary hypogonadism. Although its level fluctuates throughout the day, LH has a better representation of decreased testosterone secretion [10]. Testicular failure is diagnosed in cases of elevated LH levels.

On the contrary, a low LH level will confirm the diagnosis of secondary hypogonadism (hypogonadotropic hypogonadism). Elevated levels of the follicle-stimulating hormone are indicative of primary testicular failure and impaired spermatogenesis. FSH should be evaluated in hypogonadal men who are interested in maintaining their current fertility [36]. Comprehensive fertility testing, including a semen analysis, should be done on these patient subsets [35].

GnRH stimulation test is not frequently performed; it can be utilized to check for GnRH deficit [49]. Direct testing of GnRH concentration is challenging, mainly due to its short half-life (2–4 min) [50]. With the intravenous GnRH stimulation test, the LH and FSH should gradually increase in a hypothalamic disorder. On the contrary, a pituitary problem is diagnosed when there is no response. However, this stimulation test is more frequently used in children to distinguish between constitutional delayed puberty and idiopathic hypogonadotropic hypogonadism rather than as a routine test for male hypogonadism workup [49].

Prolactin also causes negative feedback to the hypothalamus and hypophysis; thus, it should be assessed when there is low-normal LH with low testosterone, particularly if a prolactinoma is suspected and testosterone level is <150 ng/dL [35, 51]. A repeat test is mandatory in the case of elevated prolactin levels. Cushing's syndrome should be ruled out if it is suspected [52]. If there is a complaint of gynecomastia, then serum estradiol should be checked. Additionally, serum iron and total iron-binding capacity should be evaluated to rule out hemochromatosis [35]. A genetic condition known as hereditary hemochromatosis can promote tissue iron overload, leading to gonadotroph iron toxicity and other problems, including diabetes [53].

Role of Imaging

Imaging is mainly used as an adjunct in the workup of hypogonadism. For genital evaluation, sonography is the imaging modality of choice to evaluate male genital organs. However, ultrasonography, either scrotal or transrectal sonography, should not be used routinely but only when there is a suspected pathology.

Men with hyperprolactinemia, pan-hypopituitarism, and symptoms of a space-occupying lesion (headaches, blurred vision) should have an examination of the sella turcica. If the prolactin level is normal but total testosterone levels are <150 ng/dL with low or low-normal LH, a pituitary magetic resonance imaging (MRI) should also be done to exclude a non-secreting adenoma [35]. In Kallmann syndrome, MRI might also reveal abnormal morphology or absence of the olfactory bulb. Other indications of MRI should be decided on an individual basis. Bone densitometry can be considered in men with atraumatic fractures, height loss, or low bone mass [54].

Genetic Testing

Due to the possibility of passing genetic defects to the offspring, detecting genetic abnormalities in males is essential [55]. The prioritization of genetic testing recommendations is typically determined by the clinical presentation, testing for mutations with a greater detection rate, or the inheritance pattern. Patients with nonobstructive azoospermia or severe oligospermia (sperm concentration less than five million per mL) should be offered reproductive genetic testing, which entails Y-chromosome analysis for microdeletions and karyotype testing [36].

As a common identifiable cause of primary testicular failure, KS (47 XXY) should be diagnosed using karyotyping, especially in men who have infertility, gynecomastia, very small testes, and elevated gonadotropin levels. Genetic testing should also be considered in patients with hypogonadotropic hypogonadism such as Kallmann syndrome, developmental delay, multiple congenital abnormalities, and/or dysmorphic facial features [56]. Phenotypic characteristics can be used in pattern recognition, such as anosmia in Kallmann syndrome and obesity in Prader-Willi syndrome [56]. The future widespread availability of next-generation sequencing technology could make it possible to efficiently screen several genes simultaneously as part of complete genetic panel evaluation [57].

Treatment of Male Hypogonadism

The goal of TRT in hypogonadal men is to induce and maintain secondary sex characteristics and improve symptoms of low testosterone [35]. Absolute contraindications to TRT include men with a desire for fertility in the near future, elevated hematocrit, thrombophilia, untreated severe obstructive sleep apnea, uncontrolled heart failure, recent heart attack or stroke within the past 6 months, locally advanced or metastatic prostate cancer, or breast cancer [35, 43, 44]. Relative contraindications include severe lower urinary tract or BPH symptoms [44]. Recently, there is emerging evidence that those men who have had definitive treatment of prostate cancer with a radical prostatectomy or radiation therapy and final pathology less than or equal to Gleason 7 along with an undetectable PSA can be considered for TRT. Also recent studies have demonstrated that TRT may be safe in men with BPH without increased risk of symptom progression.

There are a wide variety of formulations available for men undergoing TRT. Formulations include intramuscular injections either short or long term, transdermal patches, topical gels, subcutaneous testosterone pellets, nasal gel, buccal tablets, and oral tablets. Any of these treatment options can be initiated keeping in mind treatment goals, patient's preference, pharmacokinetics, side effect profile, and treatment cost. Table 14.2 reviews common options in testosterone replacement.

Benefits of TRT in hypogonadal men include improvement in sexual function, reduction in fat mass and increase in lean mass, improvement in insulin resistance and glycemic control in men who are hypogonadal and have type 2 diabetes, and improvement in bone density. The role of TRT in improving mood and cognition as well as vitality and physical strength still remains unclear [35, 44]. Adverse reactions from TRT include infertility, acne, oily skin, gynecomastia and breast tenderness, erythrocytosis, and decrease in high density lipoprotien levels. Other adverse reactions are dependent on the specific formulary of TRT used and include local dermatitis or pain at the injection site, fluctuation in mood or libido, transference of testosterone, alteration in taste and gum irritation, and nasal discomfort and congestion. There is no evidence from randomized clinical trials that TRT causes prostate cancer or major adverse cardiac events [35].

The goal for TRT is to maintain serum testosterone in the mid-normal range for young healthy men. While on TRT, men should undergo monitoring including symptom evaluation, testosterone level, and hematocrit at 3, 6, and 12 months after starting TRT and annually thereafter. Prostate-specific antigen (PSA), and digital rectal exam should be done at 3 months and annually after starting TRT. If hematocrit rises above 54%, then TRT should be stopped and a lower dose should be started

Table 14.2 Common options for testosterone replacement therapy

Name	Delivery method	Pharmacokinetics	Typical starting dose	Disadvantages
Testosterone cypionate or enanthate	Intramuscular injection	Supraphysiological level after injection followed by a gradual decline; low-normal level at 1–2 weeks	100–200 mg intramuscular every 1–2 weeks	Repeat injections every 1–2 weeks, most likely to cause erythrocytosis
Testosterone undecanoate	Intramuscular injection and oral tablet	Supraphysiological level after injection followed by a gradual decline; low normal level at 10–12 weeks Oral form has short half-life (2 h) and needs to be dosed twice daily	750 mg intramuscular every 10 weeks 158–396 mg oral twice daily (start 237 mg)	Unable to titrate dose to individual with injection form Oral formulation can lead to hypertension
Testosterone pellet	Subcutaneous insertion	Testosterone stays in the therapeutic range (>300 ng/dL) for 4–6 mos	450–900 mg every 3–4 months	Small incision needed to insert pellets
Testosterone gel	Topical transdermal absorption	Reaches steady state in 24 h; restores serum testosterone to physiological range	1% gel: apply 50–100 mg daily 1.62% gel: apply 20.25–81 mg daily	Small risk of transference
Testosterone patch	Topical transdermal	Restores serum testosterone to physiological range	4 mg patch daily	Skin-site irritation
Testosterone nasal	Intranasal testosterone administration	Short half-life (1.5 h) requiring dosing three times daily	5.5 mg (1 pump) into each nostril three times daily (33 mg daily)	Nasal irritation, epistaxis, rhinorrhea

after hematocrit normalizes or switching to a formulation less likely to cause polycythemia such as a gel form should ensue. If PSA rises greater than 1.4 ng/mL within 12 months, if it is higher than 4 ng/mL, or if there is abnormal DRE or worsening of lower urinary tract symptoms, then the prostate should be evaluated by a urologist [35, 43, 44].

SERMs and AIs

It is well known that an adequate level of intratesticular testosterone is needed for normal spermatogenesis to occur. Exogenously administered testosterone will suppress the HPT axis leading to inhibition of spermatogenesis, intratesticular testosterone, and testosterone synthesis. In order to raise serum and intratesticular testosterone in men who are hypogonadal and interested in fertility, selective estrogen receptor modulators (SERMs) and aromatase inhibitors (AIs) have been used off-label. In carefully selected patients, these medications can increase testosterone while maintaining spermatogenesis unlike with exogenous testosterone.

SERMs are compounds which exhibit tissue-specific estrogen receptor agonist or antagonist activity [58]. The most common SERM used in men is clomiphene citrate which has been used since the 1970s to treat men with infertility [59]. Tamoxifen is another SERM that has been used in men's health. Due to their antiestrogen properties on the hypothalamus and pituitary, clomiphene and tamoxifen lead to an increase in LH and FSH, which in turn stimulates testosterone production and spermatogenesis. Clomiphene citrate is most effective in raising the testosterone level when LH is less than or equal to 6 [60]. Clomiphene can be started at 25 mg by mouth daily and then titrated based on testosterone, LH, and estradiol levels. These should be checked 4–6 weeks after starting the medication to ensure that there is good efficacy. A semen analysis should be checked 3 months after starting the medication to determine if there has been an improvement in sperm concentration. Clomiphene has also been used for the treatment of idiopathic infertility; however, its use in this setting is controversial. Additionally, clomiphene has been used for the treatment of spermatogenesis and HPT axis recovery in men who were previously treated with exogenous testosterone [61].

More recently, clomiphene has been used as a sole therapeutic option for men with hypogonadism without an interest in fertility. Several studies have identified that clomid raises LH, FSH, and testosterone levels as well as improves symptoms of hypogonadism such as erectile function, bone mineral density, and reduction in body mass index [62]. Reports of side effects of clomid include headaches, dizziness, gynecomastia, and exacerbation of mood disorders.

AIs such as anastrozole and letrozole were originally approved for the treatment of metastatic breast cancer, but more recently they have been used off-label to increase testosterone in men with infertility and hypogonadism. AIs block the aromatase enzyme, which converts testosterone to estradiol, leading to an increase in testosterone and a decrease in estradiol. They are mainly used for certain populations of men with infertility or as an alternative to TRT for men with hypogonadism who have an altered testosterone/estradiol ratio of less than 10:1. AIs have been associated with improving sperm concentrations in men with infertility and hypogonadism. When used solely for the treatment of hypogonadism, studies do not show a significant improvement in hypogonadal symptoms as evidenced by ADAM questionnaire or improvement in body habitus or strength [63]. With long-term use, it may also lead to a decrease in bone mineral density [63]. High levels of estradiol may impact male reproductive and sexual function, but levels that are low may also have an adverse effect. Until more is known about these medications, they should be used for a short duration in men who have hypogonadism and infertility with an altered T/E2 ratio. Anastrozole can be started at 1 mg twice weekly and testosterone and estradiol levels checked after 4–6 weeks. Semen analysis can be evaluated after 3 months of treatment.

hCG and rFSH

hCG is the only nontestosterone compound that is FDA approved for the treatment of male hypogonadism. hCG is an LH analog and stimulates testosterone production from Leydig cells. It is usually most effective in the setting of hypogonadotropic hypogonadism but has also been employed to help maintain intratesticular testosterone levels and spermatogenesis in men undergoing or recovering from exogenous testosterone therapy [61, 64]. hCG is well tolerated but needs to be administered via needle injection two to three times weekly and is relatively expensive. A typical starting dose is 1500 IU–2000 IU two to three times weekly. Variations of this regimen can exist with higher doses and also with different formulations such as Ovidrel, which only needs to be injected on a weekly basis due to longer half-life. A testosterone level is repeated in a few weeks after starting to determine treatment efficacy. Semen analysis can be checked 3 months after initiation of treatment.

hCG can be administered alone or in combination with rFSH when trying to stimulate spermatogenesis in men with hypogonadotropic hypogonadism. Recombinant FSH or hMG can be used to stimulate Sertoli cells. hMG has both LH and FSH activity. Neither is a good treatment for idiopathic oligospermia.

DHEA and Other Supplements

Several testosterone-enhancing supplements have gained popularity due to ease of obtaining these supplements and direct-to-consumer advertising. However, the scientific evidence backing most of these is poor. Dehydroepiandrosterone (DHEA) is a precursor to testosterone production, and, in theory, increasing DHEA should lead to an increase in testosterone. However, it can lead to a higher estrogen level as well as cause liver toxicity. Clinical trials with DHEA have not shown a significant improvement in testosterone levels. A meta-analysis of randomized controlled trials showed that DHEA supplementation increased DHEA and estradiol levels, but there was no improvement in serum testosterone [65].

Other supplements hypothesized to increase testosterone include L-arginine, L-citrulline, and Tongkat ali. However, the scientific evidence supporting these supplements is weak at best and quality control for supplements is a big problem. The best studied supplements raise testosterone by only 50–100 points, which is something that can easily be surpassed by testosterone replacement therapy. With the issues of quality control and potential for side effects, it is best for men with hypogonadism to adhere to other methods for TRT until more evidence surrounding supplements is available.

Future Perspectives: GnRh Pumps, Stem Cells, Tissue Grafting

Several treatment options for hypogonadism are being studied and further developed. These include the use of GnRh pumps, induction of stem cells into Leydig cells, direct harvesting of Leydig stem cells for grafting purposes, and selective androgen receptor modulators. In men with hypogonadotropic hypogonadism, GnRh pumps can help restore spermatogenesis and testosterone production. These hormone pumps release GnRh in a pulsatile fashion and can restore normal levels of both FSH and LH, re-establishing HPT axis function [66]. Both human and animal stem cells in vitro can differentiate into Leydig cells, which can produce testosterone. A study by Hou and colleagues identified that human bone marrow cells cultured in a medium of gonadotropins showed that there was an increase in testosterone production compared to controls [67]. A study by Guo and colleagues demonstrated that immature Leydig cells isolated from Sprague-Dawley rats cultured in medium showed an increase in testosterone and steroidogenesis [68]. Animal models have also found that Leydig stem cells harvested from mice can be transplanted later on into castrated rats to induce testosterone production compared to placebo [69]. Selective androgen receptor modulators are analogous to SERMs and can potentially increase gonadotropins, leading to endogenous testosterone production. These are currently still in experimental phases and not ready for clinical use for the treatment of hypogonadism or infertility [70].

Conclusion

Hypogonadism is one of the most common endocrinologic abnormalities in men who have infertility but also presents a therapeutic challenge. Intratesticular testosterone is needed for spermatogenesis; however, traditional testosterone replacement therapy leads to suppression of the HPT axis and can lead to azoospermia. In this scenario, medications such as SERMs, AIs, or hCG can be utilized to raise serum testosterone while maintaining spermatogenesis. Future treatments may revolve around GnRh pumps, selective androgen receptor modulators, stem cells, and tissue grafting, but more evidence is needed before they can be widely utilized for clinical use.

References

1. Hiort O. The differential role of androgens in early human sex development. BMC Med. 2013;11:152.
2. Smith LB, Walker WH. The regulation of spermatogenesis by androgens. Semin Cell Dev Biol. 2016;201430:2–13.

3. Carnegie C. Diagnosis of hypogonadism: clinical assessments and laboratory tests. Rev Urol. 2004;6(Suppl 6):S3–8.
4. Morley JE, Kaiser FE, Perry HM, Patrick P, Morley PM, et al. Longitudinal changes in testosterone, luteinizing hormone, and follicle-stimulating hormone in healthy older men. Metab Clin Exp. 1997;46(4):410–3.
5. Harman SM, Metter EJ, Tobin JD, Pearson J, Blackman MR, Baltimore Longitudinal Study of Aging. Longitudinal effects of aging on serum total and free testosterone levels in healthy men. Baltimore Longitudinal Study of Aging. J Clin Endocrinol Metab. 2001;86(2):724–31.
6. Ahmad A, Lao M, Mechlin C, Forman M, Horvath P, et al. Prevalence of male hypogonadism in couples presenting to a reproductive endocrinology infertility clinic. Fertil Steril. 2013;100(3).
7. Soran V, Knell A, Tharakan T, Cayetano-Alcaraz A, Jayasena C, et al. Investigating the prevalence of hypogonadism and associated cardiovascular risk of males presenting with infertility: results from a diverse and multi-ethnic UK patient cohort. Endocrine abstract; 2022.
8. Giwercman YL, Giwercman A. High prevalence of hypogonadism and associated impaired metabolic and bone mineral status in sub fertile men. Clin Endocrinol. 2016;85(2):189–95.
9. Salonia A, Rastrelli G, Hackett G, Seminara SB, Huhtaniemi IT, et al. Paediatric and adult-onset male hypogonadism. Nat Rev Dis Primers. 2019;5(1):38.
10. Corradi PF, Corradi RB, Greene LW. Physiology of the hypothalamic pituitary gonadal axis in the male. Urol Clin North Am. 2016;43(2):151–62.
11. Skorupskaite K, George JT, Anderson RA. The kisspeptin-GnRH pathway in human reproductive health and disease. Hum Reprod Update. 2014;20(4):485–500.
12. Sharma A, Jayasena CN, Dhillo WS. Regulation of the hypothalamic-pituitary-testicular axis: pathophysiology of hypogonadism. Endocrinol Metab Clin N Am. 2022;51(1):29–45.
13. Grossmann M, Matsumoto AM. A perspective on middle-aged and older men with functional hypogonadism: focus on holistic management. J Clin Endocrinol Metab. 2017;102(3):1067–75.
14. Høst C, Skakkebæk A, Groth KA, Bojesen A. The role of hypogonadism in Klinefelter syndrome. Asian J Androl. 2014;16(2):185–91.
15. Samplaski MK, Lo KC, Grober ED, Millar A, Dimitromanolakis A, et al. Phenotypic differences in mosaic Klinefelter patients as compared with non-mosaic Klinefelter patients. Fertil Steril. 2014;101(4):950–5.
16. Moniez S, Pienkowski C, Lepage B, Hamdi S, Daudin M, et al. Noonan syndrome males display Sertoli cell-specific primary testicular insufficiency. Eur J Endocrinol. 2018;179(6):409–18.
17. Çömlek FÖ, Yıldız R, Seyrek F, Tütüncüler F. Leydig cell hypoplasia type 1 diagnosed in early childhood with inactivating mutation in LHCGR gene. Oxford Med Case Rep. 2021;4:1.
18. Rohayem J, Luberto A, Nieschlag E, Zitzmann M, Kliesch S. Delayed treatment of undescended testes may promote hypogonadism and infertility. Endocrine. 2017;55(3):914–24.
19. Niedzielski JK, Oszukowska E, Słowikowska-Hilczer J. Undescended testis—current trends and guidelines: a review of the literature. Arch Med Sci AMS. 2016;12(3):667–77.
20. Johansen ML, Hagen CP, Johannsen TH, Main KM, Picard JY, et al. Anti-Müllerian hormone and its clinical use in pediatrics with special emphasis on disorders of sex development. Int J Endocrinol. 2013;198698
21. Matsumoto AM, Bremner WJ. Testicular disorders. In: Melmed S, Polansky KS, Larsen PR, Kronenberg HM, editors. Williams textbook of endocrinology. 13th ed. New York: Elsevier; 2016. p. 688–777.
22. Wu H, Wang F, Tang D, Han D. Mumps orchitis: clinical aspects and mechanisms. Front Immunol. 2021;12:582946.
23. La Vignera S, Cannarella R, Duca Y, Barbagallo F, Burgio G, et al. Hypogonadism and sexual dysfunction in testicular tumor survivors: a systematic review. Front Endocrinol. 2019;10:264.
24. Okada K, Fujisawa M. Recovery of spermatogenesis following cancer treatment with cytotoxic chemotherapy and radiotherapy. World J Men's Health. 2019;37(2):166–74.
25. Dodé C, Hardelin JP. Kallmann syndrome. Eur J Hum Genet. 2009;17(2):139–46.

26. Chan YM, Lippincott MF, Butler JP, Sidhoum VF, Li CX. Exogenous kisspeptin administration as a probe of GnRH neuronal function in patients with idiopathic hypogonadotropic hypogonadism. J Clin Endocrinol Metab. 2014;99(12):E2762–71.
27. Auble BA, Bollepalli S, Makoroff K, Weis T, Khoury J. Hypopituitarism in pediatric survivors of inflicted traumatic brain injury. J Neurotrauma. 2014;31(4):321–6.
28. Majumdar A, Mangal NS. Hyperprolactinemia. J Human Reprod Sci. 2013;6(3):168–75.
29. Bawor M, Dennis BB, Samaan MC, Plater C, Worster A. Methadone induces testosterone suppression in patients with opioid addiction. Sci Rep. 2014;4:6189.
30. Stanworth RD, Jones TH. Testosterone for the aging male; current evidence and recommended practice. Clin Interv Aging. 2008;3(1):25–44.
31. Ahern T, Wu FC. New horizons in testosterone and the ageing male. Age Ageing. 2015;44(2):188–95.
32. Pivonello R, Menafra D, Riccio E, Garifalos F, Mazzella M, et al. Metabolic disorders and male hypogonadotropic hypogonadism. Front Endocrinol. 2019;10:345.
33. Corona G, Goulis DG, Huhtaniemi I, Zitzmann M, Toppari J, et al. European Academy of Andrology (EAA) guidelines on investigation, treatment and monitoring of functional hypogonadism in males: Endorsing organization: European Society of Endocrinology. Andrology. 2020;8(5):970–87.
34. Kalra S, Agrawal N, Kumar S, Sharma A. Testosterone replacement in male hypogonadism. Clin Pharmacol Adv Appl. 2010;2:149–53.
35. Bhasin S, Brito JP, Cunningham GR, Hayes FJ, Hodis HN, et al. Testosterone therapy in men with hypogonadism: an endocrine society clinical practice guideline. J Clin Endocrinol Metab. 2018;103(5):1715–44.
36. Salonia A, Bettochi C, Carvalho J, Corona G, Jones TH, et al. EAU guidelines on sexual and reproductive health. EAU; 2022.
37. Bernie AM, Scovell JM, Ramasamy R. Comparison of questionnaires used for screening and symptom identification in hypogonadal men. Aging Male. 2014;17(4):195–8.
38. Trost LW, Mulhall JP. Challenges in testosterone measurement, data interpretation, and methodological appraisal of interventional trials. J Sex Med. 2016;13(7):1029–46.
39. Brambilla DJ, O'Donnell AB, Matsumoto AM, McKinlay JB. Intraindividual variation in levels of serum testosterone and other reproductive and adrenal hormones in men. Clin Endocrinol. 2007;67(6):853–62.
40. Bremner WJ, Vitiello MV, Prinz PN. Loss of circadian rhythmicity in blood testosterone levels with aging in normal men. J Clin Endocrinol Metab. 1983;56(6):1278–81.
41. Caronia LM, Dwyer AA, Hayden D, Amati F, Pitteloud N, et al. Abrupt decrease in serum testosterone levels after an oral glucose load in men: implications for screening for hypogonadism. Clin Endocrinol. 2013;78(2):291–6.
42. Travison TG, Vesper HW, Orwoll E, Wu F, Kaufman JM, Wang Y, Lapauw B, Fiers T, Matsumoto AM, Bhasin S. Harmonized reference ranges for circulating testosterone levels in men of four cohort studies in the United States and Europe. J Clin Endocrinol Metab. 2017;102(4):1161–73.
43. Mulhall JP, Trost LW, Brannigan RE, Kurtz EG, Redmon JB, Chiles KA, Lightner DJ, Miner MM, Murad MH, Nelson CJ, Platz EA, Ramanathan LV, Lewis RW. Evaluation and management of testosterone deficiency: AUA guideline. J Urol. 2018;200(2):423–32.
44. Salonia A, Bettocchi C, Boeri L, Capogrosso P, Carvalho J, Cilesiz NC, Cocci A, Corona G, Dimitropoulos K, Gül M, Hatzichristodoulou G, Jones TH, Kadioglu A, Martínez Salamanca JI, Milenkovic U, Modgil V, Russo GI, Serefoglu EC, Tharakan T, Verze P, Minhas S, EAU Working Group on Male Sexual and Reproductive Health. European Association of Urology guidelines on sexual and reproductive health-2021 update: male sexual dysfunction. Eur Urol. 2021;80(3):333–57.
45. Rivas AM, Mulkey Z, Lado-Abeal J, Yarbrough S. Diagnosing and managing low serum testosterone. Proceedings (Baylor University. Medical Center). 2014;27(4):321–4.

46. Collier CP, Clark AF, Bain J, Godwin M, Hudson RW. Functional testosterone: biochemical assessment of hypogonadism in men—report from a multidisciplinary workshop hosted by the Ontario Society of Clinical Chemists. Aging Male. 2007;10(4):211–6.
47. Matsumoto AM, Bremner WJ. Serum testosterone assays—accuracy matters. J Clin Endocrinol Metab. 2004;89(2):520–4.
48. Shin YS, Park JK. The optimal indication for testosterone replacement therapy in late onset hypogonadism. J Clin Med. 2019;8(2):209.
49. Sun QH, Zheng Y, Zhang XL, Mu YM. Role of gonadotropin-releasing hormone stimulation test in diagnosing gonadotropin deficiency in both males and females with delayed puberty. Chin Med J. 2015;128(18):2439–43.
50. Kumar P, Sharma A. Gonadotropin-releasing hormone analogs: understanding advantages and limitations. J Human Reprod Sci. 2014;7(3):170–4.
51. Grattan DE. 60 YEARS OF NEUROENDOCRINOLOGY: The hypothalamo-prolactin axis. J Endocrinol. 2015;226(2):T101–22.
52. Luton JP, Thieblot P, Valcke JC, Mahoudeau JA, Bricaire H. Reversible gonadotropin deficiency in male Cushing's disease. J Clin Endocrinol Metab. 1977;45(3):488–95.
53. Piperno A, Pelucchi S, Mariani R. Inherited iron overload disorders. Transl Gastroenterol Hepatol. 2020;5:25.
54. Zaghouani H, Slim I, Zina NB, Mallat N, Tajouri H. Kallmann syndrome: MRI findings. Indian J Endocrinol Metab. 2013;17(Suppl 1):S142–5.
55. Zorrilla M, Yatsenko AN. The genetics of infertility: current status of the field. Curr Genet Med Rep. 2013;1(4):10.
56. Millar AC, Faghfoury H, Bieniek JM. Genetics of hypogonadotropic hypogonadism. Transl Androl Urol. 2021;10(3):1401–9.
57. Remec ZI, Trebusak Podkrajsek K, Repic LB, Kovac J, Groselj U, et al. Next-generation sequencing in newborn screening: a review of current state. Front Genet. 2021;2:662254.
58. Komm BS, Mirkin S. An overview of current and emerging SERMs. J Steroid Biochem Mol Biol. 2014 Sep;143:207–22.
59. Paulson DF, Hammond CB, de Vere WR, Wiebe RH. Clomiphene citrate: pharmacologic treatment of hypofertile male. Urology. 1977;9(4):419–21.
60. Mazzola CR, Katz DJ, Loghmanieh N, Nelson CJ, Mulhall JP. Predicting biochemical response to clomiphene citrate in men with hypogonadism. J Sex Med. 2014;11(9):2302–7.
61. Rahnema CD, Lipshultz LI, Crosnoe LE, Kovac JR, Kim ED. Anabolic steroid-induced hypogonadism: diagnosis and treatment. Fertil Steril. 2014;101(5):1271–9.
62. Wheeler KM, Sharma D, Kavoussi PK, Smith RP, Costabile R. Clomiphene citrate for the treatment of hypogonadism. Sex Med Rev. 2019;7(2):272–6.
63. Burnett-Bowie SA, McKay EA, Lee H, Leder BZ. Effects of aromatase inhibition on bone mineral density and bone turnover in older men with low testosterone levels. J Clin Endocrinol Metab. 2009;94(12):4785–92.
64. Fink J, Schoenfeld BJ, Hackney AC, Maekawa T, Horie S. Human chorionic gonadotropin treatment: a viable option for management of secondary hypogonadism and male infertility. Expert Rev Endocrinol Metab. 2021;16(1):1–8.
65. Corona G, Rastrelli G, Giagulli VA, Sila A, Sforza A, Forti G, Mannucci E, Maggi M. Dehydroepiandrosterone supplementation in elderly men: a meta-analysis study of placebo-controlled trials. J Clin Endocrinol Metab. 2013;98(9):3615–26.
66. Hao M, Mao JF, Guan QB, Tian L, Han H, Lei HE, Zheng DM, Tian ZH, Nie M, Wang X, Yu BQ, Gao YJ, Wu XY. Efficacy and safety of pulsatile gonadotropin-releasing hormone therapy in patients with congenital hypogonadotropic hypogonadism: a multicentre clinical study. Ann Transl Med. 2021;9(12):962.
67. Hou L, Dong Q, Wu YJ, et al. Gonadotropins facilitate potential differentiation of human bone marrow mesenchymal stem cells into Leydig cells in vitro. Kaohsiung J Med Sci. 2016;32:1–9.

68. Guo X, Chen Y, Hong T, et al. Induced pluripotent stem cell-derived conditional medium promotes Leydig cell antiapoptosis and proliferation via autophagy and Wnt/beta-catenin pathway. J Cell Mol Med. 2018;22:3614–26.
69. Arora H, Zuttion M, Nahar B, et al. Subcutaneous Leydig stem cell autograft: a promising strategy to increase serum testosterone. Stem Cells Transl Med. 2019;8:58–65.
70. Solomon ZJ, Mirabal JR, Mazur DJ, et al. Selective androgen receptor modulators: current knowledge and clinical applications. Sex Med Rev. 2019;7:84–94.

Chapter 15
Challenges in the Management of Nonobstructive Azoospermia

Megan McMurray and Nicholas N. Tadros

Key Points

- Nonobstructive azoospermia (NOA) is defined as an absence of sperm secondary to an impairment in spermatogenesis as opposed to obstruction.
- NOA may occur as the result of a pre-testicular cause (hypogonadotropic hypogonadism) or testicular cause (spermatogenic failure).
- Management of NOA generally consists of medical management and/or surgical sperm retrieval. Generally, medical management in the form of hormonal therapy is recommended in men with hypogonadotropic hypogonadism. Hormonal therapy in men with spermatogenic failure is controversial due to lack of strong supporting evidence; therefore, surgical sperm retrieval is typically the primary treatment modality in these men.
- Several underlying factors may predict the success of sperm retrieval.

Introduction

Infertility is estimated to affect 1 in 6 North American couples, with male factor infertility implicated in 50% of cases [1]. Azoospermia, defined as the absence of sperm in the ejaculate, is estimated to affect 1.9% of the general population and 10–20% of men with infertility [2–4]. In nonobstructive azoospermia (NOA), azoospermia is secondary to an impairment in spermatogenesis. This contrasts with obstructive azoospermia (OA), which is caused by occlusion of the ductal system or ejaculatory dysfunction.

M. McMurray (✉) · N. N. Tadros
Department of Urology, Southern Illinois University School of Medicine, Springfield, IL, USA
e-mail: mmcmurray47@siumed.edu

A. Agarwal et al. (eds.), *Current and Future Advances in Male Infertility*,
https://doi.org/10.1007/978-3-031-62648-7_15

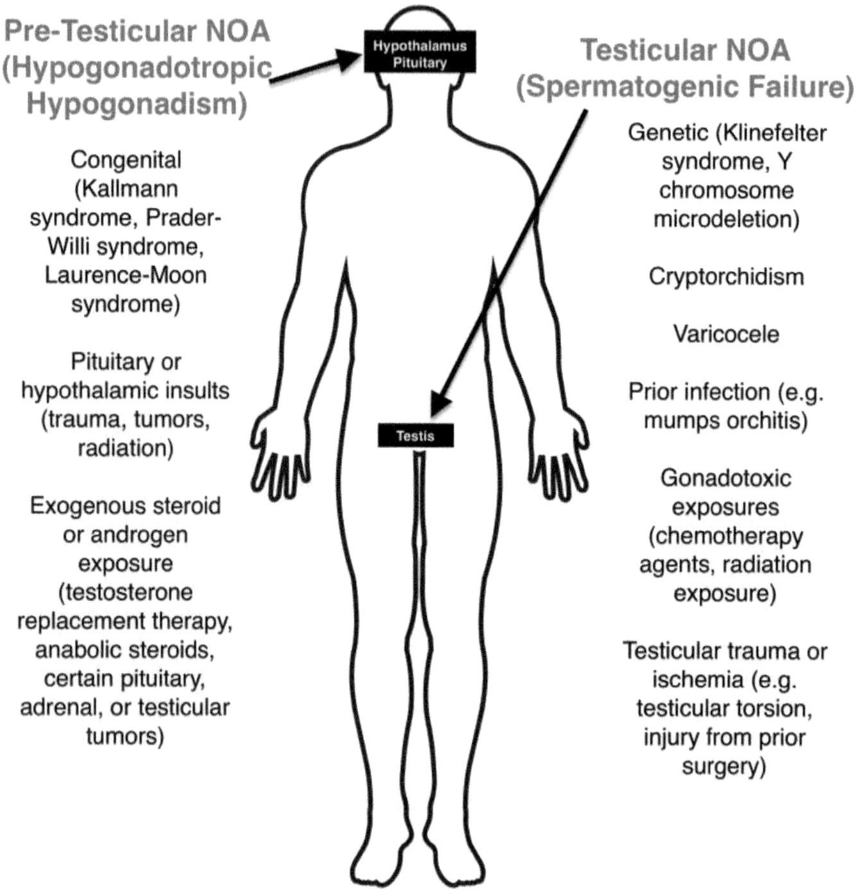

Fig. 15.1 Subtypes of nonobstructive azoospermia (NOA) and common causes

Depending on the anatomical location of the underlying problem, NOA can be classified as pre-testicular (hypogonadotropic hypogonadism) or testicular (spermatogenic failure) (Fig. 15.1). Hypogonadotropic hypogonadism (HH) refers to a hormonal abnormality that results in the inability to stimulate spermatogenesis. HH may be congenital and can be seen in Kallmann syndrome, Prader-Willi syndrome, and Laurence-Moon syndrome. Acquired causes of HH include insults to the pituitary or hypothalamus, such as trauma, tumors, or radiation. Acquired HH may also occur because of exogenous steroids or androgens, including testosterone replacement therapy, anabolic steroids, and certain pituitary, adrenal, or testicular tumors.

Spermatogenic failure (SF) may arise because of an underlying genetic abnormality such as Klinefelter syndrome or Y chromosome microdeletion. Other causes of SF include cryptorchidism, varicocele, prior infection (e.g., mumps orchitis), gonadotoxic exposures (chemotherapy agents, radiation exposure), and testicular trauma or ischemia (e.g., testicular torsion, injury from prior surgery) [5–7].

Evaluation of NOA

Evaluation of the infertility patient begins with a thorough fertility history and physical exam. Azoospermia is diagnosed via semen analysis, preferably with two concordant semen analyses obtained at least 1 month apart, showing total absence of spermatozoa, even in the centrifuged pellet. Semen volume, FSH and LH levels, and physical exam findings should aid in differentiating between OA and NOA. Men with OA can have low semen volume (<0.5–1 mL) and normal FSH levels, while men with NOA will have normal semen volume and may have an abnormal FSH level. Small testis volume may be a sign of NOA, while absence of vasa deferentia or enlarged proximal epididymis would indicate underlying OA [8].

After the diagnosis of NOA is made, hormonal evaluation should be obtained to differentiate between HH and SF. Low FSH, low LH, and low testosterone levels are seen in HH. In contrast, SF is characterized by high/normal FSH and LH and low/normal testosterone.

Karyotyping and Y chromosome microdeletion analysis are recommended in men with NOA due to SF. Azoospermia factor (AZF) microdeletions on the long arm of the Y chromosome are found in approximately 10% of men with NOA. There are three AZF regions—termed AZFa, AZFb, and AZFc—which have their own implications for fertility potential as discussed later [9].

Imaging studies may be of use in certain situations but should not be routinely performed as part of the initial evaluation of an infertile male [8]. Scrotal ultrasound may show signs of obstructive azoospermia (abnormal epididymis, dilated rete testis), varicocele, or testicular abnormalities such as microlithiasis. In cases where an abnormality in the hypothalamic-pituitary-adrenal axis is suspected, particularly in men with hyperprolactinemia, brain MRI should be considered to rule out a benign or malignant tumor [7].

Testis biopsy may be useful when it is unclear if azoospermia is obstructive or nonobstructive. However, it should not be routinely performed [8]. Potential histopathologic findings in NOA include Sertoli cell-only syndrome (no spermatogenesis), maturation arrest (incomplete spermatogenesis), hypospermatogenesis (germ cells of all stages present but reduced), seminiferous tubule hyalinization, and mixed abnormalities [10].

Management of NOA

Management of NOA is summarized in Fig. 15.2.

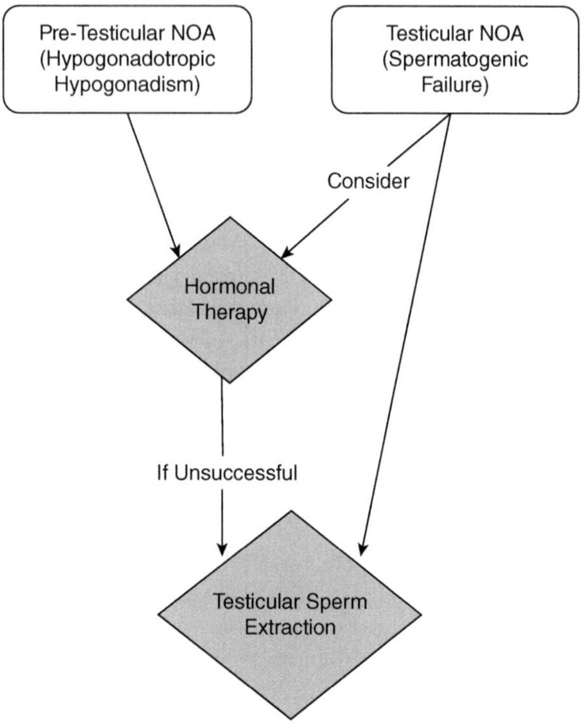

Fig. 15.2 Algorithm for the management of NOA

Hormonal Therapy

Hormonal therapy is a consideration in the management of men with NOA, predominantly in those with HH. Testosterone, particularly intratesticular testosterone (ITT), plays a pivotal role in spermatogenesis. LH and FSH also play important roles by stimulating Leydig and Sertoli cells, respectively. There are several hormonal therapy agents available, all of which ultimately aim to optimize ITT levels (Table 15.1).

Adverse effects of hormonal therapy include acne, gynecomastia, altered liver function tests, headache, loss of libido, hair loss, joint pain, cutaneous rash, lower limb swelling, ocular pruritus, depression, mastalgia, and dry mouth [11].

Hypogonadotropic Hypogonadism

HH can often be managed successfully with hormonal therapy. This condition is characterized by impaired spermatogenesis due to decreased pituitary LH production causing decreased testicular testosterone production. Therefore, management focuses on stimulating ITT production. hCG is the primary medication used in this setting, as it directly stimulates LH receptors on Leydig cells to increase

Table 15.1 Commonly utilized medications for hormonal therapy in NOA

Medication class	Medications	Mechanism of action
Gonadotrophins	Human chorionic gonadotropin (hCG)	LH analogue
	Human menopause gonadotropin (hMG)	FSH and LH analogue
	Urinary FSH (uFSH) Highly purified FSH (FSH-HP) Recombinant FSH (rFSH)	FSH analogues
	Gonadotropin-releasing hormone (GnRH)	GnRH
Aromatase inhibitors	Anastrozole Letrozole Testolactone	Blocks the conversion of testosterone to estrogen in peripheral tissues
SERMs	Clomiphene citrate Tamoxifen	Competitively inhibits estrogen receptors in the hypothalamus and pituitary → downregulates negative feedback on the hypothalamic-pituitary-gonadal axis → promotes LH and FSH secretion

testosterone production. After testosterone levels have normalized, FSH supplementation is commonly added to the hCG regimen to further stimulate spermatogenesis. There are several formulations of FSH available, including menopausal (hMG), urinary FSH (uFSH), highly purified FSH (FSH-HP), and recombinant FSH (rFSH) [12]. Alternatively, GnRH may be administered in a pulsatile manner. Unfortunately, GnRH can be expensive, and it must be administered every 2 h which makes it impractical for most patients. The success rates of GnRH therapy compared to hCG +/– FSH are generally thought to be similar [13–15]; however, GnRH may be inferior according to at least one study [16].

Spermatogenesis is achieved in 63–95% of patients with HH after receiving GnRH or hCG +/–FSH therapy [13, 14, 17–23], with one meta-analysis ascertaining a 75% success rate [15]. Pregnancy rates after hormonal therapy range from 51% to 83% [13, 14, 19, 24, 25].

One predictor of a positive response to hormonal therapy is larger pretreatment testicular volume [19, 24–26]. The timing of hypogonadism onset may also play a role; those with postpubertal HH are more likely to respond to treatment than those with prepubertal HH [15, 27, 28]. However, some studies have found no differences between congenital and acquired HH [24]. On a similar note, men who have completed sexual maturation are more likely to respond positively to hormonal therapy [25, 29].

Given the strong evidence for treating HH with hormonal therapy, the 2021 European Association of Urology (EAU) Guidelines recommend treating HH with combined hCG and FSH (or pulsatile GnRH) to induce spermatogenesis [30].

In men who have completed hormonal therapy treatment but have been unsuccessful in achieving spontaneous pregnancy, ART may be considered. Generally, this next step is recommended in patients who have completed at least 1 year of hormonal therapy and have sperm concentrations $<1 \times 10^6$/mL or patients with sperm concentrations $>5 \times 10^6$/mL who have failed to impregnate their partners over 20 months [31]. In men who did achieve spermatogenesis after hormonal therapy, 54.5–66.6% had successful ICSI [32, 33].

Androgen and Steroid Excess

In men with HH because of androgen and steroid excess, there are several considerations for management. In men on anabolic steroids or testosterone replacement therapy, the first step is discontinuation of all such hormones. Spermatogenic recovery after discontinuation of exogenous testosterone is variable. In an analysis of studies using testosterone as a short-term hormonal contraceptive, sperm recovery rates were approximately 67% at 6 months, 90% in 12 months, and 100% within 24 months [34]. However, some men may develop irreversible gonadal failure [35]. Spermatogenic recovery likely depends on several factors including age and duration of testosterone use, with higher age and longer use being associated with decreased probability of recovery of spermatogenesis [36].

Androgen excess may also result from endogenous sources. Congenital adrenal hyperplasia causes low cortisol levels, leading to increased adrenocorticotrophic hormone (ACTH), which stimulates adrenal androgen production. This induces negative feedback on gonadotropins and thereby suppresses intratesticular testosterone. Adrenal or testicular tumors, including testicular adrenal rest tumors, can also produce endogenous androgens [12]. In these men, exogenous steroid administration is typically utilized to suppress adrenocorticotrophic hormone (ACTH), potentially followed by the addition of hCG and FSH [37, 38].

Spermatogenic Failure

Hormonal therapy in men with SF is controversial. The use of hormonal therapy prior to testicular sperm extraction (TESE) in men with SF is commonly utilized despite lack of supporting evidence, particularly in men with idiopathic SF [12, 39, 40]. Due to high gonadotropin levels and abnormal testosterone-to-estradiol ratios in these patients, desensitization or downregulation of gonadotropin receptors may impact ITT levels [41, 42]. With this in mind, some groups have found that non-pulsatile administration of a GnRH analog ("gonadotropin reset") followed by hCG and FSH may be successful in inducing spermatogenesis in men with idiopathic NOA [43, 44]. Gonadotropins [41, 45], aromatase inhibitors [46–48], and SERMs [45, 49, 50] have all shown promise in this setting. However, there are no randomized controlled trials analyzing the impact of hormonal therapy in this group, and the available studies have conflicting results. Despite the physiologic rationale for hormonal therapy in this population, there is a lack of convincing evidence and no definitive protocols regarding duration, dose, or type of hormonal therapy. The 2020 American Urological Association (AUA) guidelines recommend that clinicians inform men with NOA that SERMS, aromatase inhibitors, and gonadotropins have limited data to support their use [8]. EAU guidelines also acknowledge that they cannot make conclusive recommendations regarding the use of SERMs or aromatase inhibitors in men with idiopathic infertility [30].

Men with Klinefelter syndrome are one subset of patients that will likely benefit from hormonal therapy. Predictors of successful testicular sperm extraction (TESE) in Klinefelter patients include LH <17.5 U/L, testosterone >250 ng/dL, younger postpubertal age, and normal baseline testosterone-to-estrogen ratio [51–53]. Therefore, it stands to reason that hormonal therapy before TESE may be beneficial in improving sperm retrieval rates (SRRs) in this population. In a study of 68 men with Klinefelter syndrome and low baseline testosterone levels, those who had a positive response to hormonal therapy had a 77% chance of successful TESE, compared to 55% of men who had persistent testosterone levels <250 ng/dl [52].

In men who failed initial TESE, hormonal therapy prior to redo TESE may be considered depending on pathological findings during initial TESE. In men with maturation arrest or hypospermatogenesis, salvage hormonal therapy with clomiphene, hCG, or an FSH-based hormonal therapy may be considered. Sertoli cell-only syndrome, on the other hand, is unlikely to respond to hormonal therapy [54].

Varicocele Repair

In men with NOA and a clinically apparent varicocele, varicocele repair may be considered. Varicocelectomy does improve sperm parameters including sperm concentration and progressive motility [55]. A 2016 meta-analysis looking at men with NOA and varicocele found that 43.9% of patients with NOA were found to have sperm in postoperative semen analysis after varicocelectomy, and this was significantly higher in patients with hypospermatogenesis compared to maturation arrest and Sertoli cell-only syndrome. Of the men who had return of sperm to the ejaculate, 13.6% went on to have an unassisted pregnancy and 18.9% became pregnant with the use of assisted reproductive techniques. When looking at SRR and pregnancy rates, SRR was significantly higher in men who underwent varicocelectomy (odds ratio 2.65), and pregnancy rates were higher in the varicocelectomy group but not statistically significant [56]. However, one study that was not included in the meta-analysis found a lower rate of sperm recovery in the semen (22%, with only 9.6% of men having adequate motile sperm for ICSI). Additionally, they did not find a difference in SRR in men who did or did not have a varicocelectomy, with an overall SRR of 60% in both groups [57]. Of note, previous reports suggest that 10–18% of men with NOA will have spontaneous return of sperm to the ejaculate without intervention [58], making it difficult to draw a definitive conclusion regarding the benefits of pre-TESE varicocelectomy.

Testicular Sperm Extraction

Since the introduction of intracytoplasmic sperm injection (ICSI), testicular sperm extraction (TESE) has made it possible for many men with NOA to successfully father biological children. There are several techniques for sperm extraction including testicular sperm aspiration (TESA), conventional testicular sperm extraction (cTESE), and microdissection testicular sperm extraction (micro-TESE or mTESE) (Table 15.2). TESA is performed by needle aspiration of testicular tissue. cTESE involves an open testicular biopsy, which may consist of a single large biopsy or multiple limited biopsies. In mTESE, first described by Schlegel in 1999, a 20–25× operating microscopic is used to identify the seminiferous tubules most likely to contain spermatozoa. Seminiferous tubules containing developing germ cells are generally larger and more opaque [59].

TESA is not commonly utilized in NOA due to the low likelihood of finding sperm in a random small sample in these patients. A large systematic review found that cTESE was 2.0 times more likely to have successful sperm retrieval compared to TESA (56% and 28% SRR, respectively) [60]. Compared to cTESE, mTESE is generally believed to have improved the SRR in men with NOA. In the original study by Schlegel, SRRs increased from 45% with cTESE to 63% with mTESE [59]. A large systematic review and meta-analysis found that mTESE was 1.5 times more likely to have successful sperm retrieval compared to cTESE (52% and 35% SRR, respectively) [60]. However, a separate systematic review and meta-analysis

Table 15.2 Comparison of testicular sperm extraction techniques

Surgical approach	Advantages	Disadvantages
TESA	• Minimal testicular tissue excised • Minimally invasive, does not require open biopsy • Less postoperative pain [68] • No operating microscope required	• Lowest sperm retrieval rates [60, 68] • Risk of vascular injury due to inability to visualize blood vessels
cTESE	• No operating microscope required • Less time intensive than mTESE	• More testicular tissue removed [59, 126], which may lead to testicular abnormalities (hematoma, fibrosis, testicular atrophy) [62, 63, 69, 70] • Risk of interrupting blood supply to the tunica albuginea [69]
mTESE	• Less testicular tissue removed [59, 126], lowering risk of testicular abnormalities (hematoma, fibrosis, testicular atrophy) [67] • Lower risk of vascular injury due to ability to identify blood vessels in tunica albuginea	• Operating microscope required • Careful examination of seminiferous tubules requires more operating time

TESA testicular sperm aspiration, *cTESE* conventional testicular sperm extraction, *mTESE* microdissection testicular sperm extraction found no significant difference in SRR between cTESE and mTESE, with overall SRR of 47% [61]. Other subsequent studies have also found mTESE SRR rates to be between 42% and 63% [60, 62–67].

There are several potential complications and considerations when choosing a surgical approach for sperm removal (Table 15.2). While TESA is minimally invasive, is of low cost, and excises a minimal amount of testicular tissue, it also has the lowest sperm retrieval rates [60, 68]. cTESE and mTESE are more invasive than TESA, and mTESE requires an operating microscope. In cTESE, the surgeon is unable to identify focal sperm-producing areas until after the tissue is excised, resulting in removal of more testicular tissue. This may lead to testicular abnormalities such as hematoma, fibrosis, and testicular atrophy [62, 63, 69, 70]. The surgeon is able to identify areas more likely to contain sperm under the microscope in an mTESE, allowing for removal of less testicular tissue. When comparing cTESE and mTESE complication rates, mTESE results in fewer hematomas, less testicular fibrosis, and less frequent testicular atrophy [67]. Another advantage of mTESE is the ability to visualize the testicular vessels prior to incision of the tunica albuginea, lowering the risk of vascular injury to the testicle. One potential adverse effect of TESE is decreased postoperative testosterone levels, and this appears to be a risk in both cTESE and mTESE [63]. However, at 18 months, 95% of men return to their baseline testosterone [65].

Testicular mapping via fine-needle aspiration (FNA) before TESE is an alternative approach to sperm retrieval. FNA is performed by sampling various locations (typically up to 18 sites) within the testis to identify areas of spermatogenesis. After a "heat map" is created, TESE is performed using the map as a guide. This may offer a more efficient and less invasive method for identifying areas of spermatogenesis in the testis, as specific biopsy sites can be strategically targeted. In the initial pilot study by Turek and colleagues, FNA mapping was more sensitive and equally specific in detecting sperm compared to open biopsy [71]. Sperm detection rates appear to increase with the number of FNA sites per testicle. A sperm detection rate of 35.7% was identified after using three aspiration sites per testicle [72]. In a separate study using 14 aspiration sites per testicle, sperm detection rate was 47% [73]. Another group found sperm in 58.8% of men with a mean of 15 aspiration sites (range 10–20) per testicle [74]. FNA mapping may also be useful in cases of failed mTESE. In one study, 24 out of 82 men (29%) who previously failed mTESE had at least 1 site of positive sperm on FNA mapping. Of the 24, 15 (62.5%) then underwent successful sperm retrieval [75]. Finally, FNA mapping is useful in obtaining histologic information which can help in prognostication of future TESE success. Indeed, studies have shown high concordance between FNA cytology and open biopsy histology [76–79]. The advantage of this method is that it theoretically reduces the likelihood of missing an area of spermatogenesis. However, viable sperm for ICSI are not obtained during the mapping procedure, and therefore a second TESE procedure is required in these patients, potentially delaying ICSI. Furthermore, FNA mapping may damage the testis and compromise future sperm retrieval. In one large series, 7% of patients who had sperm found on initial mapping later had failed sperm retrievals [80].

Predictors of Successful Sperm Retrieval

Patient Factors

There are several patient factors that have been evaluated as potential predictors of higher sperm retrieval rates (SRRs). A few studies have looked at the age of the patient with NOA as a potential factor with mixed results, but generally age does not appear to strongly influence SRR. One artificial neural network model found that age was a significant predictor of successful sperm retrieval [81]; however, other studies including a large meta-analysis found that age does not appear to influence SRR [61]. This may be explained by the fact that older patients are more likely to have acquired causes of NOA than congenital causes [82].

Similarly, obesity does not appear to influence SRRs [83, 84]; however, it may affect clinical pregnancy rate [84].

Studies analyzing the association between testicular volume and SRR have also had conflicting results. Ghalayini et al. found that increased testicular volume significantly increased SRR by 1.25-fold overall and by 1.31-fold for mTESE [66]. A meta-analysis of men who underwent cTESE or mTESE found that testis volume, specifically a mean volume >12.5 mL, significantly predicted SRR >60% [61]. Other studies have also identified a positive correlation between testicular size and SRR [85]. On the contrary, other studies have not found a significant correlation between testicular volume and SRR [81, 86–88], including a large meta-analysis [89]. Despite this potential correlation, reduced testis volume should not be used as an exclusion criterion for mTESE, as sperm may still be found even in testis <8 ml [61].

Clinical Factors

The etiology of NOA may also be useful in predicting the success of TESE. Idiopathic NOA is associated with an overall SRR (31.8%), but in men with a known source of NOA, we may be able to predict better or worse outcomes [90, 91].

A history of cryptorchidism treated with orchidopexy is generally considered to be a positive predictor of successful sperm retrieval in men with NOA. Men with a history of cryptorchidism have a high SRR up to 84.8% [90, 91], and SRR is significantly higher in these men than those with idiopathic NOA [92]. A predictive model developed via an artificial neural network found cryptorchidism to be a significant predictor of sperm retrieval [81]. It is unclear if age at surgery, unilateral or bilateral cryptorchidism, or testicular volume influences SRR in these patients.

Klinefelter syndrome patients have an overall SRR of 22.5–51.5% [93]. Whether the presence of Klinefelter syndrome itself is predictive of successful sperm retrieval is debated. A meta-analysis showed that SRR decreased as the number of Klinefelter syndrome patients in the population increased [61]. However, a neural computational model evaluating men with NOA found that the presence of Klinefelter syndrome significantly predicted successful sperm retrieval [81]. Several studies have evaluated whether age, testicular volume, or hormone levels influence SRR in Klinefelter patients with mixed findings [52, 53, 94, 95].

Men with Y-chromosome microdeletions have variable SRR depending on the location of the microdeletion. There are no documented cases of successful sperm retrieval in men with complete AZFa or AZFb mutations. Because of these findings, EAU guidelines recommend against TESE in men with AZFa and AZFb microdeletions [30]. Men with AZFc deletions may still have sperm present, and SRRs may be as high as 71–75% [96, 97].

Testicular pathology appears to play the most significant role in predicting success rates of mTESE. Hypospermatogenesis carries the highest SRR of 73–100%. Late maturation arrest has an SRR of 27–86%, while early maturation arrest has an SRR of 27–40%. Sertoli cell-only syndrome, on the other hand, has a lower SRR of 22–41% [67, 98]. One meta-analysis did show that hypospermatogenesis predicted successful sperm retrieval with a sensitivity of 30% and specificity of 98%, while Sertoli cell-only syndrome negatively predicted successful sperm retrieval. Maturation arrest had poor predictive accuracy in the same analysis [89]. Many men will have more than one histopathological finding, and this variety is likely associated with higher probability of sperm retrieval. In one study, SRR was 33% in men with one histologic subtype compared to 94% in men with all four histologic subtypes [99].

When considering a salvage mTESE after a previous failed surgical attempt, prior testis histology may be of use in predicting the chances of success of a repeat procedure. In men who previously underwent cTESE, salvage mTESE yielded SRRs of 39–40% in Sertoli cell-only syndrome, 36–41.7% in maturation arrest, and 75–100% in hypospermatogenesis [100, 101]. Other studies have confirmed a high SRR in men with hypospermatogenesis on repeat mTESE and lower SRR in men with Sertoli cell-only syndrome and maturation arrest [102, 103].

Hormonal Factors

Because of its role in stimulating Sertoli cells, preoperative FSH levels have been evaluated as a potential predictor of successful sperm retrieval. Some studies have demonstrated that increased FSH is associated with lower SRRs [66, 86, 104]. Other studies found little association between FSH levels and SRRs [61, 63, 81, 87, 89] or even a counterintuitive relationship showing higher FSH levels being associated with higher SRR [105]. Despite this potential correlation, high FSH is not a contraindication for mTESE as there may still be sites of sperm production in these men.

Inhibin B has also been investigated due to its role in the hypothalamic-pituitary-gonadal axis. Some studies have identified a positive correlation between inhibin B levels and SRRs [104, 106], while the majority of others have found no association [87, 107, 108]. Overall, inhibin B appears to be a poor predictor of mTESE outcome.

Testosterone may also be considered as a potential predictive factor given its important role in spermatogenesis. One analysis of several studies in men who underwent mTESE found that normal T levels were associated with higher chances of successful sperm retrieval than subnormal T levels [40]. Some studies have found similar results [109, 110], while other studies have found no correlation [111–113].

Other Factors

Surgeon experience correlates with SRR. Ishikawa et al. found that surgeons who have completed 51–100 mTESE procedures have higher SRRs than those who have completed <50 procedures (44% vs. 32%, respectively) [114].

Non-fertility Considerations

Of important note, men with infertility are at increased risks for malignancy, cardiovascular abnormalities, and overall mortality and should be counseled on these risks [115]. Indeed, the AUA guidelines state that men with abnormal semen parameters should be counseled on the health risks associated with abnormal sperm production [8].

Azoospermic men overall have a 2.2-fold increased risk of cancer, particularly those under 30 years old [116]. In some men, such as those with a history of cryptorchidism or Klinefelter syndrome, there is a known predisposition for cancer associated with the etiology of their infertility. In men with idiopathic NOA, there may be genetic and/or environmental factors increasing their risk of infertility as well as their risk of malignancy.

Emerging Technologies and Techniques

There are several areas of investigation that may aid in diagnosis and management of NOA in the future. Detailed genetic evaluation such as karyotyping for chromosomal translocations and next-generation sequencing may be useful in delineating the etiology of azoospermia [117]. Predictive modeling and artificial intelligence may be used to help predict successful sperm retrieval in men with NOA [6].

Several technologies are currently being investigated for their potential to noninvasively identify areas of spermatogenesis in the testis. Multiphoton microscopy (MPM) was successfully used by Ramasamy et al. to differentiate normal and abnormal spermatogenesis [118, 119]. However, there are limits to this technology including the narrow field of view, potential for motion artifact, and concern for the possible mutagenic potential of lasers on spermatozoa [6]. Full-field optical coherence tomography (FFOCT) may also be useful in identifying spermatozoa [120]. However, visualization is limited to a depth of 1–2 mm, and the level of detail is limited [6]. Metabolomic scanning is also being investigated. By identifying unique chemical signatures associated with various histological states of spermatogenesis, high-resolution magic angle spinning spectroscopy can be used to predict sperm presence in the testis [121]. Raman spectroscopy can also identify areas of spermatogenesis [122, 123], but requires the creation of a customized algorithm [6].

Robotic mTESE procedures have been successfully performed and may offer some advantages to conventional microscopic procedures [124]. Additionally, robotic systems offer high-resolution magnification and may be useful for incorporating MPM or FFOCT intraoperatively in the future [6].

There are several biological therapies that may also be future therapeutic options for men with NOA. Spermatogonial stem cell (SSC) transplantation is currently in the experimental phases but has shown promising results in animal models [125]. The use of embryonic and adult stem cells may also be a potential future therapeutic option; however, embryonic stem cell use is limited by ethical concerns, and adult stem cells require the use of oncogenic factors to induce differentiation into germ cells [125]. Gene therapy may also be considered; however, the exact genetic defect is typically unknown in men with NOA, which would limit the use of this technology. Additionally, there are financial, ethical, and safety concerns to overcome [125].

References

1. Agarwal A, Mulgund A, Hamada A, Chyatte MR. A unique view on male infertility around the globe. Reprod Biol Endocrinol. 2015;13(1) https://doi.org/10.1186/s12958-015-0032-1.
2. Olesen IA, Andersson AM, Aksglaede L, et al. Clinical, genetic, biochemical, and testicular biopsy findings among 1,213 men evaluated for infertility. Fertil Steril. 2017;107(1):74–82.e7. https://doi.org/10.1016/j.fertnstert.2016.09.015.
3. Jarow JP, Espeland MA, Lipshultz LI. Evaluation of the azoospermic patient. J Urol. 1989;142(1):62–5. https://doi.org/10.1016/s0022-5347(17)38662-7.
4. Willott GM. Frequency of Azospermia. Forensic Sci Int. 1982;20:9–10.
5. Cocuzza M, Alvarenga C, Pagani R. The epidemiology and etiology of azoospermia. Clinics. 2013;68:15–26. https://doi.org/10.6061/clinics/2013(Sup01)03.
6. Tharakan T, Luo R, Jayasena CN, Minhas S. Non-obstructive azoospermia: current and future perspectives. Fac Rev. 2021;10:7. https://doi.org/10.12703/r/10-7.
7. Andrade DL, Viana MC, Esteves SC. Differential diagnosis of azoospermia in men with infertility. J Clin Med. 2021;10(14):3144. https://doi.org/10.3390/jcm10143144.
8. Schlegel PN, Sigman M, Collura B, et al. Diagnosis and treatment of infertility in men: AUA/ASRM guideline part I. Fertil Steril. 2021;115(1):54–61. https://doi.org/10.1016/j.fertnstert.2020.11.015.
9. Foresta C, Moro E, Ferlin A. Y chromosome microdeletions and alterations of spermatogenesis. Endocr Rev. 2001;22(2):226–39. https://doi.org/10.1210/edrv.22.2.0425.
10. McLachlan RI, Rajpert-De Meyts E, Hoei-Hansen CE, de Kretser DM, Skakkebaek NE. Histological evaluation of the human testis—approaches to optimizing the clinical value of the assessment: mini review. Hum Reprod. 2007;22(1):2–16. https://doi.org/10.1093/humrep/del279.

11. Tharakan T, Corona G, Foran D, et al. Does hormonal therapy improve sperm retrieval rates in men with non-obstructive azoospermia: a systematic review and meta-analysis. Hum Reprod Update. 2022;28(5):609–28. https://doi.org/10.1093/humupd/dmac016.
12. Kim HH, Schlegel PN. Endocrine manipulation in male infertility. Urol Clin North Am. 2008;35(2):303–18., x. https://doi.org/10.1016/j.ucl.2008.01.003.
13. Buchter D, Behre HM, Kliesch S, Nieschlag E. Pulsatile GnRH or human chorionic gonadotropin/human menopausal gonadotropin as effective treatment for men with hypogonadotropic hypogonadism: a review of 42 cases. Eur J Endocrinol. 1998;139(3):298–303. https://doi.org/10.1530/eje.0.1390298.
14. Kliesch S, Behre HM, Nieschlag E. High efficacy of gonadotropin or pulsatile gonadotropin-releasing hormone treatment in hypogonadotropic hypogonadal men. Eur J Endocrinol. 1994;131(4):347–54. https://doi.org/10.1530/eje.0.1310347.
15. Rastrelli G, Corona G, Mannucci E, Maggi M. Factors affecting spermatogenesis upon gonadotropin-replacement therapy: a meta-analytic study. Andrology. 2014;2(6):794–808. https://doi.org/10.1111/andr.262.
16. Liu L, Banks SM, Barnes KM, Sherins RJ. Two-year comparison of testicular responses to pulsatile gonadotropin-releasing hormone and exogenous gonadotropins from the inception of therapy in men with isolated hypogonadotropic hypogonadism. J Clin Endocrinol Metab. 1988;67(6):1140–5. https://doi.org/10.1210/jcem-67-6-1140.
17. Bouloux P, Warne DW, Loumaye E. Infertility FSHSGiMs. Efficacy and safety of recombinant human follicle-stimulating hormone in men with isolated hypogonadotropic hypogonadism. Fertil Steril. 2002;77(2):270–3. https://doi.org/10.1016/s0015-0282(01)02973-9.
18. Burgues S, Calderon MD. Subcutaneous self-administration of highly purified follicle stimulating hormone and human chorionic gonadotrophin for the treatment of male hypogonadotrophic hypogonadism. Spanish Collaborative Group on Male Hypogonadotropic Hypogonadism. Hum Reprod. 1997;12(5):980–6. https://doi.org/10.1093/humrep/12.5.980.
19. Burris AS, Rodbard HW, Winters SJ, Sherins RJ. Gonadotropin therapy in men with isolated hypogonadotropic hypogonadism: the response to human chorionic gonadotropin is predicted by initial testicular size. J Clin Endocrinol Metab. 1988;66(6):1144–51. https://doi.org/10.1210/jcem-66-6-1144.
20. Delemarre-Van de Waal HA. Induction of testicular growth and spermatogenesis by pulsatile, intravenous administration of gonadotrophin-releasing hormone in patients with hypogonadotrophic hypogonadism. Clin Endocrinol (Oxf). 1993;38(5):473–80. https://doi.org/10.1111/j.1365-2265.1993.tb00342.x.
21. Group EMHS. Efficacy and safety of highly purified urinary follicle-stimulating hormone with human chorionic gonadotropin for treating men with isolated hypogonadotropic hypogonadism. European Metrodin HP Study Group. Fertil Steril. 1998;70(2):256–62. https://doi.org/10.1016/s0015-0282(98)00156-3.
22. Vicari E, Mongioi A, Calogero AE, et al. Therapy with human chorionic gonadotrophin alone induces spermatogenesis in men with isolated hypogonadotrophic hypogonadism—long-term follow-up. Int J Androl. 1992;15(4):320–9. https://doi.org/10.1111/j.1365-2605.1992.tb01131.x.
23. Yang L, Zhang SX, Dong Q, Xiong ZB, Li X. Application of hormonal treatment in hypogonadotropic hypogonadism: more than ten years experience. Int Urol Nephrol. 2012;44(2):393–9. https://doi.org/10.1007/s11255-011-0065-0.
24. Farhat R, Al-zidjali F, Alzahrani AS. Outcome of gonadotropin therapy for male infertility due to hypogonadotrophic hypogonadism. Pituitary. 2010;13(2):105–10. https://doi.org/10.1007/s11102-009-0203-1.
25. Liu PY, Gebski VJ, Turner L, Conway AJ, Wishart SM, Handelsman DJ. Predicting pregnancy and spermatogenesis by survival analysis during gonadotrophin treatment of gonadotrophin-deficient infertile men. Hum Reprod. 2002;17(3):625–33. https://doi.org/10.1093/humrep/17.3.625.

26. Miyagawa Y, Tsujimura A, Matsumiya K, et al. Outcome of gonadotropin therapy for male hypogonadotropic hypogonadism at university affiliated male infertility centers: a 30-year retrospective study. J Urol. 2005;173(6):2072–5. https://doi.org/10.1097/01.ju.0000158133.09197.f4.
27. Finkel DM, Phillips JL, Snyder PJ. Stimulation of spermatogenesis by gonadotropins in men with hypogonadotropic hypogonadism. N Engl J Med. 1985;313(11):651–5. https://doi.org/10.1056/NEJM198509123131102.
28. Kirk JM, Savage MO, Grant DB, Bouloux PM, Besser GM. Gonadal function and response to human chorionic and menopausal gonadotrophin therapy in male patients with idiopathic hypogonadotrophic hypogonadism. Clin Endocrinol. 1994;41(1):57–63. https://doi.org/10.1111/j.1365-2265.1994.tb03785.x.
29. Pitteloud N, Hayes FJ, Dwyer A, Boepple PA, Lee H, Crowley WF Jr. Predictors of outcome of long-term GnRH therapy in men with idiopathic hypogonadotropic hypogonadism. J Clin Endocrinol Metab. 2002;87(9):4128–36. https://doi.org/10.1210/jc.2002-020518.
30. Minhas S, Bettocchi C, Boeri L, et al. European Association of Urology guidelines on male sexual and reproductive health: 2021 update on male infertility. Eur Urol. 2021;80(5):603–20. https://doi.org/10.1016/j.eururo.2021.08.014.
31. Fraietta R, Zylberstejn DS, Esteves SC. Hypogonadotropic hypogonadism revisited. Clinics (Sao Paulo). 2013;68(Suppl 1):81–8. https://doi.org/10.6061/clinics/2013(sup01)09.
32. Bakircioglu ME, Erden HF, Ciray HN, Bayazit N, Bahceci M. Gonadotrophin therapy in combination with ICSI in men with hypogonadotrophic hypogonadism. Reprod Biomed Online. 2007;15(2):156–60. https://doi.org/10.1016/s1472-6483(10)60703-1.
33. Zorn B, Pfeifer M, Virant-Klun I, Meden-Vrtovec H. Intracytoplasmic sperm injection as a complement to gonadotrophin treatment in infertile men with hypogonadotrophic hypogonadism. Int J Androl. 2005;28(4):202–7. https://doi.org/10.1111/j.1365-2605.2004.00519.x.
34. Liu PY, Swerdloff RS, Christenson PD, Handelsman DJ, Wang C. Hormonal Male Contraception Summit G. Rate, extent, and modifiers of spermatogenic recovery after hormonal male contraception: an integrated analysis. Lancet. 2006;367(9520):1412–20. https://doi.org/10.1016/S0140-6736(06)68614-5.
35. Boregowda K, Joels L, Stephens JW, Price DE. Persistent primary hypogonadism associated with anabolic steroid abuse. Fertil Steril. 2011;96(1):e7–8. https://doi.org/10.1016/j.fertnstert.2011.04.029.
36. Kohn TP, Louis MR, Pickett SM, et al. Age and duration of testosterone therapy predict time to return of sperm count after human chorionic gonadotropin therapy. Fertil Steril. 2017;107(2):351–357.e1. https://doi.org/10.1016/j.fertnstert.2016.10.004.
37. Claahsen-van der Grinten HL, Otten BJ, Sweep FC, Hermus AR. Repeated successful induction of fertility after replacing hydrocortisone with dexamethasone in a patient with congenital adrenal hyperplasia and testicular adrenal rest tumors. Fertil Steril. 2007;88(3):705 e5–8. https://doi.org/10.1016/j.fertnstert.2006.11.148.
38. Patel DP, Chandrapal JC, Hotaling JM. Hormone-based treatments in subfertile males. Curr Urol Rep. 2016;17(8):56. https://doi.org/10.1007/s11934-016-0612-4.
39. Tharakan T, Salonia A, Corona G, Dhillo W, Minhas S, Jayasena C. The role of hormone stimulation in men with nonobstructive azoospermia undergoing surgical sperm retrieval. J Clin Endocrinol Metab. 2020;105(12) https://doi.org/10.1210/clinem/dgaa556.
40. Caroppo E, Colpi GM. Hormonal treatment of men with nonobstructive azoospermia: what does the evidence suggest? J Clin Med. 2021;10(3):387. https://doi.org/10.3390/jcm10030387.
41. Shiraishi K, Ohmi C, Shimabukuro T, Matsuyama H. Human chorionic gonadotrophin treatment prior to microdissection testicular sperm extraction in non-obstructive azoospermia. Hum Reprod. 2012;27(2):331–9. https://doi.org/10.1093/humrep/der404.
42. Levalle OA, Zylbersztein C, Aszpis S, et al. Serum luteinizing hormone pulsatility and intratesticular testosterone and oestradiol concentrations in idiopathic infertile men with high and

normal follicle stimulating hormone serum concentrations. Hum Reprod. 1994;9(5):781–7. https://doi.org/10.1093/oxfordjournals.humrep.a138596.
43. Foresta C, Selice R, Moretti A, et al. Gonadotropin administration after gonadotropin-releasing-hormone agonist: a therapeutic option in severe testiculopathies. Fertil Steril. 2009;92(4):1326–32. https://doi.org/10.1016/j.fertnstert.2008.07.1766.
44. Hu X, Ding Z, Hong Z, et al. Spermatogenesis improved by suppressing the high level of endogenous gonadotropins in idiopathic non-obstructive azoospermia: a case control pilot study. Reprod Biol Endocrinol. 2018;16(1) https://doi.org/10.1186/s12958-018-0401-7.
45. Hussein A, Ozgok Y, Ross L, Rao P, Niederberger C. Optimization of spermatogenesis-regulating hormones in patients with non-obstructive azoospermia and its impact on sperm retrieval: a multicentre study. BJU Int. 2013;111(3 Pt B):E110–4. https://doi.org/10.1111/j.1464-410X.2012.11485.x.
46. Del Giudice F, Busetto GM, De Berardinis E, et al. A systematic review and meta-analysis of clinical trials implementing aromatase inhibitors to treat male infertility. Asian J Androl. 2020;22(4):360–7. https://doi.org/10.4103/aja.aja_101_19.
47. Pavlovich CP, King P, Goldstein M, Schlegel PN. Evidence of a treatable endocrinopathy in infertile men. J Urol. 2001;165(3):837–41.
48. Raman JD, Schlegel PN. Aromatase inhibitors for male infertility. J Urol. 2002;167(2 Pt 1):624–9. https://doi.org/10.1097/00005392-200202000-00038.
49. Hussein A, Ozgok Y, Ross L, Niederberger C. Clomiphene administration for cases of nonobstructive azoospermia: a multicenter study. J Androl. 2005;26(6):787–91.; discussion 792-3. https://doi.org/10.2164/jandrol.04180.
50. Moein MR, Tabibnejad N, Ghasemzadeh J. Beneficial effect of tamoxifen on sperm recovery in infertile men with nonobstructive azoospermia. Andrologia. 2012;44(Suppl 1):194–8. https://doi.org/10.1111/j.1439-0272.2011.01163.x.
51. Mehta A, Paduch DA. Klinefelter syndrome: an argument for early aggressive hormonal and fertility management. Fertil Steril. 2012;98(2):274–83. https://doi.org/10.1016/j.fertnstert.2012.06.001.
52. Ramasamy R, Ricci JA, Palermo GD, Gosden LV, Rosenwaks Z, Schlegel PN. Successful fertility treatment for Klinefelter's syndrome. J Urol. 2009;182(3):1108–13. https://doi.org/10.1016/j.juro.2009.05.019.
53. Rohayem J, Fricke R, Czeloth K, et al. Age and markers of Leydig cell function, but not of Sertoli cell function predict the success of sperm retrieval in adolescents and adults with Klinefelter's syndrome. Andrology. 2015;3(5):868–75. https://doi.org/10.1111/andr.12067.
54. Shiraishi K. Hormonal therapy for non-obstructive azoospermia: basic and clinical perspectives. Reprod Med Biol. 2015;14(2):65–72. https://doi.org/10.1007/s12522-014-0193-1.
55. Baazeem A, Belzile E, Ciampi A, et al. Varicocele and male factor infertility treatment: a new meta-analysis and review of the role of varicocele repair. Eur Urol. 2011;60(4):796–808. https://doi.org/10.1016/j.eururo.2011.06.018.
56. Esteves SC, Miyaoka R, Roque M, Agarwal A. Outcome of varicocele repair in men with nonobstructive azoospermia: systematic review and meta-analysis. Asian J Androl. 2016;18(2):246–53. https://doi.org/10.4103/1008-682X.169562.
57. Schlegel PN, Kaufmann J. Role of varicocelectomy in men with nonobstructive azoospermia. Fertil Steril. 2004;81(6):1585–8. https://doi.org/10.1016/j.fertnstert.2003.10.036.
58. Flannigan RK, Schlegel PN. Microdissection testicular sperm extraction: preoperative patient optimization, surgical technique, and tissue processing. Fertil Steril. 2019;111(3):420–6. https://doi.org/10.1016/j.fertnstert.2019.01.003.
59. Schlegel PN. Testicular sperm extraction: microdissection improves sperm yield with minimal tissue excision. Hum Reprod. 1999;14(1):131–5.
60. Bernie AM, Mata DA, Ramasamy R, Schlegel PN. Comparison of microdissection testicular sperm extraction, conventional testicular sperm extraction, and testicular sperm aspiration for nonobstructive azoospermia: a systematic review and meta-analysis. Fertil Steril. 2015;104(5):1099–103.e1-3. https://doi.org/10.1016/j.fertnstert.2015.07.1136.

61. Corona G, Minhas S, Giwercman A, et al. Sperm recovery and ICSI outcomes in men with non-obstructive azoospermia: a systematic review and meta-analysis. Hum Reprod Update. 2019;25(6):733–57. https://doi.org/10.1093/humupd/dmz028.
62. Amer M, Ateyah A, Hany R, Zohdy W. Prospective comparative study between microsurgical and conventional testicular sperm extraction in non-obstructive azoospermia: follow-up by serial ultrasound examinations. Hum Reprod. 2000;15(3):653–6. https://doi.org/10.1093/humrep/15.3.653.
63. Okada H, Dobashi M, Yamazaki T, et al. Conventional versus microdissection testicular sperm extraction for nonobstructive azoospermia. J Urol. 2002;168(3):1063–7. https://doi.org/10.1097/01.ju.0000025397.03586.c4.
64. Tsujimura A, Matsumiya K, Miyagawa Y, et al. Conventional multiple or microdissection testicular sperm extraction: a comparative study. Hum Reprod. 2002;17(11):2924–9. https://doi.org/10.1093/humrep/17.11.2924.
65. Ramasamy R, Yagan N, Schlegel PN. Structural and functional changes to the testis after conventional versus microdissection testicular sperm extraction. Urology. 2005;65(6):1190–4. https://doi.org/10.1016/j.urology.2004.12.059.
66. Ghalayini IF, Al-Ghazo MA, Hani OB, et al. Clinical comparison of conventional testicular sperm extraction and microdissection techniques for non-obstructive azoospermia. J Clin Med Res. 2011;3(3):124–31. https://doi.org/10.4021/jocmr542w.
67. Deruyver Y, Vanderschueren D, Van Der Aa F. Outcome of microdissection TESE compared with conventional TESE in non-obstructive azoospermia: a systematic review. Andrology. 2014;2(1):20–4. https://doi.org/10.1111/j.2047-2927.2013.00148.x.
68. Tournaye H. Surgical sperm recovery for intracytoplasmic sperm injection: which method is to be preferred? Hum Reprod. 1999;14(Suppl 1):71–81. https://doi.org/10.1093/humrep/14.suppl_1.71.
69. Schlegel PN, Su LM. Physiological consequences of testicular sperm extraction. Hum Reprod. 1997;12(8):1688–92. https://doi.org/10.1093/humrep/12.8.1688.
70. Donoso P, Tournaye H, Devroey P. Which is the best sperm retrieval technique for non-obstructive azoospermia? A systematic review. Hum Reprod Update. 2007;13(6):539–49. https://doi.org/10.1093/humupd/dmm029.
71. Turek PJ, Cha I, Ljung BM. Systematic fine-needle aspiration of the testis: correlation to biopsy and results of organ "mapping" for mature sperm in azoospermic men. Urology. 1997;49(5):743–8. https://doi.org/10.1016/S0090-4295(97)00154-4.
72. Weiss DB, Gottschalk-Sabag S, Bar-On E, Zukerman Z, Gat Y, Bartoov B. [Seminiferous tubule cytological pattern in infertile, azoospermic men in diagnosis and therapy]. Harefuah. 1997;132(9):614–8, 680.
73. Meng MV, Cha I, Ljung BM, Turek PJ. Relationship between classic histological pattern and sperm findings on fine needle aspiration map in infertile men. Hum Reprod. 2000;15(9):1973–7. https://doi.org/10.1093/humrep/15.9.1973.
74. Lewin A, Reubinoff B, Porat-Katz A, et al. Testicular fine needle aspiration: the alternative method for sperm retrieval in non-obstructive azoospermia. Hum Reprod. 1999;14(7):1785–90. https://doi.org/10.1093/humrep/14.7.1785.
75. Jarvis S, Yee HK, Thomas N, et al. Sperm fine-needle aspiration (FNA) mapping after failed microdissection testicular sperm extraction (TESE): location and patterns of found sperm. Asian J Androl. 2018;21(1):50–5. https://doi.org/10.4103/aja.aja_68_18.
76. Aridogan IA, Bayazit Y, Yaman M, Ersoz C, Doran S. Comparison of fine-needle aspiration and open biopsy of testis in sperm retrieval and histopathologic diagnosis. Andrologia. 2003;35(2):121–5. https://doi.org/10.1046/j.1439-0272.2003.00547.x.
77. Qublan HS, Al-Jader KM, Al-Kaisi NS, et al. Fine needle aspiration cytology compared with open biopsy histology for the diagnosis of azoospermia. J Obstet Gynaecol. 2002;22(5):527–31. https://doi.org/10.1080/0144361021000003690.

78. Meng MV, Cha I, Ljung BM, Turek PJ. Testicular fine-needle aspiration in infertile men: correlation of cytologic pattern with biopsy histology. Am J Surg Pathol. 2001;25(1):71–9. https://doi.org/10.1097/00000478-200101000-00008.
79. Mahajan AD, Ali NI, Walwalkar SJ, Rege JD, Pathak HR. The role of fine-needle aspiration cytology of the testis in the diagnostic evaluation of infertility. BJU Int. 1999;84(4):485–8. https://doi.org/10.1046/j.1464-410x.1999.00169.x.
80. Turek PJ, Ljung BM, Cha I, Conaghan J. Diagnostic findings from testis fine needle aspiration mapping in obstructed and nonobstructed azoospermic men. J Urol. 2000;163(6):1709–16.
81. Ramasamy R, Padilla WO, Osterberg EC, et al. A comparison of models for predicting sperm retrieval before microdissection testicular sperm extraction in men with nonobstructive azoospermia. J Urol. 2013;189(2):638–42. https://doi.org/10.1016/j.juro.2012.09.038.
82. Ramasamy R, Trivedi NN, Reifsnyder JE, Palermo GD, Rosenwaks Z, Schlegel PN. Age does not adversely affect sperm retrieval in men undergoing microdissection testicular sperm extraction. Fertil Steril. 2014;101(3):653–5. https://doi.org/10.1016/j.fertnstert.2013.11.123.
83. Iwatsuki S, Sasaki S, Taguchi K, et al. Effect of obesity on sperm retrieval outcome and reproductive hormone levels in Japanese azoospermic men with and without Klinefelter syndrome. Andrology. 2017;5(1):82–6. https://doi.org/10.1111/andr.12281.
84. Ramasamy R, Bryson C, Reifsnyder JE, Neri Q, Palermo GD, Schlegel PN. Overweight men with nonobstructive azoospermia have worse pregnancy outcomes after microdissection testicular sperm extraction. Fertil Steril. 2013;99(2):372–6. https://doi.org/10.1016/j.fertnstert.2012.10.025.
85. Kizilkan Y, Toksoz S, Turunc T, Ozkardes H. Parameters predicting sperm retrieval rates during microscopic testicular sperm extraction in nonobstructive azoospermia. Andrologia. 2019;51(11):e13441. https://doi.org/10.1111/and.13441.
86. Colpi GM, Colpi EM, Piediferro G, et al. Microsurgical TESE versus conventional TESE for ICSI in non-obstructive azoospermia: a randomized controlled study. Reprod Biomed Online. 2009;18(3):315–9. https://doi.org/10.1016/s1472-6483(10)60087-9.
87. Tunc L, Kirac M, Gurocak S, et al. Can serum Inhibin B and FSH levels, testicular histology and volume predict the outcome of testicular sperm extraction in patients with nonobstructive azoospermia? Int Urol Nephrol. 2006;38(3–4):629–35. https://doi.org/10.1007/s11255-006-0095-1.
88. Bryson CF, Ramasamy R, Sheehan M, Palermo GD, Rosenwaks Z, Schlegel PN. Severe testicular atrophy does not affect the success of microdissection testicular sperm extraction. J Urol. 2014;191(1):175–8. https://doi.org/10.1016/j.juro.2013.07.065.
89. Li H, Chen LP, Yang J, et al. Predictive value of FSH, testicular volume, and histopathological findings for the sperm retrieval rate of microdissection TESE in nonobstructive azoospermia: a meta-analysis. Asian J Androl. 2018;20(1):30–6. https://doi.org/10.4103/aja.aja_5_17.
90. Bernie AM, Ramasamy R, Schlegel PN. Predictive factors of successful microdissection testicular sperm extraction. Basic Clin Androl. 2013;23:5. https://doi.org/10.1186/2051-4190-23-5.
91. Chen X, Ma Y, Zou S, et al. Comparison and outcomes of nonobstructive azoospermia patients with different etiology undergoing MicroTESE and ICSI treatments. Transl Androl Urol. 2019;8(4):366–73. https://doi.org/10.21037/tau.2019.04.08.
92. Kim SW, Lee J, Lee TH, Kim DS, Song S-H, Kim DK. Azoospermic men with a history of cryptorchidism treated by orchiopexy have favorable outcomes after testicular sperm extraction: a systematic review and meta-analysis. World J Men's Health. 2022;40 https://doi.org/10.5534/wjmh.210198.
93. Arshad MA, Majzoub A, Esteves SC. Predictors of surgical sperm retrieval in non-obstructive azoospermia: summary of current literature. Int Urol Nephrol. 2020;52(11):2015–38. https://doi.org/10.1007/s11255-020-02529-4.
94. Okada H, Goda K, Yamamoto Y, et al. Age as a limiting factor for successful sperm retrieval in patients with nonmosaic Klinefelter's syndrome. Fertil Steril. 2005;84(6):1662–4. https://doi.org/10.1016/j.fertnstert.2005.05.053.

95. Vernaeve V, Staessen C, Verheyen G, Van Steirteghem A, Devroey P, Tournaye H. Can biological or clinical parameters predict testicular sperm recovery in 47,XXY Klinefelter's syndrome patients? Hum Reprod. 2004;19(5):1135–9. https://doi.org/10.1093/humrep/deh253.
96. Stahl PJ, Masson P, Mielnik A, Marean MB, Schlegel PN, Paduch DA. A decade of experience emphasizes that testing for Y microdeletions is essential in American men with azoospermia and severe oligozoospermia. Fertil Steril. 2010;94(5):1753–6. https://doi.org/10.1016/j.fertnstert.2009.09.006.
97. Hopps CV. Detection of sperm in men with Y chromosome microdeletions of the AZFa, AZFb and AZFc regions. Human Reprod. 2003;18(8):1660–5. https://doi.org/10.1093/humrep/deg348.
98. Caroppo E, Colpi EM, Gazzano G, et al. Testicular histology may predict the successful sperm retrieval in patients with non-obstructive azoospermia undergoing conventional TESE: a diagnostic accuracy study. J Assist Reprod Genet. 2017;34(1):149–54. https://doi.org/10.1007/s10815-016-0812-3.
99. Punjani N, Flannigan R, Kang C, Khani F, Schlegel PN. Quantifying heterogeneity of testicular histopathology in men with nonobstructive azoospermia. J Urol. 2021;206(5):1268–75. https://doi.org/10.1097/JU.0000000000001951.
100. Kalsi JS, Shah P, Thum Y, Muneer A, Ralph DJ, Minhas S. Salvage micro-dissection testicular sperm extraction; outcome in men with non-obstructive azoospermia with previous failed sperm retrievals. BJU Int. 2015;116(3):460–5. https://doi.org/10.1111/bju.12932.
101. Tsujimura A, Miyagawa Y, Takao T, et al. Salvage microdissection testicular sperm extraction after failed conventional testicular sperm extraction in patients with nonobstructive azoospermia. J Urol. 2006;175(4):1446–9.; discussion 1449. https://doi.org/10.1016/S0022-5347(05)00678-6.
102. Xu T, Peng L, Lin X, Li J, Xu W. Predictors for successful sperm retrieval of salvage microdissection testicular sperm extraction (TESE) following failed TESE in nonobstructive azoospermia patients. Andrologia. 2017;49(4) https://doi.org/10.1111/and.12642.
103. Caroppo E, Castiglioni F, Campagna C, et al. Intrasurgical parameters associated with successful sperm retrieval in patients with non-obstructive azoospermia undergoing salvage microdissection testicular sperm extraction. Andrology. 2021;9(6):1864–71. https://doi.org/10.1111/andr.13082.
104. Bohring C, Schroeder-Printzen I, Weidner W, Krause W. Serum levels of inhibin B and follicle-stimulating hormone may predict successful sperm retrieval in men with azoospermia who are undergoing testicular sperm extraction. Fertil Steril. 2002;78(6):1195–8. https://doi.org/10.1016/s0015-0282(02)04259-0.
105. Ramasamy R, Lin K, Gosden LV, Rosenwaks Z, Palermo GD, Schlegel PN. High serum FSH levels in men with nonobstructive azoospermia does not affect success of microdissection testicular sperm extraction. Fertil Steril. 2009;92(2):590–3. https://doi.org/10.1016/j.fertnstert.2008.07.1703.
106. Ballesca JL, Balasch J, Calafell JM, et al. Serum inhibin B determination is predictive of successful testicular sperm extraction in men with non-obstructive azoospermia. Hum Reprod. 2000;15(8):1734–8. https://doi.org/10.1093/humrep/15.8.1734.
107. Mitchell V, Boitrelle F, Pigny P, et al. Seminal plasma levels of anti-Mullerian hormone and inhibin B are not predictive of testicular sperm retrieval in nonobstructive azoospermia: a study of 139 men. Fertil Steril. 2010;94(6):2147–50. https://doi.org/10.1016/j.fertnstert.2009.11.046.
108. Vernaeve V, Tournaye H, Schiettecatte J, Verheyen G, Van Steirteghem A, Devroey P. Serum inhibin B cannot predict testicular sperm retrieval in patients with non-obstructive azoospermia. Hum Reprod. 2002;17(4):971–6. https://doi.org/10.1093/humrep/17.4.971.
109. Cayan S, Orhan I, Altay B, et al. Fertility outcomes and predictors for successful sperm retrieval and pregnancy in 327 azoospermic men with a history of cryptorchidism who underwent microdissection testicular sperm extraction. Andrology. 2021;9(1):253–9. https://doi.org/10.1111/andr.12910.

110. Mehmood S, Aldaweesh S, Junejo NN, Altaweel WM, Kattan SA, Alhathal N. Microdissection testicular sperm extraction: Overall results and impact of preoperative testosterone level on sperm retrieval rate in patients with nonobstructive azoospermia. Urol Ann. 2019;11(3):287–93. https://doi.org/10.4103/UA.UA_36_18.
111. Reifsnyder JE, Ramasamy R, Husseini J, Schlegel PN. Role of optimizing testosterone before microdissection testicular sperm extraction in men with nonobstructive azoospermia. J Urol. 2012;188(2):532–6. https://doi.org/10.1016/j.juro.2012.04.002.
112. Enatsu N, Miyake H, Chiba K, Fujisawa M. Predictive factors of successful sperm retrieval on microdissection testicular sperm extraction in Japanese men. Reprod Med Biol. 2016;15(1):29–33. https://doi.org/10.1007/s12522-015-0212-x.
113. Althakafi SA, Mustafa OM, Seyam RM, Al-Hathal N, Kattan S. Serum testosterone levels and other determinants of sperm retrieval in microdissection testicular sperm extraction. Transl Androl Urol. 2017;6(2):282–7. https://doi.org/10.21037/tau.2017.02.04.
114. Ishikawa T, Nose R, Yamaguchi K, Chiba K, Fujisawa M. Learning curves of microdissection testicular sperm extraction for nonobstructive azoospermia. Fertil Steril. 2010;94(3):1008–11. https://doi.org/10.1016/j.fertnstert.2009.03.108.
115. Glazer CH, Bonde JP, Eisenberg ML, et al. Male infertility and risk of nonmalignant chronic diseases: a systematic review of the epidemiological evidence. Semin Reprod Med. 2017;35(3):282–90. https://doi.org/10.1055/s-0037-1603568.
116. Eisenberg ML, Betts P, Herder D, Lamb DJ, Lipshultz LI. Increased risk of cancer among azoospermic men. Fertil Steril. 2013;100(3):681–5. https://doi.org/10.1016/j.fertnstert.2013.05.022.
117. Punjani N, Kang C, Lamb DJ, Schlegel PN. Current updates and future perspectives in the evaluation of azoospermia: a systematic review. Arab J Urol. 2021;19(3):206–14. https://doi.org/10.1080/2090598x.2021.1954415.
118. Ramasamy R, Sterling J, Fisher ES, et al. Identification of spermatogenesis with multiphoton microscopy: an evaluation in a rodent model. J Urol. 2011;186(6):2487–92. https://doi.org/10.1016/j.juro.2011.07.081.
119. Najari BB, Ramasamy R, Sterling J, et al. Pilot study of the correlation of multiphoton tomography of ex vivo human testis with histology. J Urol. 2012;188(2):538–43. https://doi.org/10.1016/j.juro.2012.03.124.
120. Ramasamy R, Sterling J, Manzoor M, et al. Full field optical coherence tomography can identify spermatogenesis in a rodent Sertoli-cell only model. J Pathol Inform. 2012;3:4. https://doi.org/10.4103/2153-3539.93401.
121. Aaronson DS, Iman R, Walsh TJ, Kurhanewicz J, Turek PJ. A novel application of 1H magnetic resonance spectroscopy: non-invasive identification of spermatogenesis in men with non-obstructive azoospermia. Hum Reprod. 2010;25(4):847–52. https://doi.org/10.1093/humrep/dep475.
122. Liu Y, Zhu Y, Di L, et al. Raman spectroscopy as an ex vivo noninvasive approach to distinguish complete and incomplete spermatogenesis within human seminiferous tubules. Fertil Steril. 2014;102(1):54–60.e2. https://doi.org/10.1016/j.fertnstert.2014.03.035.
123. Osterberg EC, Laudano MA, Ramasamy R, et al. Identification of spermatogenesis in a rat Sertoli-cell only model using Raman spectroscopy: a feasibility study. J Urol. 2014;192(2):607–12. https://doi.org/10.1016/j.juro.2014.01.106.
124. Parekattil SJ, Gudeloglu A. Robotic assisted andrological surgery. Asian J Androl. 2013;15(1):67–74. https://doi.org/10.1038/aja.2012.131.
125. Vij SC, Sabanegh E Jr, Agarwal A. Biological therapy for non-obstructive azoospermia. Expert Opin Biol Ther. 2018;18(1):19–23. https://doi.org/10.1080/14712598.2018.1380622.
126. Amer M, Ateyah A, Zohdy W, Abd El Nasser T, Abdel-Malak G, Fakhry E. Preoperative and intraoperative factors that predict difficult testicular sperm retrieval in patients with nonobstructive azoospermia. Fertil Steril. 2002;78(3):646–7. https://doi.org/10.1016/s0015-0282(02)03273-9.

Chapter 16
Alternative Approaches to the Treatment of Male Infertility

Taymour Mostafa and Tan V. Le

Key Points

- Recent environmental, nutrition, and lifestyle changes may be related to male infertility. Modifiable risk factors for male infertility still remain an essential subject for continuous research.
- Male reproductive health may be affected by multiple factors, such as physical exercise, obesity, nutrients, alcohol, scrotal temperature, clothing, hot water, and mobile phones.
- Psychological and behavioral therapies are unquestionably necessary for the treatment of psychologically related male infertility.
- Herbal medications and acupuncture have been used to treat male infertility since ancient times, and they have been regaining favor lately. However, research about their efficacy appears to be a rediscovery of old traditional treatments.

Introduction

Management of male infertility entails several lines of treatments, including specific as well as empirical ones. These lines include hormones, antibiotics, steroids, anti-estrogens, surgical intervention, and assisted reproductive techniques (ARTs). Although several factors may affect male fertility and sperm quality, industrialization and economic growth are significant contributors due to increased exposure to pollutants, changes in diet, and unhealthy lifestyles. Aside from medical treatment, it has been addressed that changing an unhealthy lifestyle should be the first line of treatment in dealing with several medical disorders such as hypertension, diabetes,

T. Mostafa (✉)
Department of Andrology, Sexology & STIs, Faculty of Medicine, Cairo University, Cairo, Egypt

T. V. Le
Department of Andrology, Binh Dan Hospital, Ho Chi Minh City, Vietnam

Department of Andrology and Nephro-Urology, Pham Ngoc Thach University of Medicine, Ho Chi Minh City, Vietnam

A. Agarwal et al. (eds.), *Current and Future Advances in Male Infertility*,
https://doi.org/10.1007/978-3-031-62648-7_16

coronary heart disease, hypertension, arthritis, chronic obstructive pulmonary disease, and cancer [1].

Alternative medicine is defined as a set of products, practices, and theories that are perceived by their users to have the healing effects of medicine, but whose effectiveness has not been established using scientific methods [2]. Its interventions encompass a broad range of interventions that act through a variety of measurable and immeasurable mechanisms in a trial to represent valuable outcomes in many medical disorders, including male infertility management [3]. This growing attention was translated into several papers that have been published since the beginning of the twentieth century (Fig. 16.1).

This chapter aims to assess the alternative approaches to the treatment of male infertility.

Change of Lifestyle

One can ultimately modify lifestyle elements to improve overall well-being because they are within their control. Numerous factors, including the age at which paternity occurs, diet, exercise, obesity, coffee, scrotal temperature, clothing, hot water, mobile phones that might affect sperm parameters, and damage to sperm DNA, can have an impact on reproductive health [4]. Controlling the unhealthy lifestyle in male factor infertility has therefore been shown to produce promising results when combined with various treatment modalities. Couples trying to conceive should be more cognizant of and aware of the potential effects of these lifestyle factors [5].

Exercise

Frequent exercise has long been linked to health benefits for several bodily systems and may even help prevent medical disorders. For men, physical activity would have a favorable or negative impact on male infertility, depending on the type, frequency, intensity, duration, and individual physical conditions [6]. In their study, Sharma et al. [7] showed that a balanced diet and moderate exercise routine would be ideal for increasing sperm motility and morphology while reducing sperm DNA damage and reactive oxygen species (ROS) generation.

Individual health status, as well as exercise volume, intensity, and duration, appears to have an effective influence on male fertility. Some studies suggested that moderate-intensity continuous training may be more advantageous on the oxidant/antioxidant markers in seminal plasma than high-intensity continuous training and high-intensity interval training [8]. Hajizadeh Maleki et al. [9] investigated the effects of resistance exercise training on markers of reproductive performance in a group of sedentary infertile men following 24 weeks of resistance exercise. Semen samples were taken before, at 12, 24, and 7 weeks, as well as 7 and 30 days while

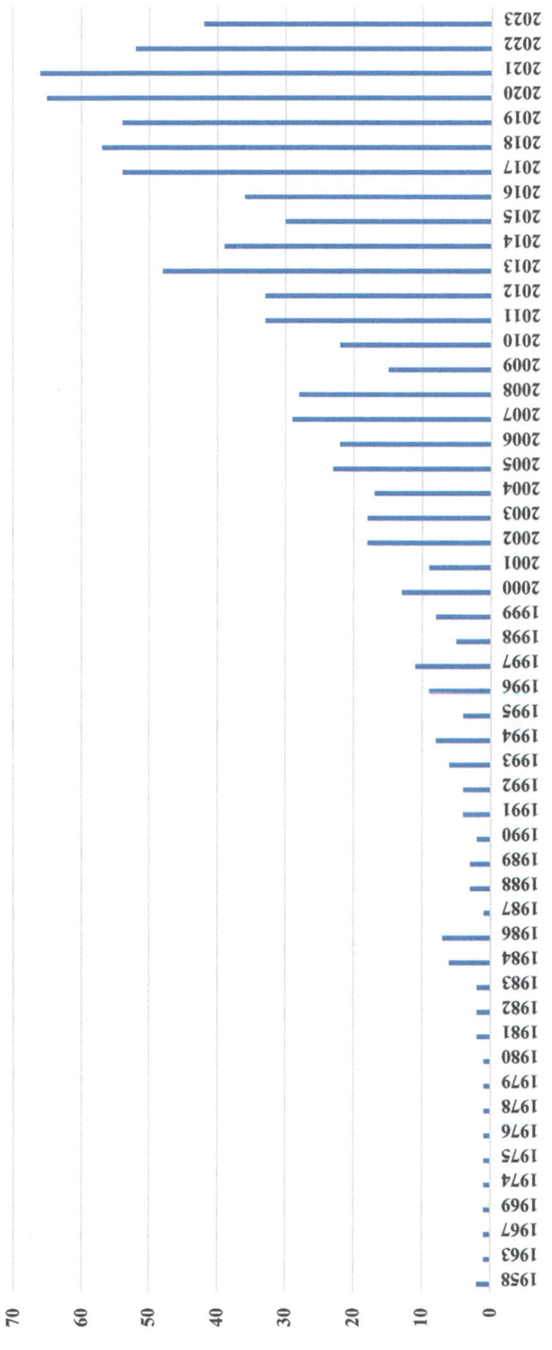

Fig. 16.1 Graphic distribution of alternative medicine studies for male infertility (1958–2023)

recovering. In these males, exercise training has positively improved semen parameters, sperm DNA integrity, and pregnancy rate while also favorably attenuating inflammation as shown by seminal cytokines OS indicators and boosted antioxidants.

In comparison to males who engage in strenuous competitive sports or elite athletes, Xie et al. [10] collectively addressed the idea that physical exercise at low to moderate levels enhances sperm concentration, total sperm count, motility, and morphology. Any intense or agonistic physical exercise may put participants at risk of deteriorating reproductive function, as demonstrated by Vaamonde et al. [11]. Matos et al. [12] also noted that high-intensity exercise is known to generate an expected drop in these parameters, which in turn has an adverse effect on testicular function. In order to effectively treat male infertility patients, it is therefore recommended to be aware of the benefits of a suitable and moderate exercise program.

Smoking

Numerous studies have confirmed that there are various harmful substances in cigarette smoke that may impair a man's ability to conceive. Smoking tobacco has been associated with decreased sperm motility, count, and normal morphology [13]. Toxic ROS found in cigarette smoke also have an adverse effect on the integrity of sperm DNA [14]. Therefore, even though smokers may not have decreased fertility overall, men who have poor-quality semen may benefit from stopping. In addition, smokers should quit because they owe it to the future generation and because tobacco smoke contains a number of toxins that might cause cancer [15].

The American Society for Reproductive Medicine's practice committee has discussed the following: (1) There is strong evidence that smoking has a detrimental impact on ART outcomes, requiring smokers to undergo nearly twice as many in vitro fertilization (IVF) cycles in order to conceive. (2) There is moderate evidence that smokers have lower semen parameters and sperm function test results than nonsmokers and that the effects are dose dependent. (3) There is strong evidence that nonsmokers who are exposed to high levels of tobacco smoke may experience reproductive repercussions comparable to those experienced by smokers.

Healthy Nutrition

Since there are clear links between male infertility, low nutritional intake, rising obesity, and environmental exposures, it is commonly accepted that nutritional status affects reproductive development and function [16]. There are no specific dietary recommendations to increase the quality of male sperm, although certain nutrients may improve or decrease male fertility. Reduced semen quality has been associated with modern Westernized diets that are high in processed foods, sugar and other refined carbs, red meat, unhealthy fats, and calories but low in nutrients [17]. Reduced consumption of fruits and vegetables, dietary fiber, polyunsaturated fatty acids (PUFAs, primarily omega-3 from fish), and different antioxidants and related cofactors (e.g., vitamins A, C, D, and E, folate, selenium, zinc, and lycopene) have been shown to aggravate nutritional status and increase a possible infertility risk [18]. Figure 16.2 lists foods that are positively or negatively linked to male fertility.

Decreased ROS to antioxidant ratios can lead to a reduction in total antioxidant capacity (TAC) when many vitamins and minerals that are essential for indirect or direct antioxidant action are deficient [19]. Better fertility results are also associated with dietary patterns rich in antioxidant-rich foods, particularly those high in β-carotenes, folate, vitamins C, D, and E, selenium, zinc, and lycopene [20]. A meta-analysis involving 1204 infertile and 8477 healthy males found an overall correlation between improved male semen parameters and dietary fruits, vegetables, vitamins, and fish [21]. Men who most closely followed the Mediterranean diet, which is abundant in green leafy vegetables and olive oil, had considerably higher sperm concentrations, progressive motility, and normal sperm morphology, according to a study by Karayiannis et al. [22].

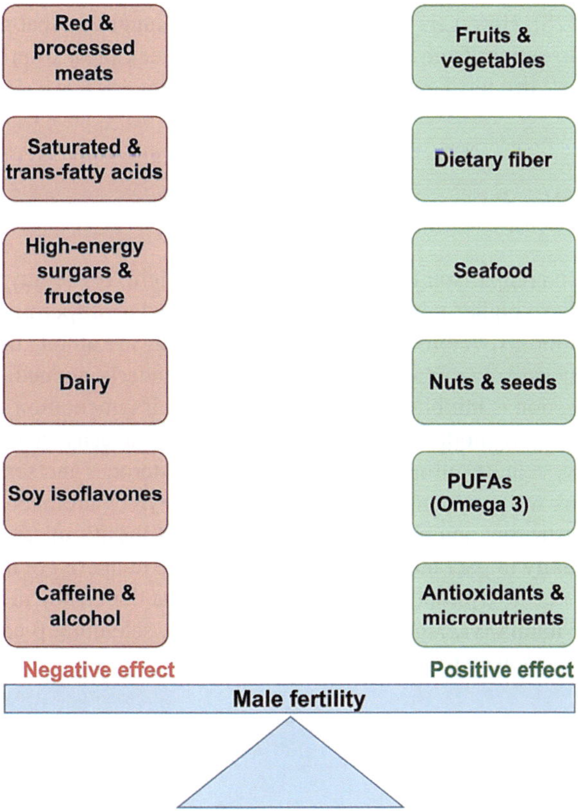

Fig. 16.2 Food groups that have a negative (red) correlation and a favorable (green) correlation with male fertility

Alcohol

There appears to be a connection between drinking alcohol and having low-quality semen [23]. Heavy drinking over an extended period has been associated with reduced gonadotropin release, testicular atrophy, decreased T, and decreased sperm production. Alcoholism and liver disease are linked, and the inability of the liver to process estrogens causes hormonal imbalances [24]. Moreover, there is a connection between acute drunkenness and alcoholism, and sexual dysfunction, which may complicate male infertility [25].

Despite the lack of significant differences in the semen characteristics between daily and infrequent drinkers, the latter group exhibited superior sperm morphology. This could be attributed to the presence of polyphenols with potential for cell protection, such as xanthohumol or resveratrol [26]. Jensen et al. [27] evaluated 8000 men from the United States and Europe who were categorized as low to moderate drinkers with no variation in the two groups' semen characteristics. It is interesting to note that there was a linear rise in serum T levels as alcohol consumption increased.

Interestingly, male partners of infertile couples using ART appear to have a positive correlation between their semen quality and moderate alcohol consumption [28]. However, Van Heertum et al. [24] suggested that male partners have to be told to refrain from alcohol use at least 1 week prior to providing a semen sample for in vitro fertilization.

Obesity

In comparison to cohorts of normal weight, obese guys have also been reported to have higher rates of oligozoospermia and azoospermia [29]. Sperm concentration, motility, viability, and proper morphology are among the semen parameters that are negatively impacted by obesity and its underlying mediators. Chromosome condensation is inhibited by obesity, and DNA fragmentation promotes apoptosis and epigenetic modifications [30]. Additionally, obesity negatively affects the endocrine system, resulting in decreased T, progesterone, and sex hormone-binding globulin, as well as increased activity of the enzymes aromatase, insulin, leptin, prolactin, estrogen, and insulin [30]. Furthermore, obesity-related physical issues may potentially impact male fertility by raising the temperature in the scrotum and leading to erectile dysfunction [31]. Furthermore, a deficiency in vital micronutrients such as vitamin B1, zinc, vitamin C, vitamin D, selenium, β-carotenes, folate, and vitamin E is linked to higher visceral obesity [32].

Other Remedies

Psychological and Behavioral Therapy

Men also have physical and psychological side effects from fertility treatments, which were noticeably worse a year after the initial fertility evaluation. These effects are similar to those experienced by women [33]. Further adding to the stress experienced by men were potentially technical procedures like ART trials (which involved waiting anxiously for the results of pregnancy tests and after cycles that failed) and tessticular sperm extraction (TESE) trials (which involved waiting for the outcomes of sperm retrieval). Additionally, male adolescents and young adults who receive a cancer diagnosis frequently have to make snap judgments regarding the cryopreservation of spermatozoa before the start of chemotherapy or radiation therapy [34].

Before now, Mitsi and Efthimiou [35] discussed how cognitive behavioral therapy (CBT) has demonstrated its superiority over other psychotherapy approaches as a successful means of reducing feelings of anxiety and depression during multiple phases of infertility care. The beneficial effects of several psychosocial methods, such as mind-body intervention, cognitive behavioral therapy, group psychotherapy, and yoga, on infertile couples were examined by Ying et al. [36].

By inhibiting sympathetic activity and stimulating neurohormonal pathways, yoga is utilized as a behavioral treatment to promote overall health and fitness and to treat particular physical and mental health disorders [37]. By lowering levels of oxidative DNA damage, lifestyle therapies like yoga and meditation can enhance the integrity of sperm DNA, as noted by Bishat et al. [38]. In their investigation of the impact of yoga on male fertility and ART outcomes, Darbandi et al. [39] found that the practice had positive stress management effects by lowering anxiety, despair, and pain.

The Development Group for the ESHRE Psychology and Counseling Guideline has recently suggested that psychosocial assistance be provided as an additional therapy during infertility treatments. The effectiveness of several psychological therapies, including progressive muscle relaxation, deep breathing, and cognitive behavioral therapy, may alter the activity of the prefrontal cortex, amygdala, hypothalamus, and hippocampus, brain areas associated with stress.

Supplements and Over-the-Counter Drugs

Although the FDA does not oversee nutritional supplements, these products, also known as food supplements or nutraceuticals, have been widely available without a prescription and are intended to improve physiological characteristics. Subjects desiring fertility may find it easy to obtain these supplements because a prescription from a doctor is not required to buy them [40]. All-natural and hence healthful, the majority of these over-the-counter drugs and supplements show antioxidant action as a treatment for male infertility caused by OS. While some writers have shown how certain supplements improve semen parameters and fertility results, others have discussed their ineffectiveness or even possibly dangerous side effects [41]. There is a list of suggested chemicals provided in Table 16.1.

Along with the extensive research on these substances, Ahmadi et al. [42] examined the impact of various oral antioxidant supplements on enhancing important semen parameters and DNA damage in addition to the substantial study conducted on these compounds. Supplements like CoQ10 and vitamin E have been shown to increase sperm count; carnitine has been shown to improve sperm motility and morphology; and taking vitamins E and C at the same time has been shown to lessen sperm DNA damage. Di Tucci et al. [43] noted that alpha lipoic acid is a chemical that shows promise because it is soluble in fat and water and functions as a "universal antioxidant." The study conducted by Abbasi et al. [44] investigated the effect of an 80-day course of alpha lipoic acid prescription on sperm progressive motility following varicocelectomy surgical repair. All things considered, Agarwal et al. [45] reported that supplementing with antioxidants enhances semen parameters.

Table 16.1 Nutraceuticals used in male infertility treatments

	Item	Function
1.	Glutathione	An intracellular antioxidant
2.	L-carnitine	Required for fatty acid metabolism with antioxidant effects
3.	Omega-3	Docosahexaenoic acid and eicosapentaenoic acid are essential to normal physiology
4.	Selenium	Provides beneficial effects to sperm
5.	Zinc	Promotes sperm quality via its antioxidant effects and a metalloenzyme cofactor in DNA transcription and protein synthesis
6.	Coenzyme Q10	Provides energy to cells with antioxidant activity
7.	Myoinositol	Improves the performance of OAT sperm in vitro and in vivo
8.	Vitamin C	Has a role in hormone production, promotion of collagen synthesis, strong antioxidant, and enzyme cofactor
9.	Vitamin E	Protects tissue polyunsaturated fatty acids against peroxidation
10.	Folic acid	Provides carbons for DNA synthesis and methylation essential for spermatogenesis and scavenging of free radicals
11.	Vitamin D	Has potential scavenger capacity
12.	Vitamin A	An essential nutrient for humans
13.	Lycopene	Most potent singlet oxygen quencher of all carotenoids reducing OS with other beneficial effects via non-oxidative mechanisms
14.	Vitamin B12	Has an essential role in red blood cell formation, cell metabolism, nerve function, and DNA production
15.	Vitamin B5	Produces energy by breaking down fats and carbohydrates
16.	Vitamin B6	Helps to create neurotransmitters, such as serotonin and dopamine
17.	Melatonin	Multifunctional hormone with antiaging, antioxidant, and anti-inflammatory functions
18.	N-acetyl cysteine	Enhances scavenging OS and stabilizes proteins with antioxidant, anti-inflammatory, and mucolytic properties

Furthermore, it offers recommendations for antioxidant therapy in some clinical situations, such as varicocele, infertility in men that cannot be explained, and cases of changed semen quality.

Though there is yet no standard for which over the counter supplement and vitamin studies have been done or the prescriptions dosed, sensible usage of supplements may be advantageous for improving sperm parameters. Considering that several studies have clarified the "antioxidant paradox" phenomenon, it may be detrimental for patients and prescribers to take these supplements over the counter [46]. Furthermore, since every product has a different ingredient at a different dose, it is challenging to experimentally address which ingredient is best for a given patient due to several circumstances. As a result, selecting the proper antioxidant dosage or antioxidant combination, which may be more potent than any one antioxidant, may be a significant issue.

The largest online survey on the topic of antioxidants and male infertility was recently conducted by Agarwal et al. [47]. The results showed that (1) there is a global recognition of the significance of this therapeutic option and (2) antioxidants are widely used to treat male infertility; however, the need for evidence-based clinical practice guidelines from professional societies is emphasized.

However, a substantial portion of dietary supplements are blends of ingredients with dubious or unknown advantages, whose use may be detrimental or even useless for infertile males. Because of this, the producers ought to thoroughly examine the data from scientific studies before releasing the formulation of any supplement. Thus, before contemplating their therapeutic usage, clinicians should assess the composition and dosage of each element.

Consequently, more studies ought to be supported to identify the right antioxidant molecules, the length of the treatment, and the optimal antioxidant dosage for use in clinical settings. An additional crucial factor to move on with micronutrient supplementation without running the risk of reductive stress is the pretreatment assessment of the seminal oxidative status.

Herbals

The active compounds in herbal medications are derived from plant parts, such as flowers, roots, or leaves. However, just because something is "natural" does not always imply that it is safe to use; if not handled properly, it could be dangerous. Although dietary supplements are not regulated by the American Food and Drug Administration, they are being utilized in some countries and are receiving increased attention as an additional or alternative therapeutic approach for a variety of illnesses, including male infertility [48].

In their investigation, Sadogh et al. [49] discussed the extracted herbal foods that famed PM physician Avicenna introduced. Among the principal foods Avicenna suggested are almond, onion, chickpea, garlic, coconut, palm date, sesame, fenugreek, carrot, fig, grapes, pistachio, hazelnut, and walnut that may have a favorable impact on T production as well as the enhancement of other sperm parameters.

Moreover, having a high concentration of various macro- and micronutrients, including vitamins, minerals, essential unsaturated fatty acids, amino acids, and phytochemicals like polyphenols, flavonoids, triterpenes, and steroids, can be thought of as the primary reasons for these foods' efficacy (a list of suggested compounds is included in Table 16.2).

There are several hypothesized pathways for these medicinal herbs' positive effects on sperm abnormalities, including their venotonic, anti-inflammatory, antioxidant, and blood T-boosting properties. Furthermore, several phytochemical groups, such as alkaloids, oxygenated volatile compounds, carotenoids, saponins, and phytosterols, appear to be in charge of their advantageous properties [50]. The T pathway is involved in the mechanisms of action, which include stimulating spermatogenesis, reducing OS, inhibiting inflammation, and activating testicular signaling pathways (PKB/ERK/PKB/TGF-β1 transformation/NF-kB signaling pathways) and nuclear factor kappa-light-chain enhancer of activated B cells [51].

For instance, taking the roots of the little evergreen shrub *Withania somnifera*, sometimes known as ashwagandha, orally has been shown to have several health benefits, including the inhibition of lipid peroxidation, the enhancement of sperm motility and count, and the regulation of reproductive hormone levels. It functions through two mechanisms: an indirect one that involves a gamma-aminobutyric acid-like mimic route that improves hormonal balance by interacting with various endocrine glands and a direct one that involves mitigating OS [52]. In oligozoospermic men, Santos et al. [53] proposed a 12-week increase in total T of 83.3 million/mL by using 5000 mg/d of powdered *Mucuna* seed and ashwagandha root (151 and 143 ng/dl, respectively).

In addition, Nasimi et al. [54] examined the effects of pentoxifylline and *Withania somnifera* on sperm parameters in 100 instances of idiopathic male infertility. For 90 days, individuals in the pentoxifylline group took six capsules containing 800 mg/daily of pentoxifylline and placebo, whereas patients in the herbal group had six capsules containing 5 g/daily of *W. somnifera* root. In comparison to the baseline, *W. somnifera* raised the mean sperm count (12.5%), enhanced sperm morphology (25.56%), and increased progressive motility (21.42%). Additionally, pentoxifylline enhanced sperm morphology (13.28%), increased mean semen volume (16.46%), and improved progressive motility (25.97%) compared to the baseline, with no significant changes observed between the two groups following treatment.

- One of the most popular herbal medications is curcumin. The turmeric rhizome yields this yellow phenolic pigment, which has anti-inflammatory, antineoplastic, and antimutagenic qualities. It is also a potent antioxidant with 300 times the potency of vitamin E [55].
- *Tribulus terrestris* belongs to the Zygophyllaceae family of herbs. The primary active phytoconstituents of this plant are flavonoids, alkaloids, saponins, lignin, amides, and glycosides. *T. terrestris* L. has been shown by Sanagoo et al. [56] to be useful in enhancing sperm motility, count, and morphology.
- Lu et al. [57] looked into the effectiveness of Huzhangdanshenyin on male immunological infertility in 90 men; 30 men received prednisone treatment for

Table 16.2 A list of herbals used in male infertility treatments

1. Acori Graminei Rhizome	19. *Crataegus monogyna*	37. *Pedalium murex* Linn.
2. Adofon	20. *Crocus sativus* Linn.	38. Pericarpium Citri Reticulate Blanco
3. Aescin	21. *Cynomorium songaricum*	39. *Petasites japonicus*
4. *Alpinia officinarum*	22. *Eurycoma longifólia*	40. *Phaleria macrocarpa*
5. *Anacyclus pyrethrum*	23. *Fagara tessmannii*	41. *Phoenix dactylifera*
6. *Andrographis paniculata*	24. Flos *Lonicerae japonicae*	42. Radix Paeoniae Rubrae
7. *Apium graveolens*	25. Fructus *Cornus officinalis*	43. *Rehmannia glutinosa* Libosch
8. Ashwagandha	26. Fructus Rubi	44. Rhizoma *Anemarrhenae asphodeloidis*
9. *Astragalus membranaceus*	27. Fructus *Schisandrae chinensis*	45. Rhizoma Cimicifugae
10. Aurantii Fructus	28. *Fumaria parviflora*	46. *Rubus coreanus*
11. Celery (*Apium graveolens*)	29. Korean red ginseng	47. Saffron
12. *Chlorophytum borivilianum*	30. *Lepidium meyenii*	48. *Satureja khuzestanica*
13. *Cinnamomum camphora*	31. *Morinda officinalis*	49. Semen Cuscutae
14. *Cinnamomum zeylanicum*	32. *Mucuna pruriens*	50. *Sesamum indicum*
15. *Corchorus depressus* Linn.	33. *Mucuna pruriens* Linn.	51. Topalaf
16. Cornus mas	34. Nelumbinis Embryo	52. *Tribulus terrestris*
17. Cortex Moudan Radicis	35. *Nigella sativa* (black cumin)	53. *Withania somnifera*
18. Cortex Phellodendri	36. Palm pollen	54. Zingiber officinale

3 months as a control group, and 60 men received Huzhangdanshenyin treatment. It was determined that Huzhangdanshenyin treats male immunological infertility better than prednisone and that it has no negative side effects and can improve sperm indices, clinical symptoms, and antisperm antibody reversing ratio.

- Infertile males in Iran and Turkey often consume *Ceratonia siliqua*, or carob, empirically because of its antioxidant qualities. Aghajani et al. [58] separated 60 infertile men into two groups and examined the effects of carob syrup twice daily or vitamin E 100 mg twice daily for 3 months on semen parameters, OS indicators, and pregnancy rate. When compared to the vitamin E-treated group, the carob group had a greater pregnancy rate and significantly better semen quality metrics and overall antioxidant capacity. These authors concluded that carob might be a useful agent for improving semen parameters because of its antioxidant qualities and role in altering T levels.
- *Aspalathus linearis*, often known as rooibos, is a significant antioxidant-rich herbal medicinal plant that originated in the fynbos of South Africa. Takalani

et al. [59] looked at how it directly affected sperm functioning in an in vitro setting. Aqueous extract of the fermented extract in sperm preparation medium (0, 0.10, 1.0, 10, and 100 μg/ml) was treated for 1 h at 37 °C with semen samples (7.5×10^6/ml), which demonstrated a decreased percentage of intact mitochondrial membrane potential and DNA fragmentation.
- The effects of *Alpinia officinarum* on semen analysis were studied by Kolangi et al. [60] in 76 individuals with idiopathic infertility ($n = 31$ received plant treatment; $n = 29$ received a placebo). For 3 months, participants were randomly assigned to receive either a placebo or 300 mg of a dried extract of *A. officinarum* rhizome per day in capsule form. Comparing the treated group with the pretreatment data, there was a substantial improvement in the mean sperm count (52×10^6/ml vs. 71×10^6/ml, $P = 0.043$) and mean sperm normal morphology (14.34% vs. 19%, $P < 0.001$).
- In treating a cohort of varicocele-associated asthenozoospermic patients, Chen et al. [61] examined the benefits of Yishen Tongluo Recipe (YTR) in combination with surgery as opposed to YTR or surgery alone. Twelve weeks into the treatment, the YTR + surgery group had a considerably better overall effectiveness rate (89.74% vs. 63.16% and 64.10%, $P < 0.05$) and progressive sperm motility (31.67 vs. 24.48 and 25.57, $P < 0.05$) compared to the YTR and the surgery group. It was determined that in individuals with varicocele-associated asthenozoospermia, the Yishen Tongluo Recipe in conjunction with surgery can greatly increase sperm quality and sperm DNA integrity. This combination is both safe and effective.
- Using Korean herbal medicine (MYOMI-14) to treat 17 infertile males with low-quality semen for 10 weeks, Jo et al. [62] investigated the results. After receiving MYOMI-14 medication, the average values of sperm concentration, sperm progressive motility, and total motile sperm count considerably improved (36.2%, 51.7%, and 55.5%; $P < 0.05$) without causing any negative side effects.

Recently, Roozbeh et al. [63] provided an overview of the research that has been done to date to ascertain the efficacy, security, and mechanism of herbal remedies in enhancing male fertility. Ultimately, a total of 20 trials with 1519 participants were examined. In these investigations, the effects on male fertility of 11 different medicinal herbs (*Mucuna pruriens*, ginseng, saffron, *Nigella sativa*, palm pollen, Adofon, Topalaf, sesame, and samba) were compared with a placebo. With the exception of one, all studies have demonstrated how useful medicinal plants are for enhancing sperm and reproductive parameters as well as male infertility. The known randomized-controlled trials (RCTs) demonstrated the beneficial benefits of medicinal plants on male fertility. Therefore, more clinical research is necessary to ascertain the optimal dose for treating male infertility in order to create a unique technique.

It is possible that variations in the medicinal plants' daily dosage led to these debates. Put another way, the kind of plant, its substance, the dosage, and the length of the intervention all affected how medicinal herbs affected male fertility. A safety assessment is also required, in addition to more thorough pharmacological research and RCTs to examine the effectiveness of promising CHM formulae for male infertility. Standardization to known active constituents and understanding polyvalent and synergistic effects, which are particularly challenging to determine because CHM formulas are composed of a mixture of different herb species, are additional challenges for the investigation of CHM formulas for their relevance in male infertility [64].

Scrotal Cooling

While scrotal temperatures between 1 and 2 °C below body temperature would naturally aid in normal spermatogenesis, raised scrotal temperature is one of the least researched risk factors for male infertility impairing spermatogenesis [65]. According to clinical research, even small changes in testicular temperature can affect spermatogenesis because testicular DNA synthesis is sensitive to temperature; its maximum point is 31 °C, while the maximum temperature for RNA and protein synthesis is 37–40 °C. A 14% decrease in spermatogenesis, with lower sperm generation and higher apoptosis, is associated with every 1 °C increase in temperature [66]. Additionally, elevated temperatures encourage the production of more ROS, which can lead to damage to the plasma membrane of sperm and specific DNA fragmentation of the mitochondrial and nuclear genomes [67]. According to Jung et al. [68], oligoasthenoteratozoospermia (OAT) patients typically had scrotal temperatures exceeding 35.5 °C even in the same ambient conditions as semen donors.

In a previous study, Robinson et al. [69] observed that seven oligozoospermic males who had scrotal cooling for 14 days had an enhanced sperm count; however, this effect did not last longer than 2 weeks. Later, Zorgniotti et al. [70] used an experimental device that uses evaporation to achieve normal testicular temperatures for as long as 20 weeks and 24 h a day to treat six infertile males with inadequate semen. Semen analysis had been improved in all cases with three pregnancies proposing scrotal hypothermia as a suitable treatment in men with varicocele, varicocelectomy failure, and/or idiopathic infertility. Zorgniotti et al. [71] reported that whereas 6/25 couples became pregnant after using an evaporative scrotal cooling device for 16 h a day for a mean of 14.5 weeks, persistent scrotal hypothermia results in different degrees of improvement over pretreatment-poor semen in 16/25 cases. But the cessation of hypothermia meant a return to the production of weak sperm. A testicular hypothermia device worn by "hardcore" was also presented by Zorgniotti et al. [72]; it lowered body temperature and improved semen parameters in some pregnancies.

Mulcahy [73] evaluated 50 men who used a package of blue ice, a gel that, when frozen, solidifies in a few hours and thaws gradually at normal temperature, causing the surrounding area to chill. The men had either oligozoospermia or asthenozoospermia. When the patient goes to bed at night, this blue ice is placed into the front of their jockey shorts to rest against their anterior scrotum. In 65% of these patients, at least a twofold increase in sperm density and similar increases in sperm motility were achieved. Furthermore, Zorgniotti et al. [74] reported that 42 patients (65.6%) who used a testicular hypothermia device worn daily for at least 16 weeks and were 64 infertile men showed improvement in one or more semen parameters.

In this regard, Jung et al. [68] reported that, during a 12-week period of usage, nocturnal scrotal cooling by an airstream led to a 1 °C drop in scrotal temperature and a statistically significant rise in total sperm output. Additionally, Jung et al. [75] used a membrane pump connected by plastic tubes to receptacles positioned in both groins to assess the effect of nightly scrotal cooling on semen quality in 20 oligozoospermia patients with a history of testicular maldescent over the course of 12 weeks. The pregenital airstream caused a 0.8 °C drop in scrotal temperature, and after 8 and 12 weeks, respectively, there was a notable rise in the total sperm count. The enhancement of sperm morphology and motility, however, was negligible.

The Scrotum Cooling Patch, introduced by Osman et al. [76], is a hydrogel pad that is nongreasy, is comfortable to apply, and contains 0.5% w/w natural menthol to offer a cooling effect without the need for refrigeration while preserving the person's privacy and dignity. According to a recent research by Zumstein et al. [77], cyclic scrotal skin cooling using special underwear is effective without interfering with day-to-day activities and considerably lowers median scrotal skin temperature by 0.7 °C. Furthermore, Benidir et al. [78] assessed infertile men's compliance with one of the two scrotal cooling devices (Snowballs or Underdog). The majority of participants (76.9%) utilized scrotal cooling for a shorter period of time than advised. According to the respondents, the devices caused discomfort (31.5%), hindered productivity (21.0%), and quickly lost cooling (14.3%). Following scrotal cooling, there were notable increases in sperm motility and vitality (from 25.4% to 29.0% and from 64.8% to 71.7%, respectively).

Systematic reviews that attempted to prove that scrotal cooling improved male fertility were unable to show any discernible increase in pregnancy rates [79]. For men who are of reproductive age, elevated scrotal sac temperature may indicate an elevated risk factor; hence, it is advised to be cognizant of this possibility. All things considered, two prospective controlled trials and a few small observational studies lacking matched control groups provide evidence for the positive impact of scrotal cooling on male fertility.

Acupuncture

With almost 4000 years of history, acupuncture is a popular adjunct therapy in traditional Chinese medicine. Frequently used as an additional therapy, acupuncture can be electrically stimulated or not. It became well known in contemporary medicine as a supplemental therapy to treat illnesses using a variety of methods, including moxibustion, hand acupuncture, electricity acupuncture, and applying pressure with the fingers to certain acupoints [80]. According to the traditional Chinese medicine (TCM) theory, blood circulation obstructions and abnormalities in the balance of vital energy are the causes of infertility. Thus, it was hypothesized that the somatic afferent neurons that innervate the skin and muscles would be activated, mediating the therapeutic effects of acupuncture [81].

With a history spanning over 4000 years, acupuncture is a frequently used supplemental therapy in TCM. Often utilized as an adjuvant therapy, acupuncture can be employed with or without electrical stimulation. It has become more well known in contemporary medicine as a supplemental therapy for treating illnesses using a variety of methods, such as finger pressure at particular acupoints, moxibustion, hand acupuncture, and electricity acupuncture [80]. Traditional Chinese medicine theory states that abnormalities in the flow of Qi energy and blood circulation lead to infertility. Therefore, it was hypothesized that the stimulation of somatic afferent neurons innervating the skin and muscle would mediate the therapeutic benefits of acupuncture. Previously, Riegler et al. [82] investigated acupuncture acupuncture's influence on 28 infertile patients with a significant increase in sperm parameters linked with no change in the performed psychological test denying placebo mechanisms. Then, Fischl et al. [83] treated 28 infertile men (10 treatments for 3 weeks) with acupuncture observing a significant improvement in sperm quality. In their study, Siterman et al. [84] assessed the effects of acupuncture on semen samples of 16 infertile patients analyzed before and 1 month after treatment (twice weekly for 5 weeks) compared with semen samples of 16 untreated infertile men. The fertility index increased significantly following improved total functional sperm fraction, percentage of viability, and total motile spermatozoa per ejaculate. Furthermore, acupuncture may be a helpful, nontraumatic treatment for males with low sperm density, particularly those who have inflammation in their genital tract. This was discussed by Siterman et al. [85]

In addition to their research, Pei et al. [86] assessed the ultramorphologic characteristics of sperm following twice-weekly acupuncture treatment for 5 weeks in 28 infertile males, in comparison with semen samples from 12 untreated controls. In the total ejaculates, there was a noteworthy rise in the proportion and quantity of sperm without ultrastructural flaws associated with better acrosome position and shape, axonemal pattern and form, and accessory fibers of sperm organelles. According to Fu et al. [87], antisperm antibodies can be regulated by acupuncture combined with herbal medication therapy. In their study, 168 infertile men were evaluated by Dong et al. [88] (85 cases and a control group of 83 cases). The primary points of treatment for the treatment group were bilateral Shengzhi points, Dicong Shenjing points, and L2 Shenjing points. Wuzi Yanzong tablets were administered orally to the control group. With increased zinc and seminal superoxide dismutase activity, the treatment group's pregnant rate of 78.8% of the patient's wife compared to 43.4% of the controls showed a significant difference ($P < 0.01$). Additionally, He et al. [89] examined 12 trials with 2177 participants and came to the conclusion that acupuncture has a unique efficacy in raising the quality of sperm. According to Kucuk et al. [90] study, acupuncture treatment twice weekly for 2 months appears to be beneficial for infertile patients with varicocele.

In individuals with idiopathic oligoasthenozoospermia, Li et al. [91] demonstrated that tamoxifen in conjunction with mid-frequency transcutaneous electrical acupoint stimulation can considerably enhance semen quality and boost levels of sex hormones. According to Jin et al. [92], sperm motility and vitality can be increased by both 2 Hz and 100 Hz TEAS, making them useful for treating asthenozoospermia. According to Gong et al. [93], infertile oligoasthenozoospermic patients' proportion of grade A sperm was dramatically increased by 100 Hz TEAS.

In their investigation, Nareswari et al. [94] presented a case diagnosed with severe OAT subjected to acupuncture therapy done at CV 3, CV 4, CV 5, CV 6, CV 7, ST 29, SP 6, SP 3, ST 36, and KI 3, alternating with KI 7 5 days/week and at LR 8 once/week, for 28 sessions. After two sets of treatments, semen analysis showed improvements, particularly in sperm motility (which had decreased from 25% to 33% to 67%). The therapeutic effects of acupuncture on idiopathic male infertility were examined by Zhang et al. [95] in 22 patients who had failed ICSI and were treated with acupuncture twice a week for 8 weeks, before undergoing intracytoplasmic sperm injection once again. Following acupuncture, quick sperm motility was considerably improved and associated with higher fertilization rates (66.2% vs. 40.2%, $P < 0.01$) when compared to that pretreatment levels.

Two to three acupuncture treatments on or around the day of embryo transfer are insufficient interventions to improve the results of IVF delivery, but they significantly reduce the stress associated with the process, as demonstrated by Hullender Rubin et al. [96]. When compared to placebo acupuncture, Coyle et al. [97] showed that acupuncture around the time of embryo transfer had no discernible impact on the success of in vitro fertilization.

However, Jerng et al. [98] addressed that the current evidence showing that acupuncture might improve poor semen quality is insufficient because of the small number of studies, inadequacy of procedures and/or insufficient information for semen analysis, high levels of heterogeneity, high risk of bias, and poor quality of reporting. According to Li et al. [99], the quality of clinical research on acupuncture treatment for oligoasthenozoospermia is relatively low, the degree of evidence currently available is low, its clinical applicability is restricted, and further research is required to confirm its therapeutic impact. Jia et al. [100] noted in their meta-analysis that when compared to placebo acupuncture, sperm motility, sperm concentration, and semen volume were not significantly improved by acupuncture alone. While sperm motility and concentration may be improved by adjuvant acupuncture, the study's heterogeneity was too great to draw firm results that would have supported the use of acupuncture as a treatment.

Conclusion

While medical interventions for male factor infertility are recommended when necessary, other therapeutic approaches have been shown to be beneficial in treating this illness. It was shown that under these situations, changing one's lifestyle could have positive effects including losing weight, quitting smoking, drinking in moderation, and maintaining a healthy diet. Furthermore, due largely to the lack of RCTs, adjuvants such as acupuncture, mind-body practices, herbal medicines, vitamins, and scrotal cooling were mentioned with inconsistent outcomes. It is therefore advised that more research be done on these things, particularly case-controlled research, in order to clarify any potential useful role that they may have.

References

1. Kushner RF, Mechanick JI. Lifestyle medicine- an emerging new discipline. US Endocrinol. 2015;11(1):36–40.
2. Tabish SA. Complementary and alternative healthcare: is it evidence-based? Int J Health Sci (Qassim). 2008;2(1):V–IX.
3. Bouychou M. Alternative medicines in medically assisted reproduction. Soins Pediatr Pueric. 2019;40(311):44–6.
4. Ilacqua A, Izzo G, Emerenziani GP, Baldari C, Aversa A. Lifestyle and fertility: the influence of stress and quality of life on male fertility. Reprod Biol Endocrinol. 2018;16(1):115.
5. Durairajanayagam D. Lifestyle causes of male infertility. Arab J Urol. 2018;16(1):10–20.
6. Di Luigi L, Romanelli F, Sgrò P, Lenzi A. Andrological aspects of physical exercise and sport medicine. Endocrine. 2012;42(2):278–84.
7. Sharma R, Biedenharn KR, Fedor JM, Agarwal A. Lifestyle factors and reproductive health: taking control of your fertility. Reprod Biol Endocrinol. 2013;11:66.
8. Hajizadeh Maleki B, Tartibian B. High-intensity interval training modulates male factor infertility through anti-inflammatory and antioxidative mechanisms in infertile men: a randomized controlled trial. Cytokine. 2020;125:154861.
9. Hajizadeh Maleki B, Tartibian B. Resistance exercise modulates male factor infertility through anti-inflammatory and antioxidative mechanisms in infertile men: a RCT. Life Sci. 2018;203:150–60.
10. Xie F, You Y, Guan C, Gu Y, Yao F, Xu J. Association between physical activity and infertility: a comprehensive systematic review and meta-analysis. J Transl Med. 2022;20(1):237.
11. Vaamonde D, Garcia-Manso JM, Hackney AC. Impact of physical activity and exercise on male reproductive potential: a new assessment questionnaire. Rev Andal Med Deport. 2017;10(2):79–93.
12. Matos B, Howl J, Ferreira R, Fardilha M. Exploring the effect of exercise training on testicular function. Eur J Appl Physiol. 2019;119(1):1–8.
13. Bundhun PK, Janoo G, Bhurtu A, et al. Tobacco smoking and semen quality in infertile males: a systematic review and meta-analysis. BMC Public Health. 2019;19(1):36.
14. Amor H, Zeyad A, Hammadeh ME. Tobacco smoking and its impact on the expression level of sperm nuclear protein genes: H2BFWT, TNP1, TNP2, PRM1 and PRM2. Andrologia. 2021;53(3):e13964.
15. Aboulmaouahib S, Madkour A, Kaarouch I, et al. Impact of alcohol and cigarette smoking consumption in male fertility potential: looks at lipid peroxidation, enzymatic antioxidant activities and sperm DNA damage. Andrologia. 2018;50(3):e12926.
16. Vanderhout SM, Rastegar Panah M, Garcia-Bailo B, et al. Nutrition, genetic variation and male fertility. Transl Androl Urol. 2021;10(3):1410–31.
17. Danielewicz A, Przybyłowicz KE, Przybyłowicz M. Dietary patterns and poor semen quality risk in men: a cross-sectional study. Nutrients. 2018;10(9):1162.
18. Aoun A, Khoury VE, Malakieh R. Can nutrition help in the treatment of infertility? Prev Nutr Food Sci. 2021;26(2):109–20.
19. Benedetti S, Tagliamonte MC, Catalani S, et al. Differences in blood and semen oxidative status in fertile and infertile men, and their relationship with sperm quality. Reprod Biomed Online. 2012;25(3):300–6.
20. Giahi L, Mohammadmoradi S, Javidan A, Sadeghi MR. Nutritional modifications in male infertility: a systematic review covering 2 decades. Nutr Rev. 2016;74(2):118–30.
21. Ricci E, Al-Beitawi S, Cipriani S, et al. Dietary habits and semen parameters: a systematic narrative review. Andrology. 2018;6(1):104–16.
22. Karayiannis D, Kontogianni MD, Mendorou C, Douka L, Mastrominas M, Yiannakouris N. Association between adherence to the Mediterranean diet and semen quality parameters in male partners of couples attempting fertility. Hum Reprod. 2017;32(1):215–22.

23. Finelli R, Mottola F, Agarwal A. Impact of alcohol consumption on male fertility potential: a narrative review. Int J Environ Res Public Health. 2022;19(1):328.
24. Van Heertum K, Rossi B. Alcohol and fertility: how much is too much? Fertil Res Pract. 2017;3:10.
25. Pendharkar S, Mattoo SK, Grover S. Sexual dysfunctions in alcohol-dependent men: a study from north India. Indian J Med Res. 2016;144(3):393–9.
26. Wogatzky J, Wirleitner B, Stecher A, et al. The combination matters - distinct impact of lifestyle factors on sperm quality: a study on semen analysis of 1683 patients according to MSOME criteria. Reprod Biol Endocrinol. 2012;10:115.
27. Jensen TK, Swan S, Jørgensen N, et al. Alcohol and male reproductive health: a cross-sectional study of 8344 healthy men from Europe and the USA. Hum Reprod. 2014;29(8):1801–9.
28. Ricci E, Noli S, Ferrari S, et al. Alcohol intake and semen variables: cross-sectional analysis of a prospective cohort study of men referring to an Italian Fertility Clinic. Andrology. 2018;6(5):690–6.
29. Bieniek JM, Kashanian JA, Deibert CM, et al. Influence of increasing body mass index on semen and reproductive hormonal parameters in a multi-institutional cohort of subfertile men. Fertil Steril. 2016;106(5):1070–5.
30. Leisegang K, Sengupta P, Agarwal A, Henkel R. Obesity and male infertility: mechanisms and management. Andrologia. 2021;53(1):e13617.
31. Cabler S, Agarwal A, Flint M, du Plessis SS. Obesity: modern man's fertility nemesis. Asian J Androl. 2010;12(4):480–9.
32. Alhashem F, Alkhateeb M, Sakr H, et al. Exercise protects against obesity induced semen abnormalities via downregulating stem cell factor, upregulating Ghrelin and normalizing oxidative stress. EXCLI J. 2014;13:551–72.
33. Mokhtari F, Torabi F, Pirhadi M. Relationship between fertility characteristics with spiritual intelligence and resilience in infertile couples. J Educ Health Promot. 2022;11:44.
34. Flynn JS, Russell KM, Lehmann V, Schenck LA, Klosky JL. Parent recommendation to bank sperm among at-risk adolescent and young adult males with cancer. Pediatr Blood Cancer. 2020;67(10):e28217.
35. Mitsi C, Efthimiou K. Infertility: psychological-psychopathological consequences and cognitive-behavioural interventions. Psychiatriki. 2014;25(4):293–302.
36. Ying L, Wu LH, Loke AY. The effects of psychosocial interventions on the mental health, pregnancy rates, and marital function of infertile couples undergoing in vitro fertilization: a systematic review. J Assist Reprod Genet. 2016;33(6):689–701.
37. Sengupta P, Chaudhuri P, Bhattacharya K. Male reproductive health and Yoga. Int J Yoga. 2013;6(2):87–95.
38. Bisht S, Banu S, Srivastava S, Pathak RU, Kumar R, Dada R, Mishra RK. Sperm methylome alterations following Yoga-based lifestyle intervention in patients of primary male infertility: a pilot study. Andrologia. 2020;52(4):e13551.
39. Darbandi S, Darbandi M, Khorram Khorshid HR, Sadeghi MR. Yoga can improve assisted reproduction technology outcomes in couples with infertility. Altern Ther Health Med. 2018;24(4):50–5.
40. Garolla A, Petre GC, Francini-Pesenti F, De Toni L, Vitagliano A, Di Nisio A, Foresta C. Dietary supplements for male infertility: a critical evaluation of their composition. Nutrients. 2020;12(5):1472.
41. Henkel R, Sandhu IS, Agarwal A. The excessive use of antioxidant therapy: a possible cause of male inferility? Andrologia. 2019;51:303–4569.
42. Ahmadi S, Bashiri R, Ghadiri-Anari A, Nadjarzadeh A. Antioxidant supplements and semen parameters: an evidence based review. Int J Reprod Biomed. 2016;14(12):729–36.
43. Di Tucci C, Galati G, Mattei G, Bonanni V, Capri O, D'Amelio R, Muzii L, Benedetti PP. The role of alpha lipoic acid in female and male infertility: a systematic review. Gynecol Endocrinol. 2021;37(6):497–505.

44. Abbasi B, Molavi N, Tavalaee M, Abbasi H, Nasr-Esfahani MH. Alpha-lipoic acid improves sperm motility in infertile men after varicocelectomy: a triple-blind randomized controlled trial. Reprod Biomed Online. 2020;41(6):1084–91.
45. Agarwal A, Leisegang K, Majzoub A, Henkel R, Finelli R, Panner Selvam MK, Tadros N, Parekh N, Ko EY, Cho CL, Arafa M, Alves MG, Oliveira PF, Alvarez JG, Shah R. Utility of antioxidants in the treatment of male infertility: clinical guidelines based on a systematic review and analysis of evidence. World J Mens Health. 2021;39(2):233–90.
46. Dimitriadis F, Symeonidis EN, Tsounapi P, Kaltsas A, Hatzichristodoulou G, Sokolakis I, Zachariou A, Takenaka A, Sofikitis N. Administration of antioxidants in infertile male: when it may have a detrimental effect? Curr Pharm Des. 2021;27(24):2796–801.
47. Agarwal A, Finelli R, MKP S, Leisegang K, Majzoub A, Tadros N, Ko E, Parekh N, Henkel R, Durairajanayagam D, Colpi GM, Cho CL, Sallam HN, Park HJ, Saleh R, Micic S, Ambar RF, Zini A, Tremellen K, Alvarez JG, Palani A, Arafa M, Gava MM, Jindal S, Amar E, Kopa Z, Moein MR, Busetto GM, Sengupta P, Kavoussi P, Maldonado I, Fikri J, Borges E, Martinez M, Bojovic D, Rajmil O, Aydos K, Parekattil S, Marmar JL, Sefrioui O, Jungwirth A, MGR P, Cordts EB, Elbardisi H, Mostafa T, Sabbaghian M, Sadighi Gilani MA, Morimoto Y, Alves MG, Spasic A, Kenic U, Ramsay J, Akande EO, Oumeziane A, Dozortsev D, Chung E, Bell EG, Allegra A, Tanos V, Fiadjoe M, Gurgan T, Abou-Abdallah M, Al-Rumaih H, Oborna I, Arab H, Esteves S, Amer M, Kadioglu A, Yuzko O, Korsak V, Shah R. A global survey of reproductive specialists to determine the clinical utility of oxidative stress testing and antioxidant use in male infertility. World J Mens Health. 2021;39(3):470–88.
48. Boroujeni SN, Malamiri FA, Bossaghzadeh F, Esmaeili A, Moudi E. The most important medicinal plants affecting sperm and testosterone production: a systematic review. JBRA Assist Reprod. 2022;26(3):522–30.
49. Sadogh A, Gorji N, Moeini R. Herbal foodstuffs in Avicenna's recommended diet to improve sperm quality and increase male fertility; an evidence-based approach. J Complement Integr Med. 2021;19(1):47–70.
50. Tahvilzadeh M, Hajimahmoodi M, Toliyat T, Karimi M, Rahimi R. An evidence-based approach to medicinal plants for the treatment of sperm abnormalities in traditional Persian medicine. Andrologia. 2016;48(8):860–79.
51. Ramgir SS, Renu K, Vellingiri B, George A, Tirupapuliyur D, Thiagarajan P, Valsala GA. Phytomedicinal therapeutics for male infertility: critical insights and scientific updates. J Nat Med. 2022;76(3):546–73.
52. Sengupta P, Agarwal A, Pogrebetskaya M, Roychoudhury S, Durairajanayagam D, Henkel R. Role of Withania somnifera (Ashwagandha) in the management of male infertility. Reprod Biomed Online. 2018;36(3):311–26.
53. Santos HO, Howell S, Teixeira FJ. Beyond tribulus (Tribulus terrestris L.): the effects of phytotherapics on testosterone, sperm and prostate parameters. J Ethnopharmacol. 2019;235:392–405.
54. Nasimi Doost Azgomi R, Nazemiyeh H, Sadeghi Bazargani H, Fazljou SMB, Nejatbakhsh F, Moini Jazani A, Ahmadi AsrBadr Y, Zomorrodi A. Comparative evaluation of the effects of Withania somnifera with pentoxifylline on the sperm parameters in idiopathic male infertility: a triple-blind randomised clinical trial. Andrologia. 2018;50:e13041–7.
55. Andrew R, Izzo AA. Principles of pharmacological research of nutraceuticals. Br J Pharmacol. 2017;174(11):1177–94.
56. Sanagoo S, Sadeghzadeh Oskouei B, Gassab Abdollahi N, Salehi-Pourmehr H, Hazhir N, Farshbaf-Khalili A. Effect of Tribulus terrestris L. on sperm parameters in men with idiopathic infertility: a systematic review. Complement Ther Med. 2019;42:95–103.
57. Lu TK, Ouyang HG, Jin GY, Hong YS, Zou Q, Lin ZY, Deng LS, Guo YB. Clinical study on the treatment of male immune infertility by Huzhangdanshenyin. Zhonghua Nan Ke Xue. 2006;12(8):750–5.
58. Aghajani MMR, Mahjoub S, Mojab F, Namdari M, Gorji NM, Dashtaki A, Mirabi P. Comparison of the effect of Ceratonia siliqua L. (Carob) syrup and vitamin E on sperm

parameters, oxidative stress index, and sex hormones in infertile men: a randomized controlled trial. Reprod Sci. 2021;28(3):766–74.
59. Takalani NB, Adefolaju GA, Henkel R, Opuwari CS. In vitro effects of aqueous extract of fermented rooibos (Aspalathus linearis) on human sperm function. Andrologia. 2021;53(8):e14114.
60. Kolangi F, Shafi H, Memariani Z, Kamalinejad M, Bioos S, Jorsaraei SGA, Bijani A, Shirafkan H, Mozaffarpur SA. Effect of Alpinia officinarum Hance rhizome extract on spermatogram factors in men with idiopathic infertility: a prospective double-blinded randomised clinical trial. Andrologia. 2019;51(1):e13172.
61. Chen X, Sun ZX, Zhao SP, Zhang XH, Chen JS, Wang R, Men B. Yishen Tongluo Recipe combined with minimally invasive surgery for the treatment of varicocele-associated asthenospermia. Zhonghua Nan Ke Xue. 2020;26(4):341–5.
62. Jo J, Lee SH, Yoon SR, Kim KI. The effectiveness of Korean herbal medicine in infertile men with poor semen quality: a prospective observational pilot study. Andrologia. 2019;51(4):e13226.
63. Roozbeh N, Amirian A, Abdi F, Haghdoost S. A systematic review on use of medicinal plants for male infertility treatment. J Family Reprod Health. 2021;15(2):74–81.
64. Jiang D, Coscione A, Li L, Zeng BY. Effect of Chinese herbal medicine on male infertility. Int Rev Neurobiol. 2017;135:297–311.
65. Hjolland NH, Bonde JP, Jensen TK, Olsen J. Diurnal scrotal skin temperature and semen quality. Int J Androl. 2000;23(5):309–18.
66. Rao M, Xia W, Yang J, Hu LX, Hu SF, Lei H, et al. Transient scrotal hyperthermia affects human sperm DNA integrity, sperm apoptosis, and sperm protein expression. Andrology. 2016;4:1054–63.
67. Aitken RJ, Baker MA. Oxidative stress, sperm survival and fertility control. Mol Cell Endocrinol. 2006;250:66–9.
68. Jung A, Eberl M, Schill WB. Improvement of semen quality by nocturnal scrotal cooling and moderate behavioural change to reduce genital heat stress in men with oligoasthenoteratozoospermia. Reproduction. 2001;121:595–603.
69. Robinson D, Rock J, Menkin MF. Control of human spermatogenesis by induced changes of intrascrotal temperature. JAMA. 1968;204:290–7.
70. Zorgniotti AW, Sealfon AI, Toth A. Chronic scrotal hypothermia as a treatment for poor semen quality. Lancet. 1980;1(8174):904–6.
71. Zorgniotti AW, Seaflon AI, Toth A. Further clinical experience with testis hypothermia for infertility due to poor semen. Urology. 1982;19(6):636–40.
72. Zorgniotti AW, Sealfon AI. Scrotal hypothermia: new therapy for poor semen. Urology. 1984;23(5):439–41.
73. Mulcahy JJ. Scrotal hypothermia and the infertile man. J Urol. 1984;132:469–70.
74. Zorgniotti AW, Cohen MS, Sealfon AI. Chronic scrotal hypothermia: results in 90 infertile couples. J Urol. 1986;135(5):944–7.
75. Jung A, Schill WB, Schuppe HC. Improvement of semen quality by nocturnal scrotal cooling in oligozoospermic men with a history of testicular maldescent. Int J Androl. 2005;28:92–8.
76. Osman MW, Nikolopoulos L, Haoula Z, Kannamannadiar J, Atiomo W. A study of the effect of the FertilMate™ Scrotum Cooling Patch on male fertility. SCOP trial (scrotal cooling patch)—study protocol for a randomised controlled trial. Trials. 2012;13:47.
77. Zumstein V, Vetterlein MW, Hoffer AP, Schmid HP, Engeler D, Betschart P. Stay cool! Special underwear for cyclic cooling significantly decreases scrotal skin temperature. Cent Eur J Urol. 2021;74(3):468–70.
78. Benidir T, Remondini T, Lau S, Jarvi K. Evaluation of patient compliance with the use of scrotal cooling devices. F S Rep. 2021;2(3):289–95.
79. Nikolopoulos I, Osman W, Haoula Z, Jayaprakasan K, Atiomo W. Scrotal cooling and its benefits to male fertility: a systematic review. J Obstet Gynaecol. 2013;33:338–42.

80. Seetharaman M, Krishnan G, Schneider RH. The future of medicine: frontiers in integrative health and medicine. Medicina (Kaunas). 2021;57(12):1303.
81. Zhou Y, Yao W, Zhang D, Yu Y, Chen S, Lu H, Jiang W, Jiang C. Effectiveness of acupuncture for asthenozoospermia: a protocol for systematic review and meta-analysis. Medicine (Baltimore). 2021;100(17):e25711.
82. Riegler R, Fischl F, Bunzel B, Neumark J. Correlation of psychological changes and spermiogram improvements following acupuncture. Urol A. 1984;23(6):329–33.
83. Fischl F, Riegler R, Bieglmayer C, Nasr F, Neumark J. Modification of semen quality by acupuncture in subfertile males. Geburtshilfe Frauenheilkd. 1984;44(8):510–2.
84. Siterman S, Eltes F, Wolfson V, Zabludovsky N, Bartoov B. Effect of acupuncture on sperm parameters of males suffering from subfertility related to low sperm quality. Arch Androl. 1997;39(2):155–61.
85. Siterman S, Eltes F, Wolfson V, Lederman H, Bartoov B. Does acupuncture treatment affect sperm density in males with very low sperm count? A pilot study. Andrologia. 2000;32(1):31–9.
86. Pei J, Strehler E, Noss U, Abt M, Piomboni P, Baccetti B, Sterzik K. Quantitative evaluation of spermatozoa ultrastructure after acupuncture treatment for idiopathic male infertility. Fertil Steril. 2005;84(1):141–7.
87. Fu B, Lun X, Gong Y. Effects of the combined therapy of acupuncture with herbal drugs on male immune infertility—a clinical report of 50 cases. J Tradit Chin Med. 2005;25(3):186–9.
88. Dong C, Chen SR, Jiang J, Xiao YH, Cai MX, Zhang YJ, Xu H, Deng LH, Li S. Clinical observation and study of mechanisms of needle-picking therapy for primary infertility of abnormal sperm. Zhongguo Zhen Jiu. 2006;26(6):389–91.
89. He Y, Chen CT, Qian LH, Xia CL, Li J, Li SQ, Liu BP. Acupuncture treatment of male infertility: a systematic review. Zhonghua Nan Ke Xue. 2015;21(7):637–45.
90. Kucuk EV, Bindayi A, Boylu U, Onol FF, Gumus E. Randomised clinical trial of comparing effects of acupuncture and varicocelectomy on sperm parameters in infertile varicocele patients. Andrologia. 2016;48(10):1080–5.
91. Li T, Xie S, Tan Y, Xie ZP, Wang WR, Li H. Mid-frequency transcutaneous electrical acu point stimulation combined with tamoxifen for the treatment of oligoasthenozoospermia. Zhonghua Nan Ke Xue. 2017;23(10):928–32.
92. Jin ZR, Liu BH, Tang WH, Jiang H, Zhang R, Han JS, Xing GG. Transcutaneous electrical acupoint stimulation for asthenozoospermia. Zhonghua Nan Ke Xue. 2017;23(1):73–7.
93. Gong Y, Li J, Wu XK. Transcutaneous electrical acupoint stimulation for the treatment of idiopathic oligoasthenospermia: a meta-analysis. Zhonghua Nan Ke Xue. 2021;27(10):917–26.
94. Nareswari I, Lestari SW, Notonegoro C. Acupuncture therapy for severe oligoasthenoteratozoospermia. Med Acupunct. 2021;33(4):302–5.
95. Zhang M, Huang G, Lu F, Paulus WE, Sterzik K. Influence of acupuncture on idiopathic male infertility in assisted reproductive technology. J Huazhong Univ Sci Technolog Med Sci. 2002;22(3):228–30.
96. Hullender Rubin LE, Anderson BJ, Craig LB. Acupuncture and in vitro fertilisation research: current and future directions. Acupunct Med. 2018;36(2):117–22.
97. Coyle ME, Stupans I, Abdel-Nour K, Ali H, Kotlyarsky M, Lie P, Tekin S, Thrimawithana T. Acupuncture versus placebo acupuncture for in vitro fertilisation: a systematic review and meta-analysis. Acupunct Med. 2021;39(1):20–9.
98. Jerng UM, Jo JY, Lee S, Lee JM, Kwon O. The effectiveness and safety of acupuncture for poor semen quality in infertile males: a systematic review and meta-analysis. Asian J Androl. 2014;16(6):884–91.
99. Li J, Wu XK, Zhang JX. Acupuncture treatment of oligoasthenozoospermia. Zhonghua Nan Ke Xue. 2018;24(1):86–90.
100. Jia W, Wang C, Yin Y. Acupuncture for oligospermia and asthenozoospermia: a systematic review and meta-analysis. Medicine (Baltimore). 2021;100(48):e27816.

Chapter 17
A Comprehensive Guide to Sperm Optimization Prior to ART

Amanda S. Setti, Daniela P. A. F. Braga, Rafael Favero Ambar, and Edson Borges Jr

Key Points

Optimizing sperm performance is crucial for improving assisted reproductive technology (ART) clinical outcomes. In this chapter, we will provide an overview of the sperm-handling approach and its outcome in ART, covering topics such as the following:

1. Sperm preparation techniques for in vitro fertilization (IVF)/intracytoplasmic sperm injection (ICSI), including simple dilution and washing, sperm migration methods, and selective washing procedures (using density gradients), and maintenance of optimal conditions during sperm handling. We will also review the processing of surgically retrieved sperm for ICSI, discussing the most appropriate types of sperm preparation techniques in cases of epididymal or testicular retrieved spermatozoa.
2. Sperm selection for conventional IVF and/or ICSI, reviewing the variety of effective techniques that have been developed for use in ART including selection based on sperm motility, selection based on nonadherence of sperm, and advanced sperm selection techniques such as motile sperm organelle morphology examination (MSOME), treatment with pentoxifylline, microfluidic sorting, selection based on sperm surface charge, selection based on non-apoptotic sperm, and selection based on sperm membrane maturity and integrity. We will

A. S. Setti · Daniela P. A. F. Braga · E. Borges Jr (✉)
Fertility Medical Group, Sao Paulo, SP, Brazil

Sapientiae Institute, Sao Paulo, SP, Brazil
e-mail: amanda@sapientiae.org.br; dbraga@fertility.com.br; edson@fertility.com.br

R. F. Ambar
Department of Urology, Centro Universitário FMABC and Andrology department at Ideia Fértil Institute, Santo André, São Paulo, Brazil

Urology department of Hospital do Servidor Público Estadual SP-IAMSPE, São Paulo, Brazil

A. Agarwal et al. (eds.), *Current and Future Advances in Male Infertility*,
https://doi.org/10.1007/978-3-031-62648-7_17

also review the selection of surgically retrieved sperm for ICSI, discussing methods for the selection of immotile spermatozoa if needed, such as mechanical touch technique, hypo-osmotic swelling test, chemical motility enhancers such as pentoxifylline and theophylline, laser-assisted immotile sperm selection, and birefringence–polarization microscopy; future advances will also be addressed.
3. Additionally, we draw attention to the promising future sperm-handling methods such as proteomic analysis, interferometric phase microscopy, confocal light absorption and scattering spectroscopy, Raman spectrometry, and peptide-based sperm selection.

Introduction

Infertility, defined as the inability of a sexually active couple without the use of contraceptive methods to establish pregnancy within 1 year, affects nearly 15% of couples at reproductive age. Thus, it is estimated that about 72 million couples [1] are subjected to fertility-related issues globally, representing a significant burden for the health system. Male infertility accounts for 50% of the infertility cases [1] generally owing to low sperm count and poor function leading to inhibited fertilization potential [2].

Lifestyle and environmental factors, genetic issues, DNA fragmentation, and advanced paternal age have been implicated in male infertility, which in turn seems to be associated with an increased risk of several malignancies. Even though advances have been made in the understanding and management of male infertility, shedding light on previously unknown topics, about 30% of male infertility incidence occurs due to idiopathic sperm abnormalities [3].

The topic of infertility has been investigated not only in the fields of science and medicine, but also socially, religiously, and philosophically. Infertility gave rise to what we now know as assisted reproductive technology (ART), which aids in the procreation procedure when other methods prove ineffective. Two different approaches can be recommended to circumvent infertility depending on the cause: artificial insemination or in vitro fertilization (IVF). Intrauterine insemination (IUI) is a simple, low-complexity technique, in which only the spermatozoa are manipulated, but success rates are lower using this method, especially for couples with male factor infertility [4]. Thus, IVF techniques are the treatment choices for these couples, which encompass conventional IVF and intracytoplasmic sperm injection (ICSI), the most widely used IVF method worldwide. In fact, it is estimated that ICSI is currently used in more than 66% [5] of IVF clinics. To perform these techniques, appropriate seminal processing must be carried out to optimize seminal quality. This chapter summarizes the sperm preparation techniques for IVF and/or ICSI, including the techniques in cases of epididymal or testicular retrieved spermatozoa, sperm selection for conventional IVF and/or ICSI including methods for the selection of immotile spermatozoa, and promising future sperm-handling methods.

Sperm Preparation Techniques for IVF/ICSI

Under in vivo conditions, during migration through the cervical mucus in the female genital tract, sperm with high fertilization potential are isolated from their immotile counterparts, debris, and seminal plasma. This process is important not only for the selection of progressive motile sperm, but also for the physiological changes related to sperm's functional competence to take place [6].

In the andrology laboratory, the objectives of sperm preparation techniques are (i) removal of toxins, contaminants, and other cellular elements from seminal plasma; (ii) selection of spermatozoa with better morphology and motility; and (iii) improvement of the fertilizing capacity of sperm for IVF/ICSI. As an alternative, sperm preparation may also be performed prognostically to assist in choosing the best IVF technique to be performed [7].

Spermatozoa must be separated from seminal plasma within 1 h after ejaculation since contaminants and leukocytes potentially present in seminal plasma can damage the plasma membrane of spermatozoa through the increased production of reactive oxygen species (ROS) [8].

Many sperm preparation procedures are available, but there are three main groups of methods. To give an overview, only the three most common techniques, classical swim-up, discontinuous density gradient centrifugation, and sperm wash, will be discussed.

Seminal Wash (Sperm Wash)

This is the fastest method, which consists of washing the seminal plasma from the final precipitate without performing sperm selection, since centrifugation results in the retrieval of all types of spermatozoa, germ cells, leukocytes, and debris. Briefly, the semen sample is diluted with a medium and centrifuged. Subsequently, the pellet is resuspended in a small amount of medium and incubated until the time of insemination [9].

Swim-up

Apart from the sperm wash, the swim-up technique is the oldest and possibly the most used sperm preparation method. Originally described by Mahadevan and Baker [10], this method is based on the active migration of spermatozoa from the cell pellet into an overlaying medium for 60-min incubation. Briefly, the washed pellet is deposited under the culture medium, and the sperm are selected through their directional progression speed capable of making them swim against the force of gravity and manage to ascend from the bottom of the tube to the layer of culture medium at the top of the conical tube (Fig. 17.1). This technique results in an extremely high percentage (>90%) of motile sperm with high incidence of normal forms, free of debris or other cells. On the other hand, motile spermatozoa may be trapped in the lower levels of the pellet and never reach the interface with the culture medium layer. In addition, the yield of spermatozoa is limited, estimated at around 20% of the neat sample; therefore, the technique is not indicated for men with moderate to severe male factor. This procedure has also been associated with a decreased percentage of normally chromatin-condensed spermatozoa [11]. As sperm are pelleted, an increased generation of ROS may occur due to close cell-to-cell contact, cell debris, and leukocytes [12], which could cause lipid peroxidation and compromise several sperm functions [13].

In the present day, this technique is performed using the liquefied semen sample, in an attempt to overcome ROS issues. Also, media layer is gently deposited over the semen layer in order to provide a cleaner yield [14].

Discontinuous Density Gradient Centrifugation

The literature has described several methods using the principle of density gradient centrifugation to split up different types of spermatozoa. Ficoll® was the first gradient material used for preparing spermatozoa [7] followed by Percoll®. Since the withdrawal of Percoll from the market for use in ART, because of its potential deleterious impact on sperm membranes due to its polyvinylpyrrolidone-coated silica content [15], various low-toxicity replacement products made of silane-coated silica particles such as IxaPrep® (MediCult, Copenhagen, Denmark), SilSelect® (FertiPro N.V., Beernem, Belgium), PureSperm® (NidaCon Laboratories AB, Gothenburg,

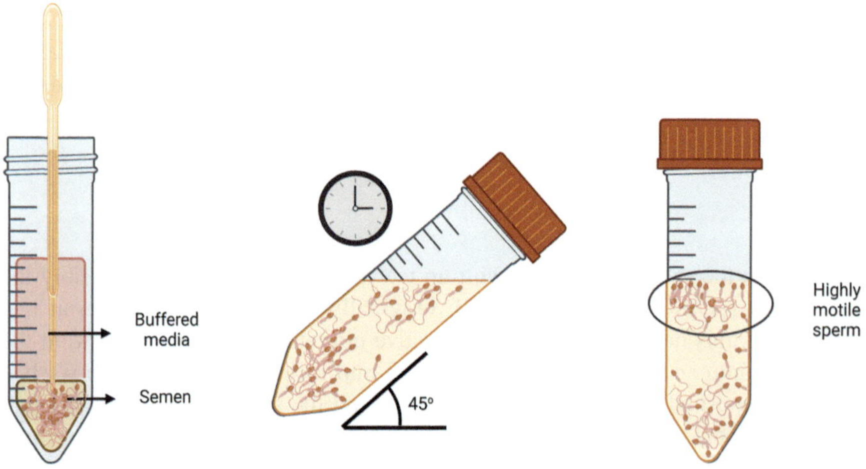

Fig. 17.1 Schematic representation of swim-up technique

Sweden), or ISolate® (Irvine Scientific, Santa Ana, CA, USA) were introduced into the market [6].

Briefly, media with different gradients are neatly stacked in a conical tube, so that the one with the lowest gradient is at the bottom of the tube and the one with the highest gradient is at the top of the tube. The sperm sample is then placed on top of the higher density media, and the tube is centrifuged. Highly motile spermatozoa move actively through the different gradients and can therefore penetrate the boundary faster than poorly motile or immotile sperm; thus, highly motile sperm cells are concentrated in the pellet at the bottom of the tube. Seminal plasma, debris, germ cells, leukocytes, and abnormal sperm, which were retained in the supernatant, are discarded, resulting in a clean final sample (Fig. 17.2). The discontinuous density gradient technique recovers a higher concentration of motile sperm when compared to the swim-up, however, with a lower final motility [16]. However, evidence indicates that the technique may increase sperm DNA fragmentation levels [17–19], which in turn could negatively impact ART reproductive outcomes.

Advantages and disadvantages for all three methods are given in Table 17.1.

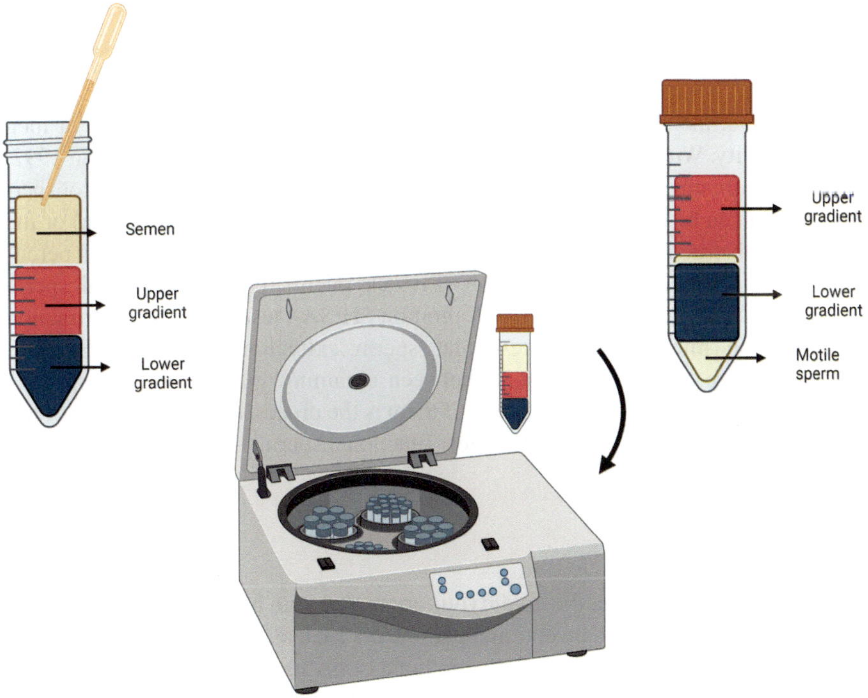

Fig. 17.2 Schematic representation of density gradient centrifugation technique: In a centrifuge tube, semen is placed on top of a gradient solution and then centrifuged. Motile spermatozoa are recovered from the bottom of the tube (pellet)

Table 17.1 Advantages and disadvantages of most used sperm preparation methods for ART

Sperm preparation method	Advantages	Disadvantages
Seminal wash	• Easy and fast to perform • Suitable for samples with severe oligozoospermia	• Retrieval of dirty final sample • Immotile sperm are recovered
Swim-up	• Easy to perform • Cost-effective • Retrieval of a clean sample of highly motile spermatozoa	• Restricted to sperm samples with high sperm count and motility • Low retrieval • Potential sperm damage by ROS • Decreased percentage of normally chromatin-condensed spermatozoa
Discontinuous density gradient centrifugation	• Clean final sample of highly motile spermatozoa • Works with very low sperm density samples • Good yield • Significant reduction of leukocytes and ROS	• Time-consuming • Expensive • Potential increase in sperm DNA fragmentation

Processing Surgically Retrieved Sperm for ICSI

Azoospermia, the absence of spermatozoa in ejaculate, affects up to 15% of men with infertility. With the advent of intracytoplasmic sperm injection (ICSI) in 1992, appropriate treatment for these men emerged. Depending on the type of azoospermia, sperm can be harvested from the epididymis (obstructive azoospermia) or the testis (nonobstructive azoospermia) [20], using different techniques such as percutaneous epididymal sperm aspiration (PESA), microsurgical epididymal sperm aspiration (MESA), testicular sperm aspiration (TESA), testicular sperm extraction (TESE), and microdissection testicular sperm extraction (micro-TESE) [21]. However, there are still many steps between obtaining sperm from azoospermic patients and achieving pregnancy. One of them is the processing and selection of not only the "best-looking" but also the most functional sperm.

Epididymal Sperm

Sperm cells retrieved from the epididymis are mixed with buffered culture medium before the assessment of conventional parameters such as count, motility, and morphology. The discontinuous density gradient centrifugation followed by double washing is generally used for preparation of those presenting with high sperm count, whereas double washing and centrifugation are used for the preparation of samples presenting with low sperm count (reviewed by Verheyen et al. [22]). An aliquot of the sperm sample preparation is placed on a petri dish and covered with mineral oil until sperm selection for ICSI. Remaining sperm can be frozen for potential successive ICSI cycles.

Testicular Sperm

Testicular aspirates are dispensed in a dry tube or in droplets of media covered with mineral oil until the time of ICSI. Different processing methods such as mechanical processing and the use of enzymes or erythrocyte-lysing buffer have been described for testicular tissue.

Mechanical sperm extraction, with rupture of seminiferous tubules by shredding and fine mincing, is the most used processing method for testicular tissue. Briefly, the testicular tissue is shredded with microscope slides, needles, or scissors, thus releasing sperm into the buffered culture medium in a petri dish. Using a phase-contrast or inverted microscope, the sample is analyzed for the presence of sperm, washed, and stored in a petri dish covered with oil, until sperm selection for ICSI [23].

Red blood cell contamination is a feature often present in the testicular tissue sample that may impede visualization of spermatozoa. After shredding procedure, the testicular tissue may be exposed to an erythrocyte-lysing buffer that may quickly improve sperm recovery and selection [24].

Enzymatic digestion, a method usually used when no sperm is identified after mechanical shredding, can be performed using collagenases type IA and IV to digest the collagen from membranes and extracellular matrix of the testicular tissue. The use of enzymes was successful in the recovery of sperm in one out of four men undergoing ICSI after sperm recovery failure post-mechanical shredding [25].

Sperm Selection Techniques for IVF/ICSI

Although some conventional sperm preparation methods can isolate highly motile spermatozoa, these techniques may not select spermatozoa based on functional competence or genetic status. Therefore, sperm selection techniques are constantly improving to aid the selection of spermatozoa with high functional competence for IVF and/or ICSI.

Sperm Selection Based on Membrane Characteristics

The sperm outer membrane plays a role in several basic processes such as cell metabolism, capacitation, oocyte binding, and acrosome reaction among others. It is targeted for the development of sperm selection methods due to its accessibility and relation with sperm vitality and quality.

Magnetic-Activated Cell Sorting (MACS)

MACS is a technique that isolates apoptotic and non-apoptotic spermatozoa based on the affinity between annexin V and phosphatidylserine (PS), a marker of apoptosis that is externalized with sperm membrane integrity loss [26]. Briefly, sperm sample is incubated with annexin V conjugated to magnetic microbeads [27], which binds to apoptotic sperm and is then removed from the sperm sample by magnets, while non-apoptotic sperm pass through the separation column (Fig. 17.3). Several studies have shown the efficacy of MACS technique in improving sperm quality in terms of motility, morphology, and viability (reviewed by Said et al. [28]). A meta-analysis of five randomized trials showed significantly higher pregnancy rates after MACS [29]. Despite being a simple and fast technique, the MACS protocol is used together with density gradient centrifugation, which includes an additional sperm sample-handling step and increases the loss of recovered spermatozoa in 15% [30]. Therefore, sperm samples should be carefully selected for the use of this sperm selection technique.

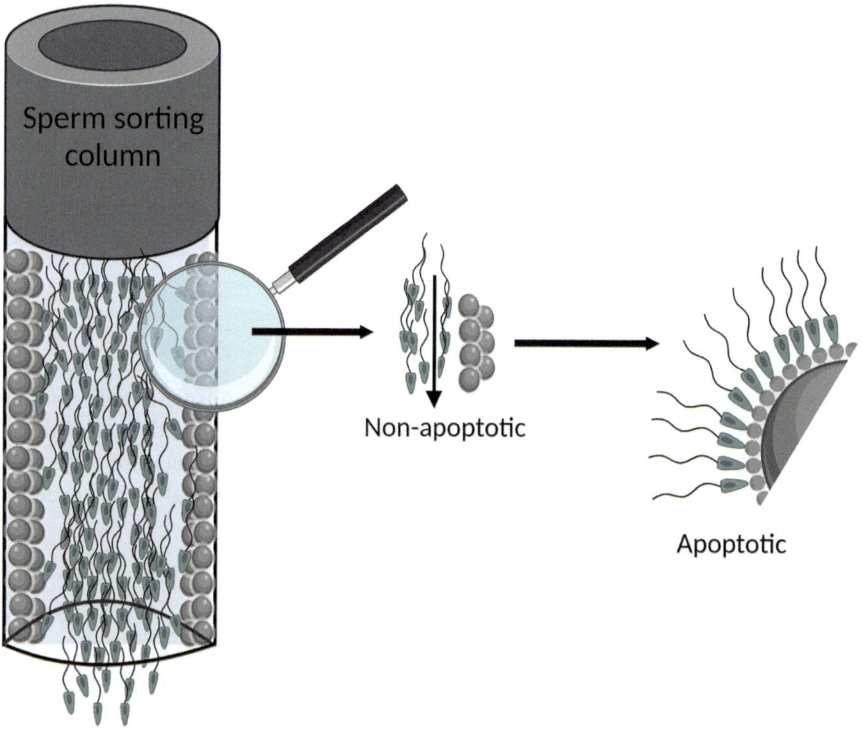

Fig. 17.3 Schematic representation of Annexin V magnetic-activated cell sorting (MACS): Semen is passed through a magnetic column, apoptotic spermatozoa are bound to magnetic beads coated with Annexin V and trapped in the column, while non-apoptotic sperm pass through the column

Hyaluronic Acid (HA) Binding

One of the main elements of the extracellular matrix surrounding the oocyte is HA, and binding sites to it are expressed by mature spermatozoa [31, 32]. Based on this spermatozoa-HA affinity, two systems of sperm selection have been developed: (i) HA-coated dishes (PICSI Sperm Selection Device, MidAtlantic Diagnostic, Origio) [32] (Fig. 17.4) and (ii) a viscous medium containing HA (Sperm Slow, MediCult, Origio) [33]. Several studies have investigated the potential benefits of using sperm selected using on HA binding methods for ICSI, and, collectively, they reveal a limited capacity of these methods for improving outcomes (reviewed by Oseguera-López et al. [34]); however, types of patients that could benefit from this procedure are yet to be confirmed by further studies.

Zeta Method

Zeta potential is a negative electrokinetic potential of around −16 to −20 mV, which is acquired by sperm membrane because of sperm surface coating with sialic acids during spermatogenesis and epididymal maturation [35]. This surface electrical charge allows the sperm to adhere to surfaces with positive charge in a protein-free medium [36]. Briefly, semen sample is washed, and the resuspended pellet is transferred to a tube, which is induced to gain positive surface charge (induction is performed by putting the tube inside a latex glove, rotating it twice or three times, and then quickly removing it from the glove). Charged sperm cells are expected to adhere with tube wall within 60 s. The remaining sample in the bottom of the tube is aspirated and discarded, and the tube wall is washed with medium to release

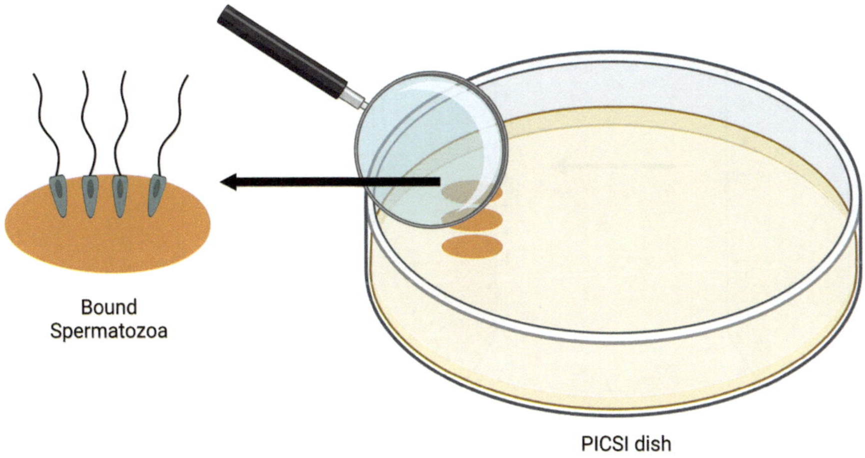

Fig. 17.4 Schematic representation of PICSI method for sperm selection based on hyaluronic acid binding. Spermatozoa are placed on a dish containing hyaluronic acid (HA) drops (orange). Matured spermatozoa bind to this HA drops and can be then used for ICSI

charged sperm [36] (Fig. 17.5). Sperm DNA fragmentation has been shown to be lower using zeta method than conventional density gradient centrifugation [37]. In addition, significantly higher fertilization, pregnancy, and implantation rates in ICSI cycles with the use of zeta method in contrast to those without the method have been observed. The zeta method is fast, simple, and low cost; however, it yields low amounts of sperm [38].

Sperm Selection Based on Morphology

Motile Sperm Organelle Morphology Examination (MSOME)

This method uses the differential interference contrast (DIC) microscopy technique, also known as Nomarski interference contrast, which allows greater depth of focus in thicker specimens observed under higher magnification [39].

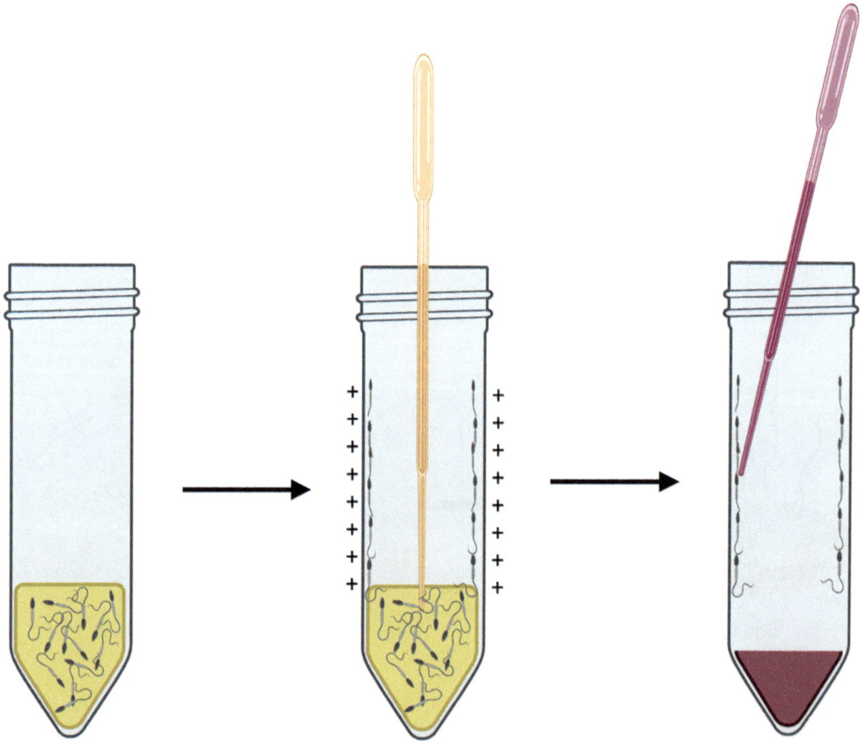

Fig. 17.5 Schematic representation of the zeta sperm selection method. Mature sperm cells remain attached to the tube walls, due to interaction between the negative electrical charge of the viable sperm membrane and the positive electrical charge of the tube. Immature sperm fraction passes freely to the bottom of the tube

The MSOME is performed under an inverted microscope equipped with high-power DIC. Briefly, an aliquot of the prepared sperm sample is transferred to a microdroplet of buffered culture medium containing polyvinylpyrrolidone in a glass-bottomed dish. A UPlan Apo x100 oil/1.35 objective lens covered by immersion oil is used to examine sperm cells. The images are captured by a high-quality image production video camera and a video monitor. The morphological examination is conducted on the monitor screen. In general, the total calculated magnification is ×6600. The MSOME allows the assessment of the acrosome, post-acrosomal lamina, neck, tail, mitochondria, and nucleus of the sperm (Fig. 17.6). MSOME could be used for the rejection of the acrosome reaction-resistant spermatozoa. In addition, vacuole-free spermatozoa seem to yield lower rates of DNA fragmentation as compared with vacuolated spermatozoa. Also, the incidence of sperm head vacuoles has been negatively correlated with chromatin condensation (reviewed by Setti et al. [40]). On the other hand, MSOME takes a long time to find suitable sperm, particularly in poor sperm quality samples. Therefore, it is somewhat unpractical and expensive.

Polarization Microscopy

Baccetti [41] has employed polarization microscopy to detect functional spermatozoa for ICSI based on the principle that, under polarized light microscopy, the head of viable spermatozoa is birefringent. Birefringence (double reflection) analysis in spermatozoa is an indicator of structural normalcy, as confirmed by transmission electron microscopy [41]. Sperm with positive birefringence present organized and compact structure, reflecting normal nucleus, acrosome, and flagellum, while those cells lacking birefringence are considered nonviable (Fig. 17.7). A recent study

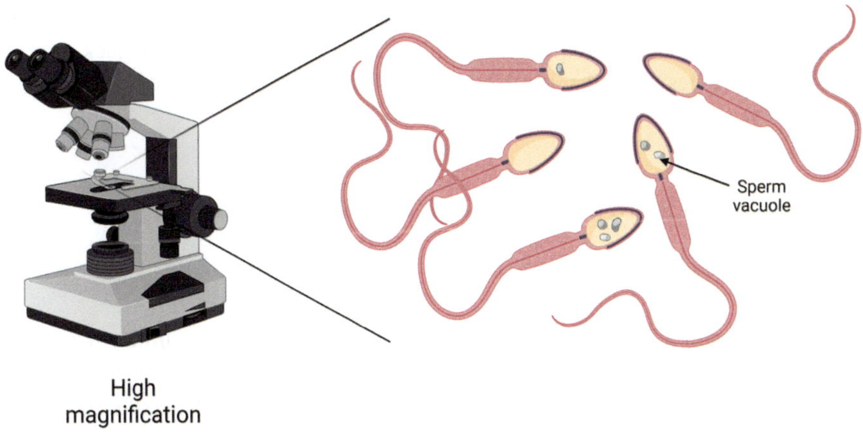

Fig. 17.6 Schematic representation of MSOME. Spermatozoa are examined under high magnification to select those with normal forms and free of vacuoles and then collected for their use in ICSI

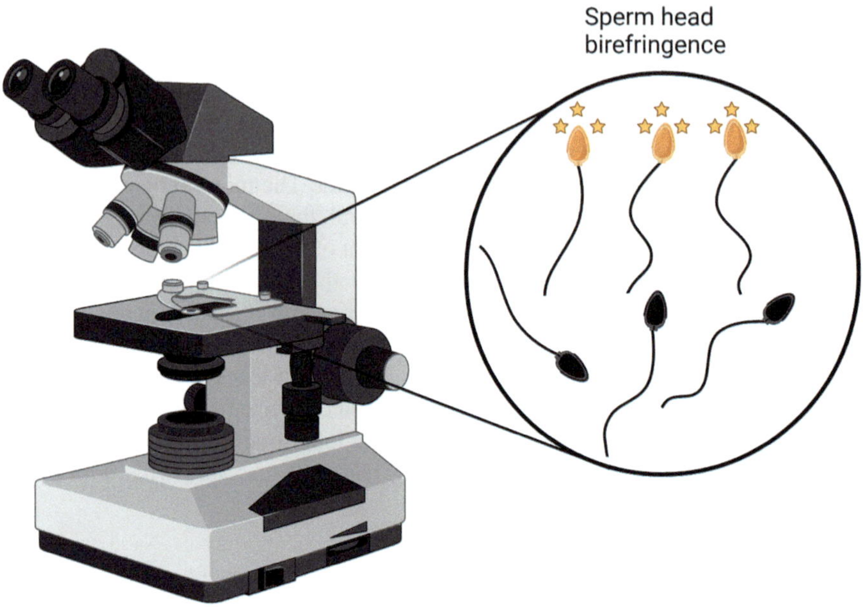

Fig. 17.7 Schematic representation of sperm selection using polarized light microscopy. Viable sperm show head birefringence (yellow), while nonviable sperm lack head birefringence (dark heads)

showed that immotile sperm cells with birefringence properties under polarized light have higher chances of inducing fertilization and embryo development compared with non-birefringent cells. In addition, a pattern of partial birefringence, associated with a reacted acrosome, was the strongest predictive factor for live birth delivery, both in ejaculated and testicular samples [42]. Nevertheless, the usefulness of selecting sperm using polarization microscopy is yet debatable (reviewed by Henkel [43]). In addition, several drawbacks preclude a more extensive use of the technique: the high-price acquisition to the embryology laboratory, the lack of reliable cutoff values, and the availability of cheaper sperm selection methods to name a few.

Sperm Selection Based on Motility and Guidance Mechanisms

Microfluidic Technology

Microfluidics allows for fast and easy sperm cell sorting, more accurately matching the natural selection method, and may be classified into three types: those that separate exclusively motile sperm, those that separate sperm without relying on sperm movement, and those that identify and choose unique sperm cells [44]. Type 1 is the most frequently used microfluidic devices that, in general, recover 100% motile sperm with superior DNA status in contrast to neat sperm.

Microfluidic technologies employ the principles of chemoattractant gradients (hyaluronic acid, cervical mucus, or acetylcholine), fluid flow (ability to pass through a streamline in a laminar flow) (Fig. 17.8), thermotactic force (responsiveness to thermal gradients), or passively driven microfluidics for sperm sorting (driven by sperm motility only) (reviewed by Olatunji and More [45]). Microfluidic devices can be considered fairly new, so the literature on the clinical effectiveness regarding sperm selection goes from significantly increased ongoing pregnancy rates [46] and improved genomic integrity [47] to no improvements at all [48].

Sperm migration within the oviducts is controlled by three key mechanisms named rheotaxis, chemotaxis, and thermotaxis; thus, sperm selection based on these guidance mechanisms has been developed.

Rheotaxis

Defined as the propensity of some living organisms to respond with motion to the mechanical stimulus of a water flow, rheotaxis makes mammalian spermatozoa guide their movement against the fluid stream directed towards them within the oviducts [49]. Nagata et al. [50] developed a technique using bull sperm as a mammalian model, in which a stream is created through a series of microchannels towards a well where the sperm sample is collected for ART use (Fig. 17.9a). Another study that compared spermatozoa selected using rheotaxis to an untreated sample and a sample subjected to density gradient centrifugation showed that rheotaxis-recovered spermatozoa presented significantly higher chromatin compaction [51]. More recently, the concept of rheotaxis has been included in

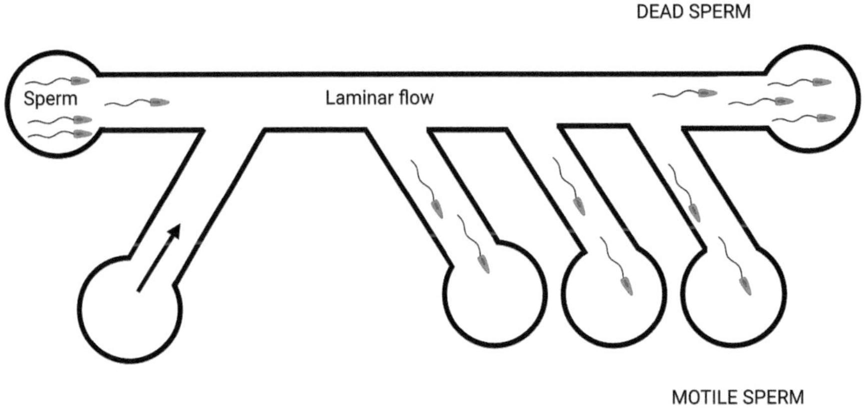

Fig. 17.8 Schematic representation of the microfluidic system. The motile fraction of sperm cells swims through the flow and is collected in separate chambers, while the immotile sperm cells arrive at the exit of the system

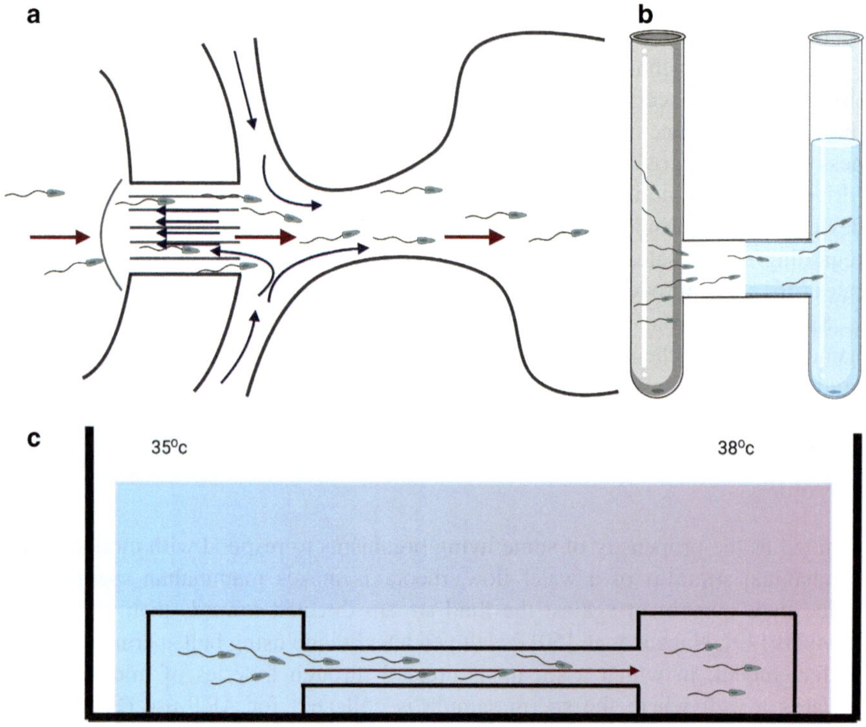

Fig. 17.9 Schematic representation of sperm selection methods based on guidance mechanisms. (**a**) Rheotaxis: a flow (blue arrows) is created through a serial of microchannels towards a well where sperm sample is retained. Sperm cells respond swimming towards it and accumulating in a receptive well (sperm migration is indicated by red arrows). (**b**) Chemotaxis: a well filled with the sperm sample is connected by a tube to a well containing the chemoattractant (blue solution). The chemoattractant generates a gradient by diffusing through the tube, and the sperm cells react by migrating towards the higher concentration and are accumulated on the opposite side of the device. (**c**) Thermotaxis: sperm sample is placed on a drop of a medium connected by a capillary to a second drop of medium. The generation of a gradient between both drops makes spermatozoa migrate from the cooler drop of medium towards the warmer temperature by thermotaxis, accumulating in the hotter drop of medium

microfluidics, thus using this rheotactic behavior to perform the sperm sorting, resulting in highly motile cells with normal morphology [52].

Chemotaxis

Defined as the movement of a microorganism towards or away from a chemical known as "chemoattractant," chemotaxis is an important mechanism that plays a vital role in guiding spermatozoa towards the cumulus-oocyte complex. Sperm cells are sensitive to chemical gradients and naturally swim towards the most concentrated areas when placed in a concentration gradient of some molecules. The progesterone hormone secreted by the cumulus cells surrounding the oocyte is used as a chemoattractant in vivo and for spermatozoa chemotaxis assays in vitro [53]. In this method, two wells are connected by a tube. One of the wells is loaded with a chemoattractant molecule medium (progesterone), and the other well is loaded with the sperm sample. A gradient is generated by the progesterone diffusion through the tube, and the spermatozoa respond with movement towards the higher concentration. Thus, chemoattracted sperm is accumulated in the initial well free of cells where they can be collected and used for ART [54] (Fig. 17.9b). These recovered spermatozoa exhibit improved morphology and reduced DNA fragmentation and apoptosis rate in contrast to those selected with density gradient centrifugation [55]. However, although chemotaxis is thoroughly mentioned as a natural sperm selection method, studies using this method to successfully sort sperm cells in microfluidics are scarce [56, 57].

Thermotaxis

With a very similar definition to the one of chemotaxis, in this mechanism, the spermatozoa can direct their movement based on a change of temperature, migrating from colder to warmer zones; thus, the driving force is a thermal gradient rather than a chemical gradient. In fact, the spermatozoa are among the most sensitive motile cells to thermal gradients [58], being able to become hyperactivated and swim up thermal gradients with temperature variation of only a few degree Celsius [59], underlying the movement of sperm cells from the fallopian tubes to the ampulla [60]. Developed by Pérez-Cerezales et al. [61], in the thermotaxis sperm selection, spermatozoa are put in a medium drop, connected to a cell-free medium drop, by a capillary. The generation of a temperature gradient between both drops, in which the cell-free drop possesses the highest temperature, makes spermatozoa migrate towards the warmer temperature by thermotaxis (Fig. 17.9c). The accumulated sperm in the second drop can be collected for ART applications. Significantly improved pregnancy rates with ICSI as compared to sperm cells selected by the swim-up method were obtained in mice [61]. Nevertheless, as with chemotaxis method, the literature is scarce to confirm the improvements in ART outcomes.

Promising Future Sperm-Handling Methods

Proteomic Analysis

Proteomic analysis of spermatozoa is difficult and might therefore be limited for various reasons such as the low protein concentration, the number of spermatozoa available for analysis specially in oligozoospermic patients, and the risk of sample contamination by leukocytes or other non-sperm cells and therefore detection of non-sperm proteins. More than 6000 sperm proteins have been identified and associated with several vital cellular functions such as motility, capacitation, sperm-oocyte binding, metabolism, apoptosis, cell cycle, or membrane trafficking, indicating the complex composition and function of the sperm cell. Differentially expressed proteins have been identified in infertile patients and in patients exhibiting seminal oxidative stress [62, 63]. However, none of the proteomic methodologies is ready to be employed for clinical use.

Interferometric Phase Microscopy (IPM)

This microscopy technique quantitatively images sperm cells without staining, generating contrast at all cell points [64]. The interferogram is generated via interference between two beams, one passing through the sample and a reference one, which is then translated into a 2D phase map image providing the sample's optical path delay at all points in the image [65]. This technique is highly correlated with the results obtained with stained sperm cells [64]. Eravuchira et al. [66] proposed a novel platform for single sperm cell selection, combining IPM with a disposable microfluidic. In order to make IPM more accessible and affordable, a compact and external interferometric module was placed at the exit of an existing imaging system. This model allows the option of assessing and selecting individual sperm cells using a single microchannel device. This automated analysis was performed in less than a second, while it is estimated that around 10 s is needed for the evaluation of a single cell by an embryologist [66]. Mirsky et al. [67] developed an automated method for sperm assessment and characterization based on a machine learning classification algorithm. Features relating to sperm morphology were extracted from the quantitative phase maps provided by IPM and used to train a support vector machine classifier to automatically classify spermatozoa according to morphology, achieving areas under (i) the receiver-operating characteristic curve and (ii) the precision-recall curve >88%, as well as precisions ≥90%. The authors believe that their automatic analysis can become the basis for single sperm cell selection in ART.

Confocal Light Absorption and Scattering Spectroscopy

This method, which is a conjugation of confocal microscopy and the principles of light scattering spectroscopy [68], has previously discriminated between apoptotic and non-apoptotic bronchial epithelial cells, by providing highly specific images of subcellular structures at submicrometer levels beyond the diffraction limit of light [68, 69].

Raman Spectrometry

Raman spectrometry can detect cells with abnormal DNA at the single-cell level through the analysis of discrete laser scattering spectra. It has been suggested that Raman microspectrometry distinguishes normal from abnormal sperm cells and that it is a valuable tool in evaluating sperm for ART [70]. Different malignancies and tumors have already been classified and diagnosed using this methodology [71] with no adverse effect on the analyzed cells [72].

Peptide-Based Sperm Selection

Enciso et al. [73] aimed at designing new peptides that bind to fragmented DNA and could potentially be used to discover DNA-damaged sperm. Thus, spermatozoa tested and noticed to be DNA damage free using this peptide-based stain technique could be used for ICSI, since these peptides do not negatively impact cell viability [74]. The authors found that the peptide had a high affinity for several types of DNA damage, and the level of DNA fragmentation was significant being highly correlated with TUNEL assay. Peptide-based sperm selection may be an inexpensive and practical substitute to the tests currently available. However, as it still requires the use of a detergent to remove the membrane, future research may let this method to be employed for the selection of viable and DNA-intact spermatozoa for ART.

Selection of Surgically Retrieved Sperm for ICSI

Since prolonged culture of surgically recovered spermatozoa up to 48 h can improve maturation and motility status, IVF centers often schedule sperm harvesting the day before the oocyte collection. In some cases, though, harvested sperm fail to achieve motility even after extended incubation period; thus, the use of add-on techniques is recommended for the selection of not only the most morphologically normal but also the most functionally available sperm (reviewed by Verheyen et al. [22]).

Mechanical Touch

This technique has been employed for detection of viable immotile spermatozoa prior to ICSI. It relies on the principle that the tail flexibility of immotile vital and non-vital sperm is different when managed with the microinjection pipette. Non-vital sperm are rigid; thus, the sperm head will move along with the tail when it is touched with the pipette. Vital sperm possess flexibility; thus, the sperm head will not follow the tail, and the tail will return to its original location.

Similar pregnancy and delivery rates were obtained when ICSI cycles using immotile testicular sperm selected with this technique were contrasted to those using motile testicular sperm [75]. The real-time, chemical- and dye-free performance allows the examined sperm to be used for ICSI, which is the major advantage of the technique. Nevertheless, it has a high inter- and intra-observer variability due to the subjectivity of the technique, and it can be time-consuming to access each sperm cell before ICSI.

Hypo-osmotic Swelling Test

Live sperm cells have intact and functional plasmatic membranes that react to hypo-osmotic solutions. Live sperm exposed to hypotonic media permit water influx and respond with tail swelling or curling, while dead sperm with unfunctional membranes will not react [22, 76, 77] (Fig. 17.10).

Chemical Motility Enhancers

Cyclic adenosine monophosphate that participates in sperm motility can be increased by phosphodiesterase inhibitors such as pentoxifylline and theophylline. It has been previously demonstrated that conjugation of pentoxifylline and theophylline to epididymal or testicular retrieved sperm resulted in the achievement of sperm motility and successful ICSI clinical outcomes (Fig. 17.11). The addition of pentoxifylline and theophylline may reduce sperm selection time; however, the toxicity of these chemical compounds could be a reason for caution. To date, there is no evidence of offspring abnormalities with the use of these components for sperm selection [22, 78].

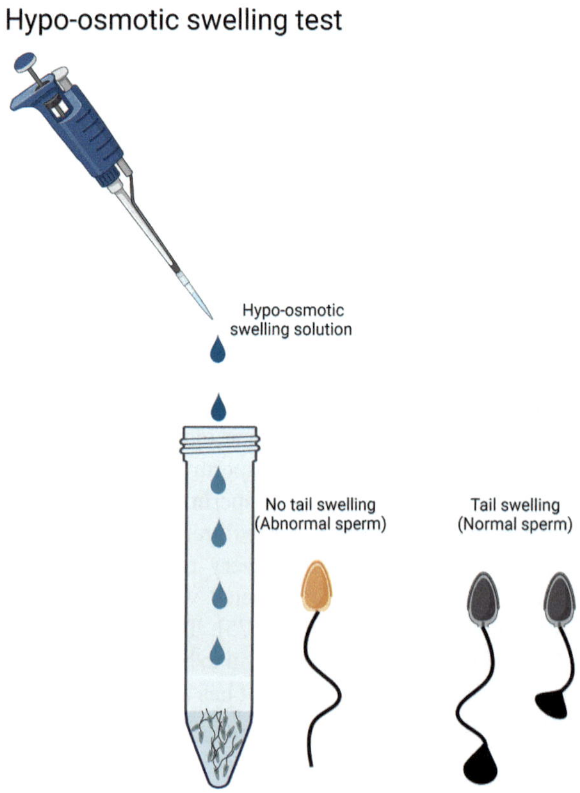

Fig. 17.10 Schematic representation of hypo-osmotic swelling test

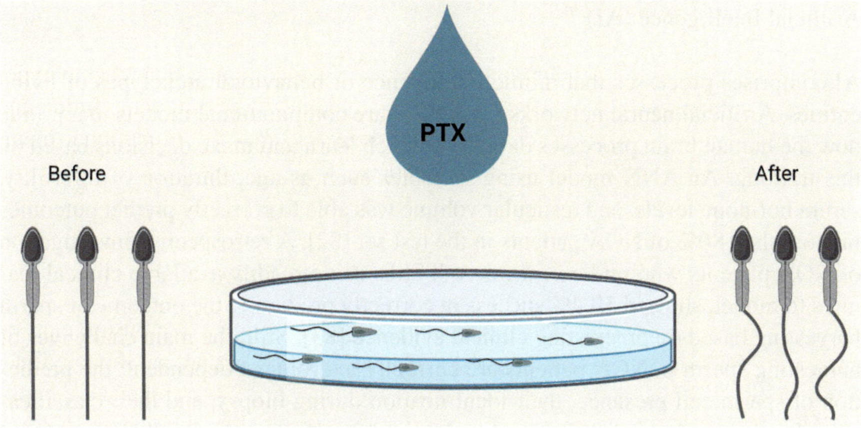

Fig. 17.11 Schematic representation of motility chemical inducers. In this case, viable motile sperms are activated by the presence of pentoxifylline

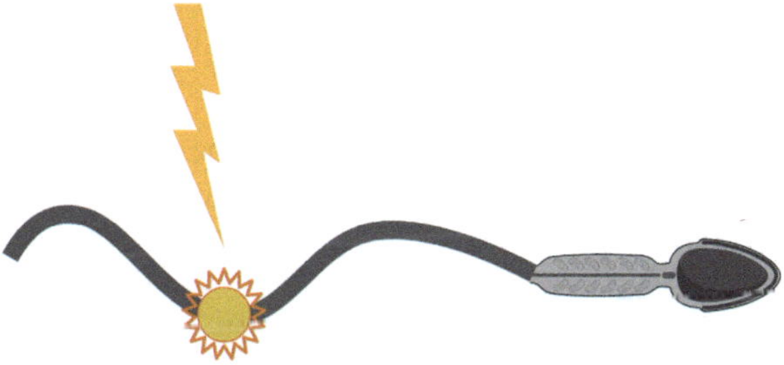

Fig. 17.12 Schematic representation of LAISS. The laser shot produces a slight tail movement in viable sperms that were initially immotile

Laser-Assisted Immotile Sperm Selection (LAISS)

As with the mechanical touch technique, LAISS also distinguishes between viable and dead immotile sperm by examining sperm tail reaction. However, the stimulus is performed by a single laser shot. Live sperm will curl their tails, while dead sperm will not dislocate their ones [79] (Fig. 17.12). LAISS is a fast, chemical-free sperm selection technique; however, the high cost of the equipment precluded its widespread application into clinical routine. Testicular sperm selected via this technique showed high fertilization potential when used for ICSI [80].

Birefringence-Polarization Microscopy

Sperm selection using this abovementioned technique was also shown to be beneficial for testicular retrieved sperm [42].

Artificial Intelligence (AI)

AI comprises processes that mimic intelligence or behavioral archetypes of living entities. Artificial neural networks (or ANNs) are computational models that mimic how the human brain processes data [81], which learn and make decisions based on this training. An ANN model using variables such as age, duration of infertility, serum hormone levels, and testicular volume was able to correctly predict outcomes in more than 80% of NOA patients in the test set [82]. A retrospective investigation of NOA patients who underwent micro-TESE, using readily available clinical features to model, showed 59.4% success in correctly predicting the outcome of sperm harvesting based on preexisting clinical evidence [83]. Still, the main challenges of harvesting sperm in NOA patients are currently andrologist dependent: the prediction of sperm cell presence, their identification during biopsy, and their classification after harvesting, but it is possible that in a near future, they will be automated with the aid of AI.

Summary

There is a margin for improvement in the evaluation and treatment of infertility as well as in the efficiency of ART, which may be achieved by further development of emerging reproductive technologies. Sperm selection techniques may represent a breakthrough in ART, especially in cases of severe male factor. The ideal sperm selection method should meet the requirements of an ART clinic, where harmony must exist between reduced timing and labor quality; it should also be fast, inexpensive, easy to learn, repeatable, and efficient in improving pregnancy rates. However, sperm selection methods available to date have not shown to be beneficial for their routine use in the clinical practice and appear to be useful only in specific cases of male infertility. None of the countless number of methods have shown remarkable results in improving pregnancy rates. Advantages and disadvantages exist for all the sperm selection methods. Although some novel methods described here have delivered promising results, they must be proved in large, randomized studies in the context of clinical practice. Therefore, at this time, one cannot claim one method to be superior to other. It is quite possible that to increase the efficiency of ART, it is necessary to use more than one method of sperm selection. Nevertheless, this hypothesis must be confirmed in appropriate trials, including semen samples of different qualities, and controlled for female infertility.

References

1. Boivin J, et al. International estimates of infertility prevalence and treatment-seeking: potential need and demand for infertility medical care. Hum Reprod. 2007;22(6):1506–12.

2. Frey K. Male reproductive health and infertility. Prim Care. 2010;37:643–52. x
3. Cavallini G. Male idiopathic oligoasthenoteratozoospermia. Asian J Androl. 2006;8(2):143–57.
4. Allahbadia GN. Intrauterine insemination: fundamentals revisited. J Obstet Gynaecol India. 2017;67(6):385–92.
5. Adamson GD, et al. International committee for monitoring assisted reproductive technology: world report on assisted reproductive technology, 2011. Fertil Steril. 2018;110(6):1067–80.
6. Henkel RR, Schill WB. Sperm preparation for ART. Reprod Biol Endocrinol. 2003;1:108.
7. Levay PF, et al. Effectiveness of various sperm processing methods in removing seminal plasma from insemination media. Hum Reprod. 1995;10(8):2056–60.
8. Henkel R, et al. Effect of reactive oxygen species produced by spermatozoa and leukocytes on sperm functions in non-leukocytospermic patients. Fertil Steril. 2005;83(3):635–42.
9. Boomsma CM, Cohlen BJ, Farquhar C. Semen preparation techniques for intrauterine insemination. Cochrane Database Syst Rev. 2019;10(10):Cd004507.
10. Mahadevan M, Baker G. Assessment and preparation of semen for in vitro fertilization. In: Wood C, Trounson A, editors. Clinical in vitro fertilization. London: Springer; 1984. p. 83–97.
11. Henkel RR, et al. Selective capacity of glass-wool filtration for the separation of human spermatozoa with condensed chromatin: a possible therapeutic modality for male-factor cases? J Assist Reprod Genet. 1994;11(8):395–400.
12. Ford W. The role of oxygen free radicals in the pathology of human spermatozoa: implications of IVF. In: Clinical IVF forum: current views in assisted reproduction. Manchester: Manchester University Press; 1990.
13. Mortimer D. Sperm preparation techniques and iatrogenic failures of in-vitro fertilization. Hum Reprod. 1991;6(2):173–6.
14. Al Hasani S, et al. Mini-swim-up: a new technique of sperm preparation for intracytoplasmic sperm injection. J Assist Reprod Genet. 1995;12(7):428–33.
15. Strehler E, et al. Detrimental effects of polyvinylpyrrolidone on the ultrastructure of spermatozoa (Notulae seminologicae 13). Hum Reprod. 1998;13(1):120–3.
16. Ng FL, Liu DY, Baker HW. Comparison of Percoll, mini-Percoll and swim-up methods for sperm preparation from abnormal semen samples. Hum Reprod. 1992;7(2):261–6.
17. Muratori M, et al. Sperm selection with density gradient centrifugation and swim up: effect on DNA fragmentation in viable spermatozoa. Sci Rep. 2019;9(1):7492.
18. Aitken RJ, et al. Potential importance of transition metals in the induction of DNA damage by sperm preparation media. Hum Reprod. 2014;29(10):2136–47.
19. Muratori M, et al. Variation of DNA fragmentation levels during density gradient sperm selection for assisted reproduction techniques: a possible new male predictive parameter of pregnancy? Medicine. 2016;95(20):e3624.
20. Male Infertility Best Practice Policy Committee of the American Urological Association Practice Committee of the American Society for Reproductive Medicine, Report on evaluation of the azoospermic male. Fertil Steril. 2006;86(5 Suppl 1):S210–5.
21. Van Peperstraten A, Proctor ML, Johnson NP, Philipson G. Techniques for surgical retrieval of sperm prior to intracytoplasmic sperm injection (ICSI) for azoospermia. Cochrane Database Syst Rev. 2008;2008(2):CD002807. https://doi.org/10.1002/14651858.CD002807.pub3. PMID: 18425884; PMCID: PMC7133779.
22. Verheyen G, Popovic-Todorovic B, Tournaye H. Processing and selection of surgically-retrieved sperm for ICSI: a review. Basic Clin Androl. 2017;27(1):6.
23. Verheyen G, et al. Comparison of four mechanical methods to retrieve spermatozoa from testicular tissue. Hum Reprod. 1995;10(11):2956–9.
24. Crabbé E, et al. Enzymatic digestion of testicular tissue may rescue the intracytoplasmic sperm injection cycle in some patients with non-obstructive azoospermia. Human Reprod (Oxford, England). 1998;13(10):2791–6.
25. Crabbe E, et al. Enzymatic digestion of testicular tissue may rescue the intracytoplasmic sperm injection cycle in some patients with non-obstructive azoospermia. Hum Reprod. 1998;13(1o):2791–6.

26. Vermes I, et al. A novel assay for apoptosis. Flow cytometric detection of phosphatidylserine expression on early apoptotic cells using fluorescein labelled Annexin V. J Immunol Methods. 1995;184(1):39–51.
27. Said TM, et al. Advantage of combining magnetic cell separation with sperm preparation techniques. Reprod Biomed Online. 2005;10(6):740–6.
28. Said T, et al. Non-apoptotic sperm selection; 2015. p. 69–79.
29. Gil M, et al. Sperm selection using magnetic activated cell sorting (MACS) in assisted reproduction: a systematic review and meta-analysis. J Assist Reprod Genet. 2013;30(4):479–85.
30. Said TM, et al. Evaluation of sperm recovery following annexin V magnetic-activated cell sorting separation. Reprod Biomed Online. 2006;13(3):336–9.
31. Cayli S, Jakab A, Ovari L, Delpiano E, Celik-Ozenci C, Sakkas D, Ward D, Huszar G. Biochemical markers of sperm function: male fertility and sperm selection for ICSI. Reprod Biomed Online. 2003;7(4):462–8. https://doi.org/10.1016/s1472-6483(10)61891-3. PMID: 14656409.
32. Huszar G, et al. Hyaluronic acid binding ability of human sperm reflects cellular maturity and fertilizing potential: selection of sperm for intracytoplasmic sperm injection. Curr Opin Obstet Gynecol. 2006;18(3):260–7.
33. Barak Y, et al. A physiological replacement for polyvinylpyrrolidone (PVP) in assisted reproductive technology. Hum Fertil. 2001;4(2):99–103.
34. Oseguera-López I, et al. Novel techniques of sperm selection for improving IVF and ICSI outcomes. Front Cell Dev Biol. 2019;7:298.
35. Chan PJ, et al. A simple zeta method for sperm selection based on membrane charge. Fertil Steril. 2006;85(2):481–6.
36. Ishijima S, Okuno M, Mohri H. Zeta potential of human X- and Y-bearing sperm. Int J Androl. 1991;14(5):340–7.
37. Zarei-Kheirabadi M, et al. Evaluation of ubiquitin and annexin V in sperm population selected based on density gradient centrifugation and zeta potential (DGC-Zeta). J Assist Reprod Genet. 2012;29(4):365–71.
38. Kheirollahi-Kouhestani M, et al. Selection of sperm based on combined density gradient and Zeta method may improve ICSI outcome. Hum Reprod. 2009;24(10):2409–16.
39. Ruzin SE. Plant microtechnique and microscopy. 1st ed. New York: Oxford University Press; 1999. p. xi. 322 p
40. Setti AS, et al. Twelve years of MSOME and IMSI: a review. Reprod Biomed Online. 2013;27(4):338–52.
41. Baccetti B. Microscopical advances in assisted reproduction. J Submicrosc Cytol Pathol. 2004;36(3–4):333–9.
42. Magli MC, et al. Birefringence properties of human immotile spermatozoa and ICSI outcome. Reprod Biomed Online. 2023;46(3):597–606.
43. Henkel R. Novel sperm tests and their importance. In: Agarwal A, Borges Jr E, Setti A, editors. Non-invasive sperm selection for in vitro fertilization. New York: Springer; 2015. p. 23–40.
44. Jameel T. Sperm swim-up: a simple and effective technique of semen processing for intrauterine insemination. J Pak Med Assoc. 2008;58(2):71–4.
45. Olatunji O, More A. A review of the impact of microfluidics technology on sperm selection technique. Cureus. 2022;14(7):e27369.
46. Gode F, et al. Comparison of microfluid sperm sorting chip and density gradient methods for use in intrauterine insemination cycles. Fertil Steril. 2019;112(5):842–848.e1.
47. Parrella A, et al. A treatment approach for couples with disrupted sperm DNA integrity and recurrent ART failure. J Assist Reprod Genet. 2019;36(10):2057–66.
48. Yetkinel S, et al. Effects of the microfluidic chip technique in sperm selection for intracytoplasmic sperm injection for unexplained infertility: a prospective, randomized controlled trial. J Assist Reprod Genet. 2019;36(3):403–9.
49. Miki K, Clapham DE. Rheotaxis guides mammalian sperm. Curr Biol. 2013;23(6):443–52.

50. Nagata MPB, et al. Live births from artificial insemination of microfluidic-sorted bovine spermatozoa characterized by trajectories correlated with fertility. Proc Natl Acad Sci. 2018;115(14):E3087–96.
51. De Martin H, et al. Positive rheotaxis extended drop: a one-step procedure to select and recover sperm with mature chromatin for intracytoplasmic sperm injection. J Assist Reprod Genet. 2017;34(12):1699–708.
52. Zhang B, Yin T, Yang J. A novel microfluidic device for selecting human sperm to increase the proportion of morphologically normal, motile sperm with uncompromised DNA integrity. Anal Methods. 2015;7(14):5981–8.
53. Oren-Benaroya R, et al. The sperm chemoattractant secreted from human cumulus cells is progesterone. Hum Reprod. 2008;23(10):2339–45.
54. Gatica LV, et al. Picomolar gradients of progesterone select functional human sperm even in subfertile samples. Mol Hum Reprod. 2013;19(9):559–69.
55. Li K, et al. Novel distance-progesterone-combined selection approach improves human sperm quality. J Transl Med. 2018;16(1):203.
56. Ko YJ, et al. Separation of progressive motile sperm from mouse semen using on-chip chemotaxis. Anal Sci. 2012;28(1):27–32.
57. Ko YJ, et al. Design, fabrication, and testing of a microfluidic device for thermotaxis and chemotaxis assays of sperm. SLAS Technol. 2018;23(6):507–15.
58. Karbalaei A, Cho HJ. Microfluidic devices developed for and inspired by thermotaxis and chemotaxis. Micromachines (Basel). 2018;9(4):149. https://doi.org/10.3390/mi9040149. PMID: 30424083; PMCID: PMC6187570.
59. Boryshpolets S, Pérez-Cerezales S, Eisenbach M. Behavioral mechanism of human sperm in thermotaxis: a role for hyperactivation. Hum Reprod. 2015;30(4):884–92.
60. Bahat A, et al. Thermotaxis of mammalian sperm cells: a potential navigation mechanism in the female genital tract. Nat Med. 2003;9(2):149–50.
61. Pérez-Cerezales S, et al. Sperm selection by thermotaxis improves ICSI outcome in mice. Sci Rep. 2018;8(1):2902.
62. Sharma R, et al. Proteomic analysis of human spermatozoa proteins with oxidative stress. Reprod Biol Endocrinol. 2013;11:48.
63. Hamada A, et al. Two-dimensional differential in-gel electrophoresis-based proteomics of male gametes in relation to oxidative stress. Fertil Steril. 2013;99(5):1216–1226.e2.
64. Girshovitz P, Shaked NT. Compact and portable low-coherence interferometer with off-axis geometry for quantitative phase microscopy and nanoscopy. Opt Express. 2013;21(5):5701–14.
65. Chan TF, Vese LA. Active contours without edges. IEEE Trans Image Process. 2001;10(2):266–77.
66. Eravuchira PJ, et al. Individual sperm selection by microfluidics integrated with interferometric phase microscopy. Methods. 2018;136:152–9.
67. Mirsky SK, et al. Automated analysis of individual sperm cells using stain-free interferometric phase microscopy and machine learning. Cytometry A. 2017;91(9):893–900.
68. Itzkan I, et al. Confocal light absorption and scattering spectroscopic microscopy monitors organelles in live cells with no exogenous labels. Proc Natl Acad Sci. 2007;104(44):17255–60.
69. Schuele G, et al. Optical spectroscopy noninvasively monitors response of organelles to cellular stress. J Biomed Opt. 2005;10(5):051404.
70. Huser T, et al. Raman spectroscopy of DNA packaging in individual human sperm cells distinguishes normal from abnormal cells. J Biophotonics. 2009;2(5):322–32.
71. Chowdary MVP, et al. Discrimination of normal, benign, and malignant breast tissues by Raman spectroscopy. Biopolymers. 2006;83(5):556–69.
72. Downes A, Mouras R, Elfick A. Optical spectroscopy for noninvasive monitoring of stem cell differentiation. J Biomed Biotechnol. 2010;2010:101864.
73. Enciso M, et al. Development of a novel synthetic oligopeptide for the detection of DNA damage in human spermatozoa. Hum Reprod. 2012;27(8):2254–66.

74. Pieczenik G, Garrisi J, Cohen J. Inhibition of human spermatozoa–zona pellucida binding by a combinatorially derived peptide from a synthetic target. Reprod Biomed Online. 2006;13(3):361–7.
75. de Oliveira NM, et al. Pregnancy with frozen-thawed and fresh testicular biopsy after motile and immotile sperm microinjection, using the mechanical touch technique to assess viability. Hum Reprod. 2004;19(2):262–5.
76. Sallam H, et al. The use of a modified hypo-osmotic swelling test for the selection of viable ejaculated and testicular immotile spermatozoa in ICSI. Hum Reprod. 2001;16(2):272–6.
77. Sallam HN, et al. The use of the modified hypo-osmotic swelling test for the selection of immotile testicular spermatozoa in patients treated with ICSI: a randomized controlled study. Hum Reprod. 2005;20(12):3435–40.
78. Loughlin KR, Agarwal A. Use of theophylline to enhance sperm function. Arch Androl. 1992;28(2):99–103.
79. Aktan TM, et al. Use of a laser to detect viable but immotile spermatozoa. Andrologia. 2004;36(6):366–9.
80. Nordhoff V, et al. Optimizing TESE-ICSI by laser-assisted selection of immotile spermatozoa and polarization microscopy for selection of oocytes. Andrology. 2013;1(1):67–74.
81. Ramesh AN, et al. Artificial intelligence in medicine. Ann R Coll Surg Engl. 2004;86(5):334–8.
82. Samli MM, Dogan I. An artificial neural network for predicting the presence of spermatozoa in the testes of men with nonobstructive azoospermia. J Urol. 2004;171(6 Pt 1):2354–7.
83. Ramasamy R, et al. A comparison of models for predicting sperm retrieval before microdissection testicular sperm extraction in men with nonobstructive azoospermia. J Urol. 2013;189(2):638–42.

Chapter 18
Artificial Intelligence in Andrology and Reproductive Medicine

Wael Zohdy and Ashok Agarwal

Abbreviations

ADHD	Attention deficit hyperactivity disorder
AI	Artificial intelligence
AIOM	Artificial intelligence optical microscopic
ANN	Artificial neural networks
ART	Assisted reproductive technique
CASA	Computer-assisted semen analysis
CNN	Convolutional neural networks
COS	Controlled ovarian stimulation
CT	Computed tomography
DL	Deep learning
EMR	Electronic medical record
GBM	Gradient boosting machines
ICD	International Classification of Diseases
ICSI	Intracytoplasmic sperm injection
IVF	In vitro fertilization
KNN	k-Nearest neighbor
micro-TESE	Microsurgical testicular sperm extraction
ML	Machine learning
MLP	Multilayer perceptron
MRI	Magnetic resonance imaging
NLP	Natural language processing
NN	Neural networks

W. Zohdy
Department of Andrology, Sexology, STIs Cairo University, Cairo, Egypt

A. Agarwal (✉)
Global Andrology Forum, Moreland Hills, OH, USA

Cleveland Clinic Foundation, Cleveland, OH, USA

A. Agarwal et al. (eds.), *Current and Future Advances in Male Infertility*,
https://doi.org/10.1007/978-3-031-62648-7_18

PET	Positron-emission tomography
RCTs	Randomized controlled trials
RF	Random forest
SCD	Sperm chromatin dispersion
SDF	Sperm DNA fragmentation
sML	Supervised machine learning
SVM	Support vector machine
SWE	Shear wave elastography
SWOT	Strengths, weaknesses, opportunities, threats
TEST	Testicular sperm extraction
WHO	World Health Organization

Key Points
- Machine learning (ML) and ANN are new avenues in the prediction of male fertility and in organizing IVF cycles.
- Deep learning has a great potential in sperm morphological assessment, sperm selection, and prediction of fertilization.
- Natural language processing (NLP) using convolutional neural network (CNN) is useful in the optimization of data extraction processes and will eventually reduce disease-coding errors in different specialties in medicine including andrology.
- AI in andrological radiology involves various aspects such as testicular cancer detection, improvement of TESE outcome, and prediction of testicular pathology.
- Robotic surgery encompasses varicocele repair, micro-TESE, and genital duct reconstruction.
- There are no standardized protocols to run the available AI models, and the majority of governing bodies do not approve their use in practice.

Introduction

What Is Artificial Intelligence?

Artificial intelligence (AI) is the development of programmed computer systems and robots that can perform tasks usually requiring human decision(s) or maneuverability [1]. It has been defined by the ISO/IEC TR 24028:2020 as the "capability of an engineered system to acquire, process, and apply knowledge and skills." Back in 1955, John McCarthy at the Dartmouth Summer Research Project on Artificial Intelligence was the first to introduce the term of AI [2].

AI improved healthcare-related outcomes and experiences through the use of algorithms retrieved from data analysis. The contemporary advances in computer science, robotics, bioinformatics, and eHealth and the need for personalized medicine have enabled the AI to play a vital role in modern healthcare [3]. All settings in

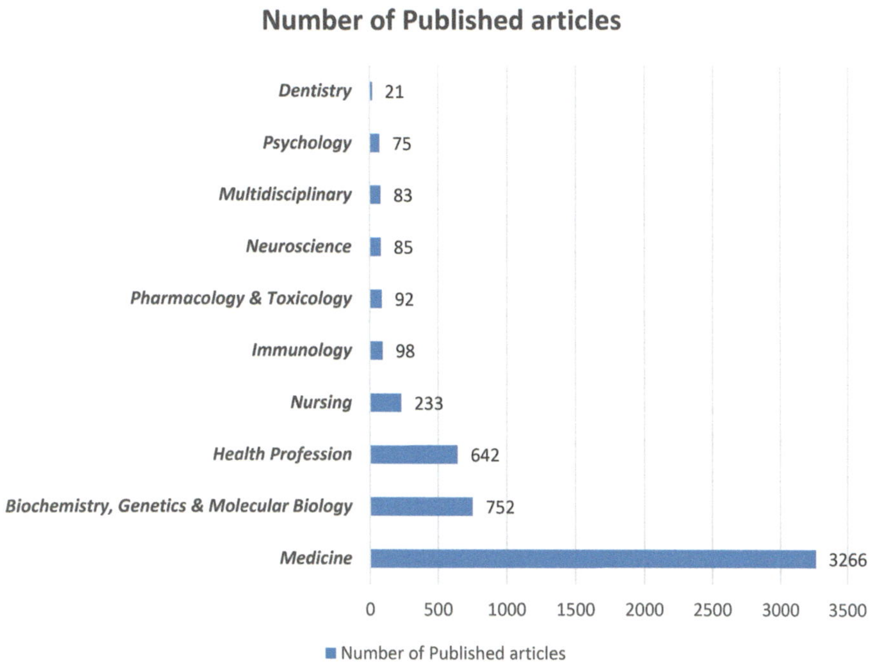

Fig. 18.1 Distribution of the published articles in various fields

the healthcare fields are supported by AI. This applies throughout many various specialties, with up to 5347 published articles as searched in February 2023. The number of articles published in various disciplines since 2000 is shown in Fig. 18.1.

AI applications, such as machine learning (ML), artificial neural networks (ANNs), and deep learning (DL), show great potential in infertility and reproductive medicine. The data resources in this field are huge and facilitate the advances in this subspecialty. The analysis of big data using the various domains of AI, such as ML, ANN, DL, natural language processing (NLP), and robotics, generates valuable and practical applications in the different areas of reproductive medicine, including sperm classification, sperm selection, oocyte, embryo selection and testing, prediction of in vitro fertilization (IVF) and intracytoplasmic sperm injection (ICSI) outcomes, robotic surgery, clinical decision systems, and cost-effectiveness [4–6]. Many of the recent reviews have highlighted the uses and implementations of AI in reproductive medicine and fertility treatment [4, 6–9]. In andrology, AI is applied in automation for evaluating sperm motility and morphology. AI can also serve as a support system in making medical decisions via supervised machine learning (sML) algorithms, which are ML-based prediction models.

AI-based prediction models and automated semen analysis are set to become valuable tools that could support and aid in diagnosing and treating male infertility and improve the accuracy of patient care. These automated, AI-based predictions could offer consistency and efficiency in terms of time and cost in infertility research and clinical management [10].

Basic Differences Between Statistics and Data Science

Statistics are based on the collection and mathematical interpretation of quantitative data. It begins with a simple model, and the data is checked to find out if it is consistent with the assumption of that model. The analysis is accomplished when the statistician is sure that all assumptions have been tested and none of them are violated. The data precision and its quality are a major concern, and mathematicians are main stakeholders involved in this field. Data science, on the other hand, involves a process of screening, meticulous inspection, presentation, and displaying of simple reports of big datasets to nontechnical people. The problems are faced by a modeling process. The latter focuses on the predictive accuracy of the model. Data scientist compares between the predictive accuracy of different machine learning methods and uses the best-fit model. They deal with big data that cannot be stored on one PC and retrieved from data warehouse. It is worth mentioning here that the precision of data collection and sources is not a primary concern in this field [11].

Machine Learning (ML)

The underlying links between inputs and outputs are explored in order to create an automated algorithm. A large dataset is vital to find complicated patterns and associations faster than traditional statistical analysis [12] with better or, at least, similar accuracy [13, 14]. In recent years, AI and ML have been extensively studied to assist physicians in diagnostic and therapeutic approaches [15–17].

Artificial Neural Network (ANN) and Deep Learning (DL)

The ANN has been inspired by the way the human brain operates. Four main components are involved in ANN (inputs, weights, bias or threshold, and output). The network deploys a training dataset, recognizes the patterns, and formulates an algorithm(s) that can be used to anticipate the outcome. The basic operation is to give a weight for each input and assign a cutoff level to decide whether the outcome is true or false. In contrast, DL is an extensive neural network with several hidden layers, hence its name "deep." It refers to the depth of layers in a given neural network that, if they consist of more than three layers inclusive of inputs and outputs, can be considered a DL algorithm [18]. Therefore, DL deals with complex problems compared to standard neural networks, for instance, image and voice recognition [19].

Decision Tree and Random Forest

Three different classes work in this mechanism, namely, supervised, unsupervised, and reinforced. In supervised learning, the input contains the data and the expected result, and the algorithm will find out the relationship, e.g., a smartphone is used to identify the owner's fingerprint [12]. A decision tree is a supervised learning algorithm that diagrammatically solves a question based on specific attributes. It looks like an inverted tree where the top (starting) point is the root node, and the branches are the outcome of decisions (leaf nodes). A random forest algorithm, on the other hand, is a collection of decision trees. Multiple trees are randomly selected, and the final question is answered based on the most selected answers by individual trees to generate the most accurate results [20].

Its shape is an inverted tree with the top/starting position being the root (root node), and the branches are the outcome of a decision (leaf nodes). A decision goes through several levels if a particular characteristic is present until a final answer is reached. A random forest algorithm is a collection of decision trees. Instead of using a single decision tree to answer a question, multiple trees are randomly selected. The final question is answered based on the most selected answers by individual trees to yield more accurate results [20].

Radiomics

It is a medical approach that aims at extracting a substantial number of quantitative features from medical images deploying a data characterization algorithm. Radiomics software are able to quantify the assigned tasks, e.g., region segmentation or conducting automated measurements. They are useful in characterization of the lesion (shape, volume, surface area, density, intensity-based feature, texture) as well as exploring its surrounding microenvironment. This makes it possible to guide the targeted agents before a procedure or to be aligned with a biopsy to maximize the clinical implications [21].

Natural Language Processing (NLP)

NLP is part of AI that focuses on building a machine or computer's ability to understand human language rather than equations or programs [22, 23]. This technology enables machines to extract classifications, such as International Classification of Diseases (ICD) diagnosis codes, from unstructured data, hence enabling physicians to write more naturally rather than having to input specific structured text or numbers for data analysis. NLP is a self-learning tool, with the more the number of datasets, the higher the utility and the prediction, therefore enabling NLP to become more "natural" and representative of the patient population [22]. Furthermore, NLP using convolutional neural network (CNN), recurrent neural network (RNN), or, as the superior algorithm, bidirectional recurrent neural network processing algorithm was shown to help optimize data extraction processes for reduced disease-coding errors in different specialties in medicine [24].

In reproductive medicine, NLP has been studied and used for research purposes, sperm classification, oocyte selection, embryo selection, clinical decision-making systems, cost-effective assessment, surgery outcome prediction, and robotic surgery development [4, 6]. For example, Osadchiy and colleagues used NLP in social media to study patients' perceptions of hypogonadism and its treatments [25]. With more research to come, the application of AI, particularly NLP, will help physicians and patients with obtaining a better diagnosis and treatment of andrological cases. Table 18.1 shows valid examples to some of the AI tools in andrology.

In the following sections, we will discuss the impact of AI on the management of infertile men, ranging across assessment, prediction of outcome, surgical treatment, and finally assisted conception.

AI in Assessment of Male Infertility

AI in Prediction of Male Fertility Potential

The noted trend of decreasing sperm count over the past couple of decades motivated some investigators to study the link between environmental factors and semen quality. Gil and colleagues utilized AI networks to explore the impact of cigarette exposure, alcohol intake, and body mass index (BMI) on semen quality. The authors retrieved the data from 100 university students by questionnaire, and through utilization of ANN, they were able to show high prediction accuracy (~86%) for sperm concentration and (73–76%) for sperm motility [34]. Semen quality could also be predicted. Candemir and colleagues suggested an algorithm that predicts semen parameters in 90% of cases through the season of analysis and genitourinary trauma [35]. Other investigators explored certain makers of fertility through AI tools, such as zinc [36, 37] and leptin [38].

Computer-Assisted Semen Analysis Systems

Semen analysis is a subjective test, and human error and intra-operator variability are expected and may result in inaccuracy and may lead the andrologist into a wrong direction. Computer-assisted semen analysis (CASA) provides reliable and objective results [39]. CASA systems are automated devices that use cameras and software to analyze and interpret the microscopic findings [40]. They are used to evaluate sperm kinematic parameters and hyper-activation, as described in the 2021 WHO lab manual for examining and processing human semen [41]. In addition, CASA assessment is more objective and reproducible than technician-based manual

Table 18.1 Basic AI techniques and some related examples

AI tool	Study	Target	References
Machine learning (ML)	Supervised ML is used to develop a scoring calculator	Predicts KS patients among men with NOA	[26]
	Varicocele repair prediction	Predicts improvement in post-varicocelectomy sperm analysis with superior performance compared to traditional logistic regression	[10]
	Sperm cell classification and selection	Shows benefit of ML for automated sperm classification, sperm selection, fertility prediction, and prediction of in vitro fertilization (IVF) outcomes	[5, 27, 28]
ANN and DL	Sperm morphology assessment	The algorithms increased the accuracy of the head, acrosome, and vacuole by 6.66%, 3.00%, and 1.33% and reached the accuracy of 84.00%, 80.66%, and 94.00% on these labels, respectively Suggested use in fertility clinics to improve the performance	[29]
-Decision tree -Random forest -SVM -Adaptive boosting -XGB	Male fertility prediction	Nine features related to lifestyle and environmental factors are utilized to develop a male fertility prediction model. Five AI tools were deployed to produce a trustworthy model, and an explainable AI is applied. The techniques are (1) LIME and (2) SHAP Finally, XGB outperformed and obtained an AUC of 0.98	[30]
Radiomics	MRI testis signals and spectroscopy to predict TESE outcome and testicular pathology	N-ADC and proton MRS are helpful in differentiating OA from NOA and predicting SR and pathological abnormality	[31–33]
NLP	Perception of hypogonadism	The authors used NLP in social media to study patients' perceptions of hypogonadism and its treatments	[25]

AI artificial intelligence, *KS* Klinefelter's syndrome, *LIME* local interpretable model-agnostic explanations, *NLP* natural language processing, *SHAP* Shapley additive explanations, *SVM* support vector machine, *XGB* conventional extreme gradient boost, *ANN* artificial neural network, *DL* deep learning

motility evaluation. It is superior to the standard methods in terms of giving objective sperm kinematic parameters, which are predictors of in vitro fertilization, alongside the sperm counts [42].

Unfortunately, some uncertainties remain to be clarified and have prevented its routine use. In this regard, a recent systematic review showed a high degree of correlation for sperm concentration and motility between manual and CASA-based semen analysis only for samples with midrange concentrations (15–60 million/mL), with residual variability dependent on the instrument used [40]. Another limitation is related to sperm morphology that remains challenging to assess with CASA due to the high number of different types of abnormalities and the various classification systems [40]. In an attempt to overcome this limitation, Thirumalarjaju et al. reported success with AI interpreting sperm morphology using an ANN. The tool was used to train and validate the network with over 3500 sperm images, and the algorithm was used to analyze nine semen samples with 100% accuracy in identifying all abnormal and normal samples [43]. It is obvious that the cumulative experience and refinement of AI will eventually overcome the barriers against digital assessment of sperm cell morphology.

In the future, artificial intelligence optical microscopic (AIOM) technologies could be helpful in also overcoming this problem, helping the CASA systems to "learn" how to classify sperm morphology correctly. Nowadays, deep learning networks can have over 100 layers and billions of nodes, far away from the first VGG-16 algorithm technologies. However, further studies are needed [44].

Identifying Chromosomal Abnormalities in Men with Azoospermia

Azoospermia is present in 10–15% of men undergoing an infertility assessment, and identifying a genetic cause is crucial [45]. Akinsal and colleagues utilized an ANN to predict the subset of azoospermic patients that should undergo further genetic testing. The authors performed a retrospective study investigating several variables and found that testicular volume and LH level have the highest power in determining those who need additional genetic workup. They found promise in deploying AI to identify a smaller cohort of men needing further evaluation, which may provide a significant cost minimization over the long run [46]. Other investigators proposed supervised ML to develop a scoring calculator that predicts KS patients among men with NOA [26].

Artificial Intelligence and Sperm DNA Fragmentation

Assessment of sperm DNA fragmentation depends on manual measurement of certain criteria under the microscope. This is applicable with Comet assay and sperm chromatin dispersion [41]. Therefore, the process is subjective [47]. AI could be useful in these techniques by rendering them more objective. A convolutional neural network (CNN) was used to predict the single-cell DNA fragmentation index in semen. This method allows for selecting sperm with the highest DNA integrity [48].

AI in Sperm Capacitation, Sperm Hyperactivation, and Fertilization Prediction

Sperm capacitation assessment is used as a complementary sperm function in certain situation. CASA, through specific gating methods, can recognize kinematic criteria of sperm motility, including sperm hyperactivation. To improve the CASA system, AI was used in order to reclassify sperm motility patterns occurring during sperm cell capacitation. The technique includes a training set of different motility tracks based on mice sperm models and uploading them into the CASA device. The system then creates SVM equations that can precisely detect the pattern of sperm motility (specific for sperm capacitation) [49]. A practical extension to this feature is the use of a machine learning algorithm to predict fertilization in normozoospermic men undergoing conventional IVF using clinical parameters and markers of capacitation [28].

AI and Sperm Selection for ART

An ideal method for sperm selection in ART is expected to be noninvasive and cost effective and yield better outcomes in terms of fertilization, embryo quality, and healthy live birth [50]. At the decision level, ML can improve the information available to the andrologist and increase the consistency of decision-making in sperm selection. The capability of ML algorithms to process substantial amounts of data helps in establishing correlations between sperm quality metrics, such as morphology, sperm DNA integrity, or chromosomal aneuploidy at the single-sperm level [5]. Sperm selection requires several steps to realize a clinical ML algorithm for this task [28, 51]. A high-speed off-axis holographic system [52] or the automated magnification switching method [53] can be useful for obtaining high-resolution images of moving sperm [5]. The application of ML is rapidly expanding within biomedical applications. The capability of this approach to process and analyze large amounts of data, particularly image data, will be particularly useful in sperm selection. Adequately trained ML algorithms could enable embryologists to improve and standardize sperm selection, increasing fertilization success rates and outcomes [5].

Skilled embryologists are able to select the blastocysts to be transferred. They rate the embryos, and this process is structured; however, it is subjective in nature. Khosravi and co-workers analyzed 10,148 embryos and formulated an AI approach termed "STORK," and their algorithm showed high performance in predicting embryo quality, outperforming individual embryologists [54]. The authors, unsuccessfully, tried to predict the live birth through grading human embryos during IVF process. They explained the failure by the subjective inconsistent assessment across various IVF centers. Nonetheless, this application shows the potential of AI in improving ART.

AI Role in IVF Clinics

AI plays a significant role in each step in IVF, from treatment regimen to gamete selection and finally to embryo selection [55]. The decision-making at the IVF clinic depends on many variables such as the age of the patient, the ovarian reserve, the male factor, and the medical history, just to name a few. The treatment cycle is aimed at maximizing the chances of pregnancy and birth of a healthy newborn [56]. The treatment protocol may therefore differ in the stimulation regimen and the fertilization choice (IVF vs. ICSI), as well as the potential for other procedures including assisted hatching and preimplantation genetic testing, among others. All the previous decisions depend heavily upon inputs from the healthcare team based on their knowledge, skills, and expertise. AI could aid them in this aspect, enabling objective decision-making in order to optimize the controlled ovarian stimulation protocol to serve the best outcome [55]. AI could be used to data-mine electronic medical records to discover novel variables that predict ICSI outcome in terms of pregnancy and live birth. The use of AI in other fields such as oncology shows promising results, with a significant reduction in time needed to formulate radiotherapy treatment plans (from days to minutes) [4, 6]. Interestingly, the use of AI to data-mine existing databases led to the identification of novel genes associated with the pathogenesis of polycystic ovarian disease [57, 58] and endometriosis [59], and incorporating AI within this domain of the IVF cycle might lead to improved success, reduce the risk of ovarian hyper-stimulation syndrome, as well as reduce the workload for the healthcare team [55]. AI does not only optimize the clinical success in IVF but will also play a vital role in the IVF day-to-day management and in the organization of busy IVF centers. Letterie and McDonald used AI in day-to-day decision-making during ovarian stimulation for IVF. They validated the algorithm against the evidence-based decisions by the clinical team. In order to accomplish this target, they retrieved data from more than 2600 IVF cycles. They deployed the algorithm in predicting four critical clinical decisions: (i) stop stimulation or continue stimulation. If the decision was to stop, then the next automated decision was to (ii) trigger or cancel. If the decision was to return, then the next key decisions were (iii) number of days to follow-up and (iv) whether any dosage adjustment was needed. The authors documented a prediction accuracy ranging from 87% to 96%. The decision algorithm and the predictive accuracy are simplified in Fig. 18.2. The authors described the first iteration of a predictive analytic algorithm that is highly accurate and will be a cornerstone in optimizing clinical decision-making during IVF [60].

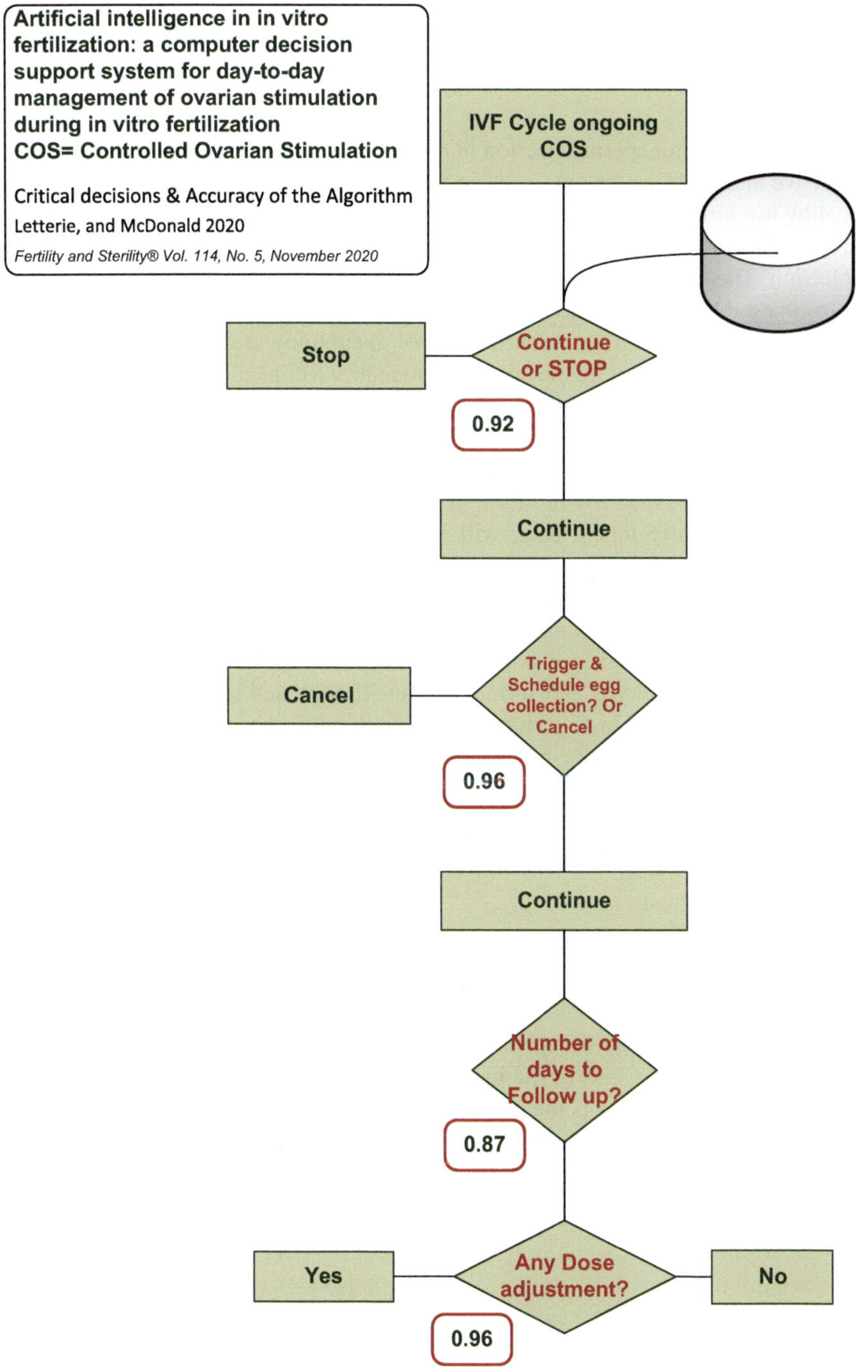

Fig. 18.2 AI in the management of IVF centers: Critical decisions and predictive accuracy [60]

AI and Gamete Selection for ART

Sperm Selection

An ideal method for sperm selection in ART is expected to be noninvasive and cost effective and yield better outcomes in terms of fertilization, embryo quality, and healthy live birth [50]. At the decision level, ML can improve the information available to the andrologist and increase the consistency of decision-making in sperm selection. The capability of ML algorithms to process substantial amounts of data helps in establishing correlations between sperm quality metrics, such as morphology, sperm DNA integrity, or chromosomal aneuploidy at the single-sperm level [5]. Sperm selection requires several steps to realize a clinical ML algorithm for this task [28, 51]. A high-speed off-axis holographic system [52] or the automated magnification switching method [53] can be useful for obtaining high-resolution images of moving sperm [5]. The application of ML is rapidly expanding within biomedical applications. The capability of this approach to process and analyze large amounts of data, particularly image data, will be particularly useful in sperm selection. Adequately trained ML algorithms could enable embryologists to improve and standardize sperm selection, increasing fertilization success rates and outcomes [5].

Skilled embryologists are able to select the blastocysts to be transferred. Although this process is structured, it is still subjective in nature. Khosravi and co-workers analyzed 10,148 embryos and formulated an AI approach termed "STORK," and their algorithm showed high performance in predicting embryo quality, outperforming individual embryologists [54]. The authors tried to predict the live birth through grading human embryos during IVF process. The model failed to predict this outcome due to the subjective inconsistent assessment across various IVF centers. Nonetheless, this application shows the potential of AI in improving ART outcomes.

Oocyte Selection

The quality of the oocytes depends on the follicle size, the morphology, and the cytoplasmic characteristics of the harvested eggs. The main barrier behind the use of AI for oocyte selection is the practice of fertilizing all available oocytes, unless, of course, AI is proved to be reliable in the prediction of blastocyst formation or more importantly live birth prior to fertilization. Such capacity appears limited based on the current literature [61].

Embryo Selection

VerMilyea and colleagues analyzed clinical data and standard static two-dimensional optical light microscope images of 8886 embryos from 11 different IVF clinics. They chose couples with known positive clinical pregnancy as measured by fetal heartbeat to provide a confidence score for prediction. The accuracy of the algorithm was determined by evaluating sensitivity and specificity. The authors used histograms of the distributions of predictions to see the overall accuracy. Comparison to embryologists' predictive accuracy was performed using a binary classification approach and a five-band ranking comparison. The model demonstrated an improved predictive ability for the evaluation of embryo viability when compared with embryologists' traditional morphological grading methods. They suggested that the proposed model could lead to improved pregnancy success rates in IVF when used in a clinical setting. They added that this cost-effective alternative may eliminate the need for complex time-lapse imaging equipment [62].

So far, the use of AI within IVF clinics is not yet a reality. This is probably due to the different AI techniques that are being proposed to be used in the daily routine of the clinics, which causes some uncertainty in their use. Fernandez and colleagues, in their systematic review, shed light on this complex scenario, by describing some of the most frequently used AI algorithms, their functionalities, and their potential use. They focused on the classification of embryonic cells and semen samples and selected 32/124 articles. From the proposed algorithms, most have achieved a satisfactory precision, demonstrating the potential of a wide range of AI techniques. However, the evaluation of these studies suggests the need for more standardized research to validate the proposed models and their algorithms. The choice of AI technique to be used is supported by a better understanding of the principles adjunct to each technique, that is, its robustness, pros, and cons. The authors provided and discussed some current and potential uses of AI on the clinic routine and explored how accurate and friendly it could be [8].

Robotic Fertility Surgery

The potential benefits of robotic fertility surgery include reduced surgeons' tremors, 3D visualization, and decreased need for surgical assistance [63]. In 2004, Schiff and his colleagues conducted the first animal model on robotic male infertility microsurgery [64]. Later on, several small retrospective studies have described robotic-assisted vasectomy reversal with comparable clinical outcomes to the traditional microsurgical approach. However, the operative time was significantly reduced with the robotic surgery ([63, 65]). In varicocele repair, robotic-assisted varicocelectomy was also reported. Still, these studies are limited by their retrospective nature, single-institution experience, and lack of comparison groups [63, 66, 67]. One robotic-assisted micro-TESE report demonstrated the safety and effectiveness of this approach; however, the details on patient characteristics, operative time, and sperm retrieval rates were not reported [68]. The studies of robotic-assisted micro-denervation of the spermatic cord were similar to robotic-assisted varicocelectomy and had the advantage of excellent visualization but did not show better results than the conventional microsurgical approach [63]. Although robotic fertility surgery procedures are evolving, no substantial clinical evidence suggests improved outcomes [68, 69]. Parekattil and Gudeloglu performed robotic TESE procedures without any complications. They stressed on the safety and feasibility of the approach in surgical sperm retrieval and described the technique as easier in tissue handling and dissection [68]. However, sperm retrieval rate and immediate and long-term complications were not reported. In the future, more rigorous studies are needed to compare robotic fertility surgery with conventional microsurgery and evaluate outcomes and cost-effectiveness.

AI in Andrological Radiology

Ultrasonography of the Testis, Epididymis, Prostate, and Seminal Vesicles

In prostate cancer, AI has been applied in transrectal ultrasonography. The diagnosis, treatment, and follow-up in men with prostatic carcinoma require accurate measurements of the prostate volume as well as boundaries' segmentation. Ultrasonography is inexpensive and does not emit radiation. However, it has a low signal-to-noise ratio and speckle noise that complicates the automatic segmentation of ultrasound images [70]. To overcome this limitation, AI has been used to achieve automatic segmentation of transrectal ultrasound images to facilitate the diagnosis of cancer, image-guided surgical planning, and even therapy planning [4, 6, 71–76].

In testicular cancer, AI may play a role in testis-sparing surgery. Favaron and colleagues used an SVM classification system on testicular contrast-enhanced ultrasound images. They classified ten benign and ten malignant lesions. The model was able to identify the disease correctly in 100% of the cases. The authors suggested that the approach is promising, but should be validated on larger dataset [77]. A therapeutic approach is increasingly used as described by Favilla and his colleagues in their systematic review [78]. Another study, using a radiomics approach, evaluated the usefulness of 44 textural features derived from the echogenicity of testicular images. Of these, 13 predicted sperm concentration, total count, and sperm motility and morphology. Moreover, many of these features predicted gonadotropin levels but not testosterone. The authors of this pilot study suggested the possibility of predicting the gonadal function of men using a subjective testicular echogenic pattern and converting it into an objective evaluation based on numerical values [79].

Computed Tomography and Magnetic Resonance Images

Applications of AI in brain magnetic resonance imaging (MRI) scans for Alzheimer's, Parkinson's, and attention deficit hyperactivity disorder (ADHD) are established and help predict the diagnosis and stage of disease [80]. In andrology, AI is combined with MRI to create algorithms that can assist the radiologist with lesion detection and classification to improve diagnostic performance and avoid unnecessary biopsies.

In computed tomography (CT) image reconstruction, AI may offer a further dose reduction through improved image quality. Similar to MRI, the methods used in CT image reconstruction are ML and DL [81]. The current international literature offers very limited data on the application of AI in andrological radiology, but the horizon perspectives of such applications are very promising. Some examples of AI applications in CT image reconstruction include abdominal and pelvic imaging. More incidental findings are identified with the rapid growth in medical imaging, especially CT. AI may help in the characterization of these lesions as benign or malignant, prioritizing this way the treatment and the follow-up evaluation of these lesions [82]. Nevertheless, further computational advances are still needed to use AI algorithms in CT image reconstruction in clinical practice.

Shear Wave Elastography

Shear wave elastography (SWE) is a medical imaging modality that displays elastic images in real time through ultrasound or MRI tracking technology. The technique is noninvasive and assesses the mechanical properties of tissues by showing the degree of tissue stiffness through different colors [83]. The ultrasound-based SWE is widely used in diagnosing breast tumors, thyroid tumors, lymph node diseases, and other superficial organ diseases as a valuable adjunct to conventional ultrasound [84].

Ultrasound-based SWE was also used to detect and quantify testicular stiffness in cases of varicocele [85], testicular microlithiasis [86], and cryptorchidism [87]. The relationship between SWE testicular stiffness and male infertility has been investigated with satisfactory preliminary results [88, 89]. In 2022, Cui and colleagues conducted a cross-sectional study on 1116 consecutive patients undergoing IVF/ICSI treatment. They concluded that ultrasound-based SWE was an effective supplement to differentiate between obstructive and nonobstructive azoospermia and also between severe oligozoospermia and nonobstructive azoospermia from other groups [90]. More studies are needed to evaluate further and perfect this new AI-based modality (Fig. 18.3).

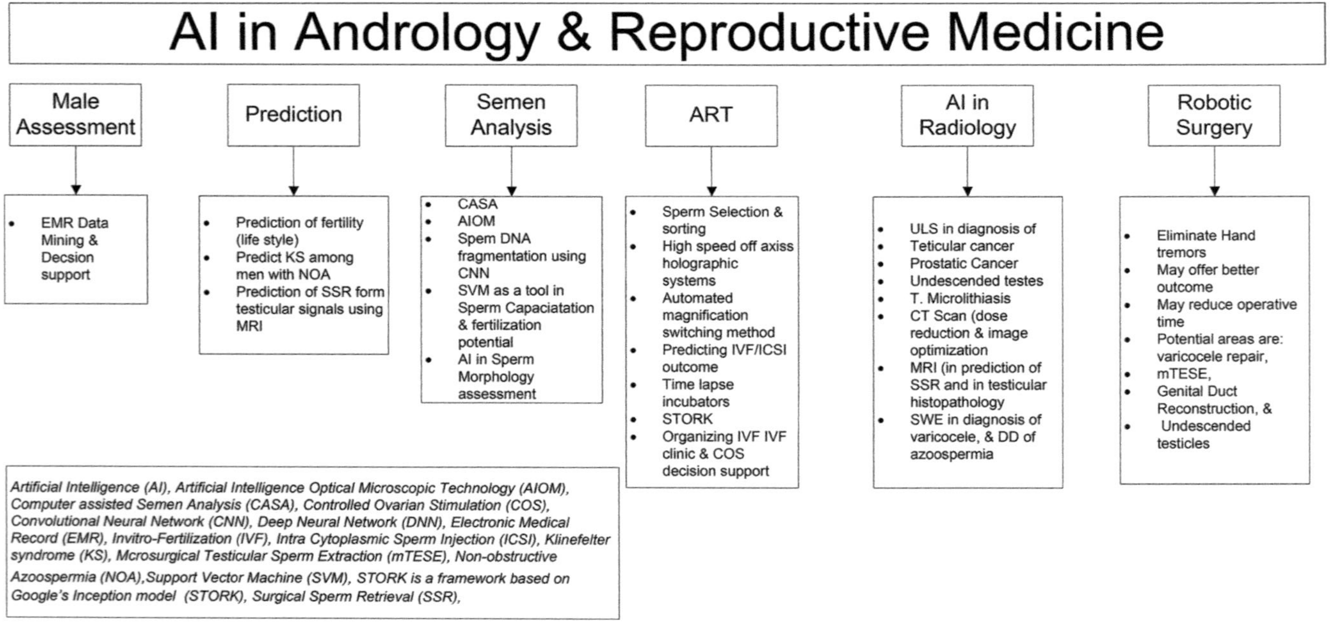

Fig. 18.3 The scope of AI in andrology, reproductive medicine, and robotic surgery

Limitations and Challenges of Artificial Intelligence in Andrology

AI has been established in many areas of technology and industry, but its use in medicine is still early [8, 91, 92]. The currently available models are still preliminary and limited. Therefore, models have to be developed for each specific application [8]. Although the utilization of AI in andrology is promising, it faces significant barriers. Data science does not focus on overcoming uncertainty; they are often inaccurate or incomplete. Second, there are no standardized protocols to run the limited number of AI models that are currently available. In addition, the approval of AI for medical applications is not standardized across governing bodies [8, 93]. Third, a recent study of healthcare providers in Germany showed a willingness to adopt AI technology in medical care [94]. However, there is worldwide concern regarding limitation of patients' autonomy. So far, most clinicians value a combination of patient-centric and evidence-based decision-making. Fourth, the cost of developing and validating an AI model in andrology is a significant challenge due to the lack of widely available funding [95]. This is particularly true given the relatively small size of the andrology specialty compared to other areas of medicine. Finally, ethical concerns are raised regarding the applicability of AI models to all patients, especially when significant individual variations are likely [96]. Generally, an ethical dilemma that can arise with the introduction of novel and expensive tools is the allocation of payment for and beneficiaries of this technology, given the disparity of insurance and financial resources across the medical landscape in many countries [95].Conflict of InterestThe authors do not have any conflict of interests regarding this manuscript.

Funding No funding was received for this chapter.

References

1. Hamet P, Tremblay J. Artificial intelligence in medicine. Metabolism. 2017;69S:S36–40. https://doi.org/10.1016/j.metabol.2017.01.011.
2. International Organization for Standardization [ISO] (2020) ISO/IEC TR 24028:2020 Information technology—artificial intelligence—overview of trustworthiness in artificial intelligence. International Organization for Standardization [ISO]. https://www.iso.org/obp/ui/#iso:std:iso-iec:tr:24028:ed-1:v1:en.
3. Kulkarni S, Seneviratne N, Baig MS, Khan AHA. Artificial intelligence in medicine: where are we now? Acad Radiol. 2020;27(1):62–70. https://doi.org/10.1016/j.acra.2019.10.001.
4. Wang R, Pan W, Jin L, Li Y, Geng Y, Gao C, et al. Artificial intelligence in reproductive medicine. Reproduction. 2019;158(4):R139–54.
5. You JB, McCallum C, Wang Y, Riordon J, Nosrati R, Sinton D. Machine learning for sperm selection. Nat Rev. 2021;18:387–403. https://doi.org/10.1038/s41585-021-00465-1.
6. Wang C, Zhu X, Hong JC, Zheng D. Artificial intelligence in radiotherapy treatment planning: present and future. Technol Cancer Res Treat. 2019;18:1533033819873922. https://doi.org/10.1177/1533033819873922.
7. Curchoe CL, Malmsten J, Bormann C, Shafiee H, Flores-Saiffe Farias A, Mendizabal G, Chavez-Badiola A, Sigaras A, Alshubbar H, Chambost J, Jacques C, Pena CA, Drakeley A, Freour T, Hajirasouliha I, Hickman CFL, Elemento O, Zaninovic N, Rosenwaks Z. Predictive

modeling in reproductive medicine: where will the future of artificial intelligence research take us? Fertil Steril. 2020;114(5):934–40. https://doi.org/10.1016/j.fertnstert.2020.10.040.
8. Fernandez EI, Ferreira AS, Cecílio MHM, Chéles DS, de Souza RCM, Nogueira MFG, Rocha JC. Artificial intelligence in the IVF laboratory: overview through the application of different types of algorithms for the classification of reproductive data. J Assist Reprod Genet. 2020;37(10):2359–76. https://doi.org/10.1007/s10815-020-01881-9. Epub 2020 Jul 11.
9. Swain J, VerMilyea MT, Meseguer M, Ezcurra D, Fertility AI Forum Group. AI in the treatment of fertility: key considerations. J Assist Reprod Genet. 2020;37(11):2817–24. https://doi.org/10.1007/s10815-020-01950-z. Epub 2020 Sep 29.
10. Ory J, Tradewell MB, Blankstein U, Lima TF, Nackeeran S, Gonzalez DC, Nwefo E, Moryousef J, Madhusoodanan V, Lau S, Jarvi K, Ramasamy R. Artificial intelligence based machine learning models predict sperm parameter upgrading after varicocele repair: a multi-institutional analysis. World J Mens Health. 2022;40(4):618–26. https://doi.org/10.5534/wjmh.210159. Epub 2022 Jan 2. PMID: 35021305; PMCID: PMC9482858.
11. Williams N, Ferdinand NP, Croft R. Project management maturity in the age of big data. Int J Manag Proj Bus. 2014;7(2):311–7.
12. Sidey-Gibbons JAM, Sidey-Gibbons CJ. Machine learning in medicine: a practical introduction. BMC Med Res Methodol. 2019;19:64.
13. Rajula HSR, Verlato G, Manchia M, Antonucci N, Fanos V. Comparison of conventional statistical methods with machine learning in medicine: diagnosis, drug development, and treatment. Medicina (Kaunas). 2020;56(9):455.
14. Choi RY, Coyner AS, Kalpathy-Cramer J, Chiang MF, Campbell JP. Introduction to machine learning, neural networks, and deep learning. Transl Vis Sci Technol. 2020;9(2):14.
15. Anagnostou T, Remzi M, Lykourinas M, Djavan B. Artificial neural networks for decision-making in urologic oncology. Eur Urol. 2003;43(6):596.
16. Hemal AK, Menon M. Robotics in urology. Curr Opin Urol. 2004;14(2):89.
17. Batko K, Ślęzak A. The use of big data analytics in healthcare. J Big Data. 2022;9(1):3. https://doi.org/10.1186/s40537-021-00553-4. Epub 2022 Jan 6.
18. Nguyen D, Nguyen H, Ong H, Le H, Ha H, Duc NT, Ngo HT. Ensemble learning using traditional machine learning and deep neural network for diagnosis of Alzheimer's disease. IBRO Neurosci Rep. 2022;13:255–63. https://doi.org/10.1016/j.ibneur.2022.08.010.
19. Gupta P, Sharma A, Jindal R. Scalable machine-learning algorithms for big data analytics: a comprehensive review. Wiley Interdiscip Rev Data Min Knowl Discov. 2016;6(6):194–214. https://doi.org/10.1002/widm.1194.
20. Amin MN, Ahmad A, Khan K, Ahmad W, Nazar S, Faraz MI, Alabdullah AA. Split tensile strength prediction of recycled aggregate-based sustainable concrete using artificial intelligence methods. Materials (Basel). 2022;15(12):4296. https://doi.org/10.3390/ma15124296. PMID: 35744356; PMCID: PMC9229664.
21. Shur JD, Doran SJ, Kumar S, Ap Dafydd D, Downey K, O'Connor JPB, Papanikolaou N, Messiou C, Koh DM, Orton MR. Radiomics in oncology: a practical guide. Radiographics. 2021;41(6):1717–32. https://doi.org/10.1148/rg.2021210037.
22. Hashimoto DA, Rosman G, Rus D, Meireles OR. Artificial intelligence in surgery: promises and perils. Ann Surg. 2018;268(1):70–6. https://doi.org/10.1097/SLA.0000000000002693.
23. Mehta N, Devarakonda MV. Machine learning, natural language programming, and electronic health records: the next step in the artificial intelligence journey? J Allergy Clin Immunol. 2018;141(6):2019–2021.e1. https://doi.org/10.1016/j.jaci.2018.02.025. Epub 2018 Mar 5.
24. Wang C, Yao C, Chen P, Shi J, Gu Z, Zhou Z. Artificial intelligence algorithm with ICD coding technology guided by the embedded electronic medical record system in medical record information management. J Healthcare Eng. 2021;2021:3293457. https://doi.org/10.1155/2021/3293457.
25. Osadchiy V, Jiang T, Mills JN, Eleswarapu SV. Low testosterone on social media: application of natural language processing to understand patients' perceptions of hypogonadism and its treatment. J Med Internet Res. 2020;22(10):e21383. https://doi.org/10.2196/21383.

26. Krenz H, Sansone A, Fujarski M, Krallmann C, Zitzmann M, et al. Machine learning based prediction models in male reproductive health: development of a proof-of-concept model for Klinefelter Syndrome in azoospermic patients. Andrology. 2022;10(3):534–44.
27. Hicks SA, Andersen JM, Witczak O, Thambawita V, Halvorsen P, Hammer HL, Haugen TB, Riegler MA. Machine learning-based analysis of sperm videos and participant data for male fertility prediction. Sci Rep. 2019;9(1):16770.
28. Gunderson SJ, Puga Molina LC, Spies N, Balestrini PA, et al. Machine-learning algorithm incorporating capacitated sperm intracellular pH predicts conventional in vitro fertilization success in normospermic patients. Fertil Steril. 2021;115(4):930–9.
29. Abbasi A, Miahi E, Mirroshandel SA. Effect of deep transfer and multi-task learning on sperm abnormality detection. Comput Biol Med. 2021;128 https://doi.org/10.1016/j.compbiomed.2020.10412.
30. GhoshRoy D, Alvi PA, Santosh KC. Explainable AI to predict male fertility using extreme gradient boosting algorithm with SMOTE. Electronics. 2023;12:15. https://doi.org/10.3390/electronics12010015.
31. Hesham Said A, Ragab A, Zohdy W, Ibrahim AS, Abd El Basset AS. Diffusion-weighted magnetic resonance imaging and magnetic resonance spectroscopy for non-invasive characterization of azoospermia: a prospective comparative single center study. Andrology. 2023.
32. Karakus C, Ozyurt R. Correlation between high choline metabolite signal in spectroscopy and sperm retrieval chance at micro-TESE. Eur Rev Med Pharmacol Sci. 2022;26(4):1125–30.
33. Tsili AC, Ntorkou A, Goussia A, Astrakas L, Panopoulou E, Sofikitis N, Argyropoulou MI. Diffusion tensor imaging parameters in testes with nonobstructive azoospermia. J MagnReson Imaging. 2018;48(5):1318–25. https://doi.org/10.1002/jmri.26050. Epub 2018 Apr 16.
34. Gil D, Girela JL, De Juan J, Gomez-Torres MJ, Johnsson M. Predicting seminal quality with artificial intelligence methods. Expert Syst Appl. 2012;39(16):12564–73.
35. Candemir C. Estimating the semen quality from life style using fuzzy radial basis functions. Int J Mach Learn Comput. 2018;8(1):44–8.
36. Fallah A, Mohammad-Hasani A, Colagar AH. Zinc is an essential element for male fertility: a review of Zn roles in men's health, germination, sperm quality, and fertilization. J Reprod Infertil. 2018;19(2):69–81.
37. Vickram AS, Kamini AR, Das R, Pathy MR, Parameswari R, Archana K, et al. Validation of artificial neural network models for predicting biochemical markers associated with male infertility. Syst Biol Reprod Med. 2016;62(4):258–65.
38. Ma Y, Chen B, Wang H, Hu K, Huang Y. Prediction of sperm retrieval in men with non-obstructive azoospermia using artificial neural networks: leptin is a good assistant diagnostic marker. Hum Reprod. 2011;26(2):294–8.
39. Tomlinson MJ, Naeem A. CASA in the medical laboratory: CASA in diagnostic andrology and assisted conception. Reprod Fertil Dev. 2018;30(6):850–9. https://doi.org/10.1071/RD17520.
40. Finelli R, Leisegang K, Tumallapalli S, Henkel R, Agarwal A. The validity and reliability of computer-aided semen analyzers in performing semen analysis: a systematic review. Transl Androl Urol. 2021;10(7):3069–79. https://doi.org/10.21037/tau-21-276.
41. World Health Organization. WHO laboratory manual for the examination and processing of human semen. World Health Organization 2021[Online]; 2021.
42. Baig AS, Shoebuddin M, Ahmed M. Comparison of manual sperm analysis with computer-assisted sperm analysis: A comparative cross-sectional study. Natl J Physiol Pharm Pharmacol. 2019;9(9):862. https://doi.org/10.5455/njppp.2019.9.0621817062019.
43. Thirumalaraju P, Bormann CL, Kanakasabapathy M, Doshi F, Souter I, Dimitriadis I, et al. Automated sperm morphology testing using artificial intelligence. Fertil Steril. 2018;110(4):e432.
44. Agarwal A, Henkel R, Huang CC, Lee MS. Automation of human semen analysis using a novel artificial intelligence optical microscopic technology. Andrologia. 2019;51(11):e13440. https://doi.org/10.1111/and.13440.

45. Majzoub A, Arafa M, Clemens H, Imperial J, Leisegang K, Khalafalla K, Agarwal A, Henkel R, Elbardisi H. A systemic review and meta-analysis exploring the predictors of sperm retrieval in patients with non-obstructive azoospermia and chromosomal abnormalities. Andrologia. 2022;54(3):e14303.
46. Akinsal EC, Haznedar B, Baydilli N, Kalinli A, Ozturk A, Ekmekçioğlu O. Artificial neural network for the prediction of chromosomal abnormalities in azoospermic males. Urol J. 2018;15(3):122–5.
47. Agarwal A, Majzoub A, Baskaran S, et al. Sperm DNA fragmentation: a new guideline for clinicians. World J Mens Health. 2020;38(4):412–71.
48. McCallum C, Riordon J, Wang Y, et al. Deep learning-based selection of human sperm with high DNA integrity. Commun Biol (Springer US). 2019;2(1):1–10.
49. Goodson SG, White S, Stevans AM, Bhat S, Kao CY, Jaworski S, Marlowe TR, Kohlmeier M, McMillan L, Zeisel SH, O'Brien DA. CASAnova: a multiclass support vector machine model for the classification of human sperm motility patterns. Biol Reprod. 2017;97(5):698–708. https://doi.org/10.1093/biolre/iox120.
50. Rappa KL, Rodriguez HF, Hakkarainen GC, Anchan RM, Mutter GL, Asghar W. Sperm processing for advanced re -productive technologies: where are we today? Biotechnol Adv. 2016;34:578–87. https://doi.org/10.1016/j.biotechadv.2016.01.007.
51. Patel DP, Gross KX, Hotaling JM. Can artificial intelligence drive optimal sperm selection for in vitro fertilization? Fertil Steril. 2021;115:883. https://doi.org/10.1016/j.fertnstert.2021.02.004.
52. Dardikman-Yoffe G, Mirsky SK, Barnea I, Shaked NT. High- resolution 4-D acquisition of freely swimming human sperm cells without staining. Sci Adv. 2020;6:eaay7619.
53. Dai C, Zhang Z, Huang J, Wang X, Ru C, Pu H, Xie S, Zhang J, Moskovtsev S, Librach C, Jarvi K, Sun Y. Automated non-invasive measurement of single sperm's motility and morphology. IEEE Trans Med Imaging. 2018;37(10):2257–65. https://doi.org/10.1109/TMI.2018.2840827. Epub 2018 May 25
54. Khosravi P, Kazemi E, Zhan Q, Malmsten JE, Toschi M, Zisimopoulos P, et al. Deep learning enables robust assessment and selection of human blastocysts after in vitro fertilization. NPJ Digit Med. 2019;2(1):21.
55. Chow DJX, Wijesinghe P, Dholakia K, Dunning KR. Does artificial intelligence have a role in the IVF clinic? Reprod Fertil. 2021;2(3):C29–34. https://doi.org/10.1530/RAF-21-0043.
56. Howie R, Kay V. Controlled ovarian stimulation for in-vitro fertilization. Br J Hosp Med. (Lond). 2018;79(4):194–9. https://doi.org/10.12968/hmed.2018.79.4.194.
57. Deepika V. Applications of artificial intelligence techniques in polycystic ovarian syndrome diagnosis. J Adv Res Technol Manag Sci. 2019;1:59–63. Back to cited text no. 13.
58. Jyothi S, Vasavi G. Polycystic ovary syndrome detection using various machine learning methods—a review. J Adv Res Dyn Control Syst. 2017;5:334–9.
59. Bouaziz J, Mashiach R, Cohen S, Kedem A, Baron A, Zajicek M, Feldman I, Seidman D, Soriano D. How artificial intelligence can improve our understanding of the genes associated with endometriosis: natural language processing of the PubMed Database. BioMed Res Int. 2018;2018:6217812. https://doi.org/10.1155/2018/6217812.
60. Letterie G, MacDonald A. Artificial intelligence in in vitro fertilization: a computer decision support system for day-to-day management of ovarian stimulation during in vitro fertilization. Fertil Steril. 2020;114(5):1026–31. https://doi.org/10.1016/j.fertnstert.2020.06.006. Epub 2020 Oct 1.
61. Prasad S, Tiwari M, Pandey AN, Shrivastav TG, Chaube SK. Impact of stress on oocyte quality and reproductive outcome. J Biomed Sci. 2016;23:36. https://doi.org/10.1186/s12929-016-0253-4.
62. VerMilyea M, Hall JMM, Diakiw SM, Johnston A, Nguyen T, Perugini D, Miller A, Picou A, Murphy AP, Perugini M. Development of an artificial intelligence-based assessment model for prediction of embryo viability using static images captured by optical light microscopy during IVF. Hum Reprod. 2020;35(4):770–84. https://doi.org/10.1093/humrep/deaa013.

63. Darves-Bornoz A, et al. Robotic surgery for male infertility. Urol Clin North Am. 2021;48(1):127–35.
64. Schiff J, Li PS, Goldstein M. Robotic microsurgical vasovasostomy and vasoepididymostomy: a prospective randomized study in a rat model. J Urol. 2004;171(4):1720–5.
65. Punjani N, et al. Technological advancements in male infertility microsurgery. J Clin Med. 2021;10(18).
66. Shu T, Taghechian S, Wang R. Initial experience with robot-assisted varicocelectomy. Asian J Androl. 2008;10(1):146–8. https://doi.org/10.1111/j.1745-7262.2008.00354.x.
67. Douroumis K, Spartalis E, Stravodimos K, Levis PK, Tsourouflis G, Dimitroulis D, Nikiteas NI. Robotic-assisted microsurgery in andrology: a systematic review. Asian J Androl. 2023; https://doi.org/10.4103/aja202295.
68. Parekattil SJ, Gudeloglu A. Robotic assisted andrological surgery. Asian J Androl [Internet]. 2013;15(1):67–74. https://doi.org/10.1038/aja.2012.131.
69. Chan P, et al. Pros and cons of robotic microsurgery as an appropriate approach to male reproductive surgery for vasectomy reversal and varicocele repair. Fertil Steril. 2018;110(5):816–23.
70. Lee H, Chen Y. Image based computer aided diagnosis system for cancer detection. Expert Syst Appl. 2015;42(12):5356–65. https://doi.org/10.1016/j.eswa.2015.02.005.
71. Zhan Y, Shen D. Deformable segmentation of 3-D ultrasound prostate images using statistical texture matching method. IEEE Trans Med Imaging. 2006;25(3):256–72. https://doi.org/10.1109/TMI.2005.862744.
72. Moradi M, Abolmaesumi P, Siemens DR, Sauerbrei EE, Boag AH, Mousavi P. Augmenting detection of prostate cancer in transrectal ultrasound images using SVM and RF time series. IEEE Trans Biomed Eng. 2009;56(9):2214–24. https://doi.org/10.1109/TBME.2008.2009766.
73. Orlando N, Gyacskov I, Gillies DJ, Guo F, Romagnoli C, D'SouzaD'Souza D, Cool DW, Hoover DA, Fenster A. Effect of dataset size, image quality, and image type on deep learning-based automatic prostate segmentation in 3D ultrasound. Phys Med Biol. 2022;67(7) https://doi.org/10.1088/1361-6560/ac5a93.
74. Loch T, Leuschner I, Genberg C, Weichert-Jacobsen K, Küppers F, Yfantis E, Evans M, Tsarev V, Stöckle M. Artificial neural network analysis (ANNA) of prostatic transrectal ultrasound. Prostate. 1999;39(3):198–204. https://doi.org/10.1002/(sici)1097-0045(19990515)39:3<198::aid-pros8>3.0.co;2-x.
75. Remzi M, Anagnostou T, Ravery V, Zlotta A, Stephan C, Marberger M, Djavan B. An artificial neural network to predict the outcome of repeat prostate biopsies. Urology. 2003;62(3):456–60. https://doi.org/10.1016/s0090-4295(03)00409-6.
76. Liu D, Tupor S, Singh J, Chernoff T, Leong N, Sadikov E, Amjad A, Zilles S. The challenges facing deep learning-based catheter localization for ultrasound guided high-dose-rate prostate brachytherapy. Med Phys. 2022;49(4):2442–51. https://doi.org/10.1002/mp.15522.
77. Favaron T, Huang D, Christensen-Jeffries K, Eckersley R, Sidhu P, Grisan E, Building A. Reduced dictionary of relevant perfusion patterns from ceus data for the classification of testis lesions. IEEE-ISBI. 2019; https://doi.org/10.1109/ISBI.2019.8759528.
78. Favilla V, Cannarella R, Tumminaro A, Di Mauro D, Condorelli RA, La Vignera S, Ficarra V, Cimino S, Calogero AE. Oncological and functional outcomes of testis sparing surgery in small testicular mass: a systematic review. Minerva Urol Nephrol. 2021;73(4):431–41. https://doi.org/10.23736/S2724-6051.21.04330-5.
79. De Santi B, Spaggiari G, Granata AR, Romeo M, Molinari F, Simoni M, Santi D. From subjective to objective: a pilot study on testicular radiomics analysis as a measure of gonadal function. Andrology. 2022;10(3):505–17. https://doi.org/10.1111/andr.13131.
80. Zhang Z, Li G, Xu Y, Tang X. Application of artificial intelligence in the MRI classification task of human brain neurological and psychiatric diseases: a scoping review. Diagnostics (Basel). 2021;11(8):1402. https://doi.org/10.3390/diagnostics11081402.
81. Zhang Z, Seeram E. The use of artificial intelligence in computed tomography image reconstruction—a literature review. J Med Imaging Radiat Sci. 2020;51(4):671–7. https://doi.org/10.1016/j.jmir.2020.09.001. Epub 2020 Sep 24.

82. Hosny A, Parmar C, Quackenbush J, Schwartz LH, Aerts HJWL. Artificial intelligence in radiology. Nat Rev Cancer. 2018;18(8):500–10. https://doi.org/10.1038/s41568-018-0016-5.
83. Sarvazyan AP, Urban MW, Greenleaf JF. Acoustic waves in medical imaging and diagnostics. Ultrasound Med Biol. 2013;39(7):1133–46.
84. Sigrist RMS, Liau J, Kaffas AE, Chammas MC, Willmann JK. Ultrasound elasography: review of techniques and clinical applications. Theranostics. 2017;7(5):1303–29.
85. Abdelwahab K, Eliwa AM, Seleem MM, El Galaly H, Ragab A, Desoky EA, Naguib M, Ali MM, Saber S, Kamel H. Role of preoperative testicular shear wave elastography in predicting improvement of semen parameters after varicocelectomy for male patients with primary infertility. Urology. 2017;107:103–6.
86. Aslan S, Ceyhan Bilgici M, Saglam D, Ozturk M. The role of ARFI elastography to evaluate microstructural changes of patients with testicular microlithiasis. Acta Radiol. 2018;59:1517–22.
87. Turna O, Alis D. A comparative study of shear wave elastography in the evaluation of undescended and retractile testes in a pediatric population. J Med Ultrason (2001). 2019;46:231–7.
88. Rocher L, Criton A, Gennisson JL, Izard V, Ferlicot S, Tanter M, Benoit G, Bellin MF, Correas JM. Testicular shear wave elastography in normal and infertile men: a prospective study on 601 patients. Ultrasound Med Biol. 2017;43:782–9.
89. Erdoğan H, Durmaz MS, Özbakır B, Cebeci H, Özkan D, Gökmen İE. Experience of using shear wave elastography in evaluation of testicular stiffness in cases of male infertility. J Ultrasound. 2020;23:529–34.
90. Cui J, Du Q, Fu W. Application of real-time shear wave elastography in the assessment of male infertility. Quant Imaging Med Surg. 2022;12(2):1505–16.
91. United States Food and Drug Administration (USFDA). Artificial Intelligence and Machine Learning (AI/ML)–enabled medical devices. [Internet]; 2021 [Site accessed 7/1/2022]. From: https://www.fda.gov/medical-devices/software-medical-device-samd/artificial-intelligence-and-machine-learning-aiml-enabled-medical-devices.
92. Iqbal JD, Vinay R. Are we ready for artificial intelligence in medicine? Swiss Med Wkly. 2022;152:w30179. https://doi.org/10.4414/smw.2022.w30179.
93. Muehlematter UJ, Daniore P, Vokinger KN. Approval of artificial intelligence and machine learning-based medical devices in the USA and Europe (2015–20): a comparative analysis. Lancet Digit Health. 2021;3(3):e195–203. https://doi.org/10.1016/S2589-7500(20)30292-2. Epub 2021 Jan 18.
94. Maassen O, Fritsch S, Palm J, Deffge S, Kunze J, Marx G, Riedel M, Schuppert A, Bickenbach J. Future medical artificial intelligence application requirements and expectations of physicians in German university hospitals: web-based survey. J Med Internet Res. 2021;23(3):e26646. https://doi.org/10.2196/26646.
95. Chen MM, Golding LP, Nicola GN. Who will pay for AI? Radiol Artif Intell. 2021;3(3):e210030. https://doi.org/10.1148/ryai.2021210030.
96. Beltramin D, Lamas E, Bousquet C. Ethical issues in the utilization of black boxes for artificial intelligence in medicine. Stud Health Technol Inform. 2022;295:249–52. https://doi.org/10.3233/SHTI220709.

Chapter 19
New Frontiers of Research and Therapy in Male Infertility

Rupin Shah and Armand Zini

Key Points
- Male infertility research is poised for a new renaissance.
- Major advances in genetic and epigenetic diagnostics and gene therapy will revolutionize our understanding and treatment of azoospermia.
- Artificial intelligence will find application in diverse areas of diagnosis and therapy of male infertility.

Introduction

The initial years following the introduction of intracytoplasmic sperm injection (ICSI) witnessed a decline in interest in the evaluation and treatment of the male partner because it was felt that ICSI rendered the male factor irrelevant. However, over time, the value of having a high-quality male gamete has been re-established, and once again, the focus is on the management of the subfertile male. In recent years, we have witnessed major advances in the understanding and management of male reproductive potential. These have been discussed in detail in the preceding 18 chapters. In this concluding chapter, we take a quick look at what is next—what will be the new areas of research that might impact clinical practice in the future.

R. Shah (✉)
Department of Urology, Lilavati Hospital and Research Centre, Mumbai, Maharashtra, India

A. Zini
St. Mary's Hospital, Montreal, QC, Canada

A. Agarwal et al. (eds.), *Current and Future Advances in Male Infertility*,
https://doi.org/10.1007/978-3-031-62648-7_19

Semen Analysis

Interpretation of Semen Analysis

As discussed in Chap. 1, the latest sixth edition of the WHO manual on semen examination has abandoned the concept of a reference range to distinguish between normal fertile and abnormal infertile semen samples [1]. This has become a source of confusion for the average clinician since most management guidelines and infertility algorithms proceed based on a "normal" or "abnormal" semen analysis. However, this is also an opportunity to redefine the utility of a semen test in the management protocol of the infertile couple. Thus, we can expect that future research will focus on developing probability-based models for interpreting semen parameters. For example, fertility potential may be quantified on a sliding scale based on the concepts of "minimal required semen parameters for fertility" at one end and "optimal semen parameters for maximum chance of fertility" at the other end of the fertility scale, with a clinical decision zone that lies in between. Future research will correlate individual and combined semen parameters with "time to pregnancy" and "probability of pregnancy" and then create a fertility potential score.

Utility of Extended and Advanced Tests

Chapter 1 also lists tests like multiple sperm defect indices, FISH, sperm DNA fragmentation, oxidative stress measurement, and many others whose clinical utility remains poorly defined. Studies are needed to assess the value of these extended and advanced tests to determine whether they should be included in future editions of the manual, whether they are of any practical predictive value to the clinician, and how they fit into our diagnostic and treatment algorithms.

Home Testing of Semen

Several home-based tests for semen evaluation have become available, and more tests, with greater accuracy, can be expected as cell phones are equipped with better cameras and possess greater processing abilities [2]. However, although there are many obvious advantages to high-quality home testing of semen, these test kits are currently not in wide use and are not available in most countries. Future research can be expected to focus on simplifying the tests, and making them less costly, while ensuring greater accuracy and reliability [3].

Incorporation of AI in Semen Testing

As discussed in Chap. 1, the sixth edition has brought back the distinction between rapidly progressive and slowly progressive sperm as being of clinical importance while also acknowledging that it is practically difficult to make this distinction accurately during manual semen testing. The incorporation of machine learning has led to a new generation of computerized semen analyzers that are very compact, quick, and simple to operate [4–6]. Future developments in these machines, and research to validate their utility and accuracy, especially for those semen parameters that are difficult to assess manually, like motility and morphology, may result in routine use of small AI-based analyzers as part of standard semen testing.

Endocrine Disruptors

The role of endocrine-disrupting chemicals (EDCs) as a cause of infertility, globally and across species [7], is widely recognized, and Chap. 2 has provided an extensive list of suspect chemicals and discussed their pharmacological impact. However, despite this wealth of data, testing for EDC is not part of routine infertility evaluation, nor is treatment to reverse the impact of EDC generally prescribed. Future research in this area needs to focus on identifying early biomarkers for the presence of significant EDC, to study the impact of exposure to single versus multiple compounds, to assess the utility of routine testing for EDC in infertile men, and to evaluate the role of protective therapeutic agents, such as antioxidants [8].

Lifestyle Modification, Supplements, and Alternative Therapies

Linked to the avoidance of EDC is also the need for a healthy lifestyle to optimize fertility. Chapter 3 presents a variety of studies supporting the value of lifestyle changes and provides detailed information on the impact of these factors and the benefit that may result from appropriate corrective measures. Chapter 16 also discusses some of these measures and further discusses the value of weight loss, psychological therapy, acupuncture, herbal preparations, and other supplements. Further research in this area is important to validate these findings, to quantify more accurately the impact of various external factors on male fertility, and to provide clear evidence of benefit from lifestyle corrective measures that can be used to motivate patients to implement appropriate lifestyle changes [9, 10].

Fertility and Testicular Cancers

Chapter 4 discusses in detail the mechanisms through which fertility is compromised in men with testicular cancer and makes a strong case for cryopreservation of available sperm prior to the start of cancer therapy. However, while prior cryopreservation is the norm at most centers, the semen sample cannot be frozen if it is azoospermic. For such cases, onco-TESE is gaining popularity, and future research must focus on the utility of this approach, especially in adolescent boys who have only immature germ cells available for cryopreservation [11]. The challenge will be to produce mature sperm through in vivo or in vitro maturation of immature germ cells that have been cryopreserved.

Sperm DNA Fragmentation

Sperm DNA fragmentation (SDF) has received significant attention in recent years since it is a clinically useful marker of sperm quality [12–15]. The sixth edition of the WHO manual has devoted a large section on SDF. The manual provides a detailed description of four different methods for testing SDF but states that clinical interpretation of SDF tests depends on the individual laboratory's reference range, since interlaboratory variability is common with these assays. Chapter 5 has provided a detailed explanation of the pathophysiology of SDF and discusses the indications for SDF testing. However, considerable confusion still exists because test results vary from laboratory to laboratory and from test to test. The SDF cutoffs also vary, and the clinical significance of borderline elevated values is disputed. The optimal treatment for elevated SDF is also unclear with choices including antioxidants, laboratory techniques for better sperm selection, and use of testicular sperm. Clarification of these issues is urgently needed and will be an important focus of research in the near future.

Oxidative Stress

Much has been written about the role of reactive oxygen species in the genesis of male infertility [16, 17]. Chapter 6 presents an exhaustive discussion of the complex ways in which oxidative stress impairs sperm function and spermatogenesis. The sixth edition of the WHO manual lists tests of oxidative stress (OS) as advanced sperm function tests. The manual describes various assays of OS and notes that the results of these tests should be interpreted with caution until their diagnostic relevance is clearly established. As discussed in Chap. 7, it has been suggested that a large proportion of so-called idiopathic male infertility may be due to oxidative stress (male oxidative stress infertility—MOSI). An important area of future research will be to evaluate the clinical utility of measuring seminal oxidants and antioxidants to provide a more accurate diagnosis and to optimize the management of infertile men with the appropriate use of antioxidant therapy and avoid overtreatment leading to induction of reductive stress [18].

Genetic and Epigenetic Testing and Gene Therapy

The role of genetic and epigenetic factors as causative factors of azoospermia, OAT, and asthenozoospermia is gaining increasing recognition [19, 20]. Chapters 8 and 9 provide an exhaustive review of the genetic and epigenetic alterations found in infertile men and discuss their clinical interpretation. However, most of these advances have yet to find application in routine clinical practice as the analysis and interpretation of results are complex. The immediate need is to use AI to integrate and analyze the huge databases of genetic abnormalities in male infertility to identify which mutations, or combinations thereof, are clinically significant and subsequently develop clinical guidelines on the use of full exome or genome screening for the detection of these abnormalities. Similarly, the clinical utility of methylation markers of epigenetic modifications causing impaired spermatogenesis needs to be validated so that the specific cause, and possible treatment, can be identified. After we gain a clear understanding of specific gene defects affecting male fertility, the next major area of research will be gene therapy to correct these disorders. Already, very exciting animal experiments have demonstrated the potential of this therapy [21], and Chap. 8 discusses some of these approaches. In the future, gene therapy for male infertility can be expected to be a critical area of research and scientific advancement.

Varicocele

Varicocele is both the most commonly diagnosed pathology related to male infertility as well as the most controversial [22]. Chapter 10 has presented the pathophysiology of varicocele in great detail, while Chap. 11 has discussed various controversies related to the clinical management of varicocele. The current level of evidence has unequivocally established that varicocele repair (VR) can improve semen parameters [23]. However, the impact of VR on live birth rates has not been established due to the paucity of randomized controlled trials [24], and this is an important area for future clinical research. Further, the role of varicocele repair in reducing SDF and improving pregnancy rates in men with significantly elevated SDF is still unclear and is an important area for future studies since clinicians are increasingly using elevated SDF as an indication for VR [25].

Male Accessory Gland Infection (MAGI) and Infertility

The association between male genital tract infection and infertility is well established [26, 27], and Chap. 12 discusses the diagnosis and treatment in detail. Despite our understanding of the field, several clinical controversies remain [28]. In particular, the significance of leukocytospermia in the presence of negative semen cultures remains a topic of debate. The importance of a positive semen culture in an asymptomatic man with no other markers of infection or inflammations is another area of uncertainty. Furthermore, the duration of antibiotic therapy and the potential role of antioxidant therapy are poorly addressed topics. All these questions need to be resolved by future research.

Hypogonadism and Infertility

Hypogonadism, both primary and secondary, is a common abnormality in the infertile male. Chapter 14 discusses the etiologies and management of this condition in detail, as well as the controversial areas that are subjects for future research. While it is a clear recommendation that testosterone should not be administered to hypogonadal men interested in fertility, new research suggests that perhaps intermittent administration of short-acting testosterone may alleviate hypogonadal symptoms without impacting gonadotropin secretion and fertility [29, 30]. Gonadotropins to raise intratesticular testosterone and induce sperm production in eugonadotropic or hypergonadotropic men with nonobstructive azoospermia are widely used clinically despite limited evidence to justify this practice [31]. Clearly, there is an urgent need for proper studies on the value of these expensive and tedious treatments.

Management of Nonobstructive Azoospermia

One of the most challenging areas in male infertility is the management of men with nonobstructive azoospermia. Chapter 15 has detailed the options available for the treatment of azoospermia due to pre-testicular and testicular causes. However, many of these men cannot be helped at present. Thus, many men with hypogonadotropic hypogonadism fail to respond to gonadotropin therapy for reasons that are yet to be elucidated. Further, the optimal dose and duration of gonadotropins for these men are still unclear as evidenced by the numerous treatment protocols available [32]. Much research still needs to be done in this area.

For men with primary testicular failure, the picture is even more dismal. We are still unable to pinpoint the genetic cause of the problem in most men with idiopathic testicular failure. Therapeutically, we rely on the relatively crude and traumatic methods of blind testicular aspiration or open parenchymal dissection to find areas of focal spermatogenesis [33]. Technical aids to help find sperm-containing tubules during surgery have been listed in Chap. 15, but none have found clinical application. The use of epigenetic markers to identify which men with NOA harbor spermatogenic foci has been discussed in earlier chapters, but these too have not yet proven their clinical utility. All these are areas for further research. Finally, there remains the question of how to help men who have no sperm production at all. Stem cell transplantation into the testes, in vitro sperm maturation, and even gene editing to restore spermatogenic genes have been performed successfully in animal models, but the application of these techniques in humans is still a long way off and represents the final frontier for future research in male infertility [34, 35].

Sperm Optimization for ART

A large proportion of couples with male factor infertility will ultimately require ART—specifically intracytoplasmic sperm injection (ICSI). In many of these cases, the semen is severely compromised, and most of the sperm in these samples are damaged—structurally, biochemically, or genetically—and lead to failed fertilization or early pregnancy loss. Chapter 17 discusses the various methods available to select the best quality sperm from a poor semen sample to ensure that the most biologically fit sperm are used for ICSI. Newer laboratory techniques continue to be described, and this will remain an active area of research as the use of ICSI for male infertility continues to grow.

Artificial Intelligence (AI) and Male Infertility

AI is poised to transform every aspect of human existence. It will have a huge impact on medicine, and its potential to transform the evaluation and management of male infertility has been elaborated upon in the final chapter of this book. Machine learning will result in small, portable but highly accurate automated semen analyzers; AI will mine through the huge genetic database to make whole-genome screening a clinically relevant test; AI-based algorithms will guide the management of infertile couples taking into consideration all biological and social variables; and AI-guided evaluation of gametes and embryos will optimize ART outcomes. The incorporation of AI in all these areas of male infertility management will be an important area of research in the next few years.

Conclusion

After decades of neglect, attention has once again shifted to the male gamete and the man behind it. We are poised at the beginning of an andrological renaissance, and a wide range of research opportunities and exciting frontiers await us.

References

1. World Health Organization. WHO laboratory manual for the examination and processing of human semen. 6th ed. Geneva: WHO Press; 2021. https://www.who.int/publications/i/item/9789240030787. Accessed 16 Feb 2023.
2. Gonzalez D, Narasimman M, Best JC, Ory J, Ramasamy R. Clinical update on home testing for male fertility. World J Men's Health. 2021;39(4):615–25. https://doi.org/10.5534/wjmh.200130.
3. Onofre J, Geenen L, Cox A, et al. Simplified sperm testing devices: a possible tool to overcome lack of accessibility and inconsistency in male factor infertility diagnosis. An opportunity for low- and middle- income countries. Facts Views Vis Obgyn. 2021;13(1):79–93. https://doi.org/10.52054/FVVO.13.1.011.
4. Agarwal A, Henkel R, Huang CC, Lee MS. Automation of human semen analysis using a novel artificial intelligence optical microscopic technology. Andrologia. 2019;51(11):e13440. https://doi.org/10.1111/and.13440.
5. Sengupta P, Dutta S, Roychoudhury S, et al. Revolutionizing semen analysis: introducing Mojo AISA, the next-gen artificial intelligence microscopy. Front Cell Dev Biol. 2023;11:1203708. https://doi.org/10.3389/fcell.2023.1203708.
6. Ghayda RA, Cannarella R, Calogero AE, et al. Global andrology forum. Artificial intelligence in andrology: from semen analysis to image diagnostics. World J Men's Health. 2024;42(1):39–61. https://doi.org/10.5534/wjmh.230050.
7. Colborn T, Dumanoski D, Myers JP. Our stolen future. New York: Penguin Group; 1997.
8. Thacharodi A, Hassan S, Acharya G, et al. Endocrine disrupting chemicals and their effects on the reproductive health in men. Environ Res. 2023;236(Pt 2):116825. https://doi.org/10.1016/j.envres.2023.116825.
9. Biggs SN, Kennedy J, Lewis SL, et al. Lifestyle and environmental risk factors for unexplained male infertility: study protocol for Australian Male Infertility Exposure (AMIE), a case-control study. Reprod Health. 2023;20(1):32. https://doi.org/10.1186/s12978-023-01578-z.
10. Rotimi DE, Singh SK. Implications of lifestyle factors on male reproductive health. JBRA Assist Reprod. 2024; https://doi.org/10.5935/1518-0557.20240007.
11. Ogouma L, Berthaut I, Lévy R, et al. Testicular sperm extraction (TESE) outcomes in the context of malignant disease: a systematic review. Asian J Androl. 2022;24(6):584–90. https://doi.org/10.4103/aja2021129.
12. Nielsen JLM, Majzoub A, Esteves S, Humaidan P. Unraveling the impact of sperm DNA fragmentation on reproductive outcomes. Semin Reprod Med. 2023; https://doi.org/10.1055/s-0043-1777324.
13. Agarwal A, Farkouh A, Saleh R, et al. Technical aspects and clinical limitations of sperm DNA fragmentation testing in male infertility: a global survey, current guidelines, and expert recommendations. World J Men's Health. 2024;42(1):202–15. https://doi.org/10.5534/wjmh.230076.
14. Farkouh A, Agarwal A, Hamoda TAA, et al. Global andrology forum. Controversy and consensus on the management of elevated sperm DNA fragmentation in male infertility: a global survey, current guidelines, and expert recommendations. World J Men's Health. 2023;41(4):809–47. https://doi.org/10.5534/wjmh.230008.

15. Lourenço ML, Moura GA, Rocha YM, et al. Impact of sperm DNA fragmentation on the clinical outcome of assisted reproduction techniques: a systematic review of the last five years. JBRA Assist Reprod. 2023;27(2):282–91. https://doi.org/10.5935/1518-0557.20220057.
16. Agarwal A, Finelli R, Selvam MKP, et al. A global survey of reproductive specialists to determine the clinical utility of oxidative stress testing and antioxidant use in male infertility. World J Men's Health. 2021;39(3):470–88. https://doi.org/10.5534/wjmh.210025.
17. Grabowska M, Duchnik E, Piasecka M. Low human sperm motility coexists with sperm nuclear DNA damage and oxidative stress in semen. Andrology. 2023; https://doi.org/10.1111/andr.13556.
18. O'Flaherty C, Scarlata E. Oxidative stress and reproductive function: The protection of mammalian spermatozoa against oxidative stress. Reproduction. 2022;164(6):F67–78. https://doi.org/10.1530/REP-22-0200.
19. Sang Q, Ray PF, Wang L. Understanding the genetics of human infertility. Science. 2023;380(6641):158–63. https://doi.org/10.1126/science.adf7760.
20. Wagner AO, Turk A, Kunej T. Towards a multi-omics of male infertility. World J Men's Health. 2023;41(2):272–88. https://doi.org/10.5534/wjmh.220186.
21. Wang YH, Yan M, Zhang X, et al. Rescue of male infertility through correcting a genetic mutation causing meiotic arrest in spermatogonial stem cells. Asian J Androl. 2021;23(6):590–9. https://doi.org/10.4103/aja.aja_97_20.
22. Arya D, Balasinor N, Singh D. Varicocoele-associated male infertility: cellular and molecular perspectives of pathophysiology. Andrology. 2022;10(8):1463–83. https://doi.org/10.1111/andr.13278.
23. Agarwal A, Cannarella R, Saleh R, et al. Impact of varicocele repair on semen parameters in infertile men: a systematic review and meta-analysis. World J Men's Health. 2023;41(2):289–310. https://doi.org/10.5534/wjmh.220142.
24. Persad E, O'Loughlin CA, Kaur S, et al. Surgical or radiological treatment for varicoceles in subfertile men. Cochrane Database Syst Rev. 2021;4(4):CD000479. https://doi.org/10.1002/14651858.CD000479.pub6.
25. Lira Neto FT, Roque M, Esteves SC. Effect of varicocelectomy on sperm deoxyribonucleic acid fragmentation rates in infertile men with clinical varicocele: a systematic review and meta-analysis. Fertil Steril. 2021;116(3):696–712. https://doi.org/10.1016/j.fertnstert.2021.04.003.
26. La Vignera S, Vicari E, Condorelli RA, et al. Male accessory gland infection and sperm parameters (review). Int J Androl. 2011;34(5 Pt 2):e330–47. https://doi.org/10.1111/j.1365-2605.2011.01200.x.
27. Everaert K, Mahmoud A, Depuydt C, et al. Chronic prostatitis and male accessory gland infection—is there an impact on male infertility (diagnosis and therapy)? Andrologia. 2003;35(5):325–30.
28. Rivero MJ, Kulkarni N, Thirumavalavan N, et al. Evaluation and management of male genital tract infections in the setting of male infertility: an updated review. Curr Opin Urol. 2023;33(3):180–6. https://doi.org/10.1097/MOU.0000000000001081.
29. Ramasamy R, Masterson TA, Best JC, et al. Effect of Natesto on reproductive hormones, semen parameters and hypogonadal symptoms: a single center, open label, single arm trial. J Urol. 2020;204(3):557–63. https://doi.org/10.1097/JU.0000000000001078.
30. Diaz P, Reddy R, Blachman-Braun R, et al. Comparison of intratesticular testosterone between men receiving nasal, intramuscular, and subcutaneous pellet testosterone therapy: evaluation of data from two single-center randomized clinical trials. World J Men's Health. 2023;41(2):390–5. https://doi.org/10.5534/wjmh.210261.
31. Schlegel PN, Sigman M, Collura B, et al. Diagnosis and treatment of infertility in men: AUA/ASRM guideline part II. Fertil Steril. 2021;115(1):62–9. https://doi.org/10.1016/j.fertnstert.2020.11.016.
32. Boeri L, Capogrosso P, Salonia A. Gonadotropin treatment for the male hypogonadotropic hypogonadism. Curr Pharm Des. 2021;27(24):2775–83. https://doi.org/10.2174/1381612826666200523175806.

33. Punjani N, Kang C, Schlegel PN. Two decades from the introduction of microdissection testicular sperm extraction: how this surgical technique has improved the management of NOA. J Clin Med. 2021;10(7):1374. https://doi.org/10.3390/jcm10071374.
34. Gul M, Hildorf S, Dong L, et al. Review of injection techniques for spermatogonial stem cell transplantation. Hum Reprod Update. 2020;26(3):368–91. https://doi.org/10.1093/humupd/dmaa003.
35. Robinson M, Sparanese S, Witherspoon L, et al. Human in vitro spermatogenesis as a regenerative therapy—where do we stand? Nat Rev Urol. 2023;20:461–79. https://doi.org/10.1038/s41585-023-00723-4.

Index

A. Agarwal et al. (eds.), *Current and Future Advances in Male Infertility*,
https://doi.org/10.1007/978-3-031-62648-7

M

N

O

GPSR Compliance

The European Union's (EU) General Product Safety Regulation (GPSR) is a set of rules that requires consumer products to be safe and our obligations to ensure this.

If you have any concerns about our products, you can contact us on ProductSafety@springernature.com

In case Publisher is established outside the EU, the EU authorized representative is:

Springer Nature Customer Service Center GmbH
Europaplatz 3
69115 Heidelberg, Germany

Batch number: 10726133

Printed by Printforce, the Netherlands